D. ZUCKER-FRANKLIN   M.F. GREAVES
C.E. GROSSI   A.M. MARMONT

ATLAS OF BLOOD CELLS
function and pathology

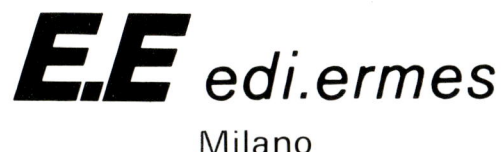
edi.ermes
Milano

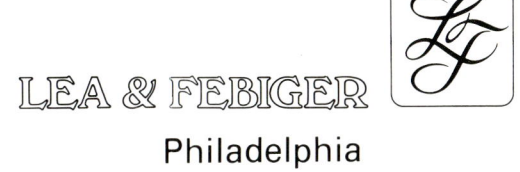
LEA & FEBIGER
Philadelphia

Edi.Ermes s.r.l.
Via Timavo, 12
20124 - Milano (Italia)

Lea & Febiger
600 South Washington Square
Philadelphia, Pa. 19106

Atlas of Blood Cells

ISBN: 88-7051-002-6 Edi.Ermes
  0-8121-0783-7 Lea & Febiger

© 1981 by Edi.Ermes s.r.l.-Milano
All rights reserved. No part of this publication may be reproduced, stored in a retrieval system, or transmitted in any form or by any means, electronic, mechanical, photocopying, recording or otherwise without written permission of the publisher.

Printed in Italy by Arti Grafiche Salea-Milano
Photolitography Farini-Milano

Hemostasis Research Lab
Mt. Sinai Medical Center
836 No. 12th Street
Milwaukee, WI 53233

MICHAEL W. MOSESSON, M.D.

ATLAS OF BLOOD CELLS

FOREWORD

"Seeing is believing", the saying goes. But "appearance may be deceiving", is another piece of worldly wisdom. So why another Atlas?

Morphology has been the bedrock of clinical hematology. When Ehrlich, after many trials, finally developed a method for staining the cells of the blood, a new era of hematology began. Ehrlich, and others who followed him, recognized for the first time the great variety of cells of the hematopoietic system, saw where they were formed at different stages of life, described changes in various physiologic and pathologic states, and learned to distinguish the immature forms of the several cell lines as well as cells typical of various forms of leukemia, multiple myeloma and other conditions. In those days atlases were deservedly popular. But what about today?

The development of electron microscopy, of a variety of cytochemical procedures, of cell markers of various kinds, of assays which reveal the reactions of cells under various circumstances, and still other recent advances have introduced a totally new world in the realm of cytology and have greatly extended our horizons. By these means we have learned about the fine structure of cells, the functions of their organelles and the ways in which cells respond in various circumstances. We have at the same time found convincing evidence that appearances may be misleading. The once enigmatic lymphocyte is an outstanding example. It is only a short time ago that the question was even asked whether this outwardly unremarkable looking cell had any function at all. A whole new world, we have found, is hidden behind its innocent appearance.

By exploiting all these new developments, the Atlas prepared by Doctors Zucker-Franklin, Greaves, Grossi and Marmont for the first time reveals what no atlas in the past was able to do. It shows in minute detail the structure of various cells and explains the role of the various organelles, illustrating how they react in a variety of circumstances. Their enzyme composition is elucidated and their antigenic capabilities and other attributes are revealed. For example, we are shown what function the microtubules of megakaryocytes serve, how the canalicular system works and how platelets adhere to one another. When morphologic alterations or functional changes are associated with disease they are illustrated. Demonstrable changes in the various lymphoproliferative diseases are shown and how these changes relate to the most commonly used classifications is explained.

This then is not the traditional geographic atlas of the blood cells and hematopoietic tissues, as the classical atlases could only be, but a dynamic and modern presentation of the hematopoietic system which illustrates the functions of the cells and shows their behaviour in response to a variety of forces that affect their growth and development.

Salt Lake City, July 1980

Maxwell M. Wintrobe

PREFACE

The medical literature abounds with hematology textbooks and "atlas style" monographs. It therefore requires a major and original incentive to produce another one. In the final analysis the motivating force for this book proved to be a need to incorporate the many diverse technical advances which have provided entirely new insight into the biology, immunology and enzymology of normal and malignant hematopoietic cells.

Conventional morphology has not become obsolete, but now demands an understanding beyond what is attainable with the Wright's stain and an oil immersion lens. The ability to identify a lymphocyte no longer suffices. Every hematologist knows that lymphocytosis requires more sophisticated characterization of the subpopulations of lymphocytes involved. This is now possible with the help of "surface markers", analysis of immunoglobulin and constitutive enzymes, tissue culture and/or cytogenetic methods. Almost all of these techniques depend on visual interpretation and, therefore, should be included in a modern atlas.

The aim of this publication is to juxtapose, for the first time, accurate color prints of traditionally-stained blood cells with electron micrographs and with illustrations indicating cell lineage, differentiation stage and, above all, cell function in health and disease. Enzymological and immunological techniques are a form of "molecular morphology" and when combined with good cytomorphology and cytochemistry provide the most reliable way to identify cell types. This has already proven to be of considerable importance in hematologic malignancies which may involve the clonal proliferation of a cell type, the precise differentiation status of which is disguised in morphological anonymity. This multidisciplinary approach has led to a reappraisal of the classification of hemopoietic cells which is both logical and relevant to the management of patients.

Since the expansion of recently acquired clinically relevant knowledge has been particularly remarkable in the area of cellular immunology and lymphoproliferative diseases, it seemed appropriate to allot somewhat more space to this cell type and to consider details which have led to one or another currently used classifications of the leukemias and lymphomas. On the other hand, major breakthroughs in the molecular biology or genetics of hemoglobins or the metabolic concomitants of neutrophil or platelet activation may seem somewhat shortchanged because they do not lend themselves to visual representation. Whenever possible these processes have been depicted in diagrams.

The Atlas is not intended to be disease-oriented. It does not consider diagnoses or treatment in great detail unless these are understood at the cellular or subcellular level. Abundant references to original and review articles should make up for the superficiality of clinical descriptions. Rather, the authors hope that this publication will supplement standard clinical texts by viewing hematology and its diseases from the vantage point of the cell.

Finally, and perhaps most importantly, the authors have been aware of the fact that many of the new methods, particularly those involving immunological assays, ultrastructural techniques, and karyotyping tend to discourage practicing hematologists. Some of these methods seem complicated or esoteric, unstandardized or shrouded in a jargon which precludes a clear understanding of their significance. It is our hope that an atlas which presents most of this new information in visual form will help to bridge this difficulty and be useful to clinicians and experimentalists alike.

We express our gratitude to all the Colleagues who have generously provided illustrations. We thank dr. A. Leprini for his drawings and illustrations. G. Grusky, Ph.D. and Susan Dittmar, B.A. provided the kind of assistance without which projects of this nature would not be possible.
Dr. Italo Grandi has encouraged us at every step of this project. He deserves the credit for the high technical standard of the printwork.

November, 1980

D. ZUCKER-FRANKLIN   M.F. GREAVES
C.E. GROSSI   A.M. MARMONT

With everlasting gratitude to Ξ
who gave me belief in myself,
and to my husband, Ed,
who stands behind me in all I do.

DZF

LIST OF CONTRIBUTORS

G. L. CASTOLDI
Division of Hematology, Department of Medicine, University of Ferrara
Ferrara, Italy

P. A. CHERVENICK
Division of Hematology-Oncology, Department of Medicine, University of Pittsburgh
Pittsburgh, U.S.A.

M. J. CLINE
Division of Hematology-Oncology, Department of Medicine, University of California
Los Angeles, U.S.A.

E. DAMASIO
Division of Hematology, S. Martino's Hospital
Genova, Italy

M. F. GREAVES
Membrane Immunology Laboratory, Imperial Cancer Research Fund
London, U.K.

C. E. GROSSI
Department of Anatomy, University of Genova
Genova, Italy

J. A. HABESHAW
ICRF Medical Oncology Unit, St. Bartholomew's Hospital
London, U.K.

L. LOMBARDI
Division of Experimental Oncology, Tumor Institute
Milano, Italy

A. M. MARMONT
Division of Hematology, S. Martino's Hospital
Genova, Italy

F. RILKE
Department of Pathology, Tumor Institute
Milano, Italy

J. D. ROWLEY
Section of Hematology-Oncology, Department of Medicine, University of Chicago
Chicago, U.S.A.

A. G. STANSFELD
Department of Pathology, St. Bartholomew's Hospital
London, U.K.

D. ZUCKER-FRANKLIN
Department of Medicine, New York University
New York, U.S.A.

CONTENTS

FOREWORD
M. M. Wintrobe

1 **CELLULAR IDENTIFICATION AND MARKERS**
M. F. Greaves

2 **IN VITRO AND IN VIVO HEMATOPOIESIS**
P. A. Chervenick, D. Zucker-Franklin

3 **ERYTHROCYTES**
G. L. Castoldi

4 **NEUTROPHILS**
A. M. Marmont, E. Damasio, D. Zucker-Franklin

5 **APLASTIC, HYPOPLASTIC AND METAPLASTIC MYELOPATHIES**
A. M. Marmont, E. Damasio

6 **EOSINOPHILS**
D. Zucker-Franklin

7 **BASOPHILS**
D. Zucker-Franklin

8 **MONOCYTES**
M. J. Cline

9 **LYMPHOCYTES**
M. F. Greaves, C. E. Grossi, J. A. Habeshaw, L. Lombardi, F. Rilke, A. G. Stansfeld

10 **MEGAKARYOCYTES AND PLATELETS**
D. Zucker-Franklin

11 **NONRANDOM CHROMOSOME CHANGES IN HEMATOLOGIC DISEASES**
J. D. Rowley

12 **TRANSPLANTATION HEMATOPOIESIS**
A. M. Marmont

Appendix
APPLICATION OF HYBRIDOMA MONOCLONAL ANTIBODIES
M. F. Greaves

1st VOLUME

1. CELLULAR IDENTIFICATION AND "MARKERS"

1. Differentiation 3
2. Cellular identity and differentiation-linked markers 4
3. "Markers" of malignancy 8
   3.1. Glucose-6-phosphate dehydrogenase (G-6-PD) isoenzymes and clonality of leukemic cells 8
   3.2. Immunoglobulin determinants and monoclonal B cell malignancy 8
References 10

2. IN VITRO AND IN VIVO HEMATOPOIESIS

1. Fetal hematopoiesis 13
2. Biology of hematopoiesis 13
3. Hematopoiesis in short term cultures 17
   3.1. Granulocyte-macrophage proliferation 17
   3.2. Erythrocyte proliferation 17
   3.3. Megakaryocyte proliferation 17
   3.4. Lymphocyte proliferation 17
4. Hematopoiesis in long term cultures 22
5. Clinical application of in vitro hematopoiesis 26
   5.1. Stem cell disorders 26
      5.1.1. Acute myelogenous leukemia 26
      5.1.2. Chronic myelogenous leukemia 26
      5.1.3. Agnogenic myeloid metaplasia 27
      5.1.4. Polycytemia vera 27
      5.1.5. Aplastic anemia 27
   5.2. Miscellaneous disorders associated with abnormal in vitro proliferation 28
      5.2.1. Myelodysplastic syndrome 28
      5.2.2. Neutropenia 28
References 29

3. ERYTHROCYTES

Part 1 General aspects of erythropoiesis

1. Introduction 35
2. Fetal erythropoiesis 35
3. Generation of erythroid cells in post-natal life 36
4. Regulation of erythroid differentiation 37
5. Morphology 39
   5.1. Light microscope cytology, cytochemistry and ultrastructure 39
   5.2. The structure of the red cell membrane 53
   5.3. The erythroblastic island 56
   5.4. Erythrocyte inclusions 59
   5.5. Physiological (reversible) changes in red cell shape 64
6. Red cell shape changes associated with pathological states 67

Part 2 Abnormalities of red cell production

1. Aplastic myelopathies 75
2. Abnormalities of DNA synthesis (megaloblastic anemias) 75
   2.1. Megaloblastic erythropoiesis 75
      2.1.1. Cytochemical and ultrastructural features 79
   2.2. Drug-induced megaloblastic changes 82
3. Disorders related to disturbances of hemoglobin synthesis 83
   3.1. Dyserythropoiesis and dyserythropoietic anemias 83
   3.2. Sideroblastic anemias 84
      3.2.1. "Synartesis" 92
   3.3. Congenital dyserythropoietic anemias 92
      3.3.1. CDA type I 92
      3.3.2. CDA type II 92
      3.3.3. CDA type III 92

3.4. Porphyrias 98
  3.4.1. Erythropoietic protoporphyria 99
  3.4.2. Symptomatic porphyrinopathies 99
3.5. Iron deficiency anemia 99
3.6. Abnormalities of the globin synthesis 101
  3.6.1. Thalassemia syndromes 101
  3.6.2. Abnormal hemoglobin: sickle cell anemia 111
  3.6.3. Unstable hemoglobins 114
4. Hyperproliferative and neoplastic erythropoiesis 114
  4.1. Acute erythremic myelosis and erythroleukemia 114
  4.2. Polycythemia vera 118

Part 3 Abnormalities of red cell destruction

1. Hereditary hemolytic anemias 123
   1.1. Hereditary spherocytosis 123
   1.2. Elliptocytosis 124
   1.3. Acanthocytosis 124
   1.4. Enzyme deficiencies 124
2. Paroxysmal nocturnal hemoglobinuria 124
3. Acquired hemolytic disorders 126
   3.1. Anemia due to infection and infestation 126
   3.2. Chemical and drug-induced anemias 130
   3.3. Autoimmune hemolytic anemias (AIHA) 131
4. The erythrocyte fragmentation syndromes 132
5. Myelophthisic anemias 134
References 137

4. NEUTROPHILS

Part 1 Normal structure and physiology

1. Differentiation and maturation 149
2. Sex chromatins 162
3. Cytoplasm and cytochemistry 163
4. Kinetics and humoral regulation of granulocytes 167
5. Chemotaxis and locomotion 167
6. Phagocytosis and degranulation 171
7. The LE phenomenon 176
8. Crystal phagocytosis 182
9. Neutrophil metabolism 183

Part 2 Neutrophil pathology

1. Abnormalities of the nucleus 185
2. Cytoplasmic abnormalities 188
   2.1. Chediak-Higashi-Steinbrink anomaly 188
   2.2. Alder-Reilly anomaly 194
   2.3. Lipid inclusions 194
3. Disorders affecting neutrophil number 194
4. Disorders of neutrophil function 196
5. Chronic myelogenous leukemia 198
   5.1. Blood and bone marrow morphology 200
   5.2. Blast transformation in Chronic Myelogenous Leukemia (CML) 205
6. The acute myelogenous leukemias 212
   6.1. General considerations 212
   6.2. Classifications of Acute Leukemia (AL) 214
   6.3. Dysmyelopoietic syndromes (DMPS) 230
7. Additional phenotypic characteristics and morphologic abnormalities associated with myelogenous leukemias 232
   7.1. The Auer body 232
8. Bone marrow morphology after therapy 235
References 236

5. APLASTIC, HYPOPLASTIC AND METAPLASTIC MYELOPATHIES

1. Acquired aplastic anemia 245
2. Pure red cell anemia (PRCA) 247
3. Agranulocytosis 250
4. The myelofibrosis-osteosclerosis syndrome (MOS) 252
5. Myelophthisis 252
References 254

6. EOSINOPHILS

1. Normal eosinophils 257
   1.1. Eosinophil structure and maturation 257
   1.2. Ultrastructure of mature eosinophils 264
   1.3. Morphologic correlates of eosinophil function 271
2. Pathology of eosinophils 276
   2.1. Malignant or primary eosinophilia 282
3. Conclusion 283
References 283

7. BASOPHILS

1. Introduction 287
2. Development 290
   2.1. Light microscopy 290
   2.2. Electron microscopy 292
3. Function 301
   3.1. Secretion-Exocytosis 301
   3.2. Endocytosis - Transport - Storage 306
3.3. Locomotion - Chemotaxis 306
4. Pathophysiology 307
   4.1. Intrinsic abnormalities 307
   4.2. "Reactive" changes in basophil numbers 308
5. Conclusions 315
References 316

8. THE MONONUCLEAR PHAGOCYTE SYSTEM - MONOCYTES AND MACROPHAGES

1. General aspects and development 321
2. Functions of the mononuclear phagocytes 330
3. Pathology of the monocyte-macrophage system 336
References 343

SUBJECT INDEX

2nd VOLUME

9. LYMPHOCYTES

Part 1 Normal lymphocytes

1. Lymphocyte heterogeneity 347
2. B lymphocytes 356
   2.1. Morphology 357
   2.2. Phenotype expression 358
      2.2.1. Surface markers 358
      2.2.2. Enzymes 367
3. T lymphocytes 369
   3.1. Morphology 369
   3.2. Phenotype expression 369
      3.2.1. Surface markers 369
      3.2.2. Enzymes 375
4. "Null" lymphocytes 380
5. Ontogenesis of lymphocytes 382
   5.1. Generation and maturation of B lymphocytes 383
   5.2. Generation and maturation of T lymphocytes 386
6. Lymphocyte activation 390
   6.1. B lymphocytes 390
   6.2. T lymphocytes 401
7. Lymphocyte-mediated cell cytotoxicity 402
References 407

Part 2 Lymphoproliferative disorders

1. Biological characterization and classification of lymphoid malignancies 409
2. Acute lymphoblastic leukemia (ALL) 412
   2.1. Morphology, cytochemistry and ultrastructure 412
   2.2. Heterogeneity and classification of ALL: immunological and enzymatic markers 420
   2.3. The ALL associated antigen: its diagnostic value and biological significance 425
   2.4. Phenotypic shift 427
   2.5. Prognostic significance of the ALL subgroups 434
3. Chronic lymphoid leukemias 436
   3.1. Chronic lymphocytic leukemia (CLL) and prolymphocytic leukemia (PLL) 436
   3.2. Leukemic reticulo-endotheliosis (LRE) or "Hairy" cell leukemia 445
4. Myeloma and the paraproteinemias 451
   4.1. Myeloma 451
   4.2. Waldenström's macroglobulinemia 464
   4.3. Heavy chain disease 465
   4.4. Amyloidosis 472
5. Lymphomas 478
   5.1. Histology and histological classification of non-Hodgkin lymphoma 478
   5.2. Immunological characterization of lymphomas 492
      5.2.1. T cell lineage lymphomas 493
      5.2.2. B cell lineage lymphomas 493
      5.2.3. Histiocytic lymphoma 496
      5.2.4. Receptor silent lymphoma 496
   5.3. Hodgkin's disease 498

6. Sézary syndrome - Lymphoma/leukemia 506
7. Summary view: lymphoid neoplasms in relation to normal lymphocyte differentiation 512
8. Non-malignant lymphoproliferative disorders 514
    8.1. Infectious mononucleosis 514
    8.2. Angioimmunoblastic lymphadenopathy 521
References 521

Part 3 Ultrastructure of non-Hodgkin malignant lymphomas

1. ML, lymphocytic, B-CLL 526
2. ML, lymphoplasmacytoid (Immunocytoma) 528
3. ML, centrocytic 532
4. ML, centroblastic-centrocytic 536
5. ML, centroblastic 542
6. ML, lymphoblastic, Burkitt's type 546
7. ML, immunoblastic 548
8. Burkitt-like ML of the adult 552
9. Malignant histiocytosis 554
References 556

10. MEGAKARYOCYTES AND PLATELETS

1. Normal megakaryocytes 559
    1.1. Nucleus 561
    1.2. Cytoplasm 561
2. Megakaryocyte pathology 570
3. Platelets 574
    3.1. Hemostasis 576
    3.2. Storage and transport 582
    3.3. Contractile system 582
    3.4. Inflammation 587
4. Platelet pathology 595
References 601

11. NONRANDOM CHROMOSOME CHANGES IN HEMATOLOGIC DISEASES

1. Introduction 605
2. Methods 605
3. Myeloproliferative disorders 610
    3.1. Ph^1-positive myelogenous leukemia 610
        3.1.1. Chronic phase of CML 610
        3.1.2. Acute phase of CML 611
    3.2. Acute nonlymphocytic leukemia 613
    3.3. Polycytemia vera 617
    3.4. Essential thrombocytosis (ET) 619
    3.5. Refractory anemia and preleukemia 620
4. Lymphoproliferative disorders 621
    4.1. Malignant lymphoma 621
        4.1.1. Hodgkin's disease 622
        4.1.2. Burkitt's lymphoma 622
        4.1.3. Poorly differentiated lymphocytic lymphoma (PDL) 623
        4.1.4. Diffuse histiocytic lymphoma 625
    4.2. T-cell dyscrasias 626
    4.3. Ataxia-telangiectasia (AT) 629
    4.4. Other lymphoproliferative diseases 630
        4.4.1. Multiple myeloma 630
        4.4.2. Acute lymphoblastic leukemia 632
5. Conclusions 633
References 633

12. TRANSPLANTATION HEMATOPOIESIS

1. General aspects 639
2. Stem cell reseeding 639
3. Evidence of engraftment 640
4. Morphological aspects of transplantation hematopoiesis 642
    4.1. Granulocyte and megakaryocyte production 642
    4.2. Erythropoiesis and erythroblastic islands 642
    4.3. Macrophage reactions 642
    4.4. Immunoreconstitution and immunodeficiency 651
References 651

APPENDIX: Applications of Hybridoma Monoclonal Antibodies 655

References 660

SUBJECT INDEX

1st VOLUME

1
Cellular identification and "markers"

M.F. GREAVES

Membrane Immunology Laboratory
Imperial Cancer Research Fund
London, U.K.

1. DIFFERENTIATION

Biologists have long argued over the precise meaning of the term *differentiation*. A mature lymphocyte or neuron has the same genetic information as the fertilized egg and differentiation must therefore be concerned with the process of *selective gene expression* which characterizes the diversity of cell types in the body. This involves a *continuous process* of progressive genetic restriction of cell lineage options which commences with a fertilized ovum and culminates in commitment to a single lineage or cell series and *maturation* to an end effector cell. Commitment of a progenitor cell to a particular cell series may be a "silent" decision in the sense that until the cell receives appropriate inducing signals and begins to mature it will not express "markers" which identify its lineage affiliation. Even then, cells committed to a particular tissue system (e.g. hemopoietic stem cells) may show no morphological or ultrastructural evidence of their "choice", this only being evident when "identity" is probed at a molecular level, e.g. antigens, enzymes. Unfortunately our knowledge of the detailed differentiation-linked phenotypes of precursor cells or tissue stem cells is rudimentary largely due to the technical problems associated with manipulation of cells occurring at very low frequencies (see Chapter 2). This has some important implications for the biology of disease states in humans and in particular for neoplasms.

Traditional pathology has a rather different perspective on differentiation. Here a differentiated state usually refers to either the social integration of a tissue in which the vast majority of component cells are performing a clear function, e.g. keratin synthesis by epidermal cells, or alternatively may refer to particular morphologic features of cells, e.g. highly condensed chromatin in small lymphocytes and plasma cells. Lymphoblastoid cells with heterodispersed chromatin and no rough endoplasmic reticulum may, for example, be considered "poorly differentiated" and yet we know from studies on polyclonal activation of lymphocytes in culture that this is a transient, cell cycle-related morphology which, in terms of gene expression, does not reflect a state of immaturity.

The traditional "single cell" terminology used by pathologists for strictly morphological reasons ignores the biological correlates of differentiation.

This may not in fact matter a great deal if subgroups of disease with "arbitrary" labels are nevertheless clinically meaningful and readily identifiable; difficulties only arise when subclasses of malignant cells are disguised by a common morphology (e.g. in acute lymphoblastic leukemia) with no clues being provided by topographical arrangements (e.g. lymphoid follicles) or when the point of interest is to understand the biology of disease.

A second though related problem concerns the concept of *de-differentiation*.
To a pathologist malignant progression is usually associated with a breakdown of normal tissue architecture and function and a dominance by cells of a "poorly differentiated character" (i.e. by anaplasia). By analogy when chronic myeloid leukemia enters its acute phase or blast crisis the picture is then dominated by "immature" or undifferentiated cells. Now the dominant cell clone in these situations may be immature and *relatively* less differentiated than the cellular components it replaces but it may be incorrect to assume that this arises by a de-differentiation or retrogressive differentiation of mature cells and that the end product is necessarily an anaplastic undifferentiated cell [1].
If, on the contrary, the original "target" cell for the malignant transformation were to be an infrequent tissue stem cell then a different evolutionary scenario can be considered in which selective events progressively compromise the capacity to mature and favor the least mature members of a malignant clone. In this way malignancies may come to reflect in part at least the phenotypic features of proliferating precursor or stem cells. This perspective of malignant cell phenotypes places considerable emphasis on the relationship between the "target" cell for the disease and the level at which maturation arrest occurs, the latter varying as the disease progresses. This view finds particularly strong support from the study of teratocarcinomas [2] and Ph^1 positive chronic myeloid leukemia [3].

Notwithstanding that with progressive aneuploidy, malignant cell clones may actually *lose* differentiated features (e.g. capacity to synthesize and secrete complete immunoglobulin molecules); it is likely that, as more refined marker systems become available, the "negative" status of the "poorly differentiated" cell can be replaced by identifying its cell lineage affiliation, "developmental" position within that lineage and proliferative status.

2. CELLULAR IDENTITY AND DIFFERENTIATION-LINKED MARKERS

Identification of cells is central to the study of the biology and pathology of the hemopoietic system. Progress in this area has been rapid in recent years and coupled with the development of functional assays for precursors (see Chapter 2) has led to an increasingly finer dissection of cellular relationships and aberrations.

Cell "markers" are now relatively commonplace in laboratories investigating blood cells and provide a more incisive, quantitative and molecular approach to the description of cell phenotypes than more traditional morphological methods. They are clearly most useful in circumstances where no clear morphological or ultrastructural correlates of cell type exist; this may be particularly pertinent in the context of hemopoietic precursors and functional subsets of lymphocytes. In leukemia and lymphoma "marker" assays have suggested new and biologically rational classifications of disease (see Chapter 9) and are now paving the way for more appropriate treatment.

The definition of a "marker" varies, some authors using it to denote the assay or reaction seen (e.g. "rosette reaction", see **Fig. 18** in Part 1 of Chapter 9), some the "probe" used (e.g. fluorescent antibody) and others the cell associated molecules (e.g. enzyme, antigen) responsible for the reaction.
Any cellular component can in principle serve as an identity tag provided it has an absolute or relative selectivity of quantitative expression when different cells of interest are compared (e.g. cells of different lineages or related cells of varying degrees of maturation).

Two major marker panels in the hemopoietic system are cell surface antigens (and other cell surface binding sites) and enzymes. The latter can be cell surface associated, lysosomal,

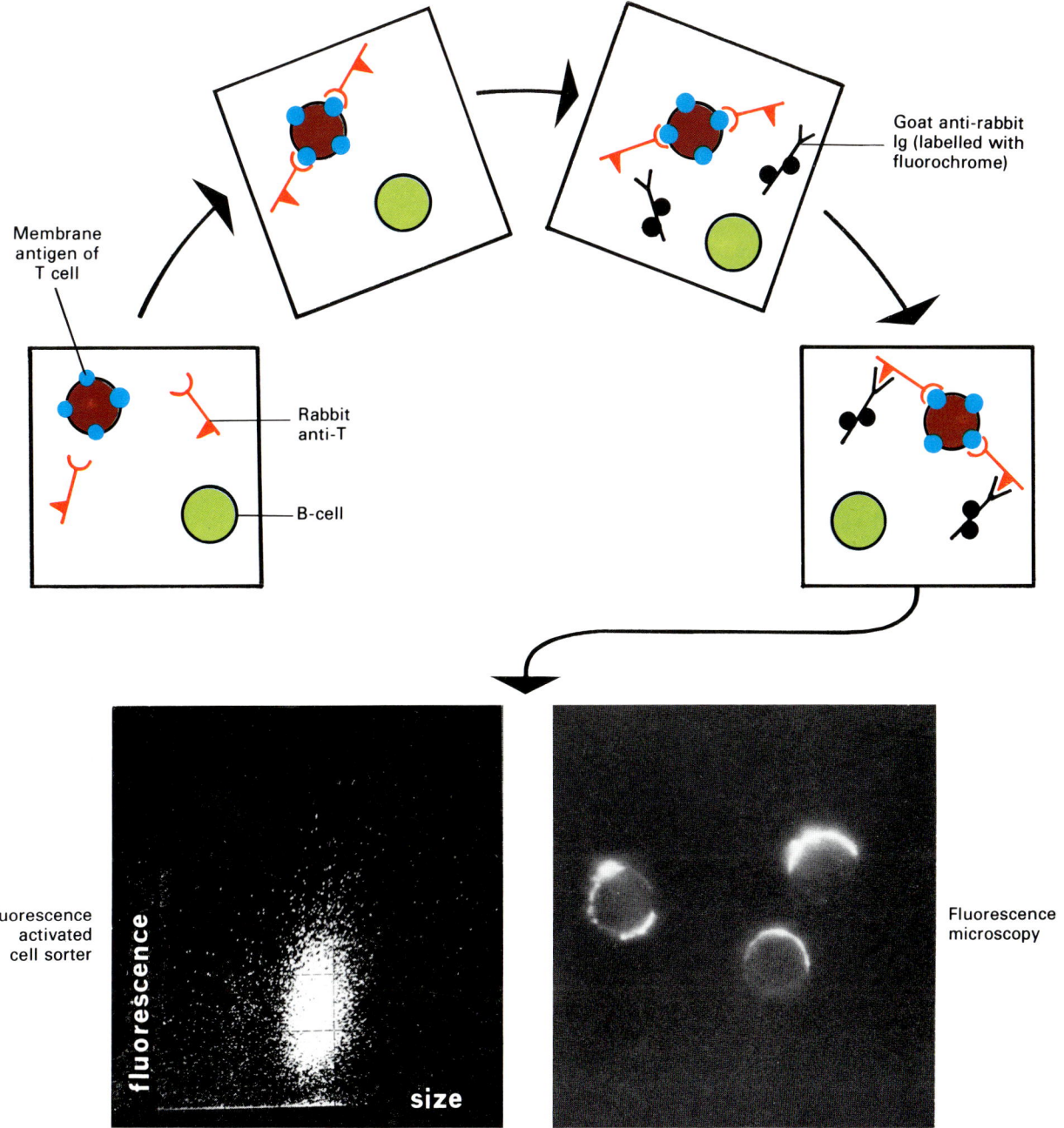

Fig. 1 *Indirect immunofluorescence technique for detecting cell surface antigens. In this schematic diagram the sequential steps in staining cells with cell surface binding antibodies are shown along with examples of the end results obtained. The stained cells show considerable redistribution of the bound fluorescent antibodies into aggregates and "caps". The Fluorescence Activated Cell Sorter profile is a polaroid photograph of the machine's oscilloscope screen. Each white dot represents the composite signal of an individual cell (10,000 cells in total) generated by fluorescence emission and light scattering. The strength of the signal detected is independent of the pattern of staining (i.e. diffuse or aggregated).*

mitochondrial, cytoplasmic or nuclear and detected by virtue of either their enzymatic activity (i.e. by cytochemistry) or their antigenicity (i.e. with a labelled anti-enzyme antibody). Enzymes that are selectively expressed in immature hemopoietic cells are particularly valuable for investigations on leukemia, e.g. myeloperoxidase in granulocytic precursors, terminal deoxynucleotidyl transferase in lymphocytic precursors (see Chapter 9).

Antibodies provide ideal markers because of their properties of specificity, diversity and stability. Antibody binding to individual cells can be visualized by immunofluorescence (i.e. fluorochrome coupled antibody), autoradiography (i.e. radio-isotope labelled antibody), enzymology (i.e. enzymes such as

peroxidase used to label antibody)
or by light (or electron) microscopy
if the antibody is made particulate
(i.e. by coupling to particles such as latex
or erythrocytes).

Two recent technical developments
(**Figs. 1, 2**) in this field promise to greatly
improve the efficiency of blood cell
analysis with antibodies. One is flow
microfluorimetry and sorting [4, 5, 6],
the other, hybridoma derived antibodies
[7, 8]. Although these both play a relatively
minor part in the data provided in this book
they are likely to become sufficiently
commonplace and important to justify
including some brief description
of the principles involved.

Flow microfluorimetry is a method
for the rapid analysis and quantitation
of individual cells in a stream of fluid.
Several different machines
with this capacity have been produced
and although fluorescence and light
scattering (roughly proportional to cell
size) are the main parameters measured,
others can be included (e.g. fluorescence
depolarization, volume) as part
of a multiparameter analysis. This is now
a mushrooming technology with large
sums of capital invested in multi-channel
analysers, data analysis by computer
and image enhancing techniques [9].
Binding of antibodies to cell surfaces
can be ideally investigated using flow
systems; quantitation of DNA, RNA
and enzymes (with fluorogenic substrates)
is becoming commonplace also.
Figure 1 illustrates a general method
used to identify selective binding
of an antibody marker to particular cells
within a mixed cell population. The labelled
cells can then be observed by fluorescence
microscopy and/or by an automated flow
system such as the Fluorescence Activated
Cell Sorter or FACS (**Fig. 1**).
FACS incorporates a 4 or 10 watt
argon lazer and can analyse 3-10,000
cells per second. Cells of interest
can also be physically sorted
under preparative, sterile conditions
by charge deflection of (cell containing)
droplets. The details of the FACS
and similar electronic analysers and sorters
have been published [4]. Examples
of the application of analysis of blood cells
by FACS can be found in individual chapters
of this book (and in reviews 5, 6).

A second important technical development
in relation to immunological markers is
the hybridoma technique (see Appendix).
The principle involved is to fuse immunized
spleen cells from mice or rats
with an immortalized myeloma cell line
from mice (or rats). The latter is selected
as a mutant or variant which does not
synthesize and secrete its own
immunoglobulin; it is also a mutant
at the locus for the enzyme hypoxanthine
phospho-ribosyl transferase (HPRT)
and can be grown under such culture
conditions that it will not survive unless
fused with a HPRT positive cell.
The resultant fused hybrid or *hybridoma*
formed between an antibody producing
normal B cell (HPRT+) and a non-secreting
(HPRT−) myeloma cell is immortal
and will secrete the antibody programmed
for by the normal (immunized) B cell
(see **Fig. 2**). If the hybrids are cloned
(as single cells) and then grown in bulk
they will produce antibody of a single
specificity (= monoclonal antibody).

Monoclonal antibodies have several
advantages over *conventional* antisera:

1. they have a highly restricted specificity
and do not require absorption; in contrast,
more conventional antisera contain
(polyclonal) antibodies of differing
specificities;

2. monoclonal antibodies can be produced
with extremely high titers and in sufficient
quantities for standardized reagents
to be made available.

The principle of antibody producing
hybridomas is illustrated in **Figure 2**.
The nature and purity of the immunizing
antigen and the efficiency of clone
screening are very important. Once clones
producing antibody of interest are identified
they can be frozen or passaged as lines
in mice (and harvested as ascitic fluid).
Hybridomas could in theory be immortal,
although in practice they may be genetically
unstable, lose chromosomes and eventually
stop making antibody.

The advent of monoclonal antibodies
at the same time as gene cloning heralds
in a new era in molecular and cellular
biology; it seems likely that these technical
innovations will lead to important advances
in our understanding of the hemopoietic
system in health and disease.

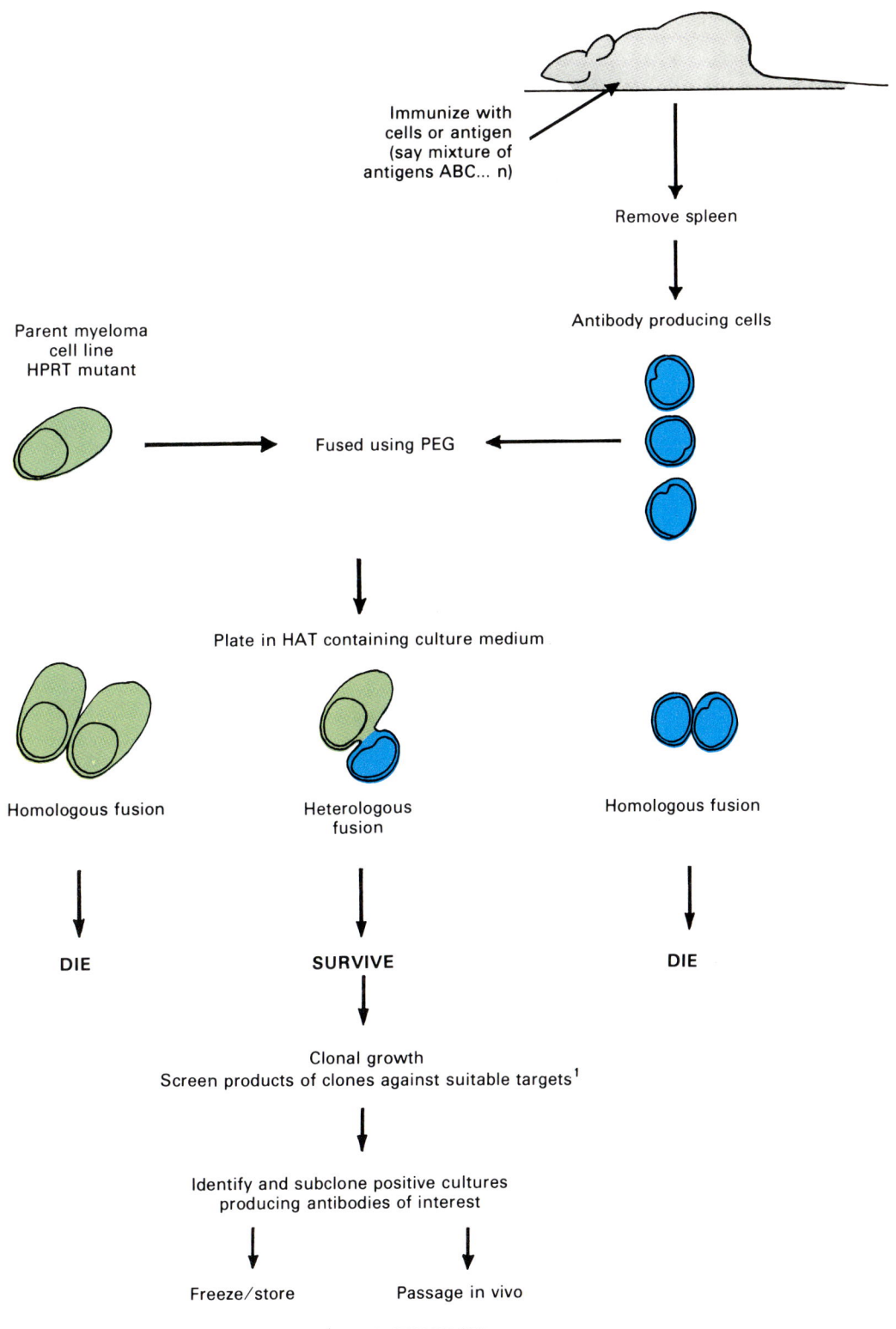

Fig. 2 Hybridoma method for producing monoclonal antibodies. Aminopterin (A) inhibits the major synthetic pathway for synthesis of purines and pyrimidines. An alternative pathway utilizes hypoxanthine for purine synthesis. HPRT mutants lack the enzyme necessary for the alternative pathway. If an HPRT − myeloma cell line is grown in the presence of Hypoxanthine, Aminopterin and Thymidine (HAT) it will die unless rescued by fusion with a normal cell (e.g. lymphocyte) that is HPRT+. Since normal immune cells survive for only a short period in vitro only hybrids will survive under these selective conditions. HPRT: hypoxanthine phosphoribosyl transferase; PEG: Polyethylene glycol; **1**, using ^{125}I or enzyme labelled anti-mouse Ig to detect binding to appropriate target antigens.
For review of hybridoma technology see ref. 8.

3. "MARKERS" OF MALIGNANCY

Malignant hemopoietic cells have been traditionally identified and classified according to morphological and cytochemical criteria which seek to relate stable or consistent features of leukemic cells to corresponding features of normal cells in blood or marrow. The same principle applies with the newer immunological and enzymatic markers although since some of these are selective for stem cell or precursor cell leukemias the correlation with normal phenotypes has not always been immediately obvious. Comparisons between leukemic cells of an immature type with normal mature blood cells (e.g. ALL with lymphocytes, AML with granulocytes) have led to erroneous conclusions and frequently to the optimistic view that a leukemia specific antigen or marker had been discovered.

To date, no unequivocal leukemia (lymphoma or myeloma) specific antigenic or enzymatic marker for human cells has been identified [3, 18]. At a single cell level the only common and consistent phenotypic features of leukemic cells which are not known to occur in equivalent normal cells are karyotypic (e.g. balanced chromosomal translocations, see Chapter 11). The non-random changes may provide important markers in particular forms of hemopoietic malignancy, e.g. (22q−) in CML, (14q+) in B lymphoma and might also play a central causal role in the malignant process [11, 12].
The presence of a common karyotype in all or most cells of a given leukemia also provides a marker for the whole cell population indicating its likely monoclonal origin [13]. Sequential analyses usually reveal the diversification of karyotype and "selection" of subclones [14]. Two other "markers" have been used to demonstrate the likely leukemic or malignant nature of a cell population; however, in contrast to the specific chromosomal changes these two are intrinsically normal markers, which can reveal the monoclonal origin of a cell population; these are glucose-6-phosphate dehydrogenase and immunoglobulin.

3.1. Glucose-6-phosphate dehydrogenase (G-6-PD) isoenzymes and clonality of leukemic cells

G-6-PD occurs in 2 major forms, A and B. These are controlled by X-linked genes. In a heterozygous female A/B, each individual cell will be either A or B type since one X chromosome is excluded in every cell (Lyon hypothesis).
As a consequence of this random selective event a normal tissue will be composed of approximately equal numbers of A cells and B cells. If, however, a single cell has a selective advantage, it will result in the appearance of a cell population that is restricted to one G-6-PD type (**Fig. 3**). This occurs in leukemia (e.g. CML, AML) and most other human neoplasms investigated and is, therefore, considered to reflect a *monoclonal* origin of disease. Whilst this may frequently be the case it cannot be ruled out that the event or events producing monoclonality were later than, and secondary to, the initial "transforming" events.

3.2. Immunoglobulin determinants and monoclonal B cell malignancy

Lymphocytes are unique cells in having a functional specificity which is highly diversified and clonally distributed so that each individual clone produces only one particular antibody either as a cell surface receptor for antigen or in response to antigenic challenge as a secreted product (of plasma cells). The genetic basis of this high degree of restriction is not fully understood (see Chapter 9).
Antibody (immunoglobulin, Ig) genes are autosomal and unique in that they undergo functional allelic exclusion wherein only products of one parental chromosome are expressed (cf. G-6-PD isoenzymes on X chromosome). Also a choice is made between 1 of the 2 sets of Ig light chain genes (kappa/κ and lambda/λ which are on different chromosomes) in order to further restrict clonal specificity.

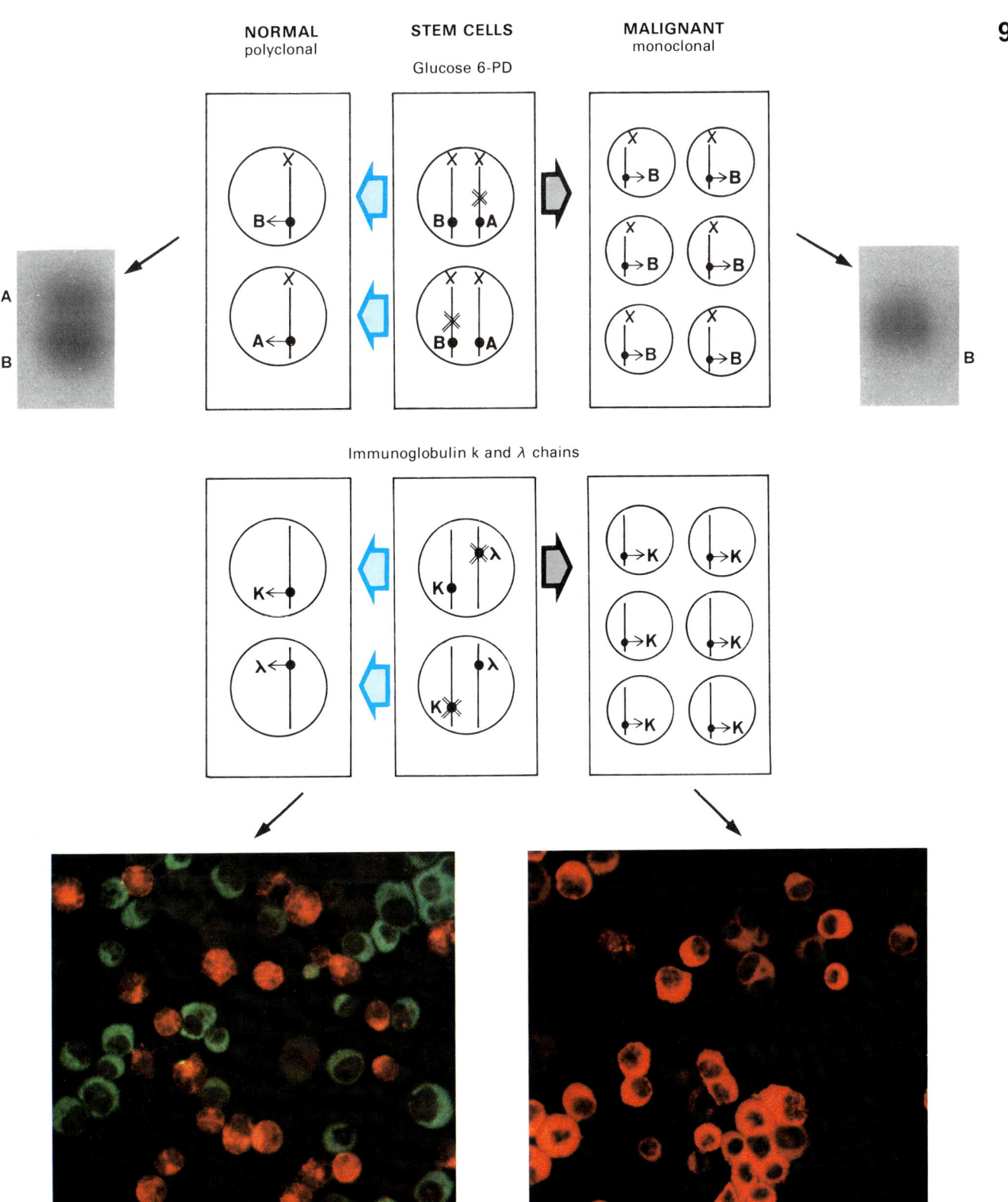

Fig. 3 *Markers of monoclonality.* Glucose-6-phosphate dehydrogenase isoenzymes. *Photographs on the right and left of the diagram (**top**) are of starch gel electrophoresis preparations showing two diffuse bands (on the left) of **A** and **B** isoenzyme from normal tissue of a Gd^B/Gd^A heterozygote and a single diffuse band of **B** isoenzyme (on the right) from malignant cells from the same patient (or any other Gd^B/Gd^A heterozygote which would also show a single **A** or **B** band).*
Immunoglobulin, κ and λ light chains. *Colored photographs on the right and left (**bottom**) show cytoplasmic staining for κ light chain (with rhodamine labelled anti-κ) and λ light chain (with fluorescein labelled anti-λ). Note that, in both normal (on the **left**) and malignant (on the **right**) tissue, individual cells produce only a single light chain type; however, as with the G-6-PD marker the normal population (on the **left**) contains a mixture of the two cell types (i.e. is polyclonal) whereas the malignant population (e.g. B immunoblastic lymphoma or myeloma) consists of a single (monoclonal) cell type.*

Antibodies can be produced against various parts of the immunoglobulin molecule (= anti-antibodies) and these provide a means to identify the restricted Ig gene product of individual B cells. Since the restriction process is essentially random, *individual* cells will produce maternal or paternal light (or heavy) Ig chain but not both and either κ or λ light chains. The whole B cell population will be a mixture of cells of the two types, not necessarily at a 1 : 1 ratio, however, since environmental antigens may selectively amplify one or the other compartment. As with the G-6-PD marker, a normal and malignant (leukemia, lymphoma, myeloma) B cell lineage population can be distinguished by virtue of the diversity of allotypes or light chain types produced (**Fig. 3**) [3, 15]. The presence of a single light chain type, for example, provides a strong indication of monoclonality; whilst this is very likely to reflect an underlying expansion of malignant cells, this is not inevitably the case since under some circumstances a self-controlled monoclonal expansion induced by an antigen might be possible. This is, however, considered to be a rare occurrence. Most immunologically activated proliferative responses are polyclonal and self-limiting. Immunoglobulins also provide another clonal antigenic marker which is operationally leukemia (lymphoma or myeloma) specific despite being encoded in normal genes. Each individual antibody whether expressed as a cell surface antigen receptor or secreted product bears its own unique antigenic determinant corresponding to the molecular region around the antibody binding site [16]. These are known as individually specific or *idiotypic* antigens and are different in principle from the Ig markers referred to above in having a clonal restriction and diversity corresponding to the potential antigenic challenge of the environment. Therefore, they provide unique clonal markers (cf. unique karyotypes).

In a chronic lymphocytic leukemia, for example, *every* cell may carry the same unique cell surface Ig idiotype. This same idiotype will probably be undetectable in normal individuals although it may well be there at a low frequency of cellular expression (say $< 1 : 10^4$). Idiotypic markers have been very important in investigating genetic control and clonal regulation of immune responses.

In lymphoid malignancies they are restricted in value as general "markers" since each patient has his or her own unique idiotype; however, if patient specific antisera are made they can provide an operationally leukemia specific probe for accurately enumerating levels of malignant cells before, during and after treatment. In view of their specificity they would also provide, in theory at least, ideal carriers of "targeted" drugs or poisons for immunotherapy.

REFERENCES

1. Foulds L.: *Neoplastic development.* Acad. Press, New York, 1969.
2. Pierce G.B., Strikes R., Fink L.M.: *Cancer. A problem of developmental biology.* Prentice Hall Publ., New Jersey, 1978.
3. Greaves M.F., Janossy G.: *Patterns of gene expression and the cellular origins of human leukemias.* Biochem. Biophys. Acta, *516*, 193, 1978.
4. Herzenberg L.A., Herzenberg L.A.: *Analysis and separation using the fluorescence activated cell sorter (FACS).* In: *Handbook of Experimental Immunology.* Vol. 2, Weir D.M. ed., Blackwell Publ., Oxford, p. 22.1, 1977.
5. Greaves M.: *Clinical applications of cell surface markers.* Progr. Hematol., 9, 255, 1975.
6. Janossy G., Roberts M.M., Capellaro D., Greaves M.F., Francis G.E.: *Use of the fluorescence activated cell sorter in human leukemia.* In: *Immunofluorescence and related staining techniques.* Knapp W., Holabar K., Wick G. eds., Elsevier/North Holland Biomed. Press, p. 111, 1978.
7. Melchers F., Potter M., Warner N.L. (eds.): *Lymphocyte hybridomas.* Current Topics in Microbiology and Immunology. Vol. 81, 1978.
8. Milstein C., Galfre G., Secher D.S., Springer T.: *Monoclonal antibodies and cell surface antigens.* Cell Biology International Reports, *3*, 1, 1979.
9. Report of the 6th Engineering Foundation Conference on Automated Cytology. J. Histochem. Cytochem., 27, 1, 1979.
10. Roberts M., Capellaro D., Greaves M.F.: *Cell surface antigens and the cell cycle. A study on leukemic and normal hemopoietic cells using microfluorimetry.* 1980 (in press).
11. Rowley J.D.: *Chromosomes in leukemia and lymphoma.* Sem. Hemat., 15, 301, 1978.
12. Kline G.: *Lymphoma development in mice and human: diversity of initiation is followed by convergent cytogenetic evolution.* Proc. Natl. Acad. Sci. (USA), 76, 2442, 1979.
13. Fialkow P.J.: *Clonal origin of human tumors.* Biochem. Biophys. Acta, *458*, 283, 1976.
14. Nowell P.C.: *The clonal evolution of tumor cell populations.* Science, 194, 23, 1976.
15. Lampson L.A., Levy R.: *A role for clonal antigens in cancer diagnosis and therapy.* J. Natl. Cancer Inst., 62, 217, 1979.
16. Möller G. (ed.): *Idiotypes on T and B cells.* Immunological Reviews, 34, 1977.

2
In vitro and in vivo hematopoiesis

P.A. CHERVENICK

Department of Medicine, University of Pittsburgh
Pittsburgh, U.S.A.

D. ZUCKER-FRANKLIN

Department of Medicine, New York University
New York, U.S.A.

1. **FETAL HEMATOPOIESIS**

Erythropoiesis begins in the yolk sac in all embryonic vertebrates during the mesoblastic period of hematopoiesis [1, 2]. At approximately 6 weeks of embryonic life, production of erythrocytes decreases in the yolk sac and begins in the embryo [1].

Erythropoiesis as well as myelopoiesis is present in the liver at 6 weeks, in the spleen by 12 weeks and in the marrow at 20 weeks [3]. Thereafter, the marrow is the major site of hematopoiesis. Fetal erythropoiesis is megaloblastic during the first 11 weeks of gestation and remains partially so until the first week of post natal life. Before erythropoiesis commences in the marrow, the circulating erythrocytes are nucleated and many of them are in mitosis (**Fig. 1**). There is evidence from studies in mice that the changing sites of hematopoiesis result from migration of stem cells through the blood [4]. Before the 20th week of fetal life, only the prehemopoietic stroma is seen in the medullary space of bones (**Fig. 2**). The earliest hematopoietic island that can be observed already shows a mixture of cells (**Fig. 3**) supporting the concept of a pluripotent stem cell in the human fetus analogous to the CFU-S in adult mice (*vide infra*). By 22 weeks of gestation, marrow hemopoiesis is very active with all cell lines represented (**Fig. 4**).

Of necessity, much of what has been learned about the dynamics of hematopoiesis in man has been deduced from *in vitro* experiments or from pathologic states with arrest or reconstitution of marrow differentiation.

2. **BIOLOGY OF HEMATOPOIESIS**

Mature blood cells of all types have a finite life span and therefore, continued production is required in order to maintain a constant level in the blood and tissues. Continuous replenishment is achieved by feed in from a normal functioning pluripotent stem cell compartment.

A pluripotent stem cell must be capable of self renewal and must also have the ability to differentiate into various progenitor cells committed to either granulopoiesis, erythropoiesis or megakaryopoiesis. A model of hematopoietic stem cell differentiation is seen in **Figure 5**. Evidence for pluripotent stem cells is derived from several sources. One is from observations of developing hemopoietic islands in the bone marrow of the human fetus where "mixed" colonies rather than cell populations made up of the same type occur from the beginning (see **Figs. 3, 4**). The second is from the spleen colony assay in the mouse, in which marrow cells containing a marker chromosome repopulate the spleen of irradiated recipients with colonies of erythrocytes, granulocytes and megakaryocytes containing the same marker chromosome [5]. The pluripotent stem cell giving rise to the various cell lines has been termed CFU-S (Colony Forming Unit-Spleen). There is no similar assay for CFU-S in man.

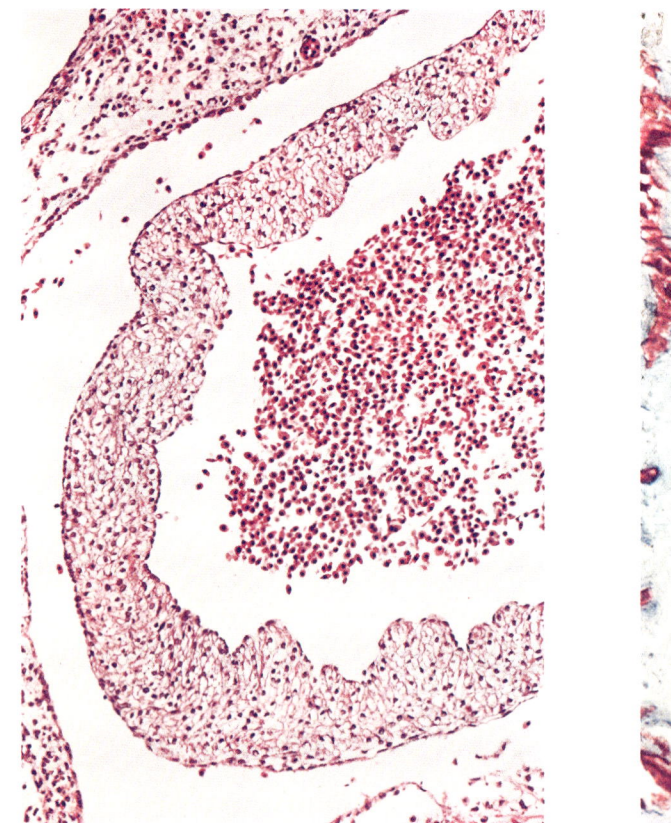
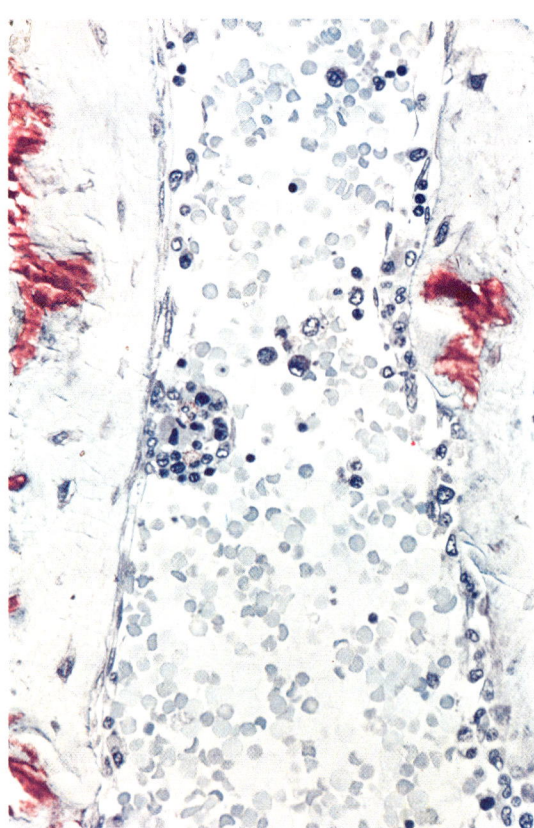

Fig. 1 Section of the heart of a 7 week old human fetus embedded in paraffin and stained with H & E. The blood at this stage of development resembles avian blood because the primitive erythrocytes are nucleated. Mitoses are also seen in the circulation at this stage.
Courtesy of Dr. W. Calvo, Department of Clinical Physiology, University of Ulm, Germany.

Fig. 2 Section through a rib of an 11 week old human fetus. The specimen was embedded in methacrylate and stained with PAS reagent. It demonstrates the prehemopoietic stage of marrow development in which only "stroma" is present. Loose connective tissue is attached to the bone trabeculae and shows large sinusoids, reticular cells and some undifferentiated mononuclear cells.
Courtesy of Dr. W. Calvo, Department of Clinical Physiology, University of Ulm, Germany.

A third observation in support of the existence of pluripotential stem cells is the distribution of the Philadelphia (Ph) chromosome in erythrocytes, granulocytes, macrophages and megakaryocytes in chronic myelogenous leukemia (CML) [6] (see Chapter 11) and a fourth is the distribution of the marker isozyme G-6-PD in myeloproliferative disorders [7] (see also Chapter 1, **Fig. 3**).

Further supporting evidence may be gleaned from studies of the marrow of transplant recipients [8]. By now it is well established that a pluripotent stem cell exists for myeloid cells. In addition, there is evidence in mice for the existence of a more primitive stem cell, a totipotent stem cell which is common for the myeloid as well as the lymphoid systems [9]. The existence of a similar cell in man can be inferred from studies of human leukemia and related diseases [10, 11, 12, 13].

Stem cells are present in low concentrations in hematopoietic tissue and number approximately one per 1,000 nucleated marrow cells [5]. There are no distinctive features which allow their certain identification, but morphologically they resemble lymphocytes [14]. Under normal circumstances, pluripotent stem cells are not actively proliferating [15] nor is it clear what regulates their proliferation. Local factors including cell-cell interaction, microenvironmental factors and humoral factors [16, 17, 18] are all considered to be of possible

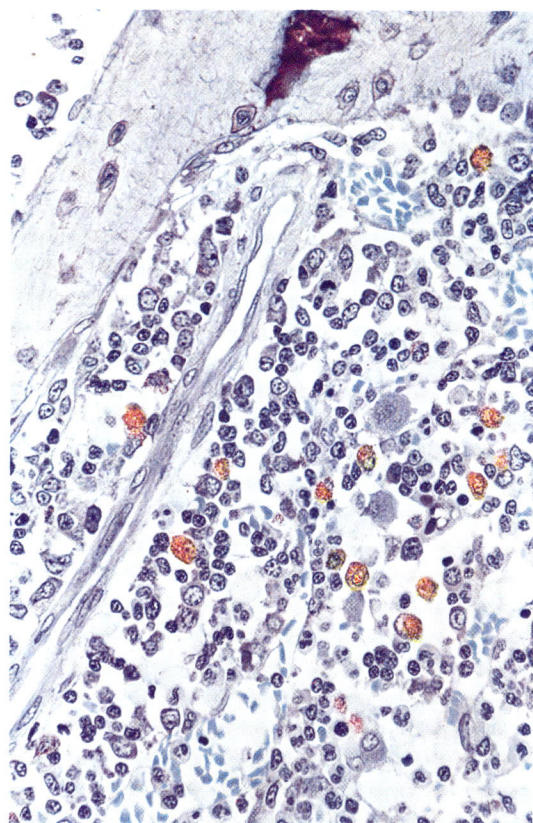

Fig. 3 Section through the humerus of a 15 week old human fetus shows the "mixed" nature of the earliest hemopoietic cells. The specimen was embedded in methacrylate and stained with Giemsa.
Courtesy of Dr. W. Calvo, Department of Clinical Physiology, University of Ulm, Germany.

Fig. 4 Section through the humerus of a 22 week old human fetus. Specimen embedded in methacrylate and stained with Giemsa. Active hematopoiesis in which all cell lines are represented now takes place in the medullary cavity. Note particularly orange-stained eosinophil precursors, one arteriole, sinusoids and bone trabeculae.
Courtesy of Dr. W. Calvo, Department of Clinical Physiology, University of Ulm, Germany.

importance in regulating their proliferation.

Pluripotent stem cells give rise to progenitor cells which are committed to differentiate along a specific pathway of hemopoiesis, i.e. to erythropoiesis, granulopoiesis or megakaryocytopoiesis (**Fig. 5**). These committed progenitor cells are detected by their ability to form colonies of specific cell types when cloned in the soft gel *in vitro* culture system described initially by Pluznik and Sachs [19] and Bradley and Metcalf [20] and adapted for human marrow culture by Pike and Robinson [21].

Cells giving rise to colonies of granulocyte-macrophages are referred to as CFU-GM, those giving rise to erythrocytes, CFU-E and those giving rise to megakaryocytes, CFU-MEG. Cell proliferation within each colony is regulated by specific growth regulators such as colony stimulating factor (CSF) (also referred to as colony stimulating activity, CSA), a glycoprotein which stimulates granulocyte and macrophage precursors and erythropoietin (EP) which stimulates erythroid precursors.

Committed progenitor cells are also infrequent in marrow with approximately 1 cell per 500 nucleated cells being a granulocyte-macrophage progenitor (CFU-GM). They differ from pluripotent stem cells in size and density and by a larger fraction being in an active generative cycle [15, 22]. Morphologically they resemble medium size lympocytes [23] (**Fig. 6**).

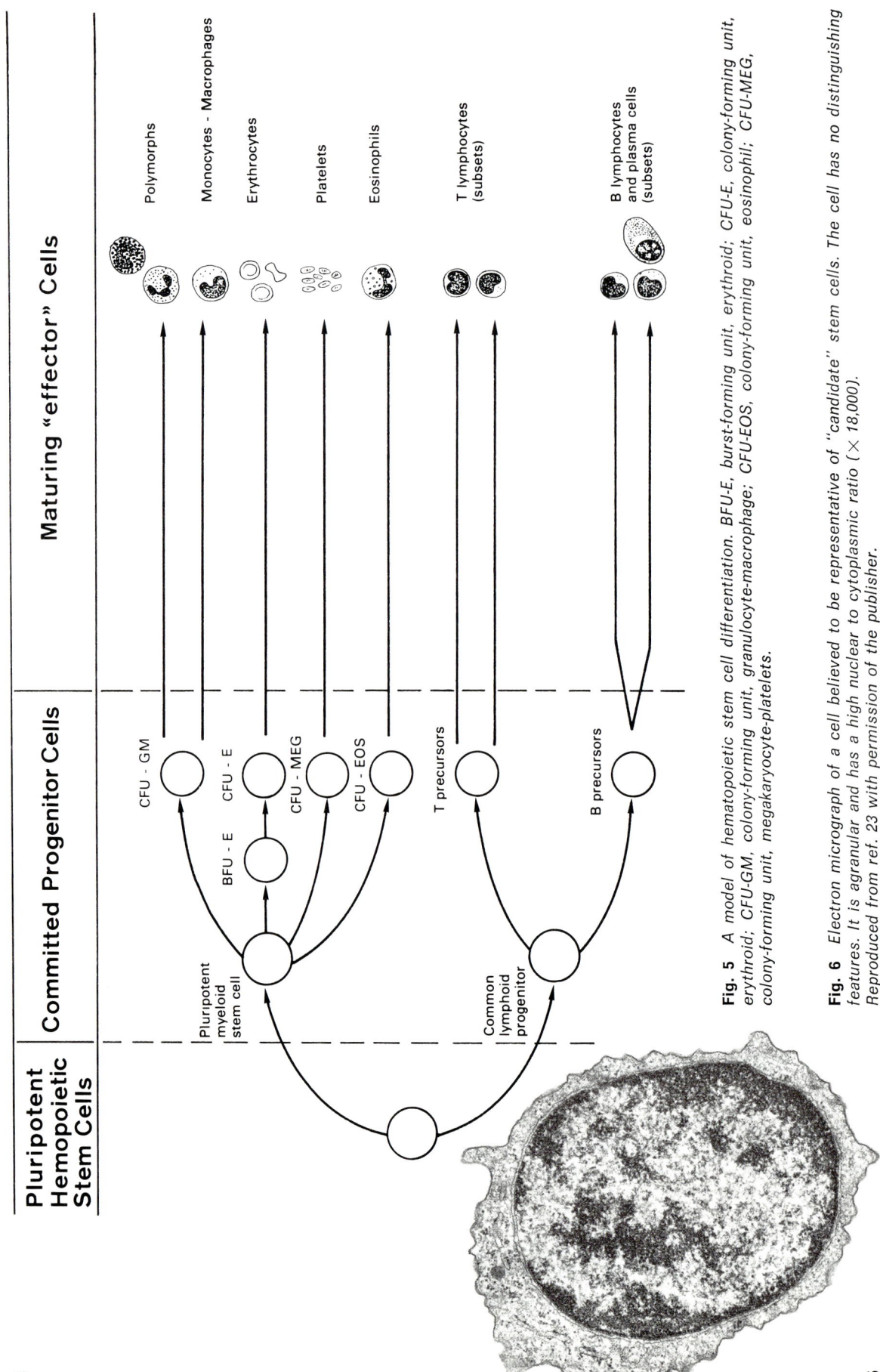

Fig. 5 A model of hematopoietic stem cell differentiation. BFU-E, burst-forming unit, erythroid; CFU-E, colony-forming unit, erythroid; CFU-GM, colony-forming unit, granulocyte-macrophage; CFU-EOS, colony-forming unit, eosinophil; CFU-MEG, colony-forming unit, megakaryocyte-platelets.

Fig. 6 Electron micrograph of a cell believed to be representative of "candidate" stem cells. The cell has no distinguishing features. It is agranular and has a high nuclear to cytoplasmic ratio ($\times$ 18,000). Reproduced from ref. 23 with permission of the publisher.

3. HEMATOPOIESIS IN SHORT TERM CULTURES

3.1. Granulocyte-macrophage proliferation

When marrow or nucleated blood cells are cultured in the presence of CSF, granulocyte macrophage progenitor cells (CFU-GM) proliferate and differentiate to form colonies of 50-2,000 cells after 10-14 days in culture (**Figs. 7-8**). Morphologically these colonies consist of either eosinophils, monocytes, neutrophils or macrophages [24, 25] (**Figs. 8 a-d** and **9-11**). It is presumed that CFU-GM give rise to the earliest recognizable granulocyte, the myeloblast. Eosinophils arise from progenitor cells (CFU-EOS) which differ from CFU-GM [26, 27] and respond to a specific CSF [26, 28] (see Chapter 6). CSF active on human cells is derived from several sources, including blood monocytes [29, 30, 31], activated lymphocytes [32], human embryo kidney [33], human placenta [34] and several established cell lines [35]. Granulocyte-macrophage proliferation *in vitro* is also modulated by inhibitors released from granulocytes [36] and by prostaglandins [37].

3.2. Erythrocyte proliferation

A method for culturing erythroid cells in mice was developed by Stephenson et al. [38] and later adapted for the culture of human cells [39, 40]. In this culture system, erythroid progenitor cells proliferate to form colonies of erythrocytes if erythropoietin is present. Two distinct populations of erythroid progenitor cells are recognized; one gives rise to colonies which attain a maximal size of 8-150 cells after 7-8 days in culture, then mature and degenerate. Progenitor cells giving rise to these colonies are termed CFU-E (Colony Forming Unit-Erythroid) (**Fig. 12 a**). A second and more primitive progenitor cell is relatively insensitive to EP. In the presence of large amounts of EP, much larger colonies of erythroid cells are present after 14 days in the form of clusters or "bursts" (**Fig. 12 b**) and arise from a progenitor cell termed BFU-E (Burst Forming Unit-Erythroid). CFU-E are considered to be progeny of BFU-E and presumably give rise to the earliest recognizable erythroid cell, the pronormoblast (see Chapter 3). Erythroid colony formation is also influenced by enhancing activity termed "burst promoting activity" (BPA) obtained from T-lymphocytes [41], monocytes and macrophages [42, 43]. Several hormones including dexamethasone, growth hormone and thyroid hormone enhance the effect of erythropoietin [44, 45].

3.3. Megakaryocyte proliferation

Megakaryocyte progenitor cells (CFU-MEG) proliferate to form colonies of megakaryocytes with platelet formation when cultured *in vitro* [46, 47, 48 a] (**Figs. 13, 14**). CFU-MEG proliferate in response to materials which presumably contain thrombopoietin and are provided by mitogen stimulated lymphocytes for murine cells [46] and high concentrations of erythropoietin for humans [48]. Human megakaryocyte colonies attain a size of 2-30 cells after 10-12 days in culture and then degenerate. Recently Fauser and Messner [48 b] have introduced a Colony Forming Technique in soft agar which detects the common progenitor of erythroblasts, neutrophils, eosinophils, macrophages and megakaryocytes.

3.4. Lymphocyte proliferation

Lymphocytes can also be cloned in the soft gel *in vitro* culture system. In the presence of appropriate stimulation, lymphocytes from blood, marrow, spleen and lymph nodes proliferate to form colonies of thymus dependent (T) or bone marrow derived (B) lymphocytes [49, 50]. Stimulation with phytohemagglutinin (PHA) or concanavalin A (Con A) is required for clonal proliferation of T cell colonies and pokeweed mitogen (PWM) and PHA for B cell colonies. Colonies reach a maximum size of 200-500 cells after 3-5 days in culture. The frequency of lymphocyte colony forming cells varies between 0.05% and 1% of blood lymphocytes. In addition to colony formation from normal cells, lymphocytes from patients with lymphoma and CLL can also be induced to form colonies *in vitro* [51, 52].

Fig. 7 a) Light microscopic photograph of unstained granulocyte and monocyte-macrophage colonies from human marrow. Marrow cells were cultured for 14 days in methylcellulose. **b)** Diffuse and compact granulocyte-macrophage colonies are seen at low magnification. **c)** High magnification showing spreading of granulocyte colony. **d)** High magnification showing large diffuse neutrophil colony and a small dense compact eosinophil colony (**arrow**).

Fig. 8 Light microscopic photograph of cells from granulocyte, monocyte and macrophage colonies grown from human marrow. Cells were aspirated from individual colonies after 14 days in culture and stained with Wright's stain. **a)** Cells from an eosinophil colony. **b)** Portion of a monocyte colony. **c, d)** Cells from a neutrophil colony showing maturing neutrophils. **e)** Large cells from a macrophage colony. Macrophages often accumulate lipid droplets which cause the cells to appear "foamy".

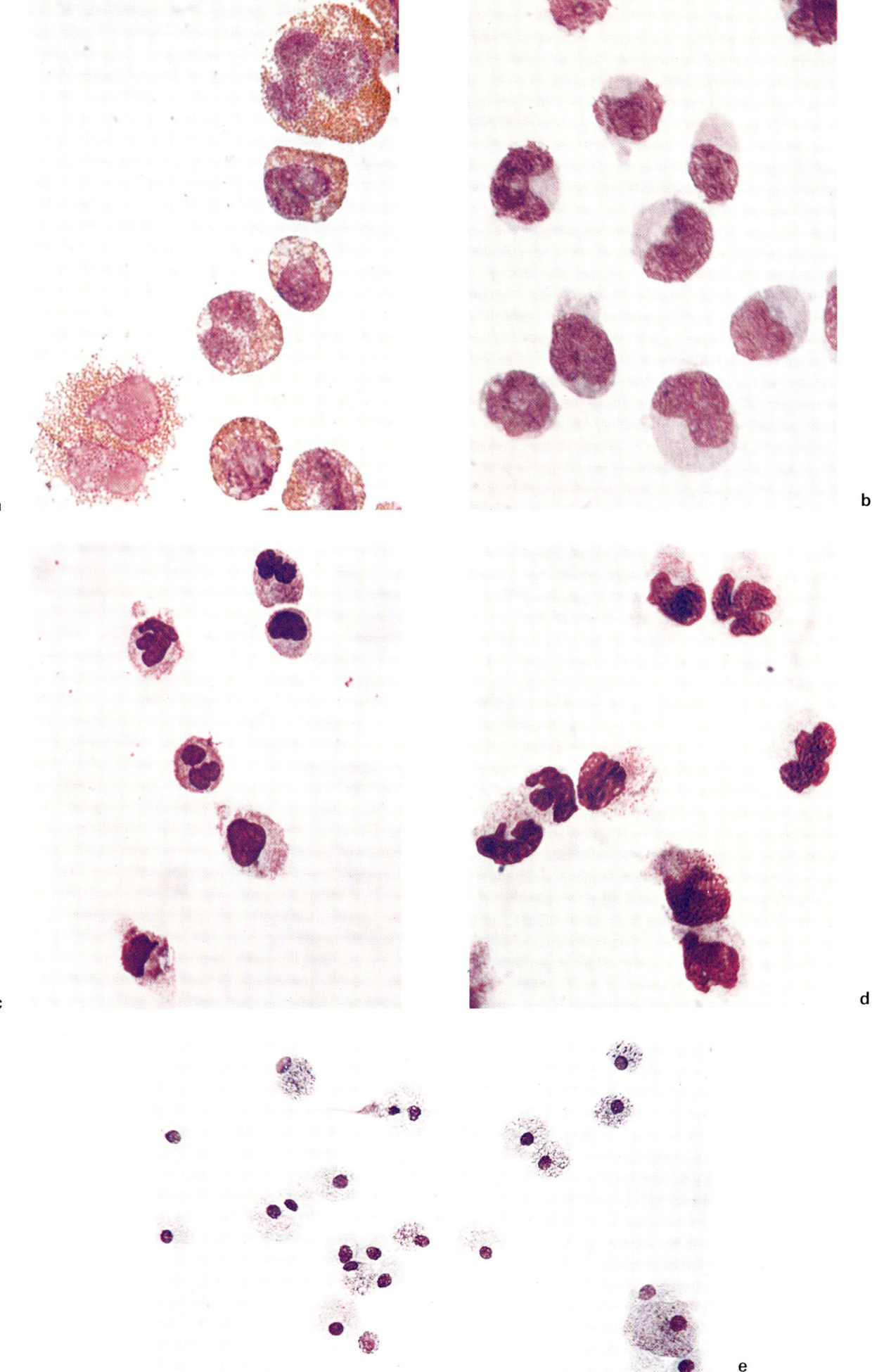

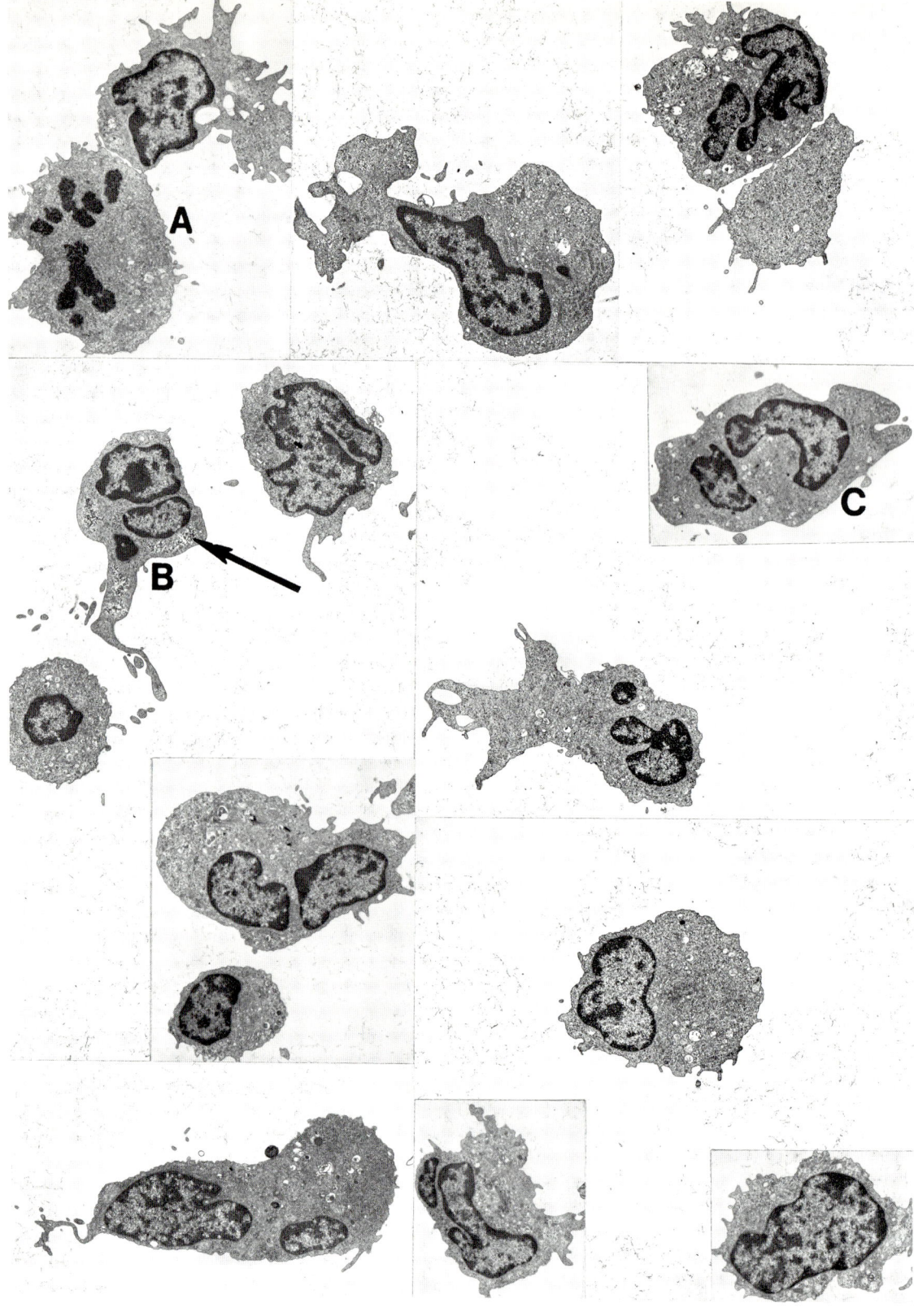

Fig. 9 Electron micrograph of representative cells in a neutrophil colony after 14 days in soft agar culture. Since these colonies appear "loose" by light microscopy, the cells are too far apart to permit a survey electron micrograph encompassing the entire colony. Therefore, cells photographed individually or in groups have been reassembled here in a fashion that closely resembles their original distribution in the intact colony. Note that the majority of cells have reached the metamyelocyte stage of development although some mitoses are still evident (**A**). The nuclei of some cells are fully segmented and may have reached an "end stage" as judged by their heterochromatin distribution (**B**). The mature appearing cells have an abundance of glycogen (**arrow** in **B**). The cell labelled **C** is seen at higher magnification in **Fig. 10** ($\times$ 4,000).

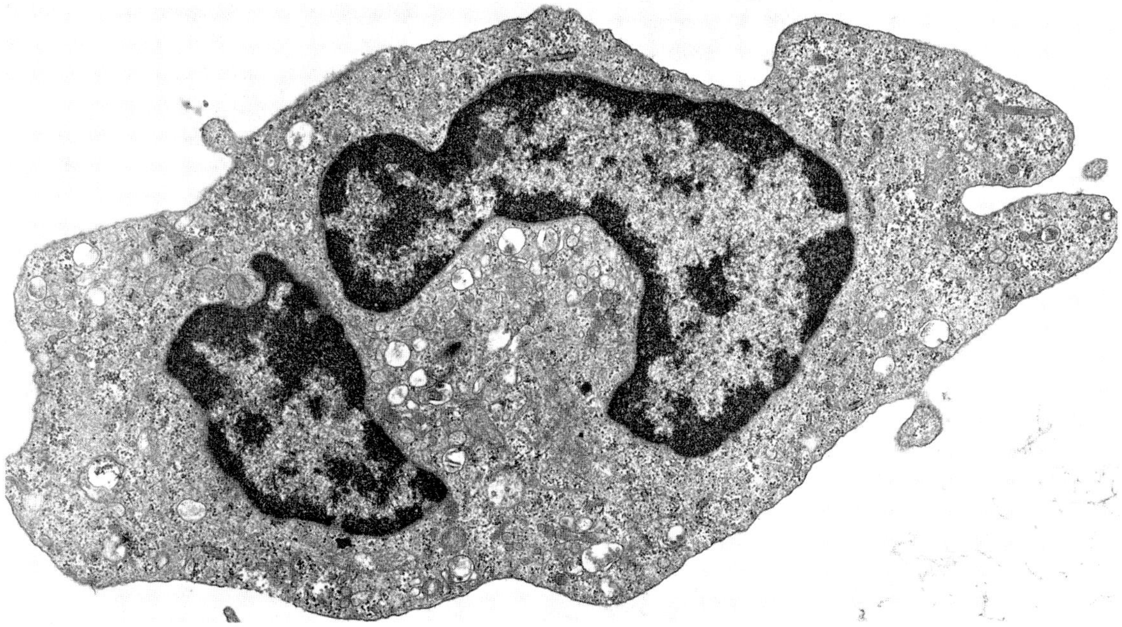

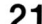

Figs. 10 and **11** Two cells from a neutrophil colony after 14 days in soft agar culture.
These two cells probably represent the same stage i.e. metamyelocyte stage of development. Note that the cell illustrated in **Fig. 11** still contains many profiles of rough endoplasmic reticulum (**RER**) and that the granules are relatively small (**G**). The cell in **Fig. 10** has a larger number of granules, less RER and a greater abundance of small black dots which represent glycogen. **Fig. 10** ($\times$ 14,000); **Fig. 11** ($\times$ 22,000).

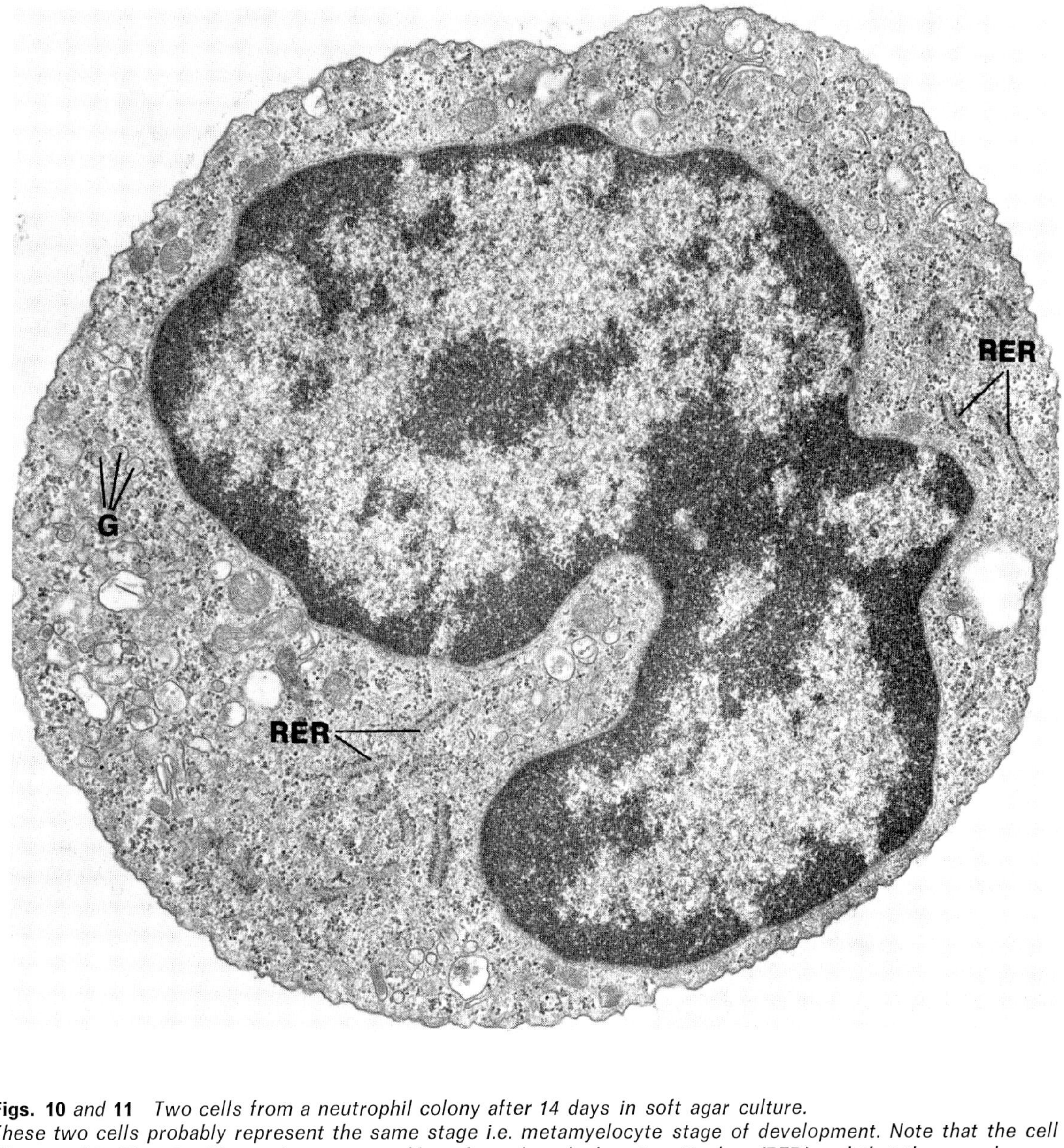

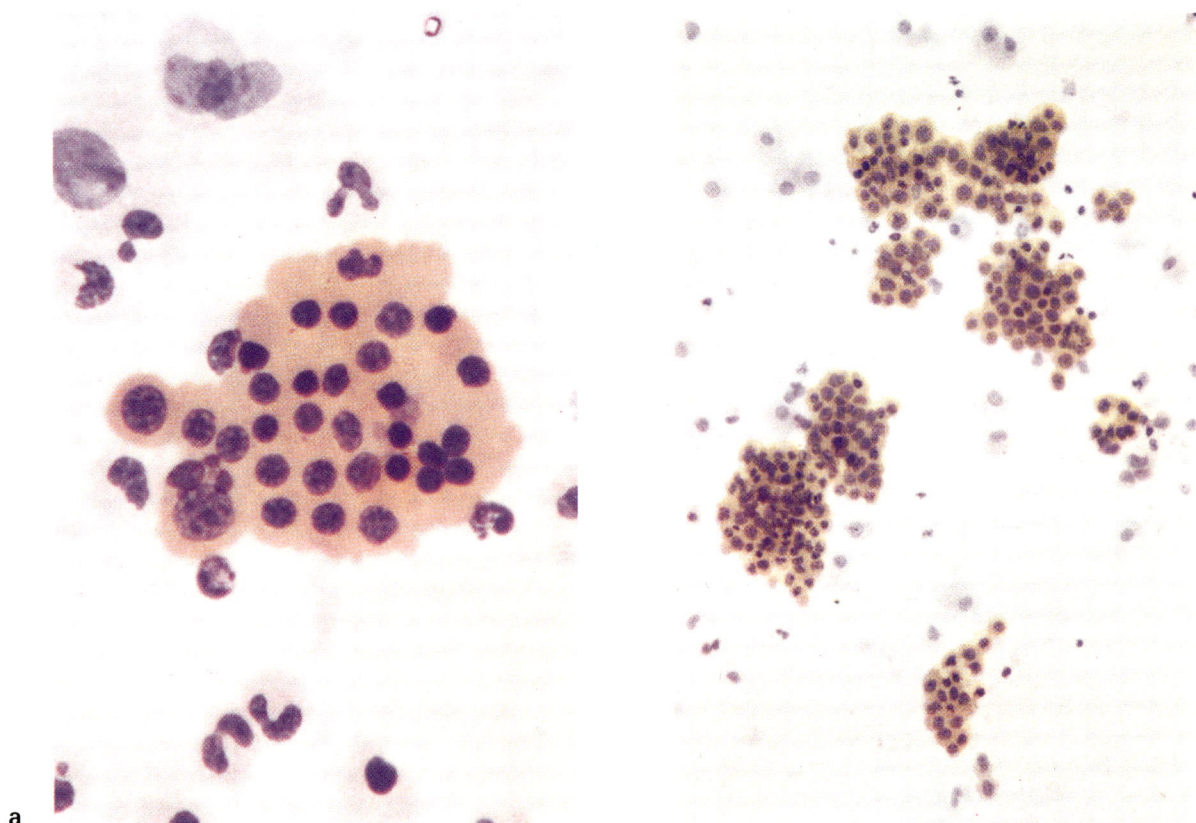

Fig. 12 Light microscopic photograph of erythroid colonies grown from human marrow in plasma clot.
a) Small, single colony arising from CFU-E.
b) Large clusters (bursts) of erythroid colonies arising from the more primitive precursor, BFU-E.

4. HEMATOPOIESIS IN LONG TERM CULTURES

In addition to the availability of *in vitro* systems for assaying the clonal proliferation of hematopoietic cells, Dexter et al. [53] more recently described a method for maintaining hematopoietic cells in long term culture. This system not only allows for the proliferation of pluripotent stem cells (CFU-S) but also supports extensive proliferation of granulocytes and their progenitor cells (CFU-GM), megakaryocytes and their precursor cells (CFU-MEG) and committed erythroid progenitor cells (BFU-E and CFU-E).

The maintenance of stem cells and their progeny in the continuous culture system is dependent upon a suitable marrow derived adherent cell population.

An adherent layer is established after 1-3 weeks in culture and consists of a heterogeneous population of cells including endothelial cells, giant fat containing cells, and macrophages [54] (**Figs. 15-17).** These cells support the proliferation and differentiation of CFU-S and their progeny for as long as 3-4 months in mice [55], for greater than 1 year in prosimian cultures [56], but for only 6-8 weeks in humans [55].

The potential clinical value as well as basic research interest of an *in vitro* maintained source of self-replicating pluripotential stem cells is obvious.

2 HEMATOPOIESIS

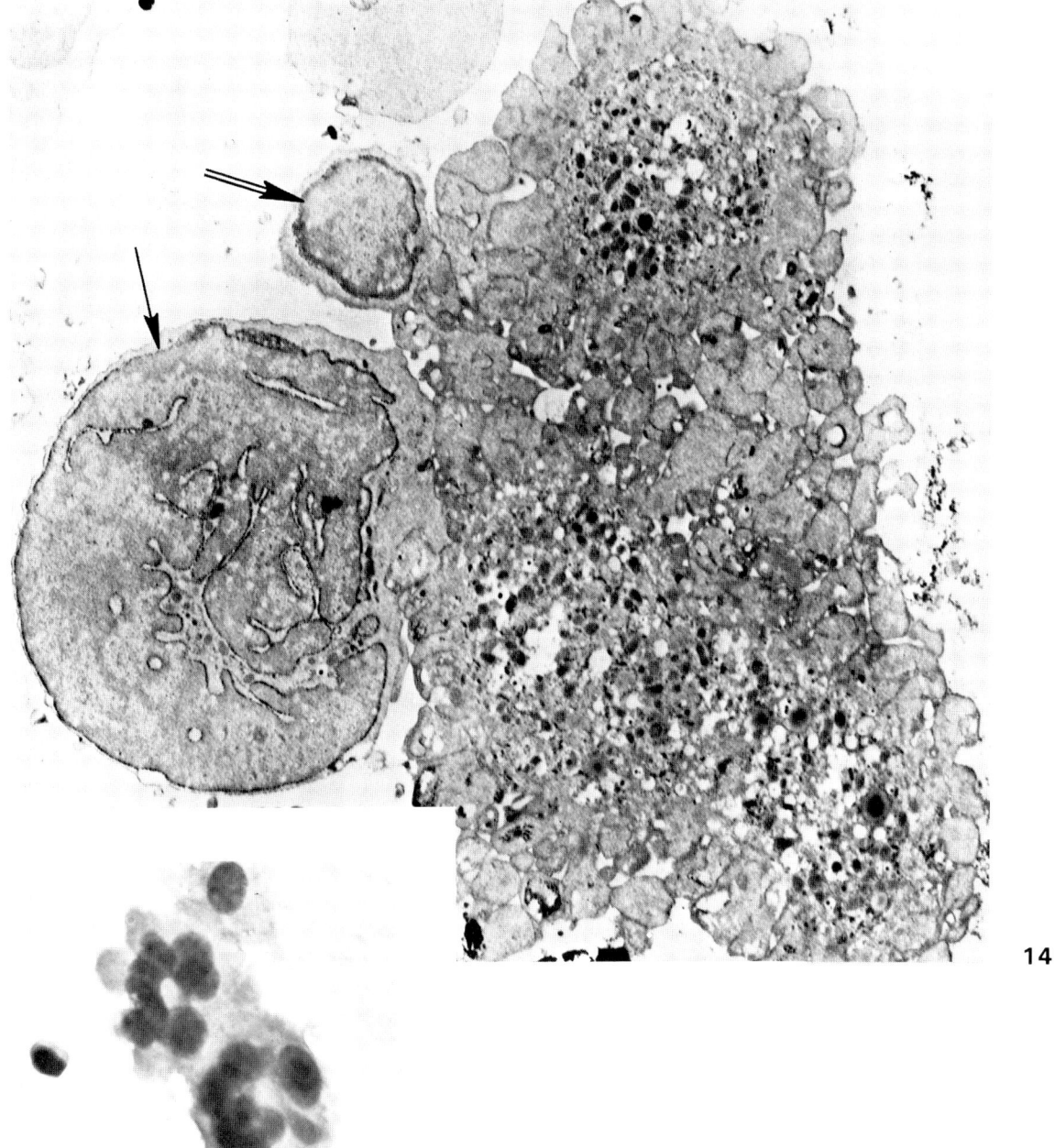

Fig. 13 Light microscopic photograph of two megakaryocytes in a colony. The macrophage with the round nucleus and a lymphocyte permit appreciation of the size and the typical multilobed nucleus of the megakaryocyte.

Fig. 14 Electron micrograph of a naked megakaryocyte nucleus (**arrow**) that has probably "shed" its platelets (**right**). The large folded nucleus as well as the small round nucleus (**double arrow**) are identified by the black reaction product indicative of platelet peroxidase in the perinuclear space. Taken from a 14 day old colony initiated with neonatal blood.
Courtesy of Dr. Breton-Gorius; reproduced from ref. 48 a.

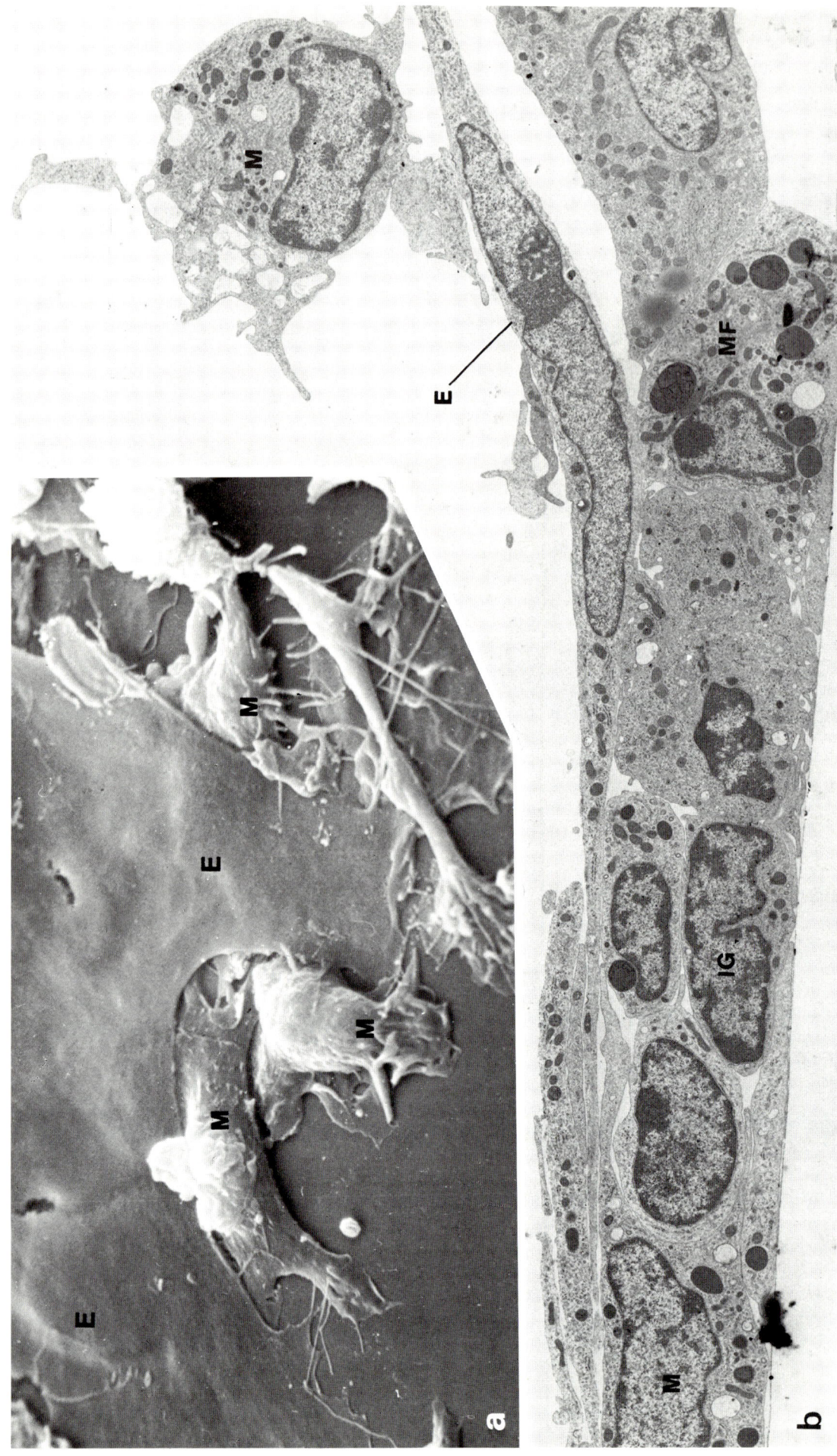

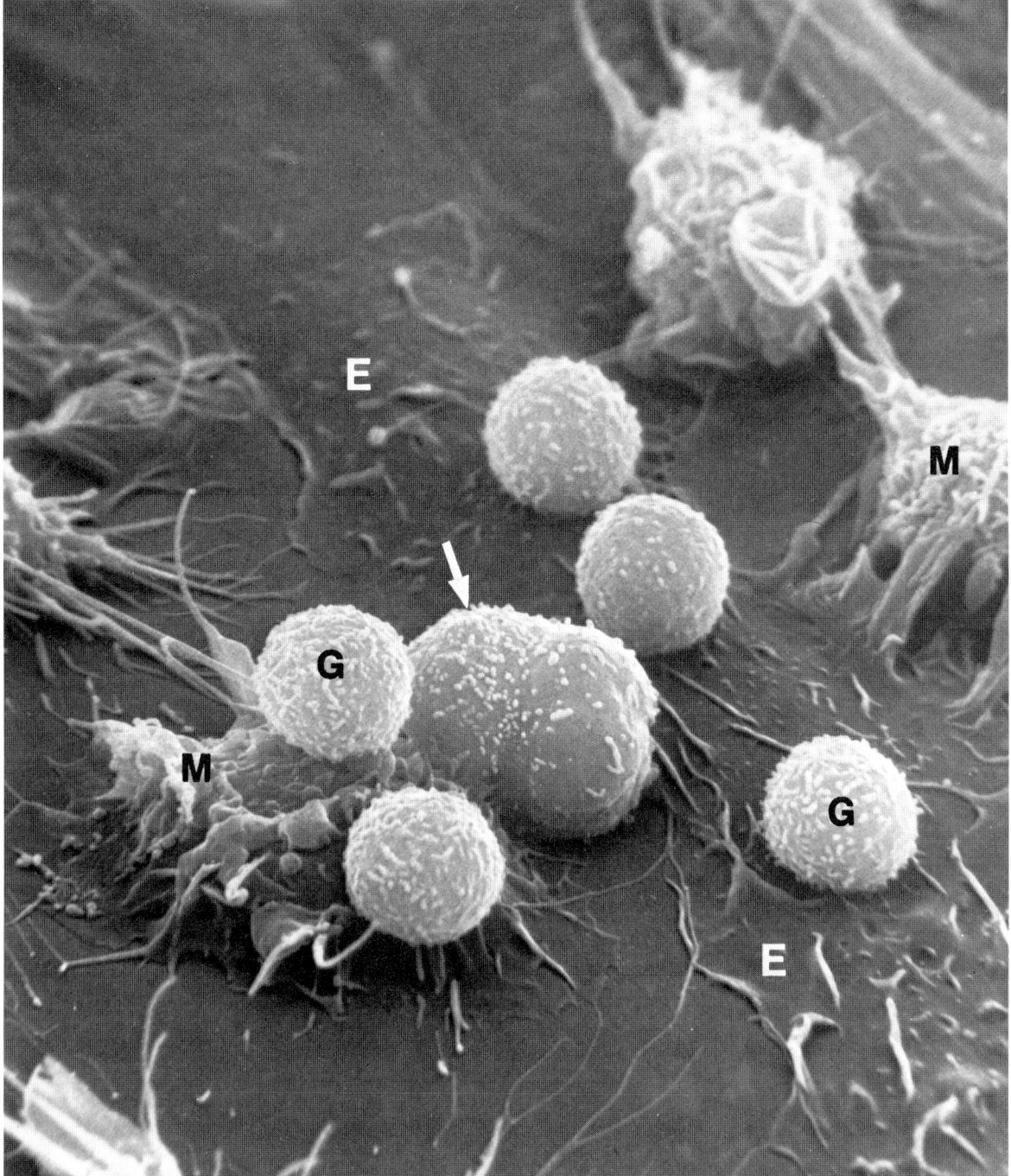

Fig. 16 Scanning electron micrograph of hematopoietic cells cultured by the same method as illustrated in Fig. 15 a. The cells are seen on the surface of flattened endothelial cells (E). Spherical granulocytes (G) and monocytes with many processes (M) are seen. Dividing granulocyte in center (arrow) ($\times$ 3,800).

Fig. 15 a) Scanning electron micrograph showing a detail of a long term marrow culture prepared by the method described in ref. 53. The adherent layer is two to three cells deep in most places. The edge of the sheet of epithelioid (endothelial-derived) cells (E) partially covers several monocytes (M) ($\times$ 2,400).
b) Transmission electron micrograph of a section cut at right angles to the culture. A monocyte (M) is attached to the upper surface of a flattened endothelial-derived cell (E) which covers in turn the remainder of the cells present: monocytes (M), immature granulocyte (IG), a monocyte with accumulated fat droplets (MF) ($\times$ 7,000).
Courtesy of Dr. T.D. Allen, Christie Hospital, Manchester, UK.

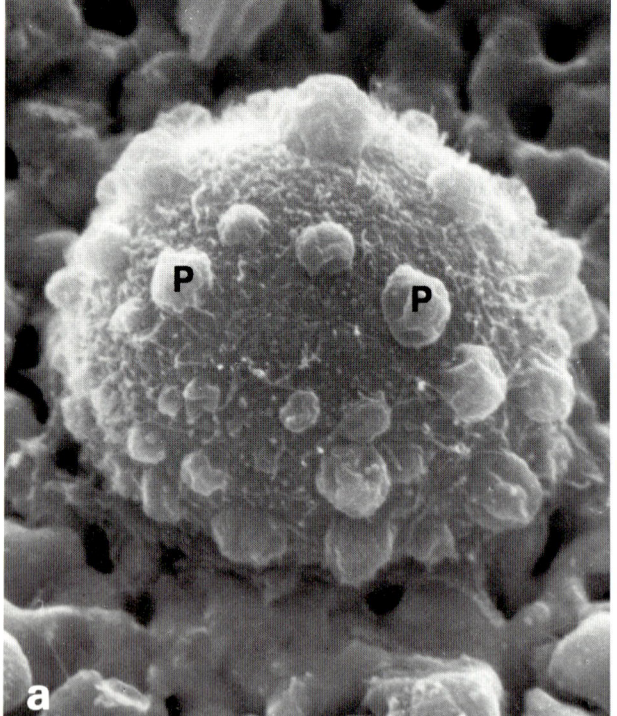
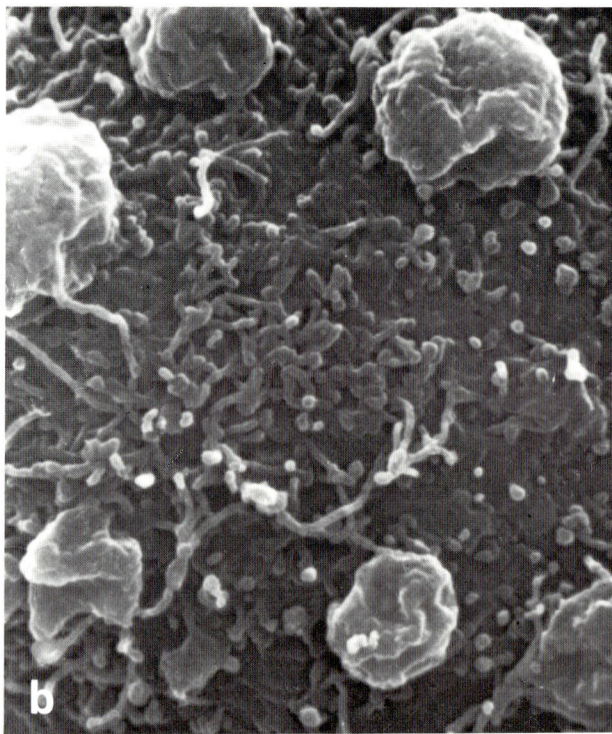

Fig. 17 a) *A scanning micrograph of a megaryocyte from long term culture as described in ref. 53. The exoplasmic bullae are believed to represent budding platelets (**P**) (× 3,000).*

b) *Higher magnification of a detail of the megakaryocyte shows the individual platelets to better advantage (× 10,000).*

5. CLINICAL APPLICATION OF IN VITRO HEMATOPOIESIS

5.1. Stem cell disorders

A number of diseases are now recognized as stem cell disorders and among these are included acute and chronic myelogenous leukemia, agnogenic myeloid metaplasia, polycythemia vera, paroxysmal nocturnal hemoglobinuria, and aplastic anemia. These disorders may manifest abnormal proliferative characteristics in the *in vitro* culture system.

5.1.1. In *Acute Myelogenous Leukemia (AML)* and its variants (monocytic, myelomonocytic, promyelocytic) cells proliferate abnormally in culture [57, 58, 59, 60]. In most instances, proliferation is either in the form of clusters (< 50 cells) (**Fig. 18**) or no proliferation is observed. In a smaller number of patients, abnormal proliferation is manifest by a decreased number and size of colonies, and in a few, colony formation resembles that of normals. In nearly all instances, cellular maturation is abnormal. Progenitor cells (CFU-GM) forming clusters and colonies differ from normal in that they are of a lighter buoyant density [61] and often have abnormal morphology when examined by electron microscopy. However, their proliferation in culture is dependent on the presence of colony stimulating factor (CSF) similar to normal cells. During a chemotherapy induced remission, colony formation returns to normal.

5.1.2. *Chronic Myelogenous Leukemia (CML)* cells form colonies *in vitro* which are similar to normal in size and morphology, but are present in greater frequency in marrow and blood [61, 62]. The leukemic nature of the cells is indicated by the presence of the Ph[1] chromosome [63] (also see Chapter 11). As in AML, colony forming cells in CML are of lighter buoyant density than normal and are entirely dependent on the presence

Fig. 18 Light microscopic appearance of unstained culture showing cluster formation in acute myeloblastic leukemia (**AML**). Note that no colonies are present (a colony is usually defined as having more than 50 cells). The illustration shows the characteristic appearance for myeloid leukemic CFU-GM proliferation in vitro.

of CSF for proliferation and differentiation [61]. When transformation to the acute phase (blast crisis) occurs, proliferation takes the pattern of that seen in AML. Abnormal *in vitro* proliferation in CML may be seen for months before clinical and morphologic changes of blast transformation are recognized in the marrow and blood.

5.1.3. In *Agnogenic Myeloid Metaplasia (AMM)* granulocyte colony formation resembles that of normal in size and morphology [64]. However, as in AML and CML, CFU-GM are of an abnormally light buoyant density [65]. Characteristically, the number of CFU-C and CFU-E is increased in the blood even though blood leukocytes may not be elevated [64, 66], indicating that more progenitor cells are released from the marrow or from other areas into the circulation. In instances where the disease transforms into leukemia, proliferation becomes abnormal and is similar to the pattern seen in AML.

5.1.4. In *Polycythemia Vera (PV)* granulocyte colony formation is normal in marrow and blood, and in contrast to AML, CML, and AMM, CFU-GM are of normal buoyant density [65, 67]. Two populations of CFU-E exist in PV [68, 69]. One population is extremely sensitive to erythropoietin (EP), forms erythroid colonies in the absence of exogenous EP and probably represents the abnormal clone. A second demonstrates a normal response to EP and presumably represents the normal CFU-E population. As the disease progresses, the abnormal clone increases and suppresses normal erythroid progenitor cells [70].

When patients with PV develop myelofibrosis, increased numbers of CFU-GM and CFU-E circulate in the blood [64, 66]. Therefore, the number of colonies formed may be indicative of the stage of the disease.

5.1.5. *Aplastic Anemia (AA)* is characterized by marrow hypoplasia with resultant pancytopenia [71]. In most instances, it results from damaged pluripotent stem cells with decreased output into the granulocytic, erythrocytic and megakaryocytic cell lines.

The establishment of marrow grafts in the majority of patients supports the concept that the basic defect is an abnormal stem cell [72]. Marrow progenitor cells, CFU-GM and CFU-E, are decreased in nearly all instances [73, 74]. Immune mechanisms due to the presence of a population of suppressor lymphocytes may be responsible for AA in a small number of patients [75, 76].

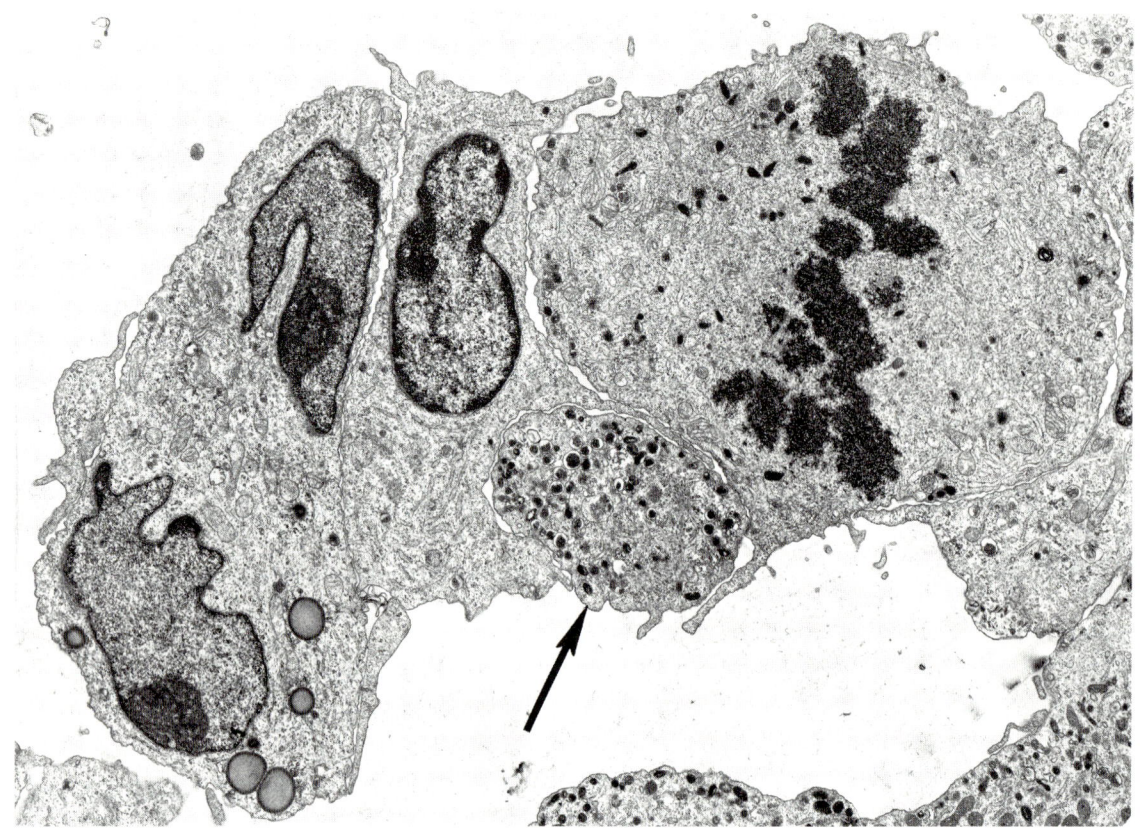

Fig. 19 Detail of a 15 day old myeloblast/promyelocyte colony prepared from the marrow of a patient with Kostman's type infantile neutropenia. The nuclei are primitive and display abnormally large nucleoli. Rough endoplasmic reticulum is abundant. The large number of granules in the cell indicated by the **arrow** suggests that this colony probably consists of aberrant neutrophil precursors ($\times$ 5,000). Reproduced from ref. 89.

5.2. Miscellaneous disorders associated with abnormal in vitro proliferation

5.2.1. The *myelodysplastic syndrome* also referred to as *"preleukemia"* [77] is characterized by abnormalities in proliferation of one or more hematopoietic cell lines which, after a number of months or years, may terminate in acute leukemia. This syndrome is observed in two situations. In one, the abnormalities occur in the absence of any recognized disease and is therefore considered idiopathic. The second is associated with disorders such as refractory sideroblastic anemia or paroxysmal nocturnal hemoglobinuria (PNH). Common to all of these disorders is the presence of anemia, although variable degrees of neutropenia and thrombocytopenia may also be present. Blasts are not increased in the marrow and erythroid precursors may be megaloblastic. In many of these patients chromosome abnormalities are present. The soft agar culture system may be helpful in establishing a diagnosis, since the granulocyte macrophage progenitor cells (CFU-GM) are abnormal in many of these patients [59, 78, 79]. Cultures are characterized by either a decrease in colony number or by an increase in cluster formation similar to that observed in acute leukemia. Cultures may be abnormal for months prior to the development of overt leukemia.

5.2.2. *Neutropenia*. The *in vitro* culture of marrow from patients with unexplained neutropenia may also be helpful. The patterns are varied and reflect the variable etiologies of the neutropenia encountered in patients. In drug-induced neutropenia associated with marrow hypoplasia, the number of CFU-GM is decreased. Subjects with idiopathic neutropenia manifest a wide range of CFU-GM reflecting the heterogeneity of this group of individuals [80].

In Felty's syndrome (neutropenia, arthritis, splenomegaly), CFU-GM are either normal or decreased and merely reflect the rate of marrow production of neutrophils in this disorder [81].

Congenital neutropenia has been reported under a variety of titles [82, 83, 84, 85, 86, 87]. With the help of studies on neutrophil kinetics and *in vitro* cultures, at least three forms can be distinguished [88].

Hereditary autosomal dominant neutropenia is characterized by neutropenia in the absence of anemia and thrombocytopenia and patients are free of severe infection. Marrow neutrophils and CFU-GM are reduced.

Patients with chronic benign neutropenia of childhood are also free of severe infection. The marrow is cellular and appears normal except for a decrease in segmented neutrophils but band forms are plentiful. CFU-GM are increased in the marrow of these patients and colony size and morphology are normal.

On the other hand, Kostman's type of neutropenia (infantile genetic agranulocytosis) is characterized by severe infections and early death. The marrow reveals a decreased M-E ratio with a reduced mass of neutrophils and neutrophil precursors. At times, no neutrophils are seen beyond the myeloblast or promyelocyte stage. CFU-GM are increased in the marrow and colony size is normal. The morphology of these colonies appears grossly normal by light microscopy, but by electron microscopy it becomes apparent that maturation of neutrophils in this disorder is abnormal and that the neutrophils are intrinsically defective (**Fig. 19**) [89].

REFERENCES

1. Bloom W., Bartlemez G.W.: *Hematopoiesis in young human embryos.* Am. J. Anat., *67*, 21, 1940.
2. Downey H.: *Handbook of Hematology.* New York, PB Hoeber Inc., 1938.
3. Knoll W.: *Die Blutbildung beim Embryo.* Acta Hematol., *2*, 369, 1949.
4. Moore M.A.S., Metcalf D.: *Ontogeny of the hematopoietic system. Yolk sac origin of in vivo and in vitro colony forming cells in the developing mouse embryo.* Brit. J. Hemat., *18*, 279, 1970.
5. Becker A.J., Mc Culloch E.A., Till J.E.: *Cytological demonstration of the clonal nature of spleen colonies derived from transplanted mouse marrow cells.* Nature, *197*, 452, 1963.
6. Whang J., Frei E. III, Tjio J.H., Carbone P.P., Brecher G.: *The distribution of the Philadelphia chromosome in patients with chronic myelocytic leukemia.* Blood, *22*, 664, 1963.
7. Adamson J.W., Fialkow P.W.: *The pathogenesis of myeloproliferative syndromes.* Brit. J. Hemat., *38*, 299, 1978.
8. Marmont A.M.: *Transplantation hemopoiesis. Morphologic bone marrow studies after allogeneic marrow transplantation in man for severe aplastic anemia and acute leukemia.* Nouv. Rév. Franç. Hemat., *21*, 133, 1979.
9. Abramson S., Miller R.G., Phillips R.A.: *The identification in adult bone marrow of pluripotent and restricted stem cells of the myeloid and lymphoid systems.* J. Exp. Med., *145*, 1567, 1977.
10. LeBien T.W., Hozier J., Minowada J., Kersey J.H.: *Origin of chronic myelocytic leukemia in a precursor of pre-B lymphocytes.* New Engl. J. Med., *301*, 144, 1979.
11. Greaves M.F., Verbi W., Reeves B.R. et al.: *"Pre-B" phenotypes in blast crisis of Ph^1 positive CML: evidence for a pluripotential stem cell "target".* Leukemia Res., *3*, 181, 1980.
12. Fialkow P.J., Denman A.M., Jacobson R.J., Lowenthal M.N.: *Chronic myelocytic leukemia. Origin of some lymphocytes from leukemic stem cells.* J. Clin. Invest., *62*, 815, 1978.
13. Boggs D.R.: *Hematopoietic stem cell theory in relation to possible lymphoblastic conversion of chronic myeloid leukemia.* Blood, *44*, 449, 1974.
14. van Bekkum D.W., van Noord M.J., Maat B., Dicke K.A.: *Attempts at identification of hematopoietic stem cell in mouse.* Blood, *38*, 547, 1971.
15. Iscove N.N., Till J.E., Mc Culloch E.A.: *The proliferative states of mouse granulopoietic progenitor cells.* Proc. Soc. Exp. Biol. Med., *134*, 33, 1970.
16. Fried W., Gurney C.W.: *Regulation mechanism of the stem cell compartment.* J. Lab. Clin. Med., *71*, 948, 1968.
17. Wolf M.S., Trentin J.J.: *Hemopoietic colony studies. V. Effect of hemopoietic organ stroma on differentiation of pluripotent stem cells.* J. Exp. Med., *127*, 205, 1968.
18. Lord B.I., Mori K.J., Wright E.G.: *A stimulator of stem cell proliferation in regenerating bone marrow.* Biomed., *27*, 223, 1977.
19. Pluznik D., Sachs L.: *The cloning in normal "mast" cells in tissue culture.* J. Cell. Comp. Physiol., *66*, 319-324, 1965.
20. Bradley T.R., Metcalf D.: *The growth of mouse bone marrow cells in vitro.* Aust. J. Exp. Biol. Med. Sci., *44*, 287, 1966.
21. Pike B.L., Robinson W.A.: *Human bone marrow colony*

growth in agar gel. J. Cell Physiol., 76, 77, 1970.
22. Haskill J.S., McNeil T.A., Moore M.A.S.: *Density distribution analysis of in vivo and in vitro colony forming cells in bone marrow*. J. Cell Physiol., 75, 167, 1970.
23. Zucker-Franklin D., Grusky G., L'Esperance P.: *Granulocyte colonies derived from lymphocyte fractions of normal human peripheral blood*. Proc. Natl. Acad. Sci., 71, 2711, 1974.
24. Chervenick P.A., Boggs D.R.: *In vitro growth of granulocytic and mononuclear cell colonies from blood of normal individuals*. Blood, 37, 131, 1971.
25. Zucker-Franklin D., Grusky G.: *Ultrastructural analysis of hematopoietic colonies from human peripheral blood*. J. Cell Biol., 63, 855, 1974.
26. Metcalf D., Parker J., Chester H.M., Kincade P.W.: *Formation of "eosinophilic like" granulocytic colonies by mouse bone marrow cells in vitro*. J. Cell Physiol., 84, 275, 1974.
27. Dao C., Metcalf D., Bilski-Pasquier G.: *Eosinophil and neutrophil colony-forming cells in culture*. Blood, 50, 833, 1977.
28. Ruscetti F.W., Cypess R.H., Chervenick P.A.: *Specific release of neutrophilic and eosinophilic stimulating factors from sensitized lymphocytes*. Blood, 47, 757, 1975.
29. Chervenick P.A., Lo Buglio A.F.: *Human blood monocytes: stimulators of granulocyte and mononuclear colony formation in vitro*. Science, 178, 164, 1972.
30. Moore M.A.S., Williams N.: *Physical separation of colony stimulating cells from in vitro colony forming cells in hematopoietic tissues*. J. Cell. Physiol., 80, 195, 1972.
31. Golde D.W., Cline M.J.: *Identification of the colony-stimulating cell in human peripheral blood*. J. Clin. Invest., 51, 2981, 1972.
32. Cline M.J., Golde D.W.: *Production of colony stimulating activity by human lymphocytes*. Nature, 248, 703, 1974.
33. Brown C.H., Carbone P.D.: *In vitro growth of normal and leukemic human bone marrow*. J. Natl. Canc. Inst., 46, 989, 1971.
34. Burgess A.W., Wilson E.M.A., Metcalf D.: *Stimulation by human placental conditioned medium of hemopoietic colony formation by human marrow cells*. Blood, 49, 573, 1977.
35. Di Persio J.F., Brennan J.K., Lichtman M.A., Speiser B.L.: *Human cell lines that elaborate colony stimulating activity for the marrow cells of man and other species*. Blood, 51, 507, 1978.
36. Broxmeyer H.E., Smithyman A., Eger R.R. et al.: *Identification of lactoferrin as the granulocyte derived inhibitor of colony stimulating activity (CSA) production*. J. Exp. Med., 148, 1052, 1978.
37. Kurland J., Moore M.A.S.: *Modulation of hemopoiesis by prostaglandin*. Exp. Hematol., 5, 357, 1977.
38. Stephenson J.R., Axelrad A.A., McLeod D.L., Shreeve M.M.: *Induction of colonies of hemoglobin-synthesizing cells by erythropoietin in vitro*. Proc. Natl. Acad. Sci., 68, 1542, 1971.
39. Tepperman A.D., Curtis J.E., McCulloch E.A.: *Erythropoietic colonies in cultures of human marrow*. Blood, 44, 659, 1974.
40. Gregory C.J., Eaves A.C.: *Human marrow cells capable of erythropoietic differentiation in vitro: definition of three erythroid colony responses*. Blood, 49, 855, 1977.
41. Nathan D.G., Chess L., Hillman D.G., Clarke B., Breard J., Merler E., Housman D.E.: *Human erythroid burst forming unit: T-cell requirement for proliferation in vitro*. J. Exp. Med., 147, 324, 1978.
42. Aye M.T.: *The enhancement of erythroid colony formation by leukocyte conditioned medium*. Blood, 46, 1022, 1975.
43. Gordon L.I., Branda R.F., Zanjani E.D., Jacob H.S.: *Stimulation of erythroid colony (EC) formation by bone marrow (BM) macrophages*. Blood, 52 (Suppl.), 1, 204, 1978.
44. Adamson J.W., Popovic W.J., Brown J.E.: *Hormonal control of erythropoiesis*. In: *Hematopoietic Cell Differentiation*. Golde D.W., Cline M.J., Metcalf D. eds., New York Academic Press, p. 53, 1978.
45. Golde D.W., Bersch N., Li C.H.: *Growth hormone species specific stimulation of erythropoiesis in vitro*. Science, 196, 1112, 1977.
46. Nakeff A., Daniels-McQueen S.: *In vitro colony assay for a new class of megakaryocyte precursor: Colony-forming unit megakaryocyte (CFU-M)*. Proc. Soc. Exp. Biol. Med., 151, 587, 1976.
47. Williams N., McDonald T.P., Rabellino E.M.: *Maturation and regulation of megakaryocytopoiesis*. Blood Cells, 5, 43, 1979.
48 a. Vainchenker W., Bouquet J., Guichard J., Breton-Gorius J.: *Megakaryocyte colony formation from human bone marrow precursors*. Blood, 54, 940, 1979.
48 b. Fauser A.A., Messner H.A.: *Identification of megakaryocytes, macrophages and eosinophils in colonies of human bone marrow containing neutrophilic granulocytes and erythroblasts*. Blood, 53, 1023, 1979.
49. Rozenszajn L.A., Shoham D., Kalechman I.: *Clonal proliferation of PHA stimulated lymphocytes in soft agar culture*. Immunology, 29, 1041, 1975.
50. Radnay J., Goldman I., Rozenszajn L.A.: *Growth of human B lymphocyte colonies in vitro*. Nature, 278, 351, 1979.
51. Sutherland D.C., Dalton G., Wilson J.D.: *T-lymphocyte colonies in malignant disease*. Lancet, 2, 1113, 1976.
52. Foa R., Catovsky D.: *T-cell colonies in normal blood, bone marrow and lymphoproliferative disorders*. Clin. Exp. Immunol., 36, 488, 1979.
53. Dexter T.M., Allen T.D., Lajtha L.G.: *Conditions controlling the proliferation of hemopoietic stem cells in vitro*. J. Cell Physiol., 91, 335, 1977.
54. Allen T.D.: *Ultrastructural aspects of in vitro hematopoiesis*. In: 2nd *Symposium of the British Society for Cell Biology on Stem Cells and Tissue Homeostasis*. Lord B.I., Potter C.S., Cole R.J. eds., Cambridge University Press, p. 217, 1978.
55. Moore M.A.S., Sheridan A.P.C.: *Pluripotential stem cell replication in continuous human, prosimian and murine bone marrow culture*. Blood Cells, 5, 297, 1979.
56. Moore M.A.S., Sheridan A.P.C., Allen T.D., Dexter T.M.: *Prolonged hematopoiesis in a primate bone marrow culture system. Characteristics of stem cell production and the hematopoietic microenvironment*. Blood, 54, 775, 1979.
57. Moore M.A.S., Spitzer G., Williams N.: *Agar culture studies in 127 cases of untreated acute leukemia: The prognostic value of reclassification of leukemia according to in vitro growth characteristics*. Blood, 44, 1, 1974.
58. Paran M., Sachs L., Barak Y., Resnitsky P.: *In vitro induction of granulocyte differentiation in hematopoietic cells from leukemic and non-leukemic patients*. Proc. Natl. Acad. Sci., 67, 1542, 1970.
59. Greenberg P.L., Nichols W., Schrier S.L.: *Granulopoiesis in acute myeloid leukemia and preleukemia*. New Engl. J. Med., 284, 1225, 1971.
60. Curtis J.E., Cowan D.H., Bergsagel D.E. et al.: *Acute leukemia in adults: assessment of remission induction with combination chemotherapy by clinical and cell culture criteria*. Can. Med. Assoc. J., 113, 289, 1975.
61. Moore M.A.S., Williams N., Metcalf D.: *In vitro colony formation by normal and leukemic human hematopoietic cells. Characterization of the colony forming cell*. J. Natl. Cancer Inst., 50, 603, 1973.
62. Moberg C., Olofsson T., Olsson I.: *Granulopoiesis in chronic myeloid leukemia. In vitro cloning of blood and bone marrow cells in agar culture*. Scand. J. Hemat., 12, 381, 1974.
63. Chervenick P.A., Ellis L.D., Pan S.F., Lawson A.L.: *Human leukemic cells. In vitro growth of colonies containing the Philadelphia (Ph¹) chromosome*. Science, 174, 1134, 1971.
64. Chervenick P.A.: *Increase in circulating stem cells in patients with myelofibrosis*. Blood, 41, 67, 1973.
65. Moore M.A.S., Spitzer G.: *In vitro studies in myeloproliferative disorders*. In: 8th *Leukocyte Culture Conference*. Lindahl-Kiessling K., Osoba D. eds., New York, Academic Press, p. 431, 1974.
66. Chikkappa G., Carsten A.L., Chanana A.D., Cronkite E.P.: *Increased granulocytic, erythrocytic, and megakaryocytic*

progenitors in myelofibrosis with myeloid metaplasia. Am. J. Hemat., 4, 121, 1978.
67. Greenberg P., Mara B., Bax I., Brossel R., Schrier S.: *The myeloproliferative disorders: correlation between clinical evaluation and alterations of granulopoiesis*. Am. J. Med., 61, 878, 1976.
68. Prchal J.F., Adamson J.W., Murphy S., Steinman L., Fialkow P.J.: *Polycythemia vera: the in vitro response of normal and abnormal stem cell lines to erythropoietin*. J. Clin. Invest., 61, 1044, 1978.
69. Zanjani E.D., Lutton J.D., Hoffman R., Wasserman L.R.: *Erythroid colony formation by polycythemia vera bone marrow in vitro*. J. Clin. Invest., 59, 841, 1977.
70. Zanjani E.D., Kaplan M.E., Ascensao J.L., Banisadre M., Roodman G.D., Wasserman L.R.: *Normal stem cell suppression in polycythemia vera*. Blood, 54 (Suppl.), 1, 147 A, 1979.
71. Williams D.M., Lynch R.E., Cartwright G.E.: *Drug-induced aplastic anemia*. Sem. in Hematol., 10, 195, 1973.
72. Thomas E.D., Fefer A., Buckner C.D., Storb R.: *Current status of bone marrow transplantation for aplastic anemia and acute leukemia*. Blood, 49, 671, 1977.
73. Kurnick J.E., Robinson W.A., Dickey C.A.: *In vitro granulocytic colony forming potential of bone marrow from patients with granulocytopenia and aplastic anemia*. Proc. Soc. Exp. Biol. Med., 137, 917, 1971.
74. Hansi W., Rich I., Heimpel H., Heit W., Kubanek B.: *Erythroid colony forming cells in aplastic anemia*. Brit. J. Hemat., 37, 483, 1977.
75. Kagan W.A., Ascensao J.A., Pahwa R.N. *et al.*: *Aplastic anemia: presence in human bone marrow of cells that suppress myelopoiesis*. Proc. Natl. Acad. Sci., 73, 2890, 1976.
76. Hoffman R., Zanjani E.D., Lutton J.D., Zalusky R., Wasserman L.R.: *Suppression of erythroid colony formation by lymphocytes from patients with aplastic anemia*. New Engl. J. Med., 296, 10, 1977.
77. Linman J.W., Bagby G.C.: *The preleukemic syndrome*. Cancer, 42, 854, 1978.
78. Verma D.S., Spitzer G., Dicke K.A., McCredie K.B.: *In vitro agar culture patterns in preleukemia and their clinical significance*. Leukemia Research, 3, 41, 1979.
79. Senn J.S., Pinkerton P.H., Price G.B., Mak T.W., McCulloch E.A.: *Human preleukemia. Cell culture studies in sideroblastic anemia*. Brit. J. Cancer, 33, 299, 1976.
80. Greenberg P.L., Schrier S.L.: *Granulopoiesis in neutropenic disorders*. Blood, 41, 753, 1973.
81. Srodes C.H., Hyde F., Chervenick P.A., Boggs D.R.: *Neutrophil kinetics in Felty's syndrome*. Blood, 40, 950 A, 1972.
82. Kauder E., Mauer M.A.: *Neutropenias of childhood*. J. Pediatrics, 69, 147, 1966.
83. Zuelzer W.W., Bajoghli M.: *Chronic granulocytopenia in childhood*. Blood, 23, 359, 1964.
84. Cutting H.O., Lang J.E.: *Familial benign chronic neutropenia*. Ann. Int. Med., 61, 876, 1964.
85. Kostmann R.: *Infantile genetic agranulocytosis*. Acta Paediatr., 45 (Suppl.), 105, 1, 1956.
86. Olofsson T., Olsson I., Kostmann R., Malstrom S., Thilen A.: *Granulopoiesis in infantile genetic agranulocytosis*. Scand. J. Hemat., 16, 18, 1976.
87. Barak Y., Paran M., Levin S., Sachs L.: *In vitro induction of myeloid proliferation and maturation in infantile genetic agranulocytosis*. Blood, 38, 74, 1971.
88. Joyce R.A., Boggs D.R., Chervenick P.A.: *Neutrophil kinetics in hereditary and congenital neutropenias*. New Engl. J. Med., 295, 1385, 1976.
89. Zucker-Franklin D., L'Esperance P., Good R.A.: *Congenital neutropenia: an intrinsic cell defect demonstrated by electron microscopy of soft agar colonies*. Blood, 49, 425, 1977.

3
Erythrocytes

G.L. CASTOLDI

Department of Medicine, University of Ferrara
Ferrara, Italy

Part 1 GENERAL ASPECTS OF ERYTHROPOIESIS

1. INTRODUCTION

The circulating red cells and their precursors may be considered as a functional unit as suggested by Boykott who introduced the term *erythron* in 1929 [1]. The series of cells which constitutes the erythron is usually restricted to a group of elements clearly recognizable in the marrow starting with the pronormoblasts and terminating with the mature red cells in the peripheral blood. However, since there is a direct developmental connection between progenitor cells and mature cells, the erythron should also include the morphologically non identifiable elements which consist of the committed precursors of the erythroid line.

The existence of the latter cells has been amply demonstrated (see Chapter 2) by biological assays, but their morphology and other phenotypic characteristics are still largely unknown.
In terms of kinetics, the proliferation of the cells within the erythron is accomplished by two main steps corresponding to two distinct sequential compartments [2]: pre-amplification and amplification phase respectively [3, 4]. Although this distinction may be considered empirical in terms of an ongoing continuous process, it may be appropriate in a discussion of the biological characteristics which distinguish the two compartments.

2. FETAL ERYTHROPOIESIS

Fetal erythropoiesis may be considered in three main periods of hemopoietic activity which involve, sequentially, the yolk sac, the liver, and the bone marrow (see Chapter 2).

Available data support the concept that fetal erythropoiesis takes place in these sites by seeding of primitive cells which migrate from the yolk sac rather than as a consequence of a local differentiation of stem cells under the influence of various inductive processes [5].

The first period begins between the 14-19th day of development [6] and continues until the end of the third month. This phase is characterized by the differentiation in the wall of the yolk sac of mesenchymal elements (*mesoblastic phase*) which are grouped in solid masses (*blood islands*) (see Chapter 2).

The cells in these aggregates develop along two different lines, the endothelial cells at the periphery of the blood islands and the primitive blood cells in the center [7].

The earliest recognizable cells within the islands have a basophilic cytoplasm and large nuclei with nucleoli. They differentiate into primitive erythroblasts which look like megaloblasts. Their nuclei are retained throughout their life span.

After the first embryonic month, erythropoiesis is prominent in the liver, the spleen and for a limited period in the thymus [8]. The liver remains the principal anatomical site for erythropoiesis from the third to the sixth month (*hepatic phase*) and continues to perform this function until the first week of post-natal life.

Erythroblasts, often surrounding reticulum cells laden with nuclear remnants ("fetal erythroblastic islands") [9], are concentrated extravascularly within the hepatic parenchyma and, apart from an initial megaloblastic phase, show normoblastic features including anucleated cells which are slightly larger than adult red cells (**Fig. 1**) [10].
The *myeloid phase* of fetal erythropoiesis begins during the fifth month of gestation (see Chapter 2). In the early phase of activity the fetal bone marrow gives rise mainly to granulocytic elements, but, in the last three months of pregnancy it becomes the major site of erythropoiesis and shows a predominance of normoblasts [11].

During intrauterine life, erythropoiesis is associated with the production of embryonic hemoglobin. The mesoblastic phase is characterized by hemoglobins Gower I and Gower II, an A-like hemoglobin defined as hemoglobin Portland and fetal hemoglobin (Hb α_2-γ_2). Hb F predominates during the hepatic phase and constitutes about 90% of the hemoglobin molecules synthesized during the last period of gestation.

3. GENERATION OF ERYTHROID CELLS IN POST-NATAL LIFE

Pronormoblasts are the earliest recognizable erythroid cells in the bone marrow. They do not constitute a self maintaining population of cells [12]. The existence of morphologically non-identifiable erythroid stem cells has been deduced from studies on *in vivo* and *in vitro* colony forming methods [13, 14]. The generation of erythroid cells in post-natal life is accomplished via a sequence of differentiation steps starting with the multipotential stem cell (CFU-s – "Colony Forming Unit-spleen") and the committed precursors (pERC and ERC – "Erythropoietin Responsive Cells") down to the erythroblastic phase and ending with the fully developed mature forms [15] (see Chapter 2).

ERC's are not a homogeneous population of cells as demonstrated by quantitative assays *in vitro* [16]. Correlation between the number of clusters of hemoglobin synthesizing cells in the presence of different concentrations of erythropoietin and the number of cells originally plated has led to the definition of an "Erythroid Colony Forming Unit" (CFU-E) which is clonal, i.e. arises from a single progenitor cell. Since the CFU-E has limited growth capacities, it is probably more differentiated than the multipotent stem cell (CFU-s) (see Chapter 2).

There is accumulating evidence to indicate that the differentiation of hemoglobin synthesizing cells from primitive committed erythroid precursors may involve several more discrete steps [17, 18].

Axelrad *et al.* [19] observed that very high concentrations of erythropoietin in the culture medium, would result in large aggregates of hemoglobin synthesizing cells ("Erythroid bursts"). The cells giving rise to the bursts were referred to as "Burst Forming Units" (BFU-E). Erythroid bursts are usually fewer in number than CFU-E, but endowed with a substantially greater proliferative capacity.
Based on the timing of colony maturation and the size of the colony, at least three classes of erythropoietic progenitors have been defined [20]. They have been termed *day-8 BFU-E* (progenitors of late bursts formed by four or more clusters and seen after 8-10 days of culture), *day-3* BFU-E (progenitors of early bursts containing four or more clusters and seen after 3-4 days), and *CFU-E* (progenitors of single or paired clusters seen after 2 days). These classes of cells appear

3 ERYTHROCYTES

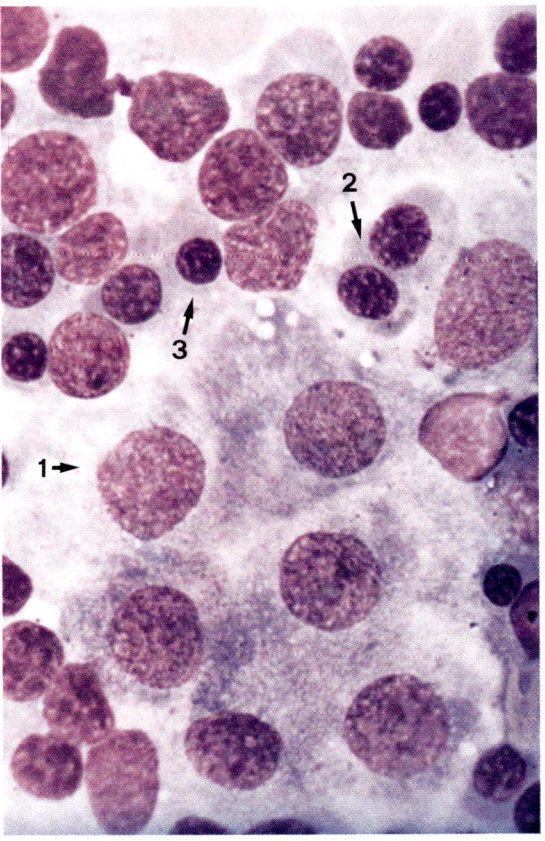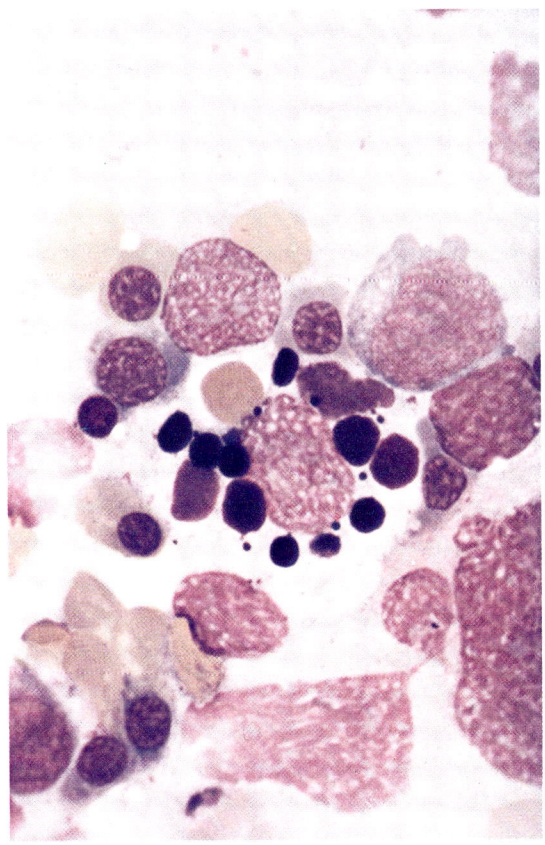

Fig. 1 *Liver imprints from a human embryo at eight weeks of gestation.* **a)** *Erythroblasts with normoblastic features are distributed among the hepatocytes.* **1**, *Hepatocyte;* **2**, *Early polychromatic normoblast;* **3**, *Late polychromatic normoblast.*
b) *A macrophage engulfing several nuclei derived from erythroblast breakdown.*

to be sequentially related in order of maturation. Cells moving from one compartment to the next exhibit a progressive decrease in proliferative activity and a parallel increase in the capacity to respond to erythropoietin.

Day-8 BFU-E appear to be relatively independent of erythropoietin since the cells of this class of progenitors do not proliferate in response to variations in the concentration of this hormone. By contrast erythropoietin does seem to be necessary for the maintenance and proliferation of the latter class of progenitor cells [21].

The differentiation and proliferative activity of the different erythroid compartments is probably regulated by several "humoral" factors acting as specific inhibitors or promotors. These may be elaborated by elements of the erythron itself or other cells, e.g. histiocytes, endocrine cells [22, 23]. An outline of the principal characteristics expressed by the cells involved in the different phases of erythropoiesis is shown in **Figure 2**.

4. REGULATION OF ERYTHROID DIFFERENTIATION

Erythroid differentiation is stimulated primarily by the action of erythropoietin (Ep), a glycoprotein with a molecular weight of about 46,000 daltons [24]. Erythropoietin is thought to be generated by the interaction of a renal erythropoietic factor (REF or "Erythrogenin") with a serum component which is probably

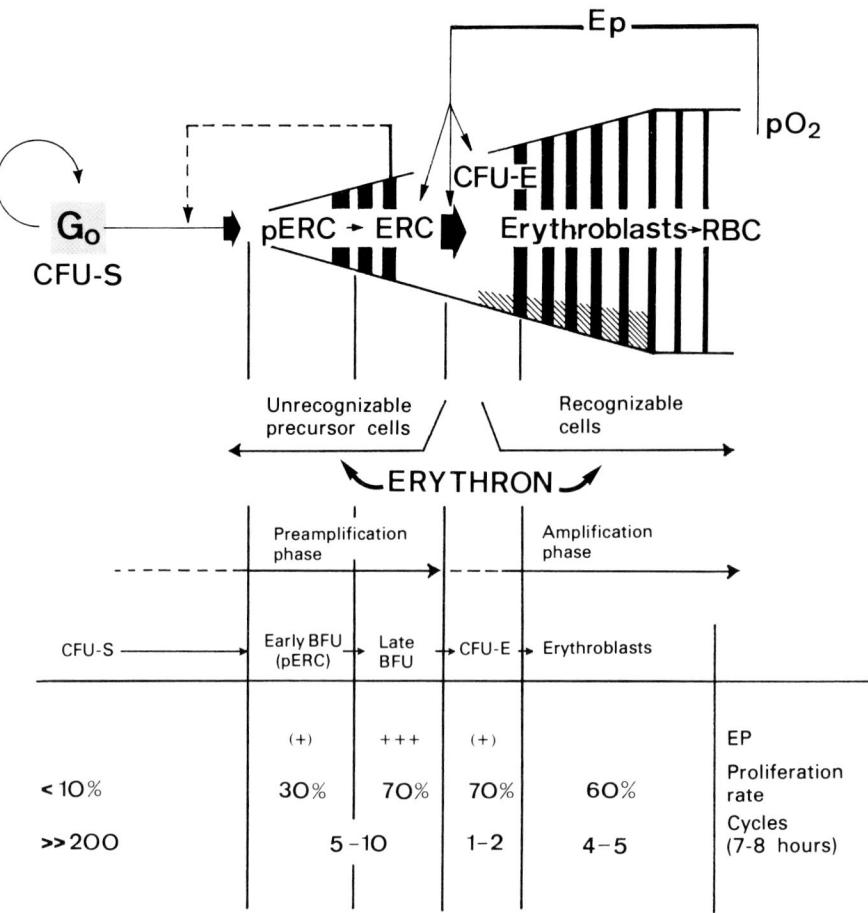

Fig. 2 *Schematic drawing of the differentiation steps of the erythropoietic cell line. The effects of erythropoietin (Ep) on cell proliferation as well as some biological characteristics of the various cell populations are illustrated. Ineffective erythropoiesis is dashed within the erythroblastic compartment.*
Adapted from refs. 2, 3, 22.

derived from the liver [25]. The principal stimulus for the production of erythropoietin is tissue hypoxia, although some influence may also be exerted by the acid-base equilibrium [26] and by the endocrine system [27, 28].
Ep induces three major responses [29-32]:
a) stimulation of Ep-sensitive cells to differentiate into pronormoblasts;
b) initiation of hemoglobin synthesis (enhancement of globin mRNA between the proerythroblast and the basophilic erythroblast stage of differentiation) [33];
c) increase in the rate of self-renewal of morphologically unrecognizable precursors.
Ep probably does not have to enter the target cells in order to elicit its effects: an interaction with a protein-like cell surface receptor as well as translocation of a membrane signal to a cytoplasmic cell mediator which directly or indirectly induces a marked increase of a heterogeneous RNA (mRNA, rRNA, tRNA) are postulated to work in concert with other cell surface receptor systems (e.g. hormones, neurotransmitters, antigens) [34, 35] (**Fig. 3**).

Increase in heterogeneous RNA is detectable within 15-30 minutes after exposure of the cells to Ep. The increase in tRNA and rRNA following mRNA synthesis in the nucleus occurs in concert with the elaboration of enzymes (e.g. ALA-synthetase) involved in heme synthesis and an increased rate of cell division. Ep may also be required to support heme synthesis in the postmitotic compartment and therefore may be involved in the last phase of maturation.

3 ERYTHROCYTES

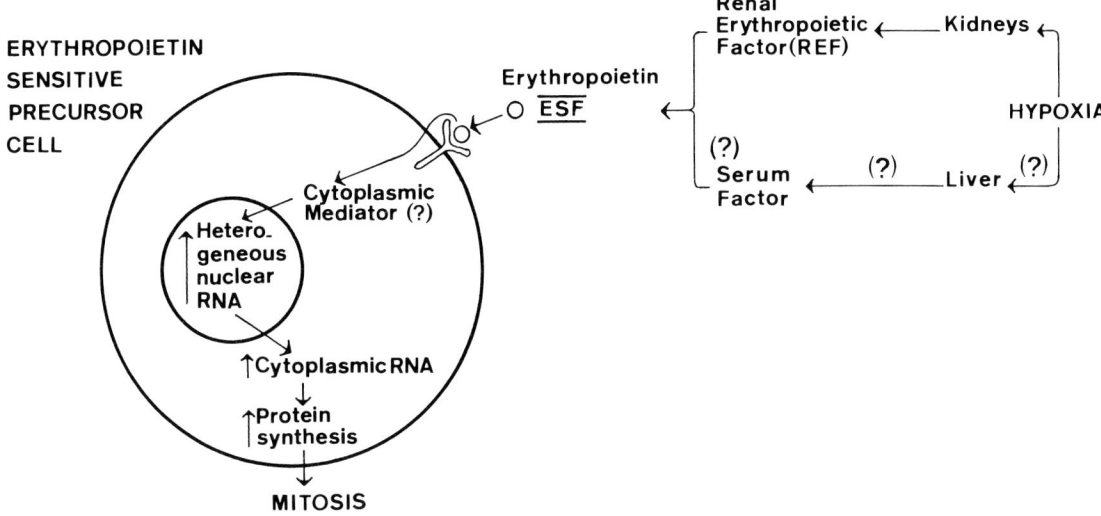

Fig. 3 *Hypothetical, schematic representation for the Ep regulation of erythropoiesis.*

Finally Ep may exert an effect on the release of reticulocytes from the bone marrow as suggested in experimental models. Ep probably influences the expansion of the perisinusoidal adventitial cells which regulate the exposure of the endothelial wall to the penetration by the newly formed reticulocytes in the marrow (see **Fig. 1**, p. 641) [36].

5. MORPHOLOGY

5.1. Light microscope cytology, cytochemistry and ultrastructure

The first recognizable cell in the erythroid series is the pronormoblast (see **Figs. 6 a and b**). Normally these cells undergo further division giving rise to four generations of daughter cells which are classified as *basophilic normoblasts* (two steps) followed by *early* and *late polychromatophilic normoblasts* (**Fig. 4**) [37, 38]. Maturation stages of normoblasts may be classified as E_1, E_2, E_3, E_4, E_5, a classification that is based on their nuclear diameters [39].

While the cells between the pronormoblast and the early polychromatophilic normoblast are proliferating cells, the late polychromatophilic normoblast is a non dividing cell. It develops into a reticulocyte after extrusion of its nucleus and crossing of the sinusoidal barrier of the bone marrow [40-44]. Circulating reticulocytes develop further into fully mature red cells.

Most of the steps involved in the differentiation and maturation of erythroid cells are reflected by biochemical changes of both nuclear and cytoplasmic components (e.g. linear decrease in RNA from the pronormoblast on and the appearance of hemoglobin in the basophilic elements with an increasing rate in the more mature cells [45-47]. The structural changes in nuclear chromatin and cytoplasmic organelles (e.g. ribosomes, mitochondria, Golgi apparatus) may be documented by ultrastructural studies [48-50]. Whilst the different stages of normoblast maturation are recognizable by light microscopy, the corresponding ultrastructural changes are less well defined because they are too gradual. The developmental sequence of erythroid maturation involves the following major features (**Fig. 5**): a) progressive

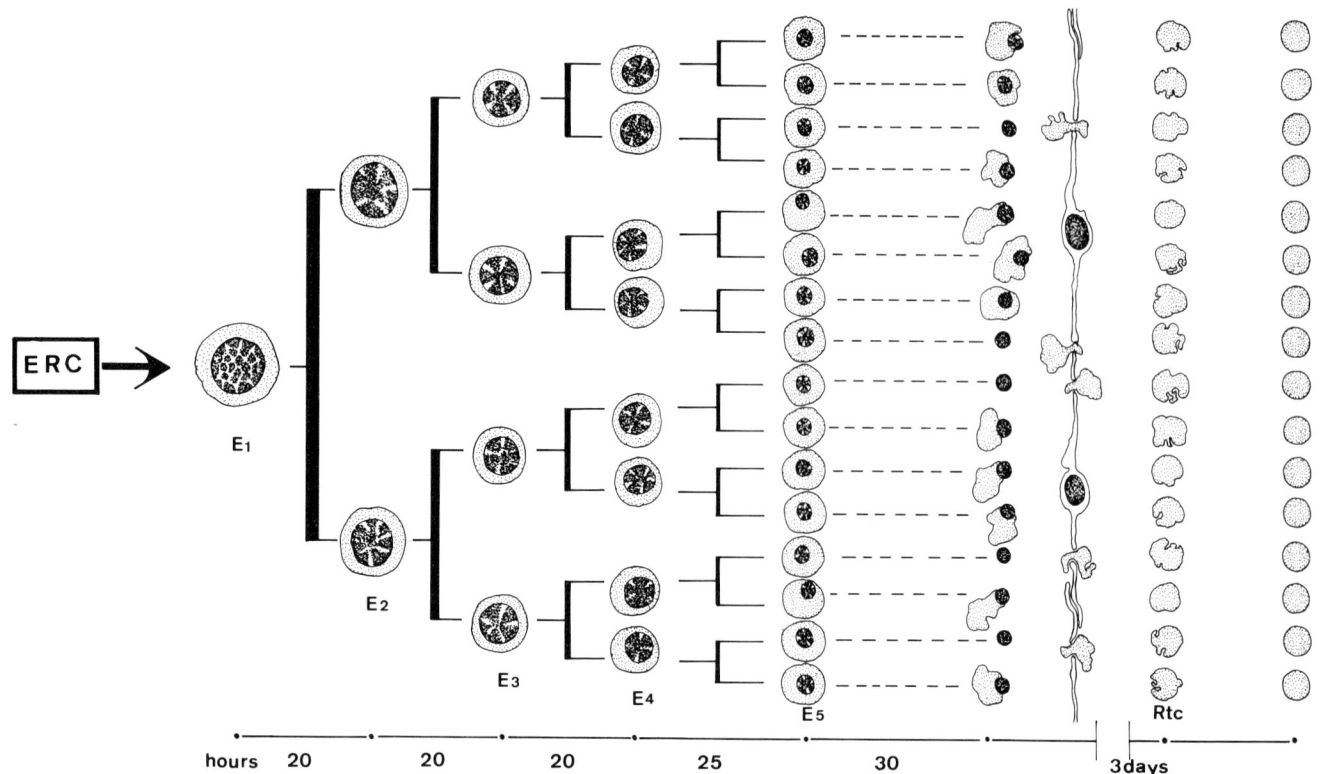

Fig. 4 Maturation sequence of the erythroid cells in normal bone marrow ($E_1 \rightarrow E_5$). Seven days are required to reach full erythrocyte maturation, as suggested by the time which the red cells require for the utilization of an injected dose of Fe^{59}. Denucleation of the late polychromatophilic normoblasts takes place within the marrow and the newly formed reticulocytes migrate into the circulation after having actively penetrated the endothelial cells in the proximity of their junctional zones [42-44].

condensation of chromatin; b) reduction in the number of nucleoli; c) decrease in the number of ribosomes and mitochondria; d) gradual increase in the electron density of the cytoplasm which corresponds to hemoglobin accumulation; e) increase in ferritin molecules within the cytoplasm in the form of aggregates or bound to the plasma membrane.
The detailed morphological patterns of erythropoietic cell maturation both in conventionally stained smears (May Grünwald - Giemsa) and in ultrastructural preparations are illustrated in **Figures 6-12**.

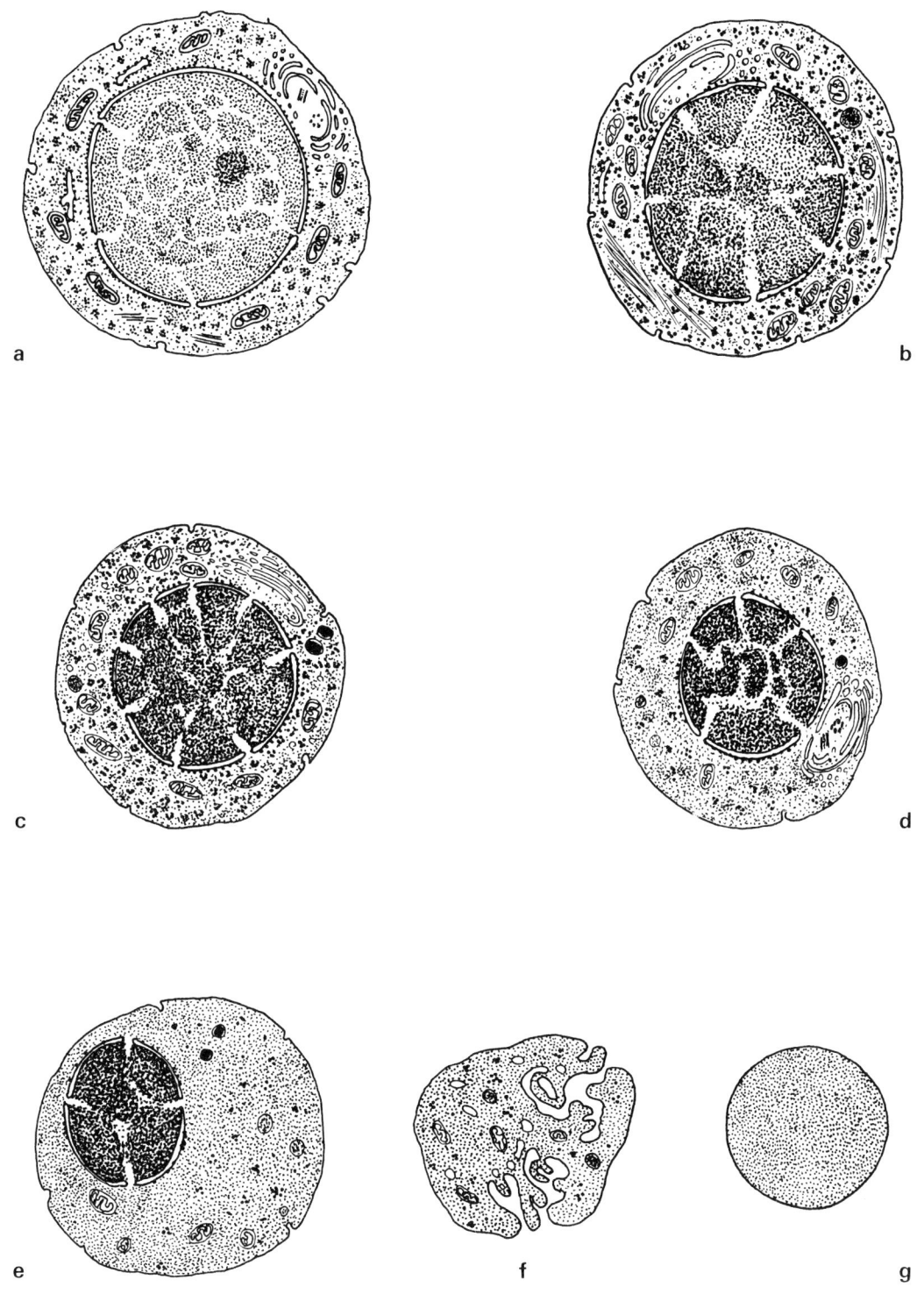

Fig. 5 Schematic representation of the principal ultrastructural changes (**a** to **g**) during the developmental sequence from the pronormoblast to the mature red cell (progressive condensation of nuclear chromatin, decrease in the cytoplasmic content of ribosomes and mitochondria with increasing maturation and increased cytoplasmic electron density).

BLOOD CELLS

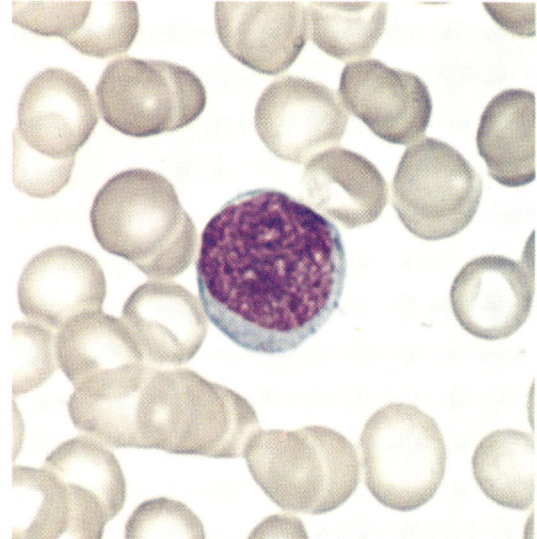

Fig. 6 a) The pronormoblast (**) is the first of the red cell series recognizable in conventional bone marrow smears. It shows a round or slightly oval shape with a diameter of 12-20 µm. The nucleus is large with finely dispersed chromatin and one or more nucleoli. The cytoplasm is scanty and stains deep blue. In most of these cells a juxtanuclear clear zone corresponds to the Golgi apparatus (arcoplasmic area).

(**) "Normoblastic erythropoiesis" is a morphological definition for all erythroid cells with features resembling those of nucleated red cell precursors in normal adult bone marrow [37].

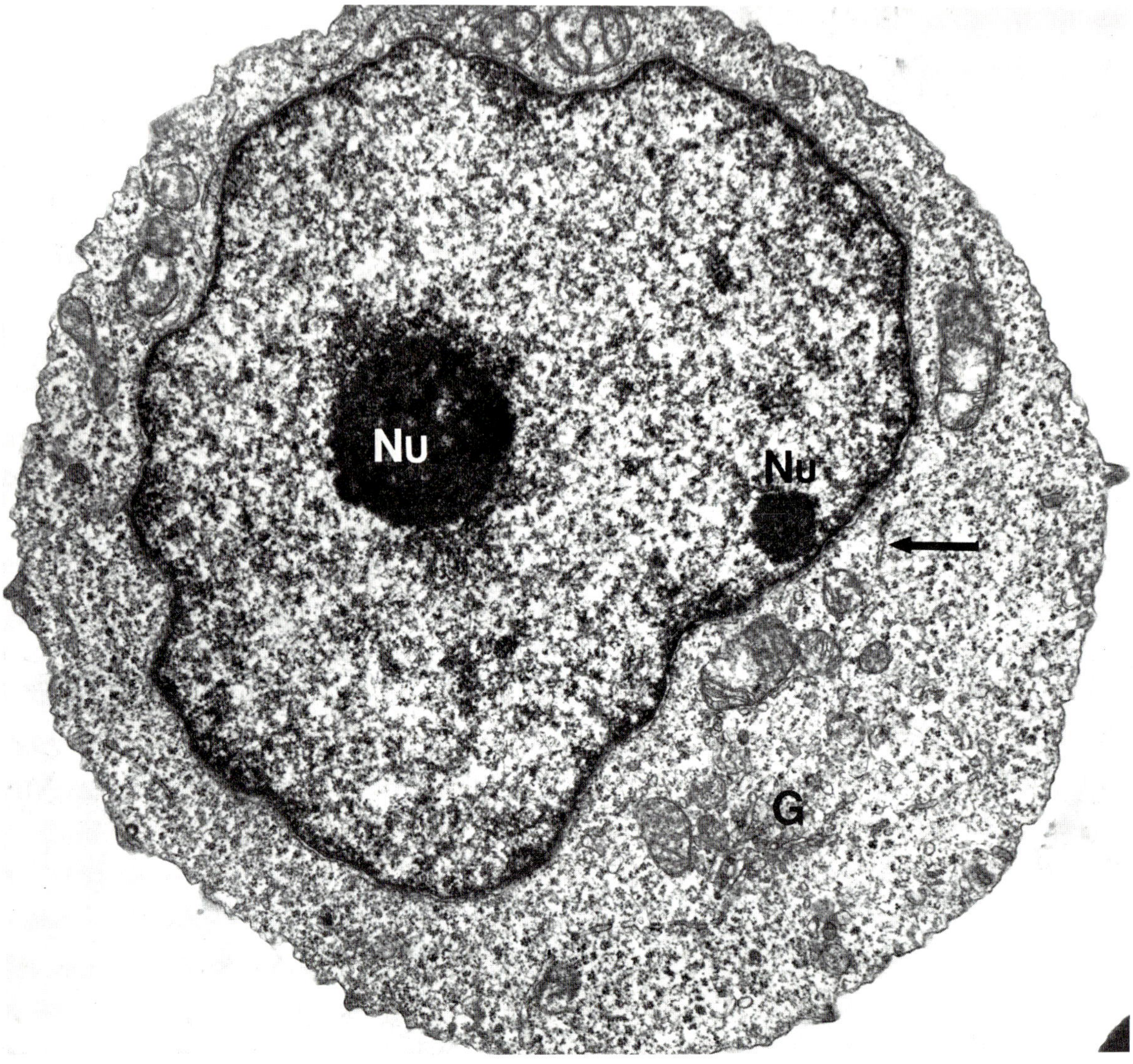

6 b

3 ERYTHROCYTES

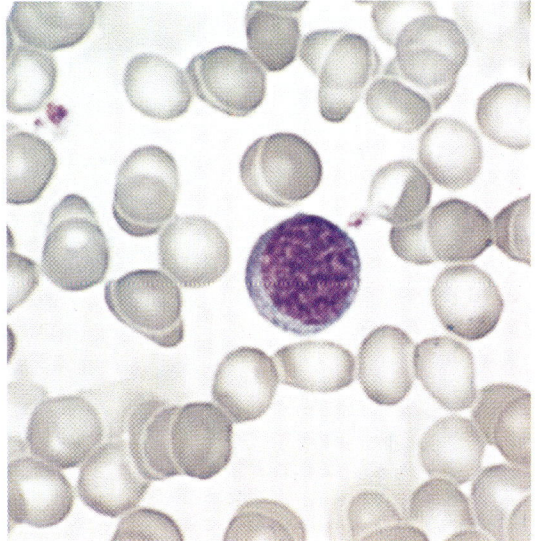

Fig. 7 a) Basophilic normoblast which is smaller than the pronormoblast ranging in diameter from 10 to 18 μm. The nuclear to cytoplasmic ratio is also lower than that of the pronormoblast. The cytoplasm is strongly basophilic. The chromatin pattern is rather coarse and shows small condensed masses adjacent to the nuclear membrane. The nucleoli are inconspicuous or absent.

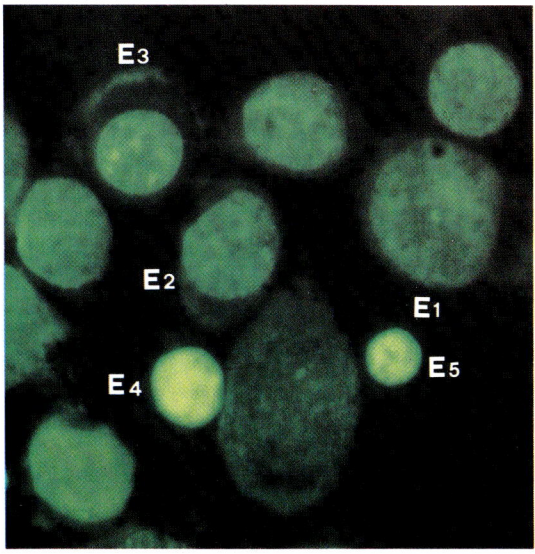

Fig. 7 b) The progressive chromatin condensation with increasing maturity of the erythroid cells is easily demonstrated when the cells are stained with fluorochromes (e.g. quinacrine) and increasing brightness becomes apparent. All stages from the pronormoblast (E_1) to the late polychromatophilic normoblast (E_5) are shown.

Fig. 6 b) Pronormoblast, illustrating the fine chromatin pattern of a "primitive" nucleus with two nucleoli (**Nu**). The cytoplasm also lacks differentiation. There is a small Golgi zone (**G**) and only few profiles of endoplasmic reticulum (**arrow**). The abundance of polyribosomes accounts for the basophilia of the cell seen on light microscopy ($\times$ 14,000).
Courtesy of Dr. D. Zucker-Franklin, Department of Medicine, New York University.

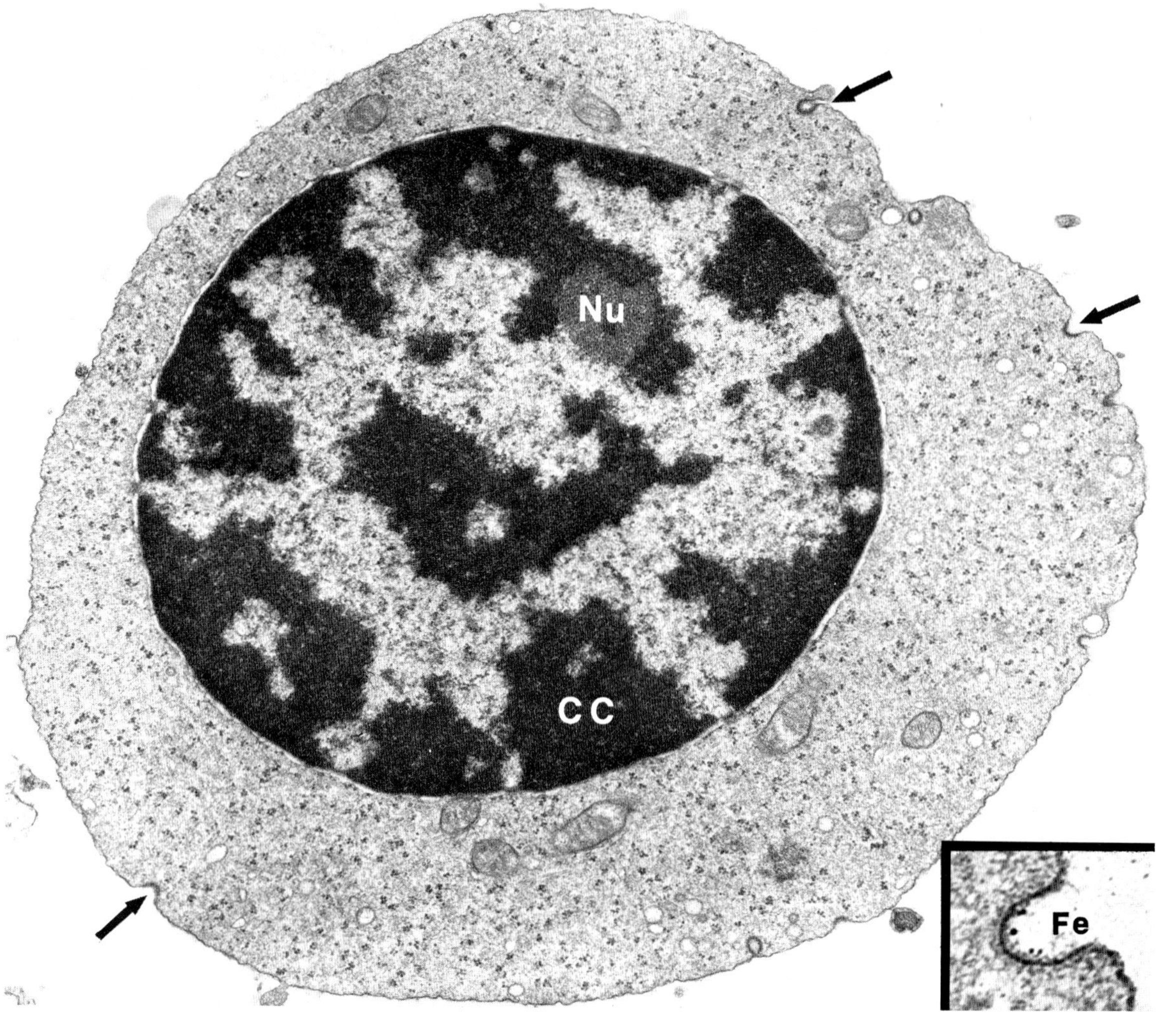

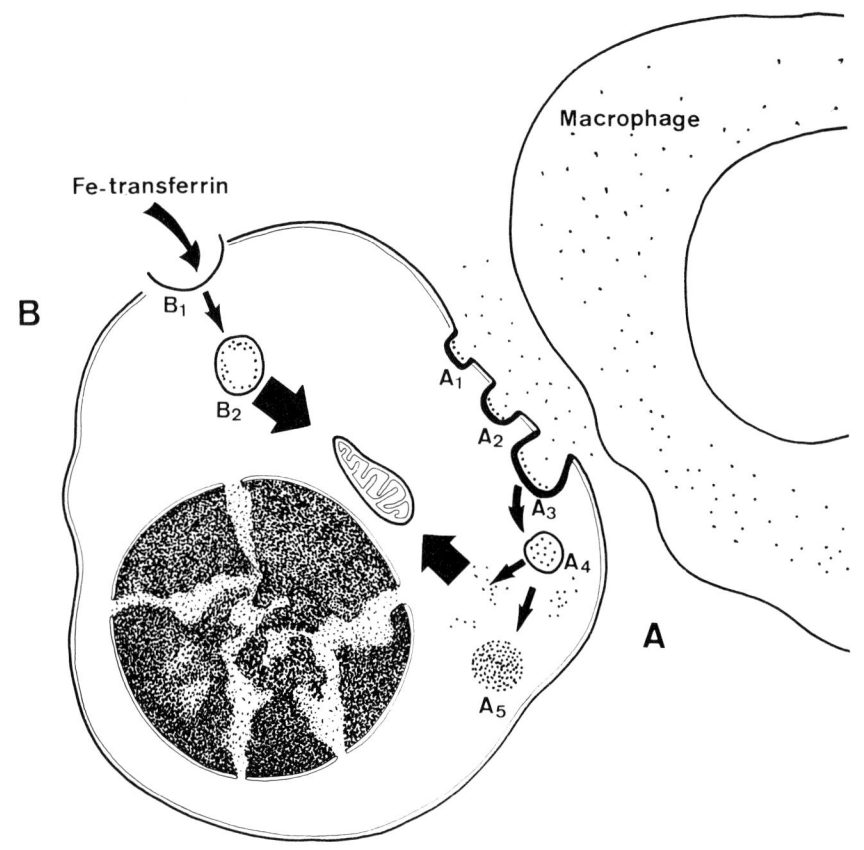

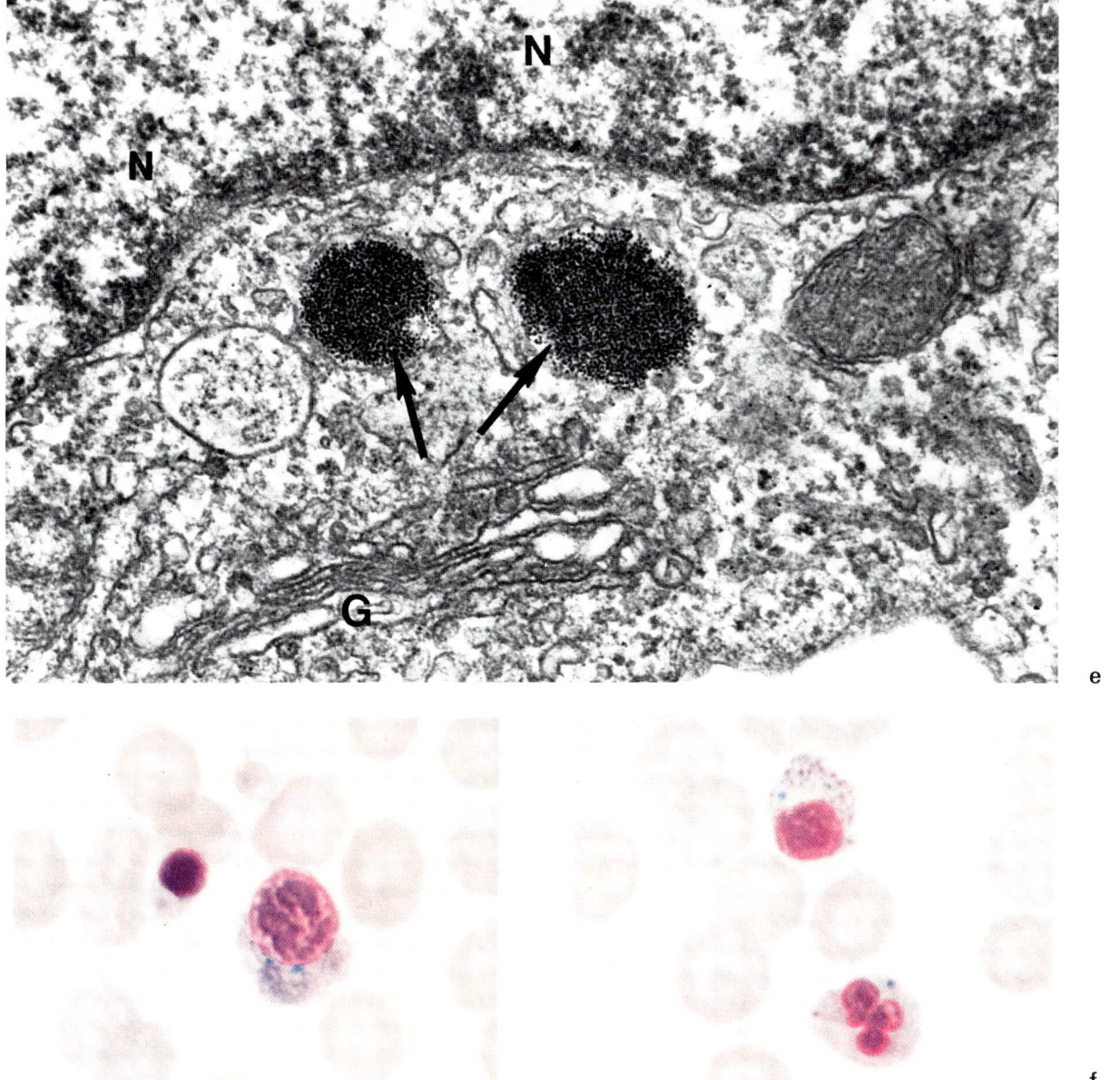

Fig. 7 **c)** Basophilic erythroblast with clumps of condensed chromatin (**CC**) and only a vestigial nucleolus (**Nu**). Although the cytoplasm is still replete with polyribosomes which would account for the degree of basophilia on light microscopy, the grey background indicates the presence of hemoglobin. Several pinocytotic vesicles are detectable at the level of the cytoplasmic membrane, mainly related to absorption of iron in the form of ferritin molecules ("rhopheocytosis") ($\times$ 18,000; Inset: $\times$ 40,000). **Fe**, iron.
Courtesy of Dr. D. Zucker-Franklin, Department of Medicine, New York University.

d) Iron absorption in developing normoblasts. The mechanisms by which iron is delivered to the mitochondria of the developing normoblasts for the incorporation into heme, are still controversial. Two principal patterns are illustrated in this schematic drawing, where the stipples represent ferritin. According to pattern **A**, iron is transferred as preformed ferritin from a histiocyte (the "nursing" cell) to the adjacent normoblast. Bessis et al. have illustrated all the stages of this process which correspond to an invagination of the cell membrane progressively enclosing ferritin molecules ($A_1 \longrightarrow A_5$) [51, 52]. According to pattern **B** iron is selectively taken up by absorption to the erythroid cell surface of transferrin molecules, probably via specific receptors [53, 54]. Endocytosis of iron laden transferrin molecules or of transferrin-receptor complexes ($B_1 \longrightarrow B_2$) leads to the internalization of iron for heme synthesis. Ferritin accumulates in the cytoplasm in the form of dispersed molecules or aggregates which may be either free or contained in membrane-bound vacuoles (see **e**). Ferritin aggregates costitute a yellow-brown pigment known as hemosiderin and are responsible for positive staining of the erythroblasts with the Prussian blue reaction (Perls' reaction) [55] (see **f**).

e) Detail of an erythroblast from a patient with anemia of chronic disease associated with "ineffective" erythropoiesis. Note the large membrane-bound inclusions containing ferritin (**arrows**). **G**, Golgi apparatus; **N**, Nucleus ($\times$ 63,000).
Courtesy of Dr. D. Zucker-Franklin, Department of Medicine, New York University.

f) Erythroblasts containing iron granules stained with Prussian blue dye (sideroblasts). Granules stain deep blue and show different size. Usually no more that three or four granules are recognizable by light microscopy under normal conditions.

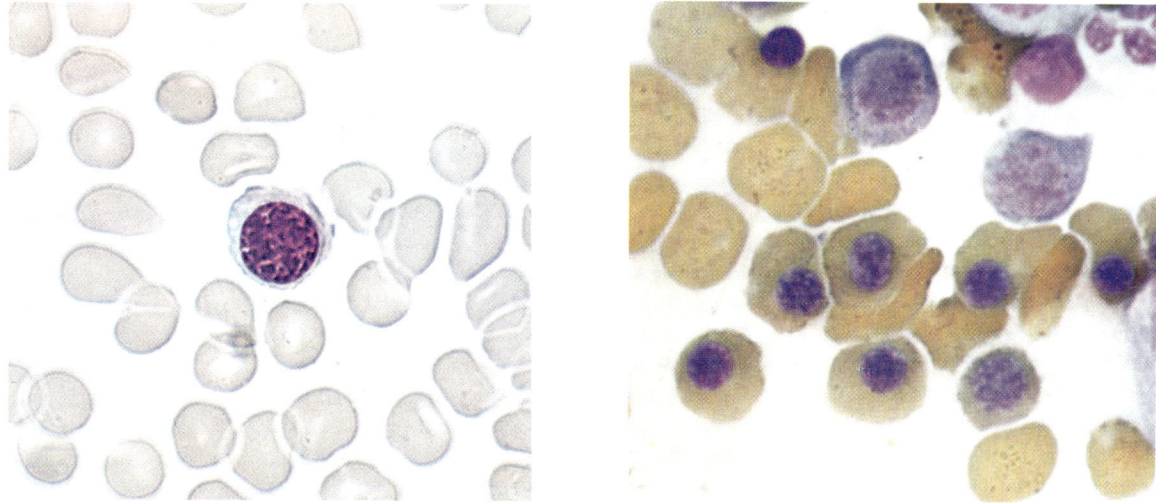

Fig. 8 a) In the early polychromatophilic normoblast the nuclear to cytoplasmic ratio is further decreased. The diameter ranges from 10 to 15 μm. The nucleus shows a coarsely clumped chromatin pattern. The cytoplasm exhibits polychromatophilic staining because of beginning hemoglobinization. This is the last cell of the erythroblastic line capable of mitotic activity. The hemoglobin may act as a regulator of the DNA synthesis, the latter being inhibited when a critical concentration of hemoglobin is reached within the cell [56-58].

b) Benzidine staning for hemoglobin. Early polychromatophilic normoblasts show grey-brown staining because of incomplete hemoglobinization. Late polychromatophilic normoblasts demonstrate fully hemoglobinized cytoplasm.

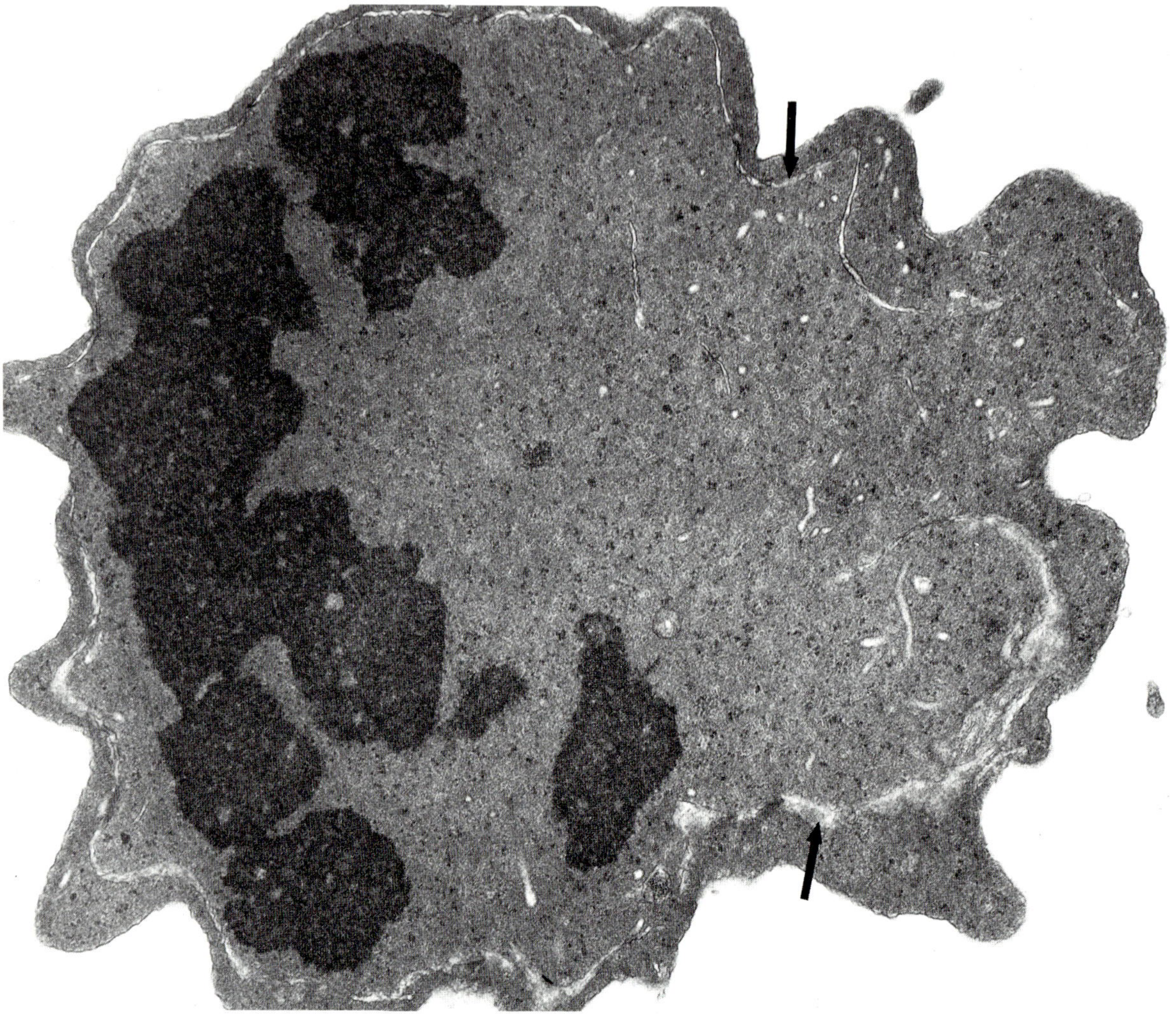

Fig. 8 c) Polychromatophilic normoblast in mitosis. The degree of electron density of the cytoplasm reflects the high hemoglobin content. Obtained from a patient with accelerated erythropoiesis due to hemolysis. Note the disintegration of the nuclear membrane (**arrows**) (× 22,000).
Courtesy of Dr. D. Zucker-Franklin, Department of Medicine, New York University.

3 ERYTHROCYTES

Fig. 9 a) Late polychromatophilic normoblast. This non dividing cell measures 10-12 μm in diameter. The nucleus is small and contains heavily condensed chromatin. The most mature cells may show pyknotic, deeply staining nuclei which are often eccentrically placed before their extrusion. The cytoplasm is acidophilic due to increasing hemoglobinization. Although these cells have been designated as "orthochromatophilic" normoblasts because of the similarity of the staining of their cytoplasm with the erythrocytes, they are in most instances still polychromatophilic.

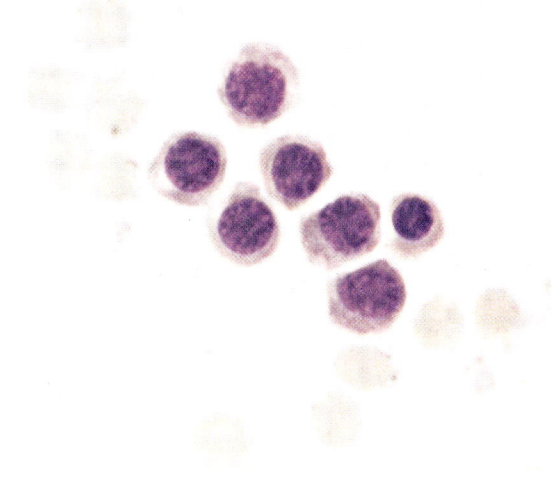

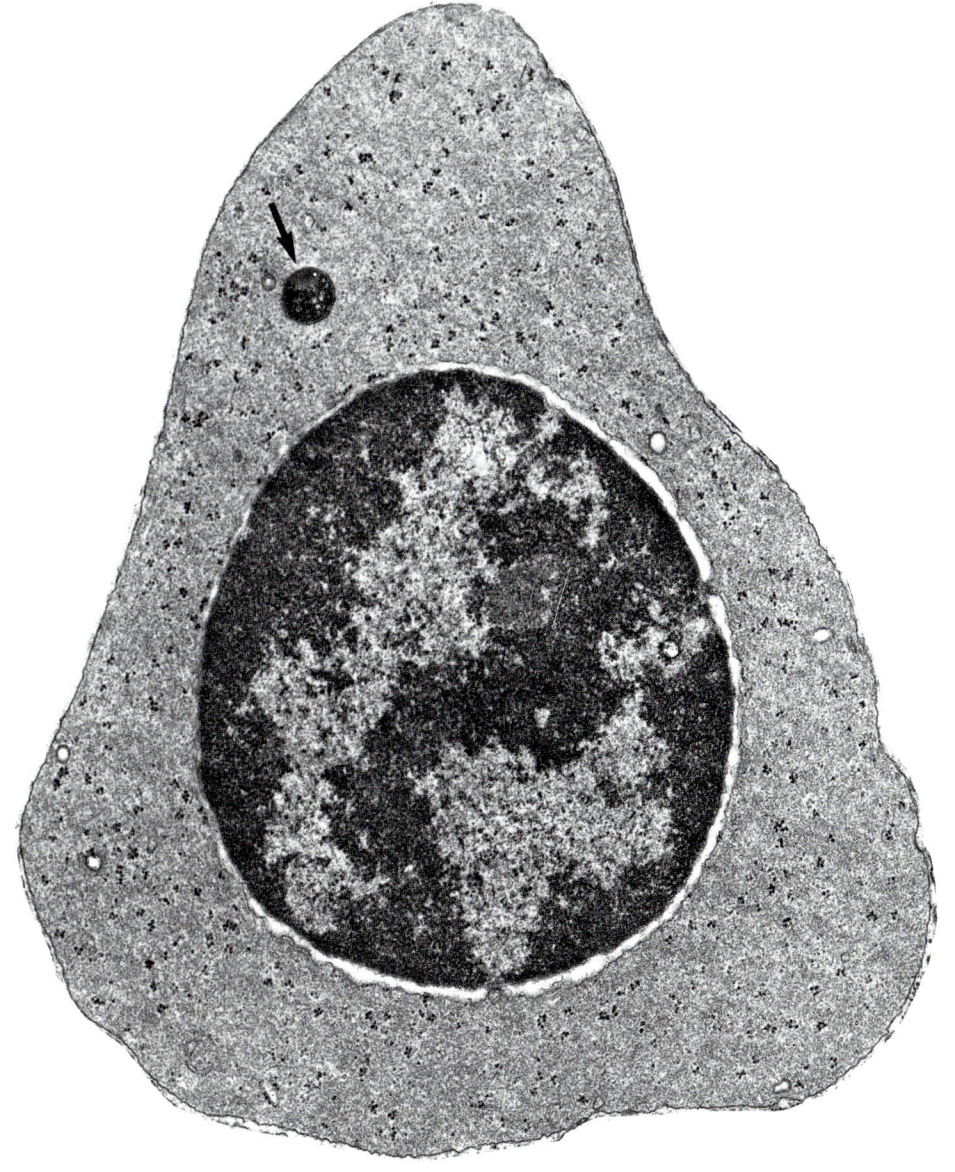

Fig. 9 b) The ultrastructure of the late polychromatophilic normoblast shows large masses of condensed nuclear chromatin. There is an increase in the electron density of the cytoplasm related to the accumulation of hemoglobin. The polyribosomes as well as the number of mitochondria are markedly decreased **(arrow)** (× 22,000).
Courtesy of Prof. E. Reale, Department of Electron Microscopy, Medical School, Hannover.

Fig. 10 *This series of illustrations shows:*

a) Nuclear extrusion and birth of the reticulocyte. The late polychromatophilic normoblast becomes a reticulocyte after extruding its nucleus. Although observations in some pathological conditions have suggested the possibility that nuclear fragmentation (karyorrhexis) is the mechanism by which the nuclei are lost, the alternative process of active expulsion of the nucleus (denucleation) seems to be more likely [59, 60]. Bessis and Bricka [59]) have shown by means of microcinematographic studies that the denucleation process is preceded by a bulge on the erythroblast surface and active contraction of the cell which promotes extrusion.

b) Denucleation process observed by fluorescence microscopy after acridine-orange staining. Red stained cytoplasm shows a contraction around the midportion of the cell until the nucleus is expelled.
Courtesy of Prof. A.M. Marmont, S. Martino's Hospital, Genova.

*c) Bone marrow erythroblasts showing sequential stages of nuclear extrusion (**1** to **4**). In **3**, the extruded nucleus is in close contact with two mononuclear cells. In **4**, a denuded nucleus displays adherent cytoplasmic remnants (**arrow**) (**1**, × 11,000; **2**, × 11,000; **3**, × 16,000; **4**, × 13,000).*
Courtesy of Dr. D. Zucker-Franklin, Department of Medicine, New York University.

3 ERYTHROCYTES

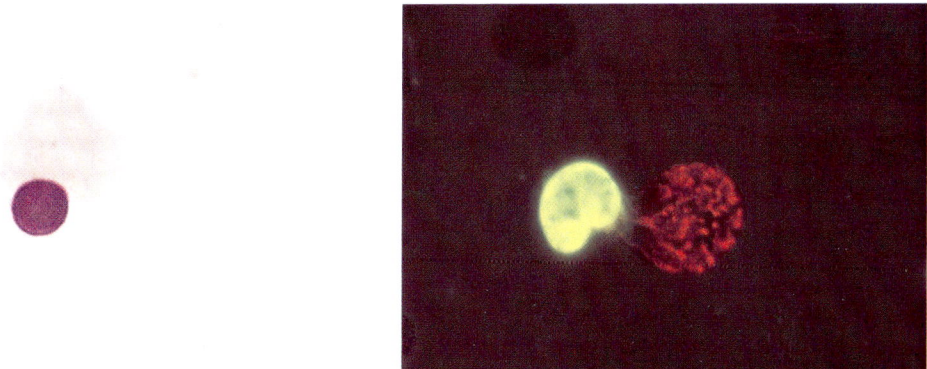

a

b

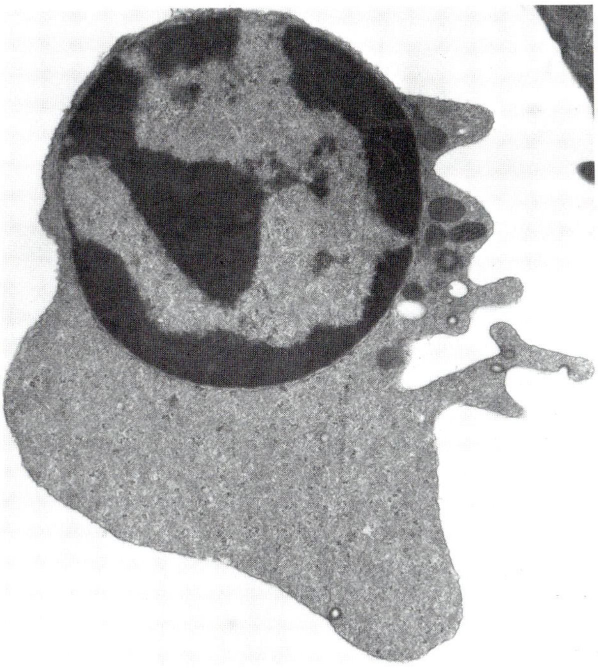

c₁

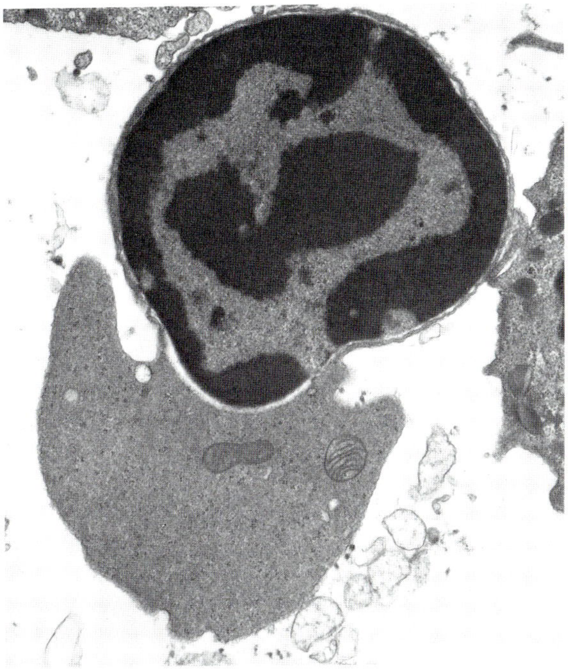

c₂

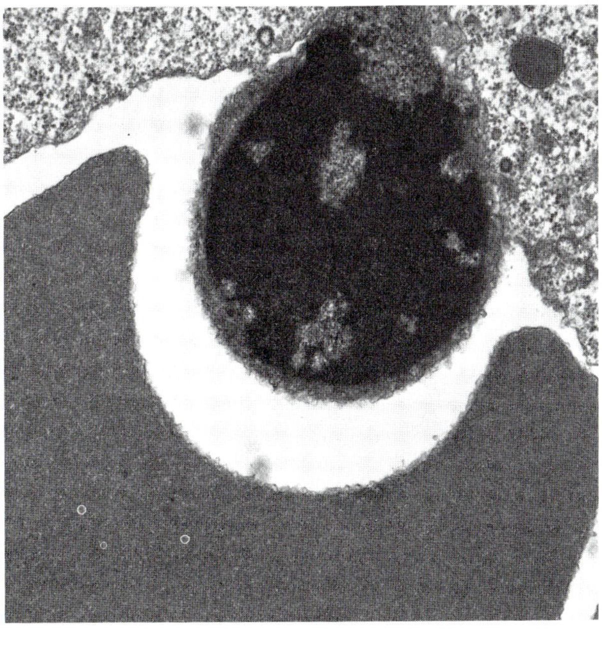

c₃

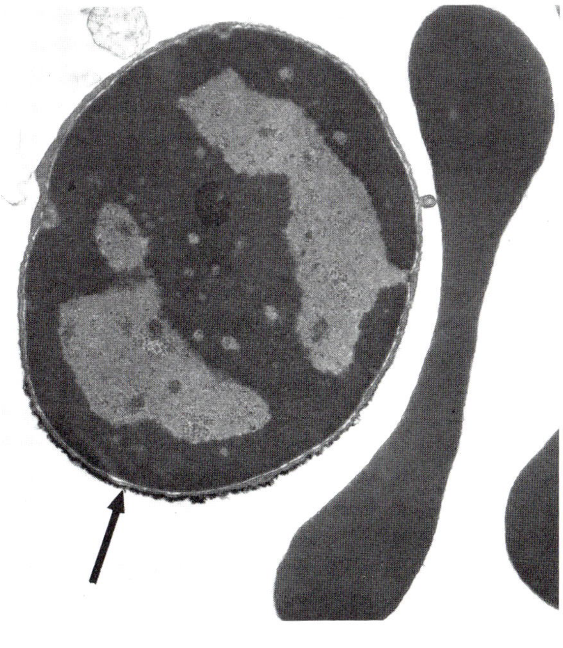

c₄

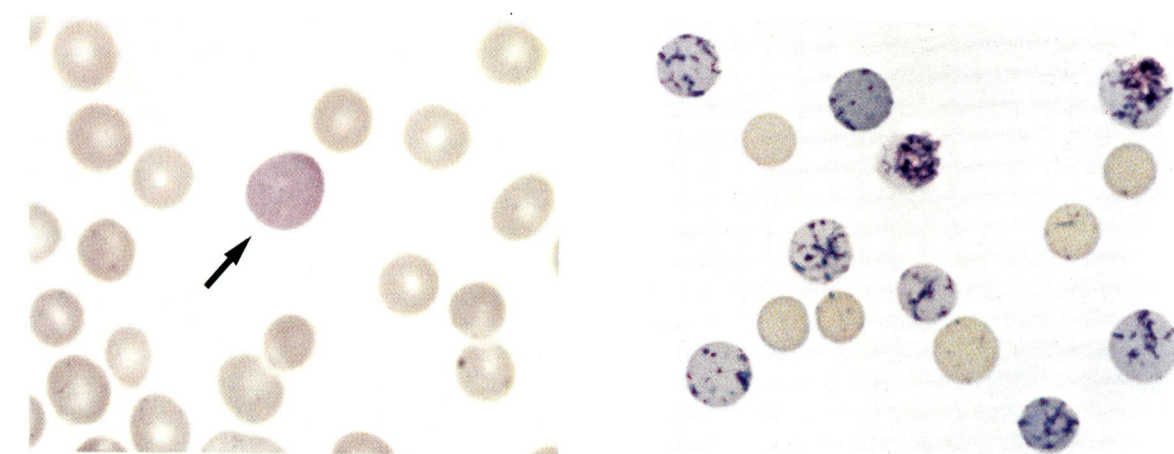

Fig. 11 a-f) *Illustrate various aspects of reticulocytes, i.e. young erythrocytes that have lost their nuclei, but are not fully mature.*

a) *The* **arrow** *indicates a cell that measures about 10 μm in diameter and has an irregular circumference. It is polychromatophilic because it does not yet have its full complement of hemoglobin (which stains pink) and still retains residual RNA (which stains blue). Based on the degree of maturation, several classes of reticulocytes have been recognized [61, 62]. The earlier forms of this maturation series stay in the marrow, while the more mature ones circulate in the blood where they constitute 1-2% of the red cell count. To facilitate the reticulocyte count certain dyes e.g. methylene blue are used to precipitate the residual RNA [63]. Such precipitates form clumps or a fine network illustrated in* **b**.

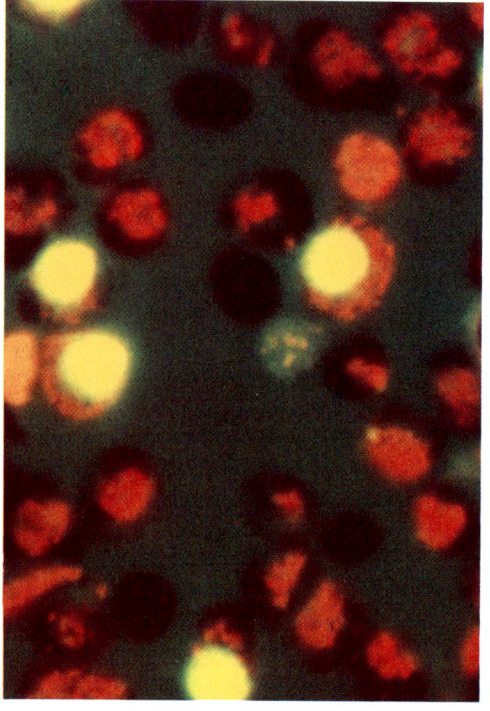
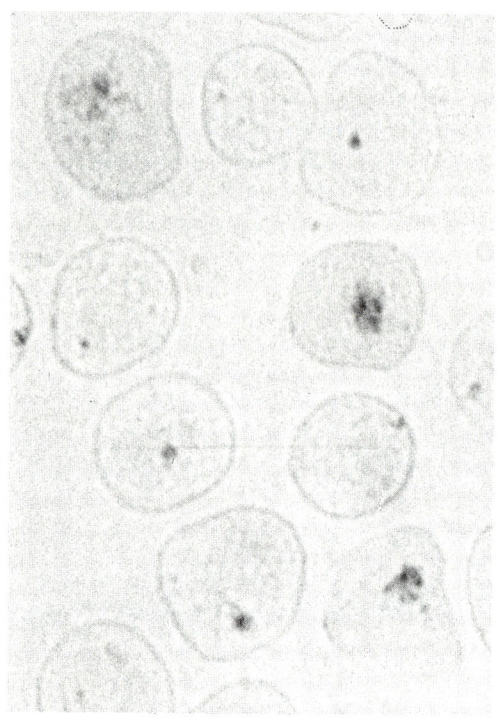

Fig. 11 c) *The reticulocyte maturation as assessed by means of the subdivision into four classes on the basis of the ribosome precipitates ("substantia granulofilamentosa") may be more accurately estimated by determination of the relative amount of RNA in the different elements after acridine-orange (AO) staining [64-66]. Preliminary alcohol fixation prevents precipitation of the AO-RNA complex which emits a red fluorescence.*
Courtesy of Prof. A.M. Marmont, S. Martino's Hospital, Genova.

d) *Since reticulocytes possess some enzymes which are lost in mature red cells, cytochemical techniques may also be valuable for their identification. Non specific esterases and several dehydrogenases have been used for this purpose [67]. In* **d** *the reaction product for dihydro-orotic acid dehydrogenase is illustrated to distinguish reticulocytes from mature erythrocytes.*

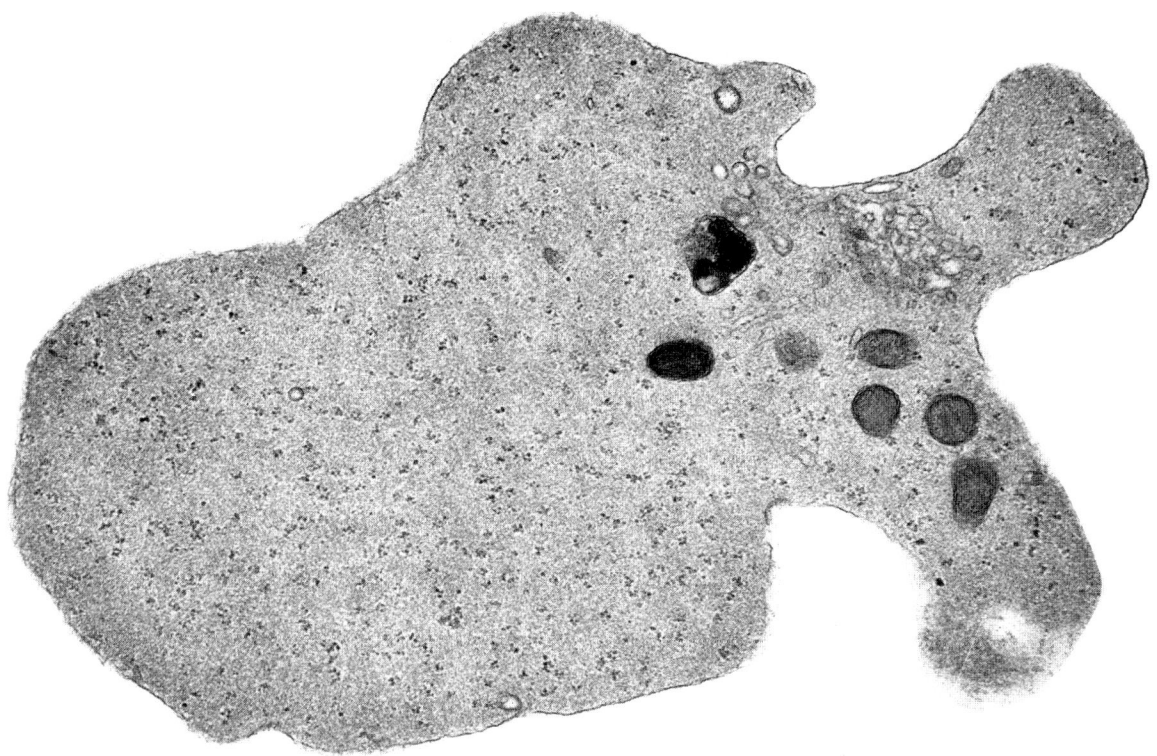

Fig. 11 e) Ultrastructure of a reticulocyte. This cell shows irregular surface, with several indentations, possibly due to active movements. Within the cytoplasmatic matrix some remnants of the Golgi complex, few mitochondria, polyribosomes and sometimes ferritin aggregates are recognizable ($\times$ 22,000).
Courtesy of Prof. E. Reale, Department of Electron Microscopy, University of Hannover.

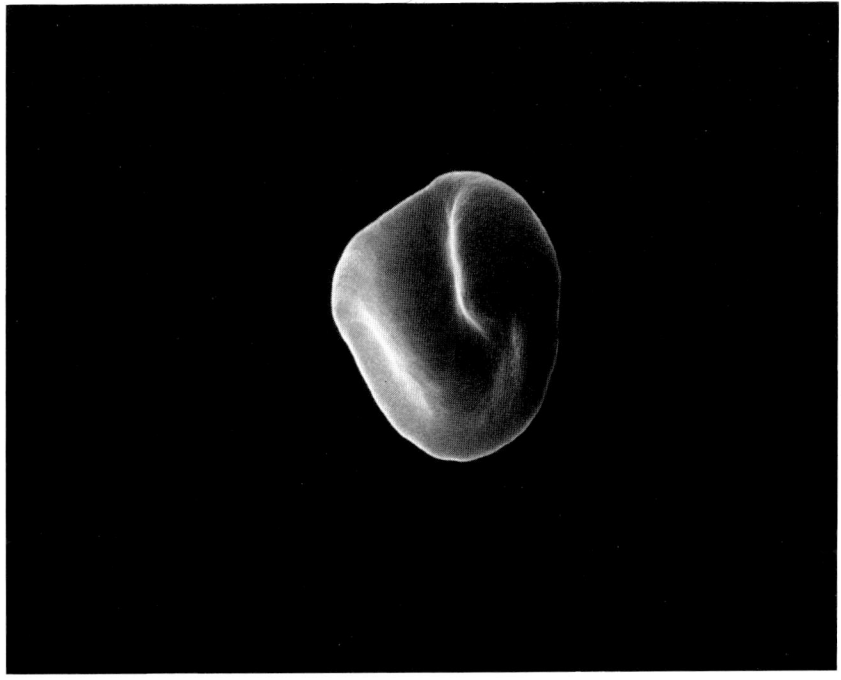

Fig. 11 f) SEM observation of a reticulocyte. Its surface is lobulated or irregularly indented reflecting active cellular movements ($\times$ 5,200).

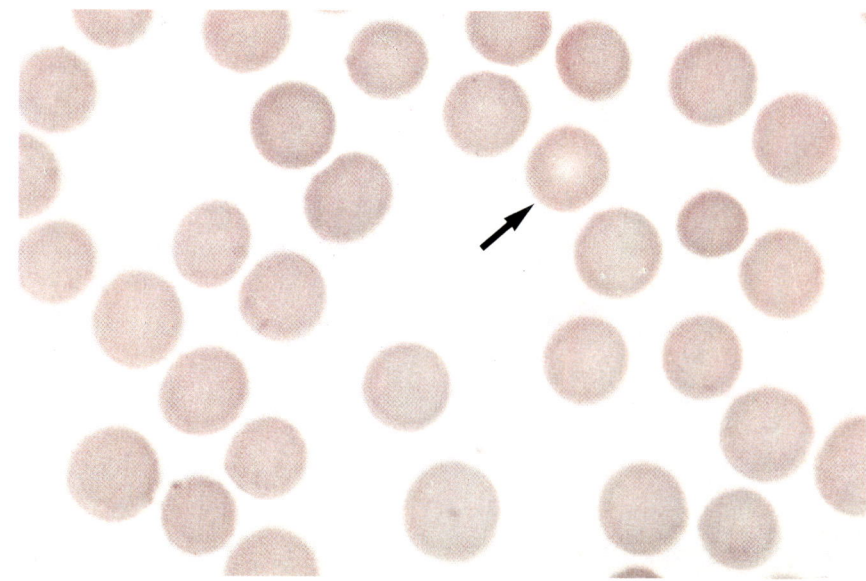

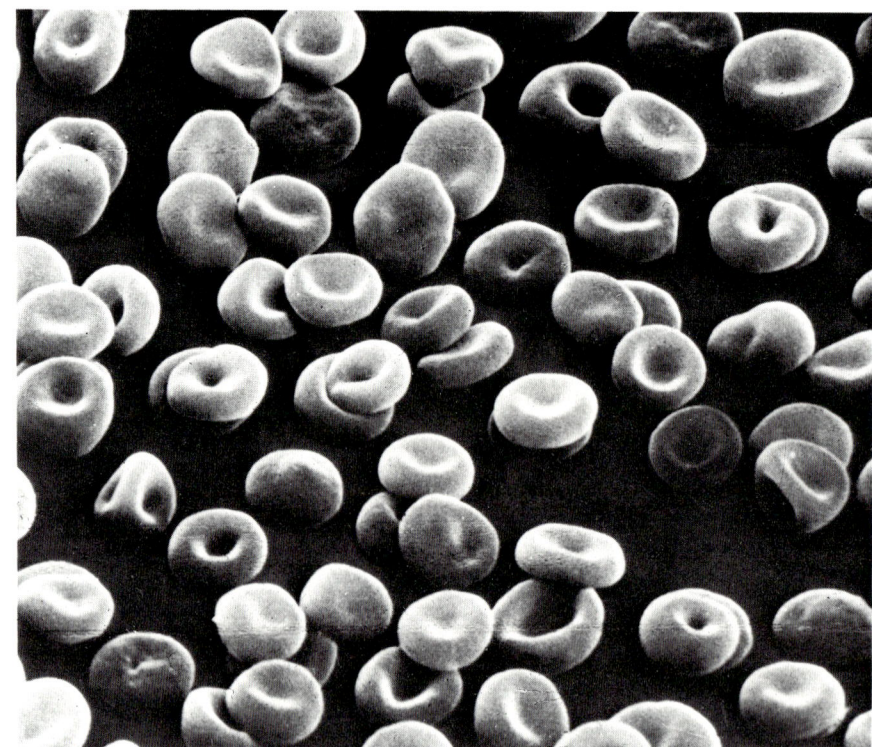

Fig. 12 a, b) Erythrocyte. This cell stains deep orange in normally prepared smears (a) and appears as a biconcave disc (discocyte) by scanning electron microscopy (b). Its diameter measures 7-8 μm. The **arrow** indicates a normal erythrocyte which illustrates a clear center due to the biconcavity of the cell (Hb concentration less dense).

The young erythrocyte, as it is released from the bone marrow, is subjected to some surface remodeling due to numerous events while in the circulation. Immunological reactions or repeated mechanical stresses [68, 69] may irreversibly alter membrane structure. The gradual loss of membrane fragments leads to the formation of a relatively rigid spherocyte, devoid of active metabolic properties. This is easily trapped by the reticuloendothelial cells (mainly in the spleen) (see also **Fig. 25 k-m**).

b) Courtesy of Dr. H. Kayden, New York University.

3 ERYTHROCYTES

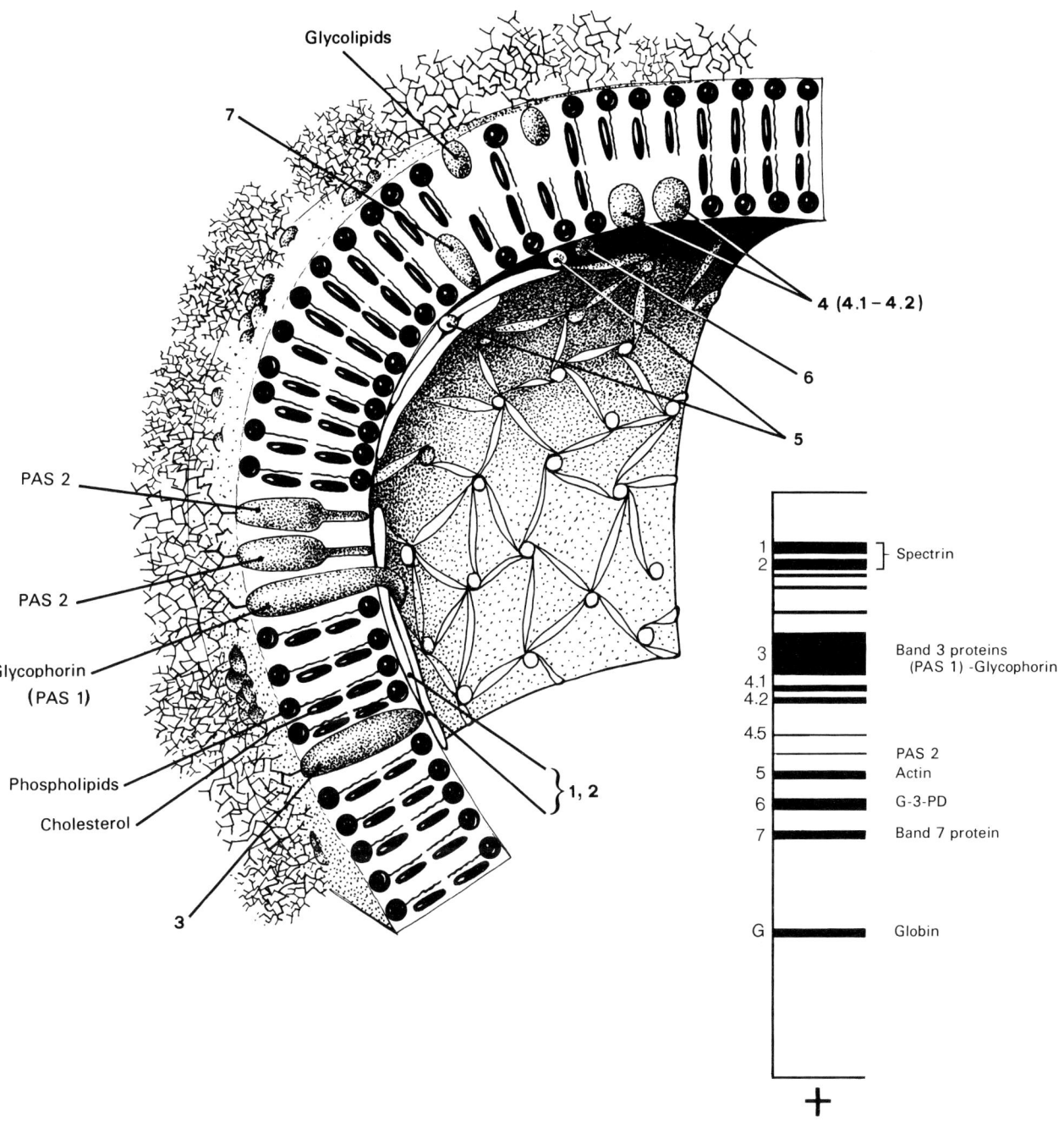

Fig. 13 a) *Diagrammatic model of the human erythrocyte membrane showing the major membrane proteins, numbered according to their sequence in SDS-PAGE pattern after Coomassie blue staining (**inset**).*
1-2: Spectrin; **3**: Band 3 protein(s); **4.1** and **4.2**: band 4.1 protein and band 4.2 protein; **5**: actin; **6**: glyceraldehyde-3-phosphate dehydrogenase; **7**: band 7 protein. Glycophorin migrates within band **3** in the SDS-PAGE system.

5.2. The structure of the red cell membrane

The structure of the red blood cell membrane is represented diagrammatically in **Figure 13** as a lipid bilayer arranged according to the Singer-Nicolson fluid mosaic model [70] with insertion of protein components [71-74]. The concept of single protein components is based on their identification by polyacrylamide gel electrophoresis after solubilization with sodium dodecyl sulfate (SDS-PAGE) [75-77]. Some proteins are embedded in the hydrophobic core of the membrane (*integral proteins*), whereas others, such as spectrin, are extrinsic but may be associated with the sites of protrusion

Table 1 PLASMA MEMBRANE CHARACTERISTICS OF THE ERYTHROID SERIES

1. *Blood group antigens*: e.g. A, B, H, Rh(D), I and i, etc. present on normoblasts [81, 82]; status on precursors cells uncertain.
2. *HLA expression*: present on precursor cells and lost at the reticulocyte stage.
3. *HLA-DR/Ia-like antigen*: expressed on colony forming erythroid precursors (BFU-E, CFU-E).
4. *Glycophorin*: a major transmembrane glycoprotein of the red cells associated with the appearance of hemoglobin in normoblasts and lacking in pronormoblasts [83].
   Carbohydrate residues responsible for MN blood groups and binding of lectins and influenza virus.
5. *Spectrin*: submembranous component.
6. *Erythropoietin receptors* on BFU-E and CFU-E: functionally detected but not yet directly demonstrated on single cells.

of the former molecules (*peripheral proteins*). Some integral proteins traverse the whole membrane (*transmembrane proteins*) and contact the spectrin components (1 and 2) on the inner side of the membrane. The outward facing hydrophobic N-terminal regions of transmembrane proteins are heavily glycosylated. The sugar residues of oligosaccharide sequences have been identified as binding sites for viruses and lectins and as antigenic determinants (e.g. MN blood group antigens) [74]. Glycophorin (major sialoglycoprotein, MN-glycoprotein, either in a dimeric-PAS-1 or monomeric form-PAS-2) represents one of the best characterized integral membrane (glyco)proteins.

Component 3 is represented by a transmembrane protein associated with cation transport and containing the enzyme acetylcholinesterase. A fraction of band 3 (about 15%) is linked to the erythrocyte cytoskeleton through association with "ankyrin" which represents the membrane attachment protein for spectrin in human erythrocyte membranes [78].

Another enzyme is present in band 6 (glyceraldehyde-3-phosphate dehydrogenase) and is localized at the inner surface of the membrane.

Spectrin is composed of two bands (1 and 2) and has myosin-like properties; it interacts with actin (5) making a complex network at the internal surface [79]. The polymerization of spectrin is important for spectrin-actin interaction, as well as for its phosphorylated state. Dephosphorylation of spectrin induces aggregation of this membrane component with alteration of the network and of some membrane properties (as the "contraction" of the membrane in the discocyte-echinocyte transition) [80].
Most of the components of the red cell membrane are expressed in the course of erythroblast maturation [81].
These biological properties are important markers in defining the phenotype of the cells in several disorders and may be usefully studied for diagnostic purposes. In **Table 1** the principal membrane characteristics of the erythroid series are listed.

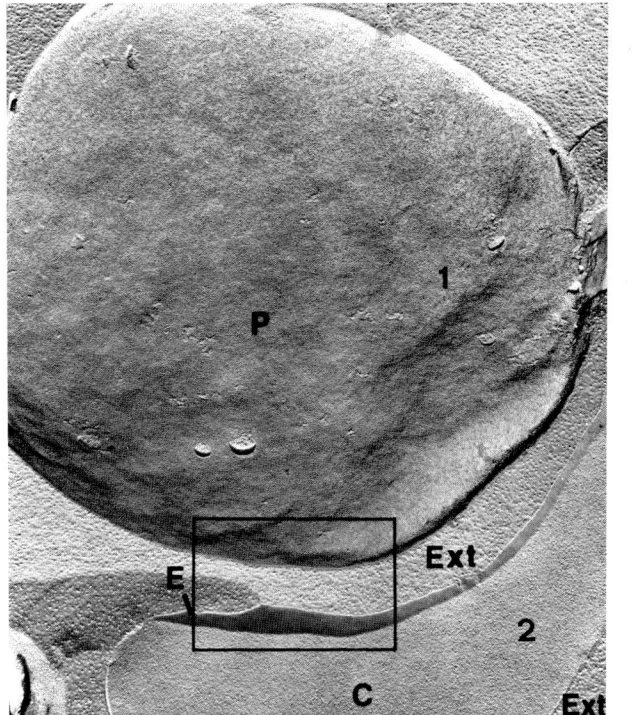

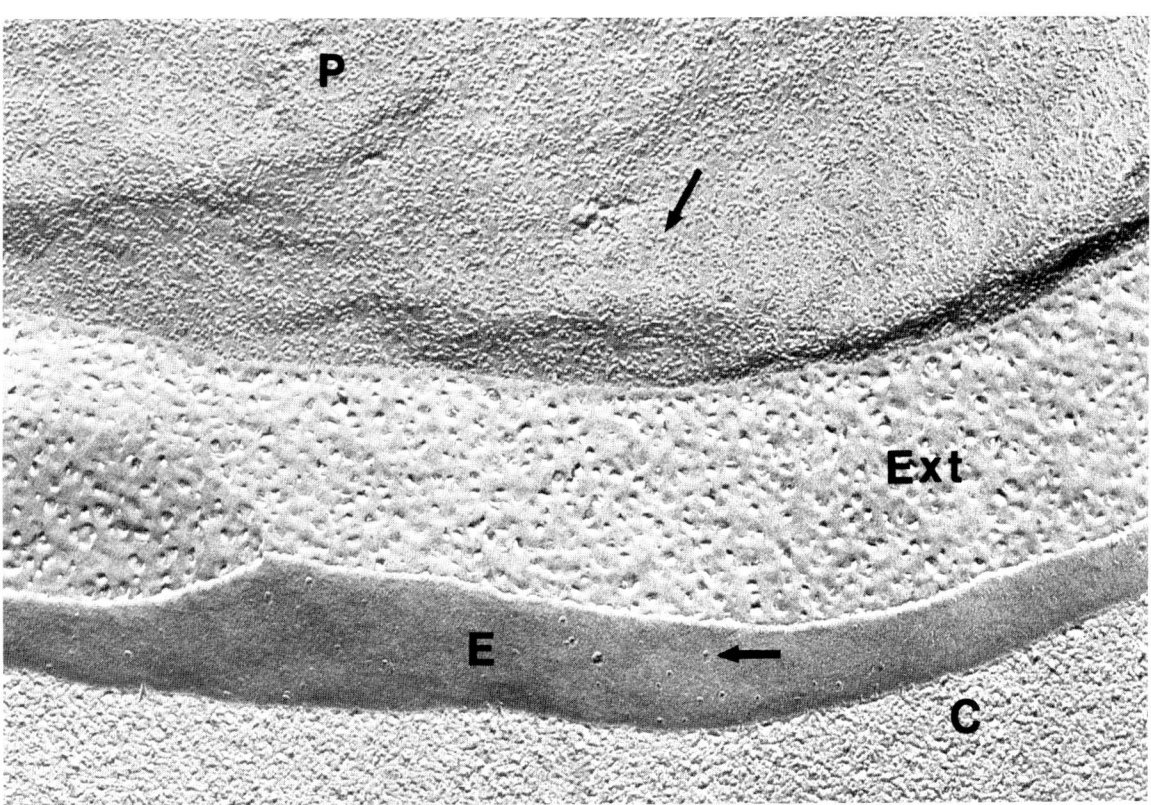

Fig. 13 b) Replica of two adjacent freeze-fractured erytrocytes (**1** and **2**). In the top cell the cleavage plane has revealed the protoplasmic leaflet of the membrane, P face (**P**). The fracture then crossed extracellular space (**Ext**) after which it cleaved the membrane of the lower cell exposing its cytoplasm (**C**) and a small part of its external leaflet, E face (**E**). The area delimited by the rectangle is seen at higher magnification in **c** ($\times$ 15,000).

c) The area delimited by the rectangle in **b** shown at higher resolution to illustrate the difference in the number and distribution of intramembranous particles (**arrows**). The particles are extremely dense on the P face of the erythrocyte membrane. Aggregation of the particles has been observed as a result of treatment with antisera and other in vitro manipulations. However, the function of the IMP's and their relationship to the membrane proteins remains to be elucidated ($\times$ 73,000).

Courtesy of Dr. D. Zucker-Franklin, Department of Medicine, New York University.

Fig. 14 Erythroblastic island. Several erythroblasts cluster around a central macrophage ("nursing cell") which exhibits elongated projections of cytoplasm between the erythroid cells. Erythroblasts show various degrees of chromatin condensation.

Fig. 15 Prussian blue staining of an erythroblastic island. Some erythroblasts located at the periphery exhibit a close connection with cytoplasmic portions of the central reticulum cell. These heavily stained fragments may keep a firm attachment to the erythroblastic cells, even when they are detached from the "nursing" histiocyte by mechanical procedures.

5.3. The erythroblastic island

The erythroblastic island is believed to be the anatomical unit [84] which supports the amplification phase of erythropoietic proliferation. Erythroid aggregates surrounding a central reticulum cell have been described in various pathological conditions [85, 86], but their physiological significance in normal erythropoiesis [3] and in the regenerating bone marrow following transplantation [87] has attracted attention only recently. The erythroblastic island is composed of one or two histiocytes (macrophages) surrounded by concentric layers of maturing erythroblasts (**Fig. 14**).

The central histiocyte extends thin processes in between the erythroblasts. The processes stain deeply with Prussian blue (**Fig. 15**). The close association between the cytoplasmic appendages of the histiocytes and even the most peripherally located erythroblasts suggests the possibility that "trophic" factors may be released by the central cell (nursing cell) which induce or influence the development of the erythropoietic pattern within the island (**Fig. 16**).

Fig. 16 a) Schematic drawing of the ultrastructural features of an erythroblastic island. Several erythroblasts cluster around the central macrophage which exhibits elongated projections of cytoplasm embracing the erythroid cells. Erythroblasts show various degrees of chromatin condensation and contain polyribosomes and mitochondria. The same relationship between macrophage and erythroblasts is shown in the picture (**top right**).
b) Erythroblastic island viewed by scanning electron microscopy, showing several erythroblasts (**Eb**) which are concentrically placed around the "nursing" reticulum cell (**RC**).
Courtesy of Prof. P. Motta, University of Rome.

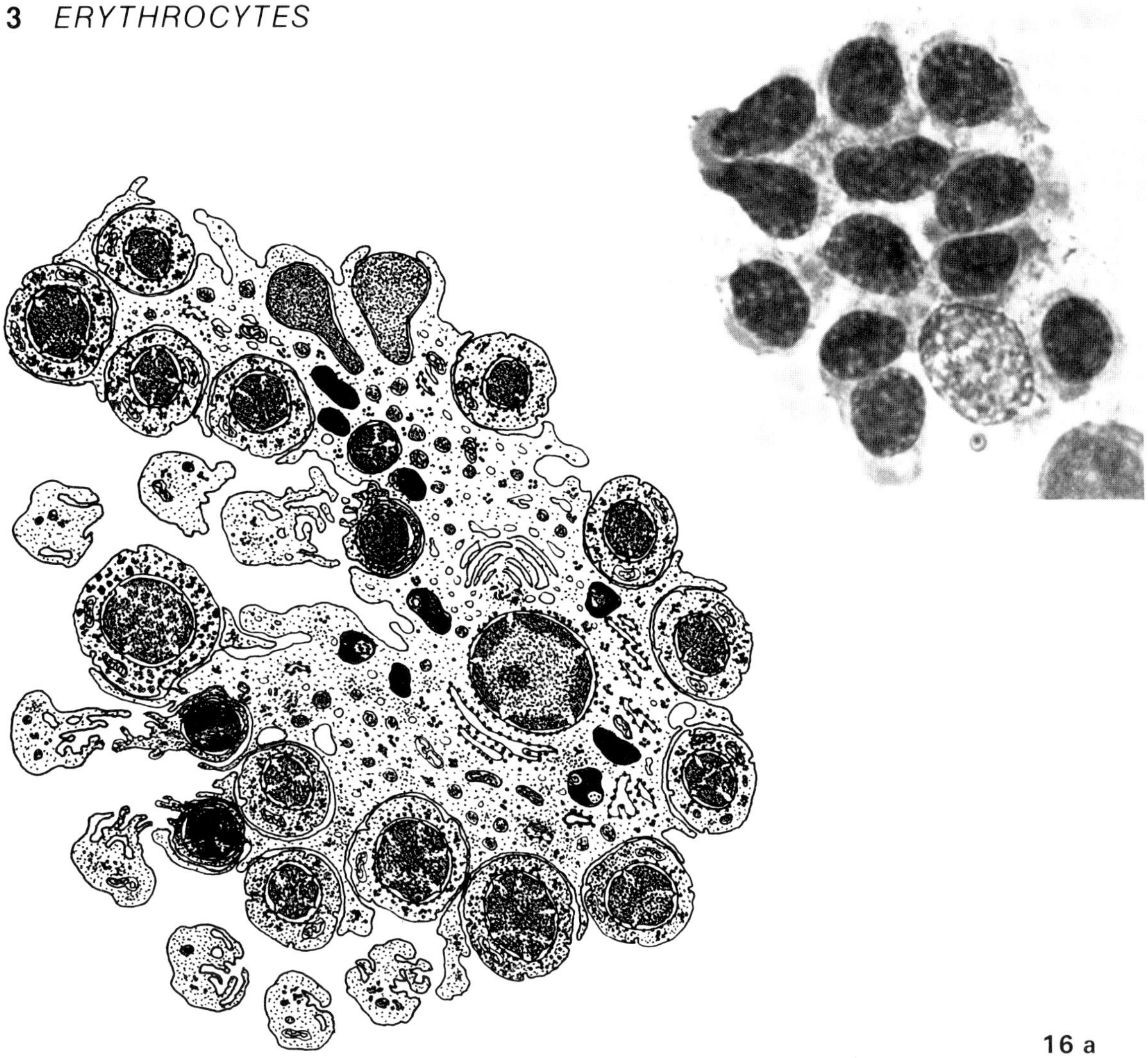

3 ERYTHROCYTES

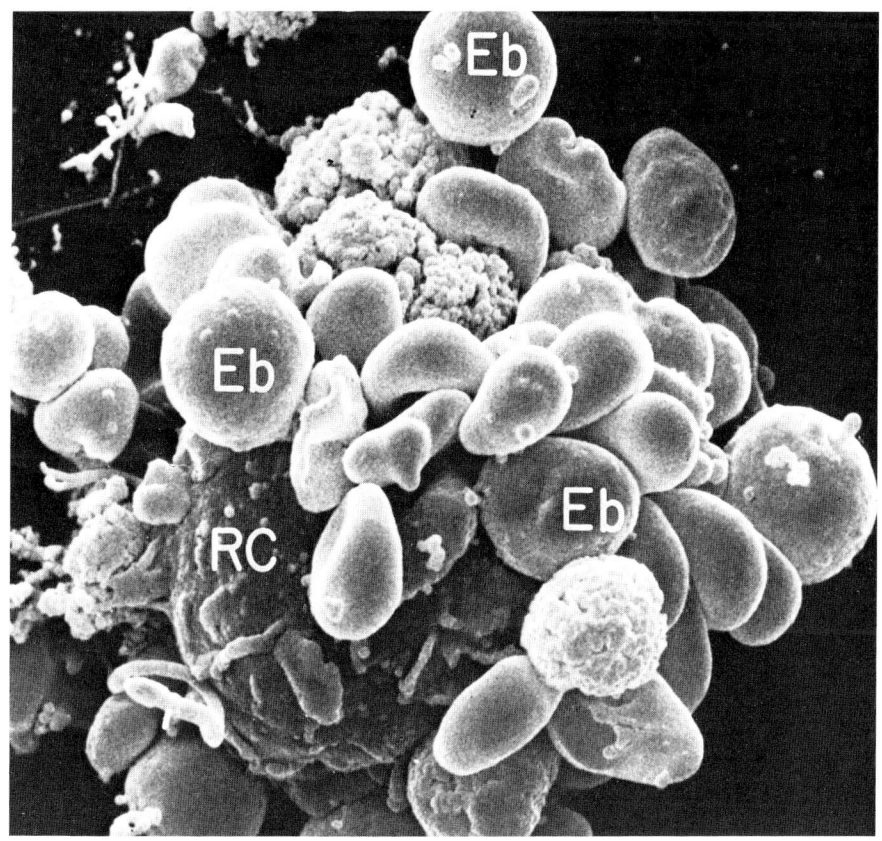

16 a

b

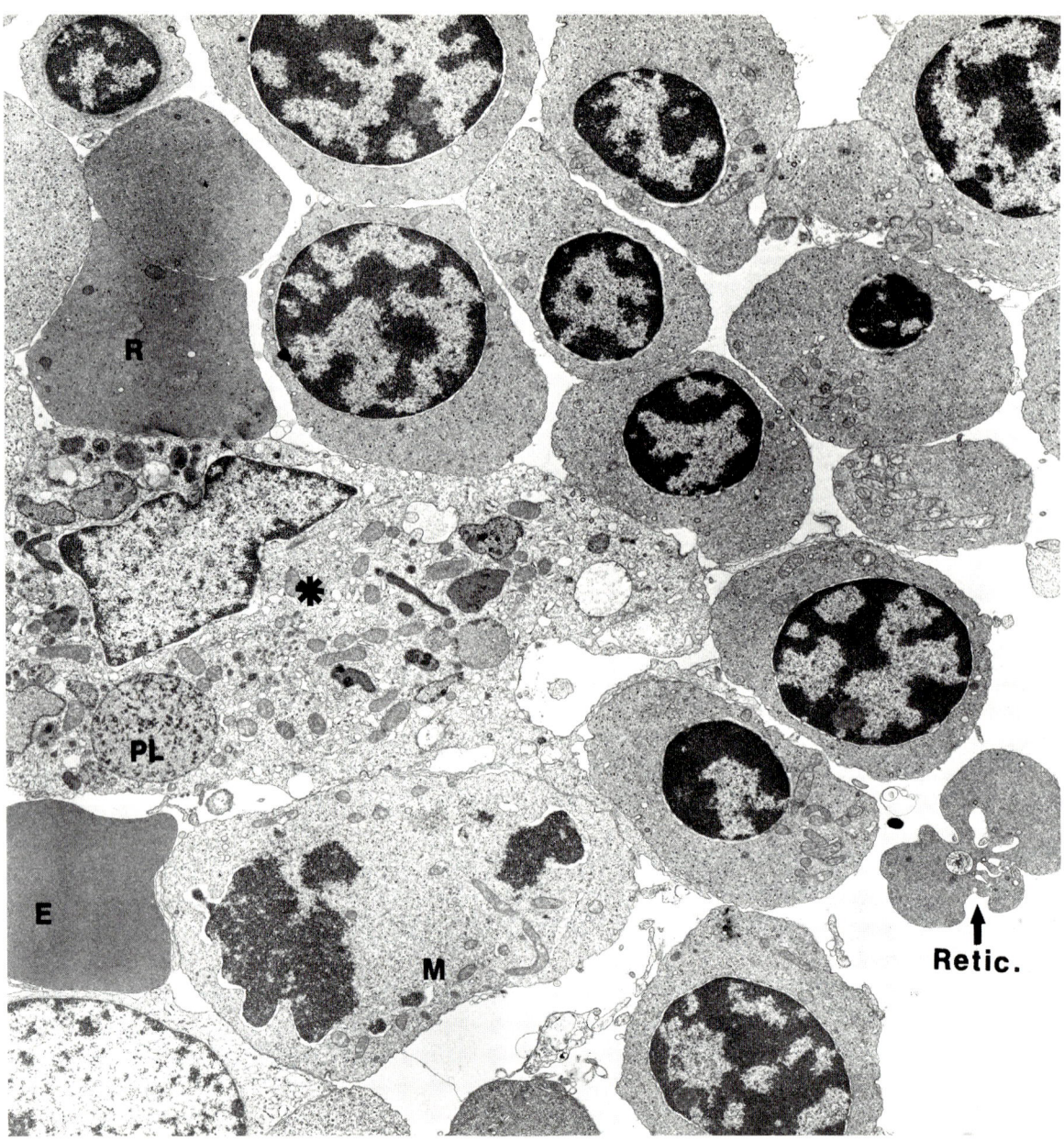

Fig. 16 c) Detail of an erythroblastic island. A reticulum cell (*) containing many inclusions probably representing phagolysosomes **(PL)** is surrounded by erythroid elements at all stages of differentiation and maturation. Note the erythroblast in mitosis **(M)**, the young reticulocyte **(Retic)** shortly after nuclear extrusion, older reticulocytes **(R)** with a smoother contour, more electron dense cytoplasm but some residual organelles, and the mature erythrocyte **(E)** devoid of organelles, and even more electron dense cytoplasm reflecting almost complete hemoglobinization ($\times$ 5,500).
Courtesy of Dr. D. Zucker-Franklin, Department of Medicine, New York University.

It is likely that, in part, this function may be accomplished by the passage of substances, such as ferritin molecules, into the developing erythroblasts, as has been demonstrated by ultrastructural studies ("rhopheocytosis") [88, 89]. The central histiocyte, moreover, appears to engulf and degrade the extruded erythroblastic nuclei of the island. This feature is commonly observed in the hepatic phase of fetal erythropoiesis (see **Fig. 1**) and has been documented in regenerating marrows after experimental aplasia [90] and after bone marrow engraftment [87]. This well documented activity of the central histiocyte may represent a specific function which prevents the disorganization of the island and facilitates maturation of the surrounding cells [3].

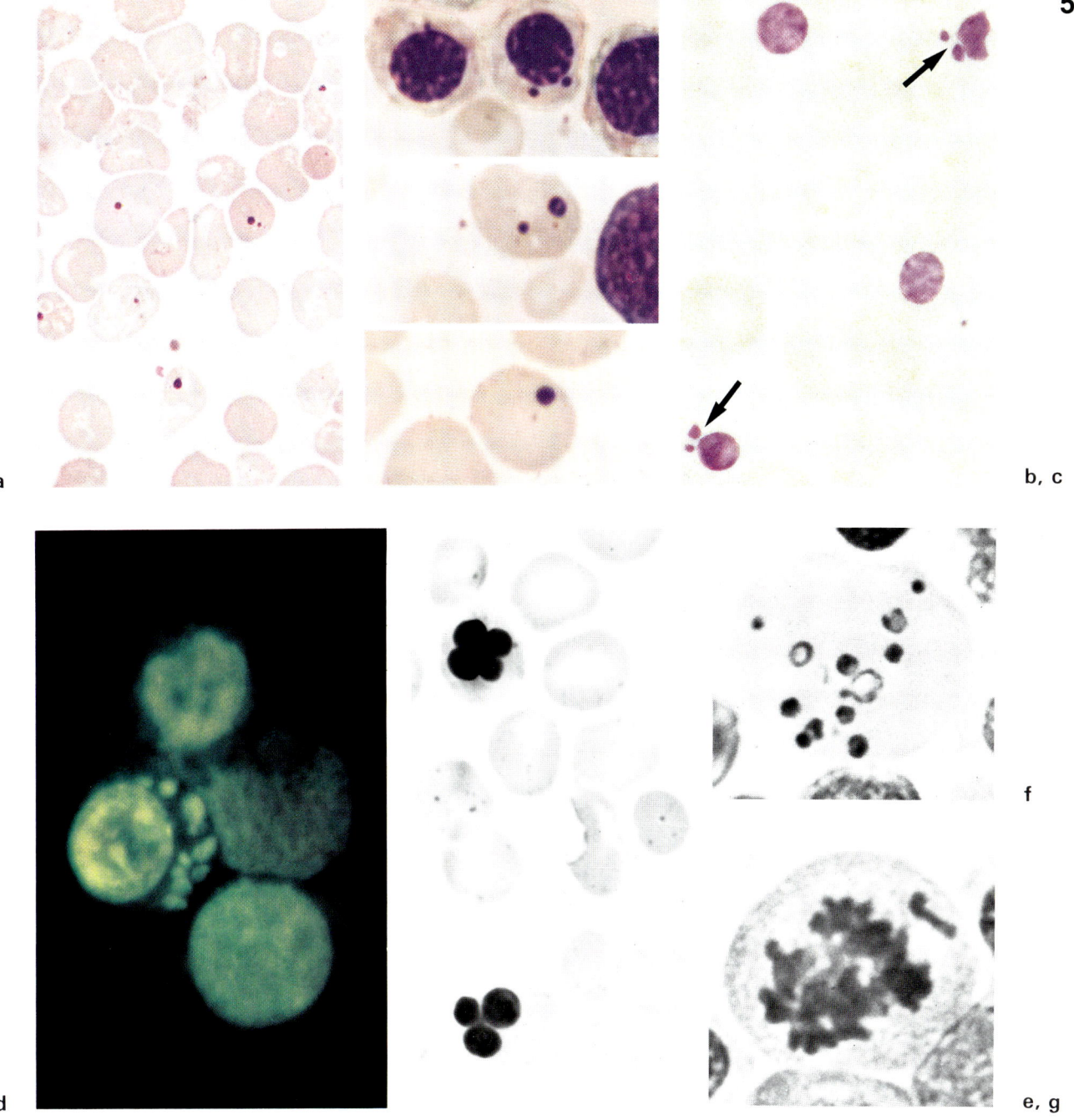

Fig. 17 a-g) Howell-Jolly bodies appear as spherical inclusions of 0,5-1 µm in diameter [92], which stain deep purple like the pyknotic nuclei of late polychromatophilic erythroblasts (**a, b**). The structures are remnants of nuclear chromatin and are, therefore, delineated by the Feulgen technique (**arrows in c**) [93]; when stained with quinacrine, Howell-Jolly bodies are brightly fluorescent (**d**).
Usually, there is only one body per cell, but in some dyserythropoietic anemias, numerous bodies may be seen within the same cell. In myeloproliferative disorders nuclear fragmentation (karyorrhexis) or incomplete nuclear extrusion may give rise to multiple inclusions (**e, f**) [94]. Alternatively the bodies may arise from premature separation of some chromatin material from the mitotic spindle (**g**) [95].
Splenectomy is the most common cause for the appearance of Howell-Jolly bodies in the blood, for in healthy individuals such nuclear remnants would be removed by spleen macrophages.

5.4. Erythrocyte inclusions

Nuclear or cytoplasmatic remnants may constitute the origin of some inclusions seen in reticulocytes or even in some young red cells. Although most of these inclusions arise as a consequence of physiological processes, they are frequently observed in pathological conditions, such as severe or long-standing anemias or in disorders characterized by a reduced clearing activity of the spleen (**Figs. 17-21**).

Fig. 18 a-c) Cabot rings *are thin strands of material which stain red violet with Romanowsky dyes and appear concentrically within erythrocytes. In some instances the ring may be twisted or associated with other inclusions, such as basophilic stippling (*a*). The ring may be single or, less frequently, multiple. No definitive agreement has been reached on the mechanisms which may be involved in the formation of these structures [96, 97].*
In **b** *a mitotic division is shown in which a purple filamentous connection (possibly originating from the spindle fibers) joins the newly formed erythroblasts.*
In **c** *a separated erythroblast is still retaining a convoluted filamentous projection.*

Fig. 19 Basophilic stippling *refers to an accumulation of granules which stain deep blue. The granules vary in size and number and are thought to derive from clumping of ribosomes [98]. The intracellular aggregates may also include mitochondria and siderosomes. Basophilic stippling is observed mainly in disorders characterized by altered hemoglobin synthesis.*

Fig. 20 Pappenheimer bodies *stain purple with Romanowsky stains [99] and are usually located in the periphery of the cells. They represent ferritin aggregates and stain positively with the Prussian blue reagent. Therefore, such cells are also referred to as siderocytes. In splenectomized patients erythrocytes containing Pappenheimer bodies are commonly observed [100].*

3 ERYTHROCYTES

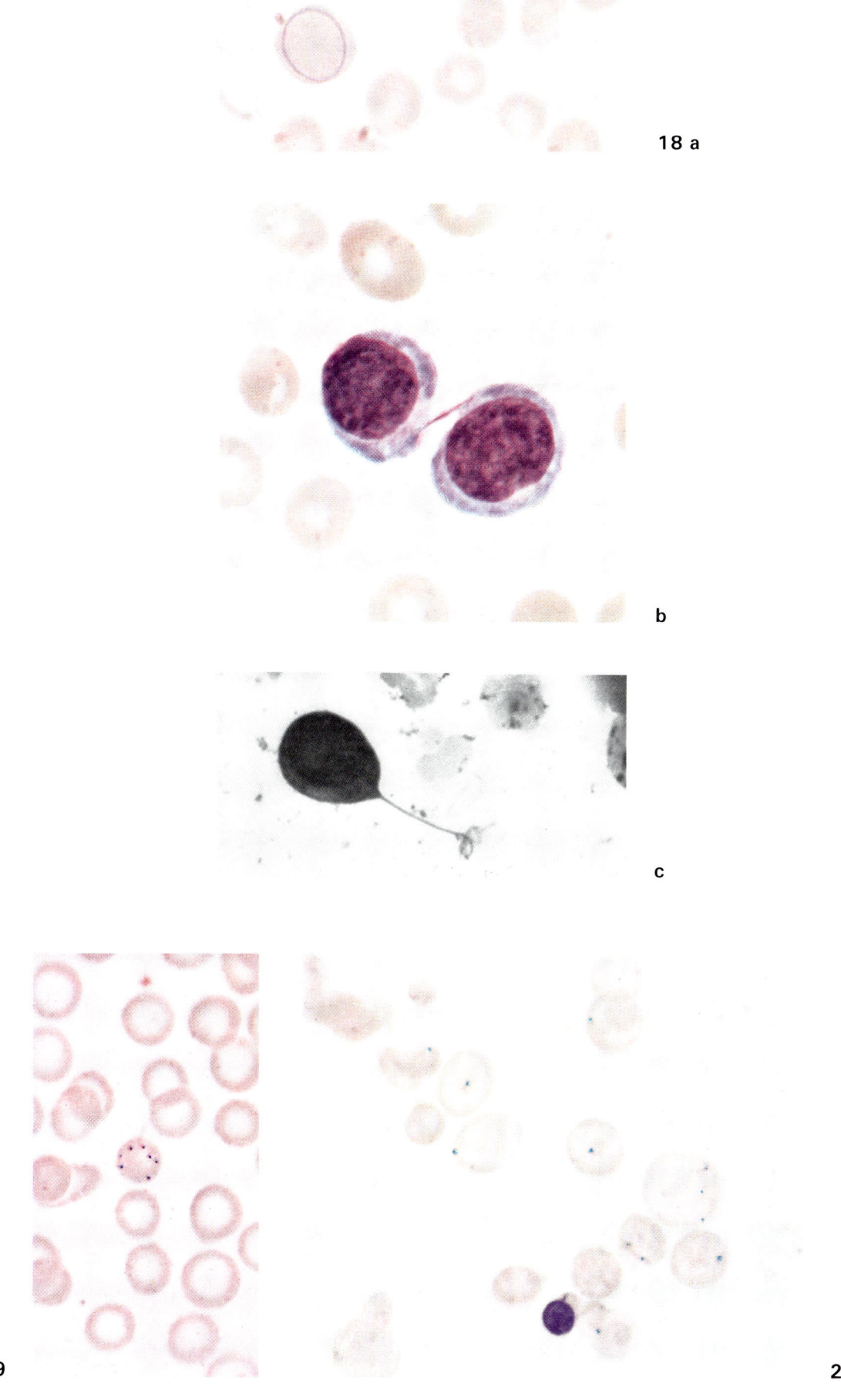

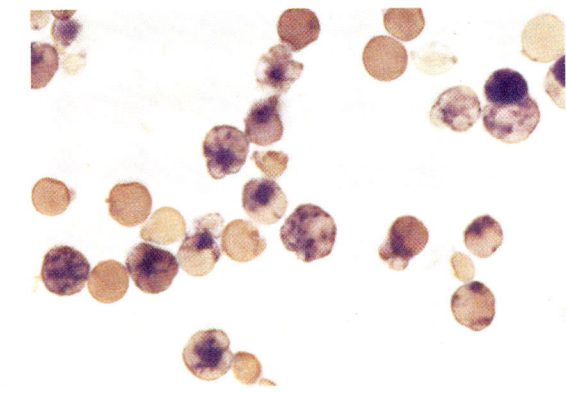

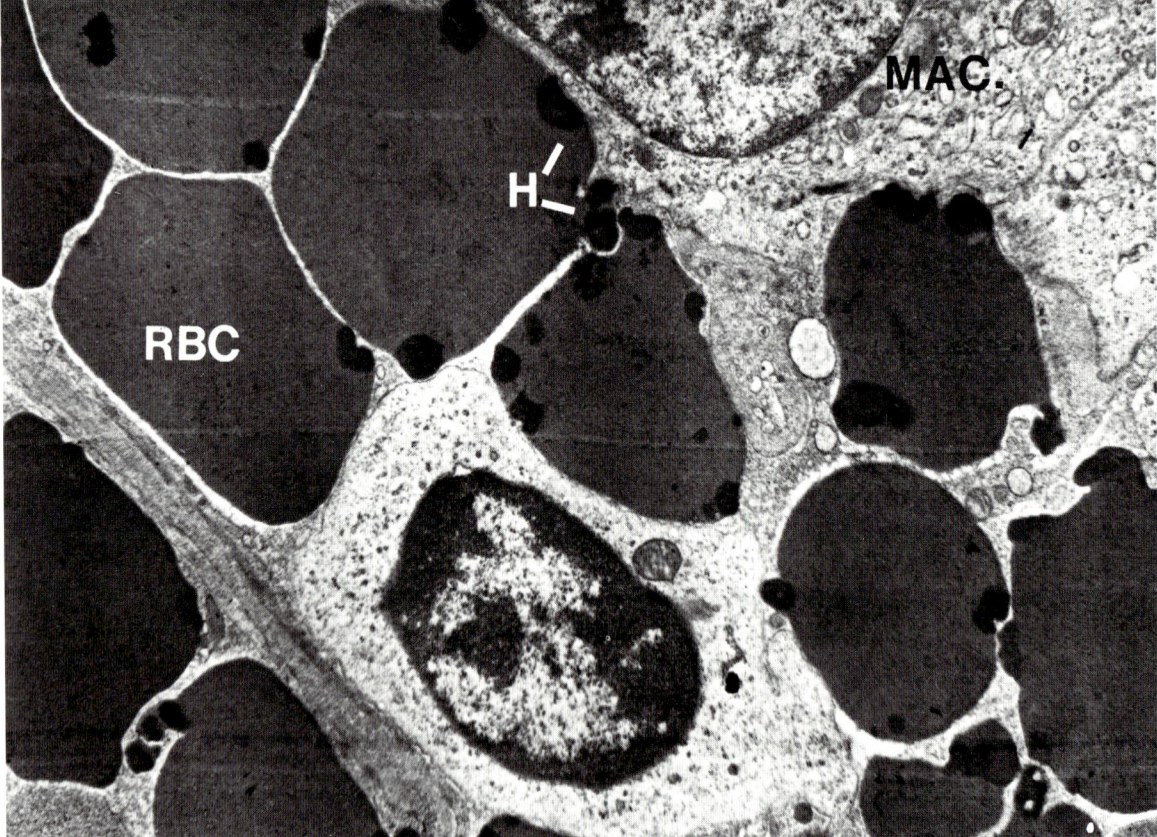

Fig. 21 a-d) Heinz bodies *appear as purple violet inclusions of various sizes, usually located at the erythrocyte periphery, after supravital staining with Nile blue sulfate or other basic dyes such as methylviolet or brilliant cresyl blue. They consist of aggregates of denatured hemoglobin, which show a firm attachment to the red cell membrane, as revealed by electron microscopy [101, 102].*

A decreased concentration of reducing enzymes may cause the formation of hemoglobin precipitates. Thus Heinz bodies may be encountered in aged cells [103], in splenectomized patients, or more frequently, in patients with enzyme defects (notably glucose-6-phosphate dehydrogenase deficiency). This leads to an increased susceptibility to oxidative injury (as after phenylhydrazine) of unstable hemoglobins, and in hemoglobin H disease (α-thalassemia) [104, 105].

a) *Single or multiple refractile granules of precipitated hemoglobin are seen in a wet preparation after supravital staining with Nile blue sulfate in presence of phenylhydrazine in a case of β-thalassemia intermedia (splenectomized patient).*

Although the red cells may exhibit some intrinsic protease activity capable of degrading the hemoglobin subunits produced in excess [106], the spleen appears to play a major role in removing the Heinz bodies ("pitting fuction") [107] (see **b***).*

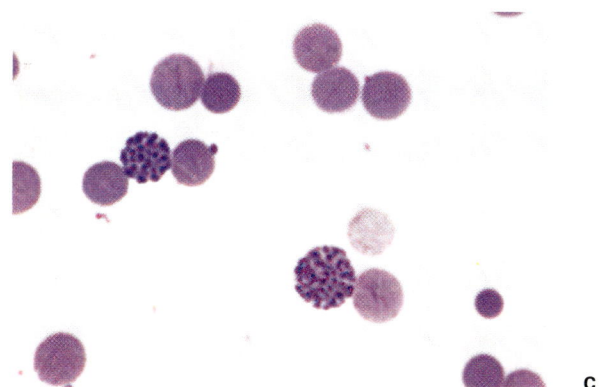

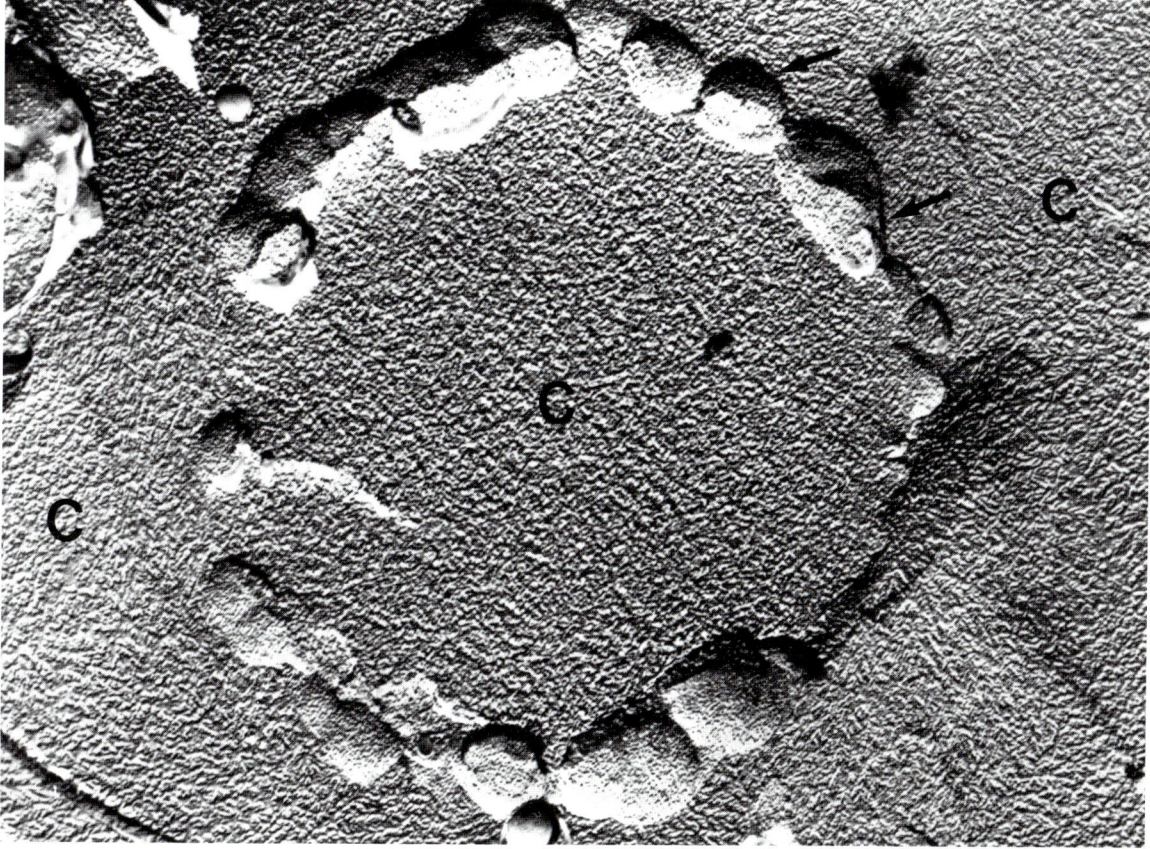

Fig. 21 b) Section of spleen (Billroth cord) actively sequestering Heinz body-containing red cells; from a rabbit given acetylphenylhydrazine to induce a hemolytic process analogous to hemolysis in patients with G6PD deficiency. Two splenic macrophages (**MAC**) are seen. The Heinz bodies (**H**) are located just beneath the red cell plasma membrane ($\times \pm 10{,}000$).
Courtesy of Dr. Richard Rifkind, Columbia University College of Physicians and Surgeons, New York.

c) A diffuse stippling of red blood cells ("golf balls") after incubation with brilliant cresyl blue, showing β4 chain precipitates (Hb H) in a case of α-thalassemia.
Courtesy of Prof. G. Castaldi, Ferrara.

d) Freeze fracture replica of an erythrocyte from a patient with α-thalassemia. The cell has been fractured through its cytoplasm (**C**). Its membrane has been cleaved only in regions where it passed over inclusions presumed to be Heinz bodies (**arrows**). Here the P-face i.e. the internal or cytoplasmic leaflet of the membrane has been exposed as evidenced by the density of intramembranous particles. The external leaflet would have fewer particles ($\times 15{,}000$).
Courtesy of Dr. G. Zavagli, Department of Medicine, University of Ferrara.

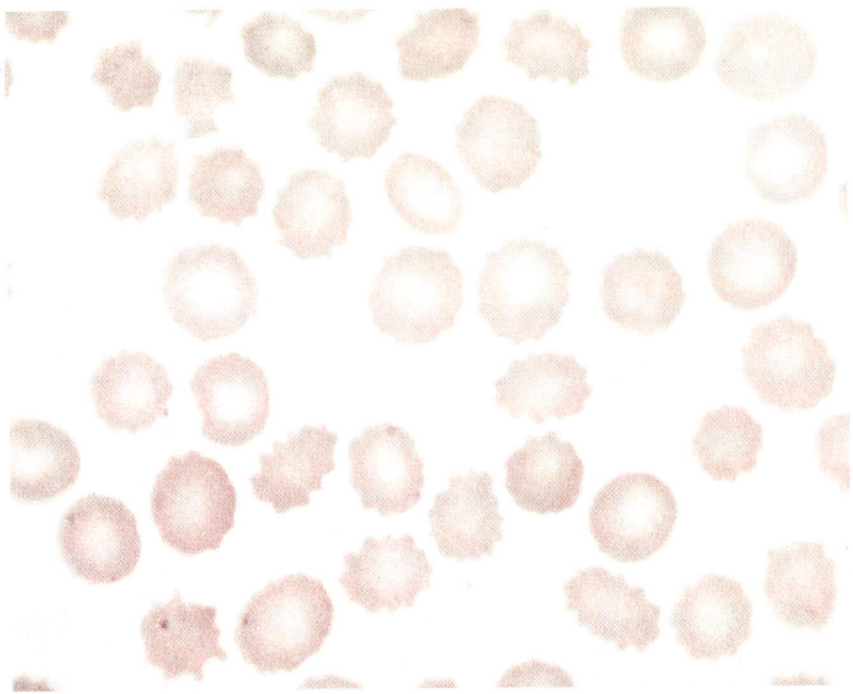

Fig. 22 a) Spiculated erythrocytes representing artifacts due to poor technique in preparing smears.

5.5. Physiological (reversible) changes in red cell shape

Extensive studies by Bessis and his collaborators [48, 108, 109] have drawn attention to modifications of the shape of red cells under the influence of various factors *in vivo* and *in vitro*.

Although some changes have been recognized for some time in conventionally stained smears [110-112], a physiologically oriented classification of these reversible changes in red cells has only been possible with the help of scanning electron microscopy (SEM) [113]. In this section reference will be made only to key forms of the so called *discocyte-echinocyte-stomatocyte equilibrium*. More extensive illustrations are available in ref. 113. The discocyte may undergo two different and, to some extent, reversible changes, i.e. the *echinocytic* and the *stomatocytic* forms; the alterations are determined by the pH of the medium, the intrinsic metabolic state of the cells (ATP depletion, Ca^{++} turnover [114, 115]) and the use of some chemical substances.

The *discocyte-echinocyte transformation* (**Fig. 22**) is characterized by the formation of cells exhibiting several short, regularly spaced, spicules on their surface and a spherocytic shape. Among the factors known to be "echinocytogenetic" are fatty acids, lysolecithins [116], biliary acids, barbiturates, detergents, anti-A sera [117] and an elevated pH of the medium (9-10) [118].

The *discocyte-stomatocyte transformation* (**Fig. 23**) shows a similar sequence giving rise to cup-shaped red cells with a spherocytic appearance in the last step. "Stomatocytogenetic" factors are considered the phenothiazines [119], anti-histaminic drugs, local anesthetics, propanolol, papaverine, chloroquine, Tween 80, inhibitors of thiol groups (such as AET,2,aminoethyl-isothiouronium bromide [120]), some cytostatic drugs (vincristine, vinblastine) and a low pH of the medium (2.0).

Fig. 22 b, c) *The discocyte-echinocyte transformation (b ⟶ c) is characterized by the progressive appearance of regularly spaced spicules on the surface of the cells which gradually assume an ovoidal form. According to empiric criteria, three stages, echinocyte I, II, and III, are distinguished on the basis of the prominence and the number of the spicules. The ransformation is largely reversible, unless toxic concentrations of the echinocytogenic substances are used and a fully developed spherocytic form is reached ("sphero-echinocyte") (SEM observation) (× 4,600).*
Courtesy of Dr. H. Kayden, New York University.

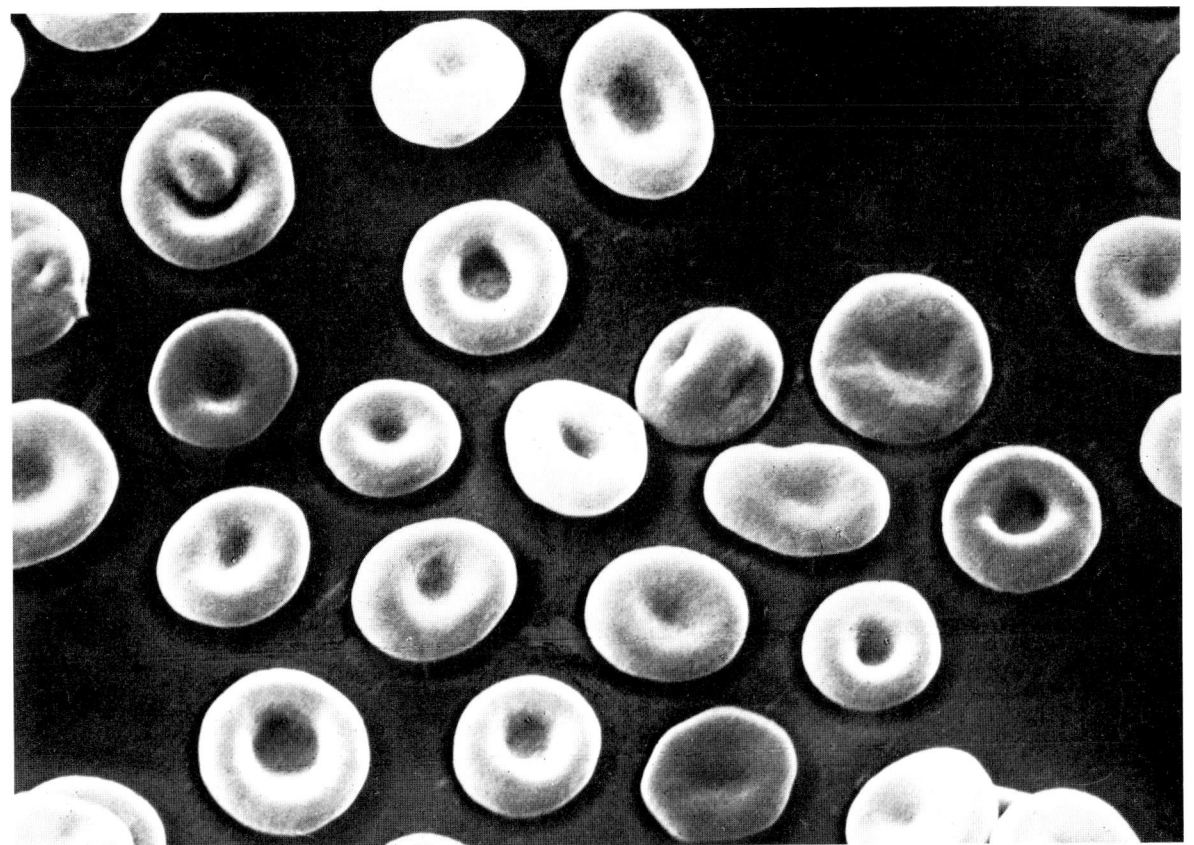

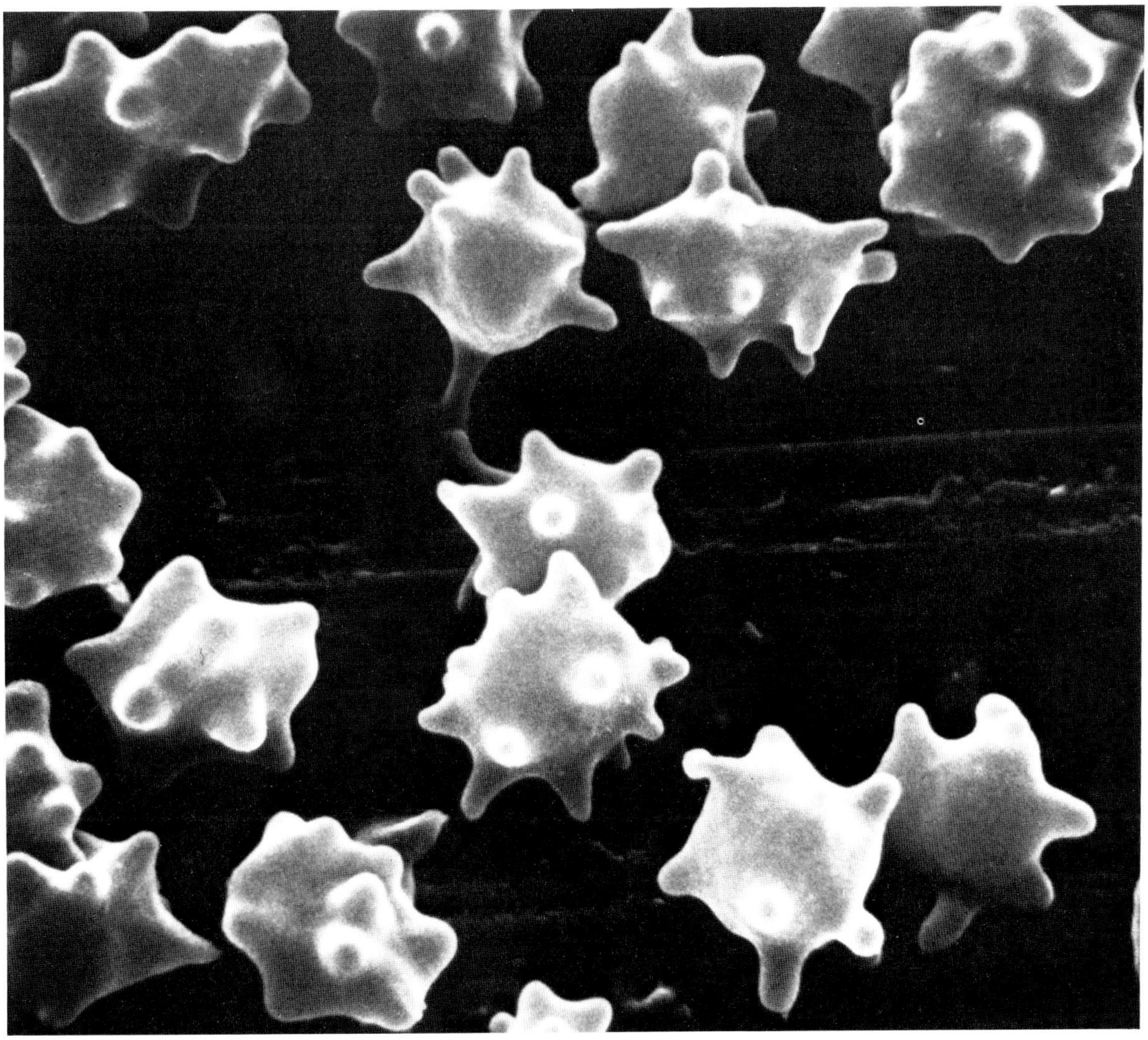

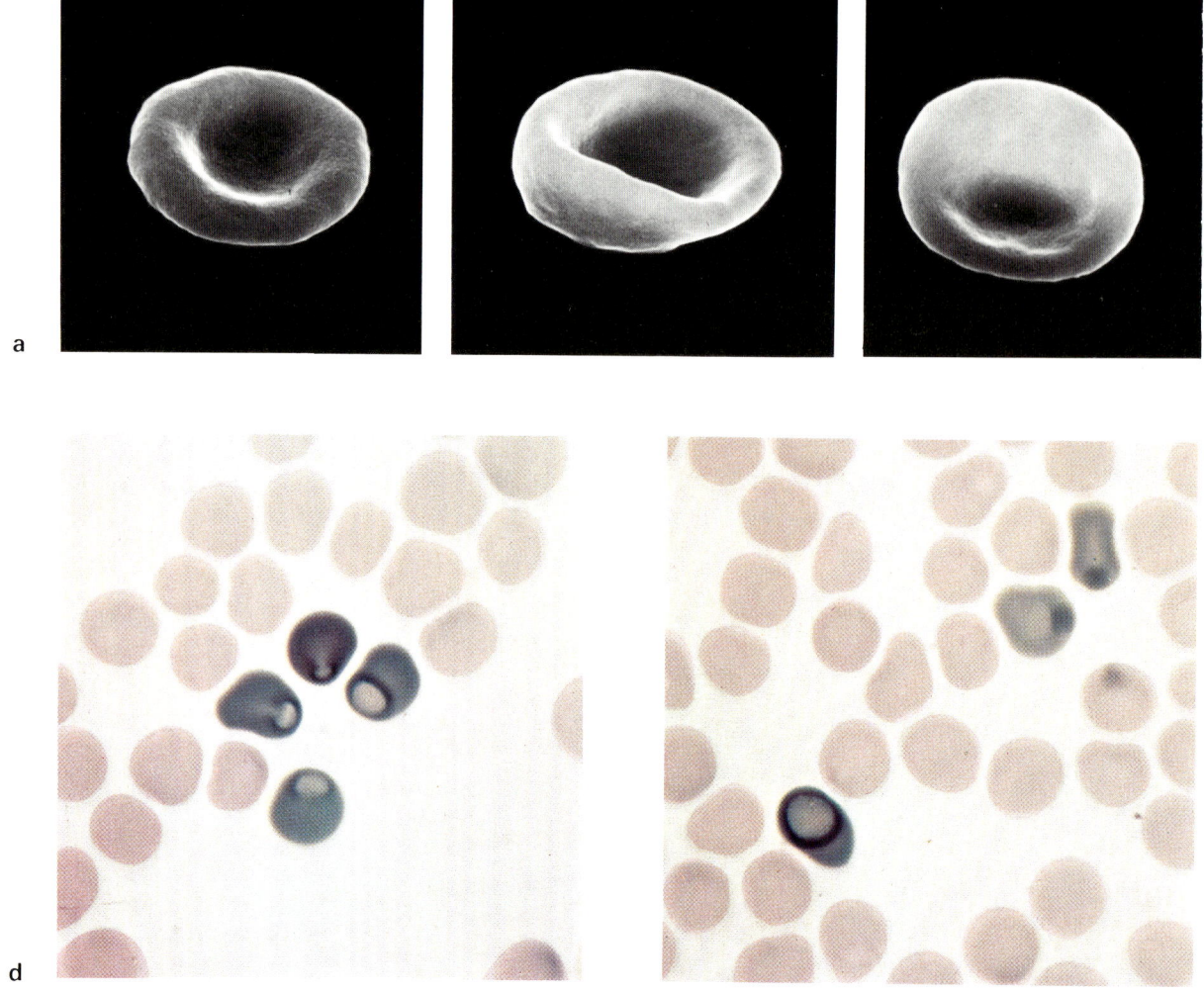

Fig. 23 In the discocyte-stomatocyte transformation (**a-c**) the red cells assume a bowl-shaped form with progressive loss (through three morphologically recognizable stages, stomatocyte I, II, and III) of the concavity, as the spherocytic form, which is a non reversible condition, is approached.
Similar stomatocytic forms have been observed in blood smears treated with mordant solutions (Na molybdate) at low pH (2.0) and stained with Amido Black B 10. All the passages from cup-shaped elements to irreversibly transformed sphero-stomatocytes are observed (**d-e**) (**a, b, c**: SEM observation, × 5,200).

3 ERYTHROCYTES

6. RED CELL SHAPE CHANGES ASSOCIATED WITH PATHOLOGICAL STATES

Modification of size or shape of the red cells represents one of the most common morphological abnormalities occurring in pathological conditions.
The study of these features offers a key to the interpretation of some underlying diseases in many patients. Since single morphological abnormalities are shared by different pathological conditions [121], a review of the principal features with reference to the disorders in which they occur is illustrated in the following pictures (**Fig. 24**). The nomenclature used here is the one proposed by Bessis [122] to describe the three dimensional shape of the cells as observed with the scanning electron microscope (**Fig. 25**). It is worth recalling that the spleen plays a major role in removing most of these altered cells (see **Figs. 25 k-m**).

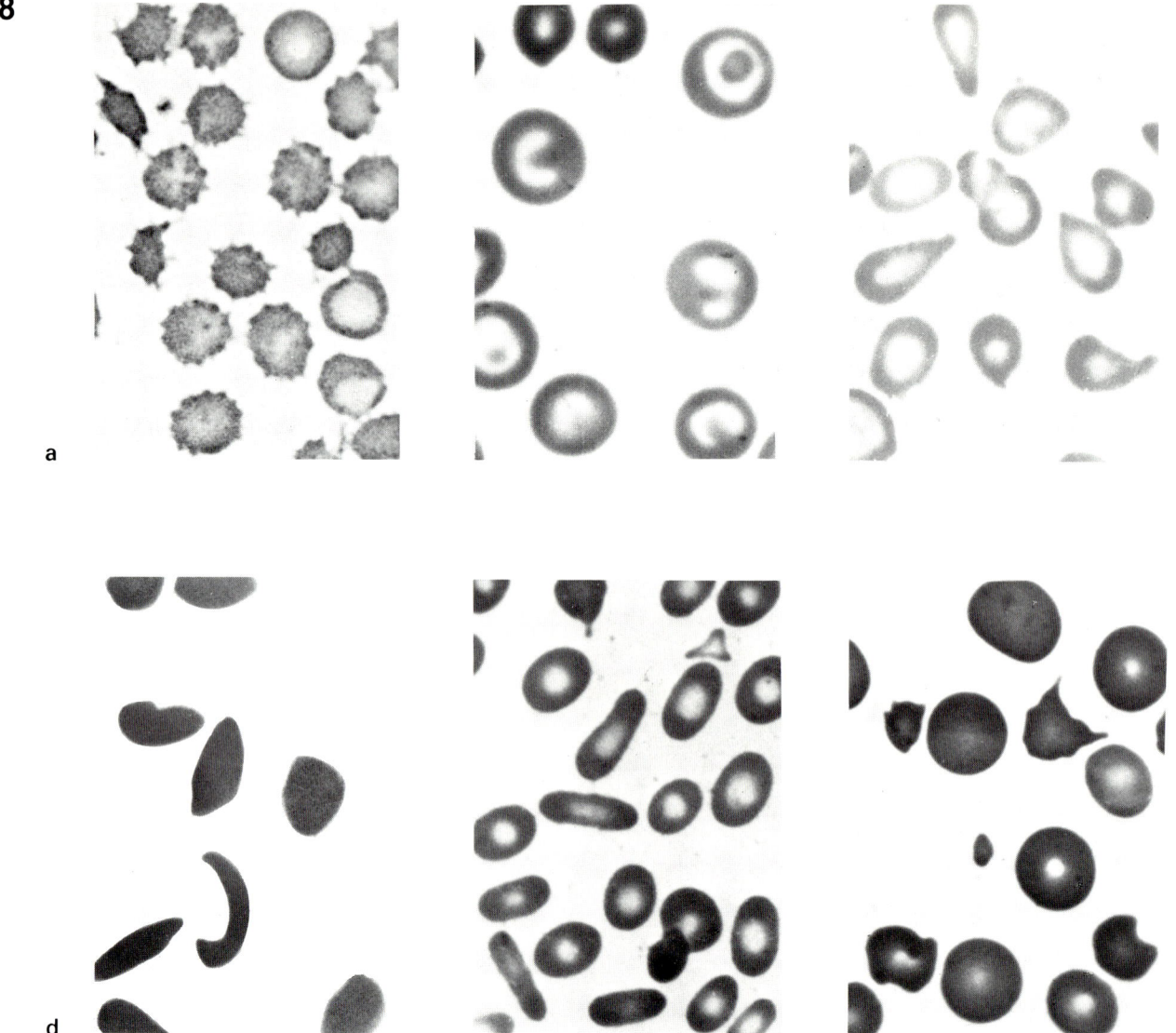

Fig. 24 a) Acanthocytes (ákanta = spine) are erythrocytes possessing several thorn-like projections spaced unevenly over the surface. These are usually smaller than normal red cells. They are observed in congenital abetalipoproteinemia, in liver disease (alcoholic cirrhosis), after splenectomy and even after heparin administration. Acanthocytes are to be distinguished from echinocytes ("crenated cells", "spur cells") which present fairly regularly spaced projections and which may be induced by a variety of substances and conditons (see **Fig. 22 a**).

b) Codocytes (kódon = bell) = Target cells are cup-shaped erythrocytes characterized by considerable reduction in thickness, showing a darkly staining central density surrounded by a peripheral hemoglobin ring with an interposed achromic zone. The intense staining of the central area is believed to be due to contact of the two opposing plasma membranes. Codocytes occur frequently in hypochromic anemias (thalassemias, hemoglobinopathies, sideropenic anemias), in liver disease often associated with biliary obstruction, in hereditary deficiency of lecitin-cholesterol acyl-transferase (LCAT), after splenectomy and even as consequence of improper preparation.

c) Dacrocytes (dákryon = tear) = Tear drop cells are erythrocytes which exhibit an elongated projection at one pole. This feature is associated with the "pitting function" of the spleen. They are most frequently observed in thalassemia, myelofibrosis, Heinz body anemias, bone marrow metastases.

d) Drepanocytes (drepánon = sickle) = Sickle cells are erythrocytes deformed by the precipitation of polymerized Hb S. The final form is that of crescent cells with filamentous processes (see **Fig. 59**).

e) Elliptocytes (elleiptikós = elliptic) include a morphological spectrum of red cells which show a progressive deformation ranging from oval cells (ovalocytes) to cells with true elliptocytic features (cigar-shaped erythrocytes). Oval red cells are found in hereditary elliptocytosis, in megaloblastic anemias, thalassemias, iron deficiency and in normal conditions (less than 1%).

f) Keratocytes (kéras = horn) are characterized by the presence of two projections which become thinner at the extremities, giving rise to horned features. The cells have also been referred to as "helmet cells". The spicules result from a disruption of a vacuole near the periphery of the erythrocyte. It has been suggested

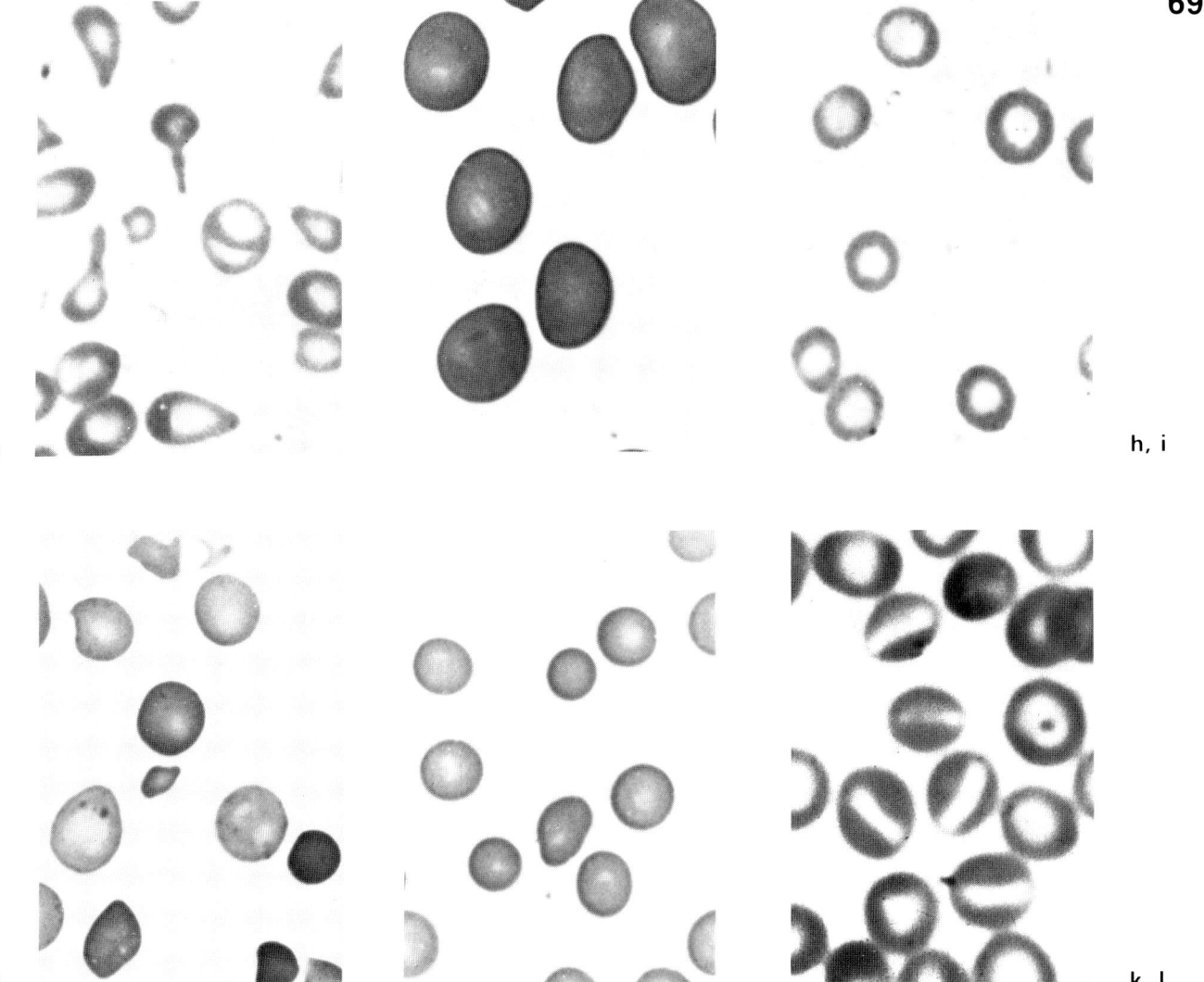

that these cells may arise from repeated collisions in disturbed circulatory conditions such as disseminated intravascular coagulation, cavernous hemangiomas or hemolytic anemias due to mechanical trauma.

g) Knizocytes *(gnúzos = dimple)* are difficult to recognize in ordinary smears. The cells appear to contain a central stick. This feature is due to the presence of two or more invaginations of the membrane. All the conditions which are associated with spherocytosis may present such cells in the peripheral blood.

h) Megalocytes *(mégas = giant)* are erythrocytes with increased volume (> 95 μm³) and with larger diameters than their normal counterparts (> 8.5 μm). Most megalocytes have a tendency to be ovalocytic. Such cells are rarely seen in the absence of anisocytosis of the blood picture. By definition these cells are encountered in patients with megaloblastic marrows.

i) Microcytes *(micrós = small)* are cells with a reduced volume (< 85 μm³) and a diameter less than 6 μm. Most of these exhibit an achromic center with a thin peripheral rim of hemoglobin. They are often associated with reduced thickness of the cells (microleptocytes; *leptós = thin*). These cells are seen in several conditions characterized by iron deficiency. Their diagnostic significance is rather limited.

j) Schizocytes *(skisis = cleft)* Helmet cells are irregular cell fragments arising from erythrocyte damage. These cells are seen in several hemolytic disorders, such as microangiopathic hemolytic anemia and diseases associated with intravascular deposition of fibrin. Fibrin filaments may play an important role in cell disruption.

k) Spherocytes *(sfáira = a sphere)* are thicker than normal, since they have lost their biconcave configuration. They appear as rounded elements with a decreased surface to volume ratio. In normal preparations they appear as small dark cells, although the volume is nearly normal because of their increased thickness. Spherocytes are found in hereditary spherocytosis (sphero-stomatocytes) and in certain hemolytic anemias (immune hemolytic anemia, Heinz body hemolytic anemia, fragmentation hemolysis).

l) Stomatocytes *(stóma = mouth)* are cup-shaped erythrocytes which exhibit a slot-like central pale area. They are associated with hereditary stomatocytosis, liver desease, neoplastic conditions, hemolytic disorders characterized by altered permeability of the membrane to sodium, but they may also be observed in normal specimens as a consequence of improper physico-chemical conditions.

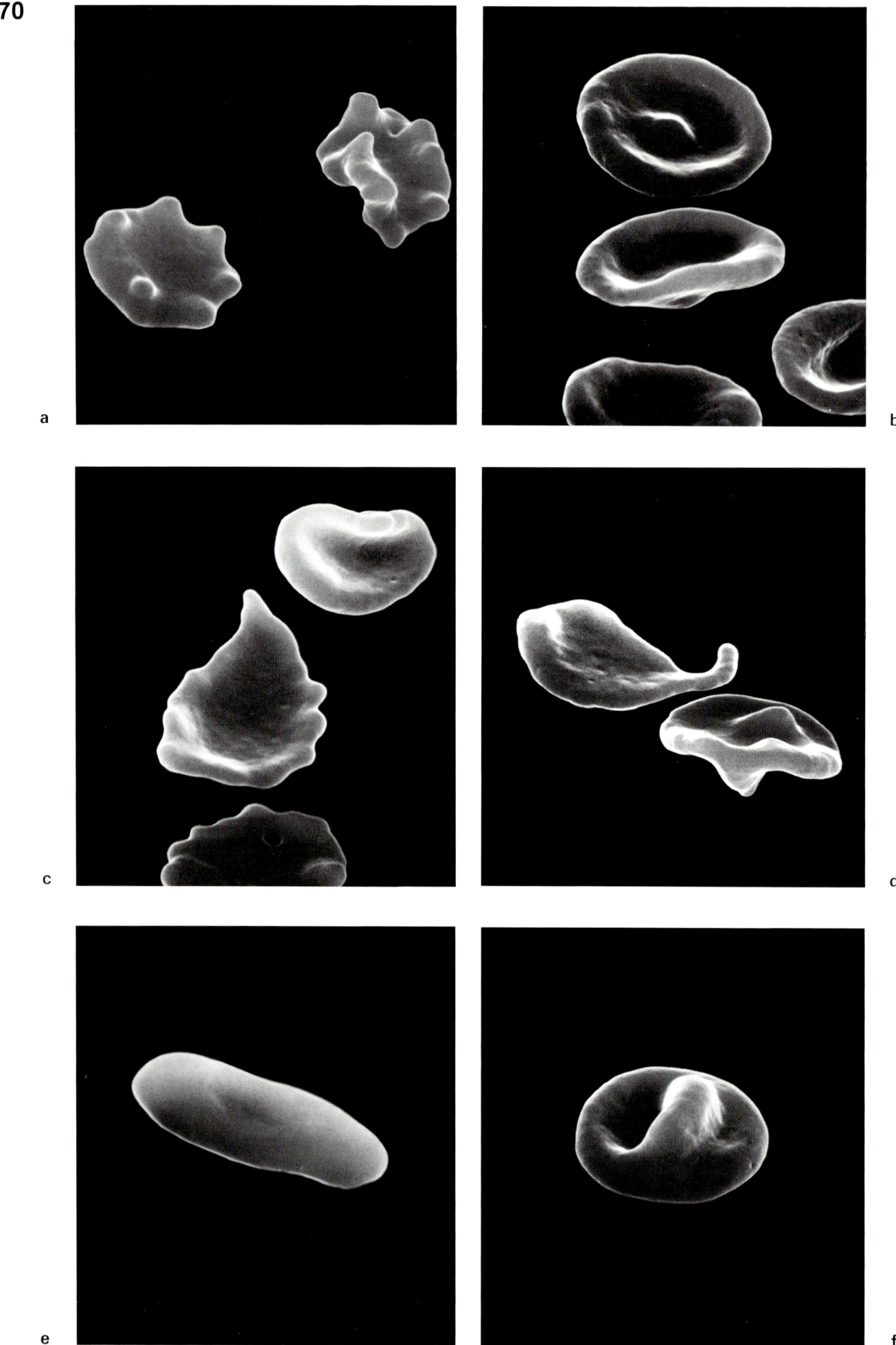

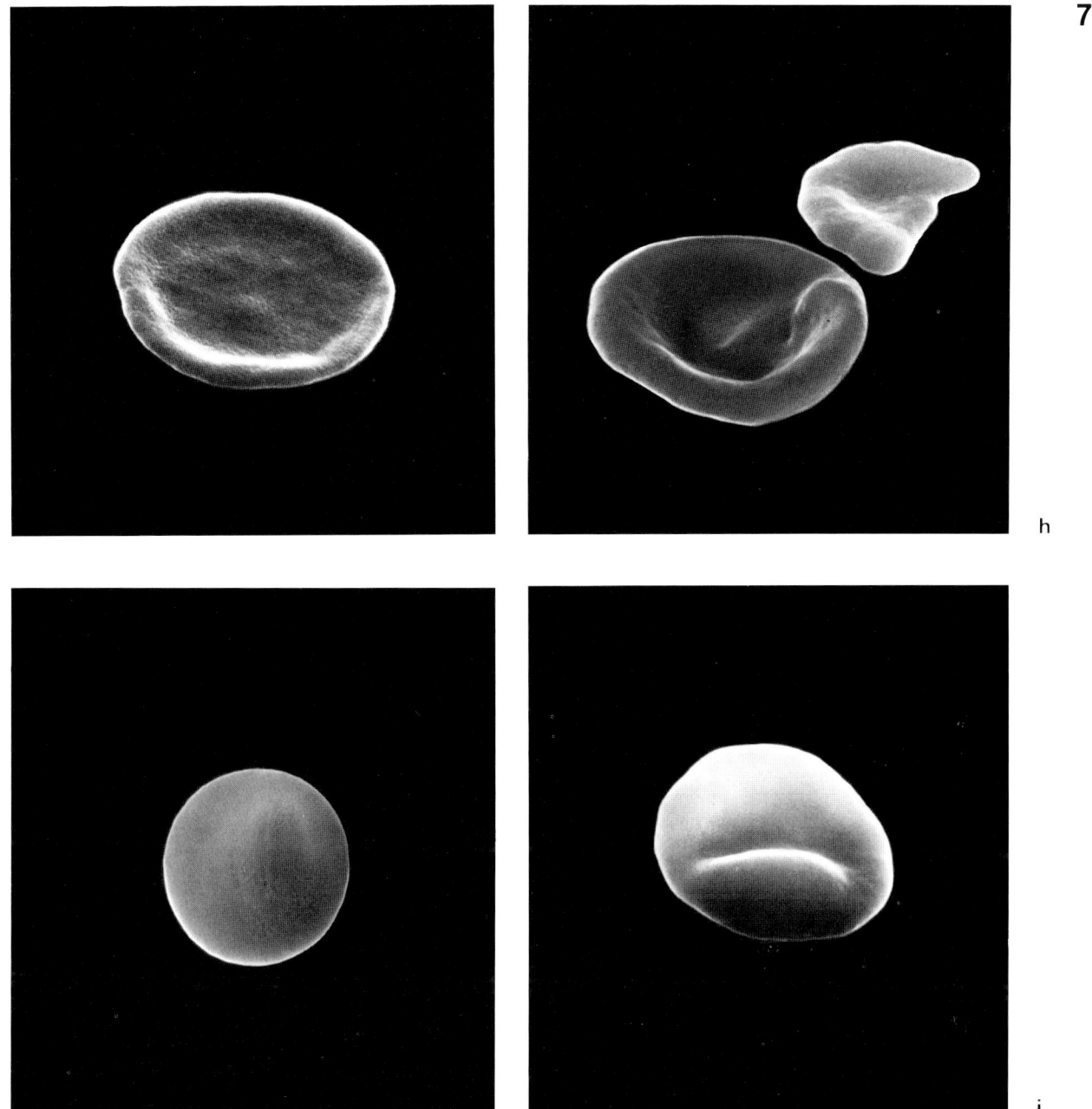

Fig. 25 a-j) Illustrate the most commonly encountered shapes that erythrocytes may assume under a variety of physiological or pathological conditions. SEM, (× 5,200). These should be compared with **Fig. 24 a-l**.
a) echinocytes; **b)** lepto-codocytes or target cells; **c, d)** dacryocytes; **e)** ellyptocyte; **f)** knizocyte; **g)** leptocyte; **h)** schizocyte (keratocyte); **i)** spherocyte; **j)** sphero-stomatocyte.

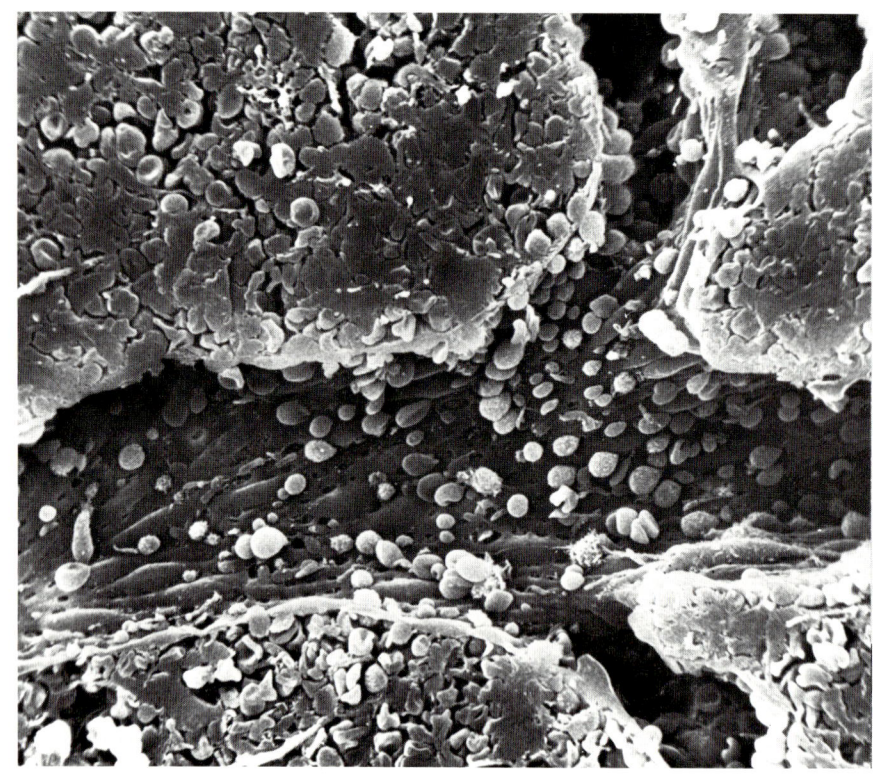

Fig. 25 k) Scanning electron micrograph of a freeze-fractured specimen of normal rat spleen (low magnification). The packed cell mass represents the splenic cords and the canal-like structures in the center the splenic sinuses.
l) Photomicroghaph of a splenic sinus in the normal rat spleen (high magnification). A number of deformed red cells traversing the slits can be seen.
m) A deformable normal rat red cell traversing an endothelial slit.
Courtesy of Drs. A. de Boisfleury and N. Mohandas (from: Antibody induced spherocytic anemia: II. Splenic passage and sequestration of red cells. Blood Cells, 3, 197, 1977).

3 ERYTHROCYTES

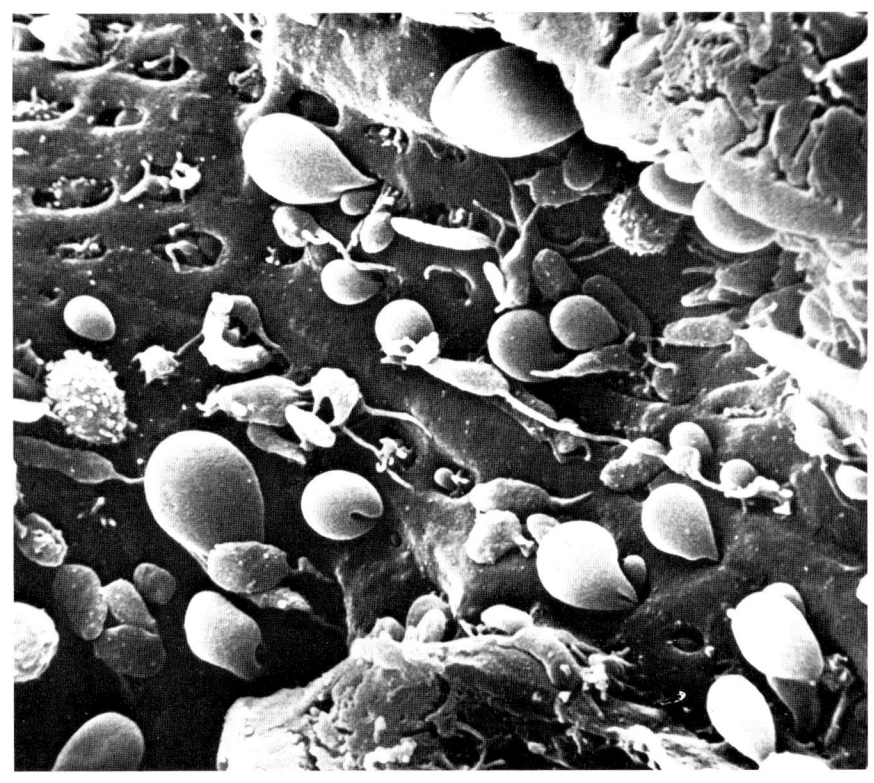

l

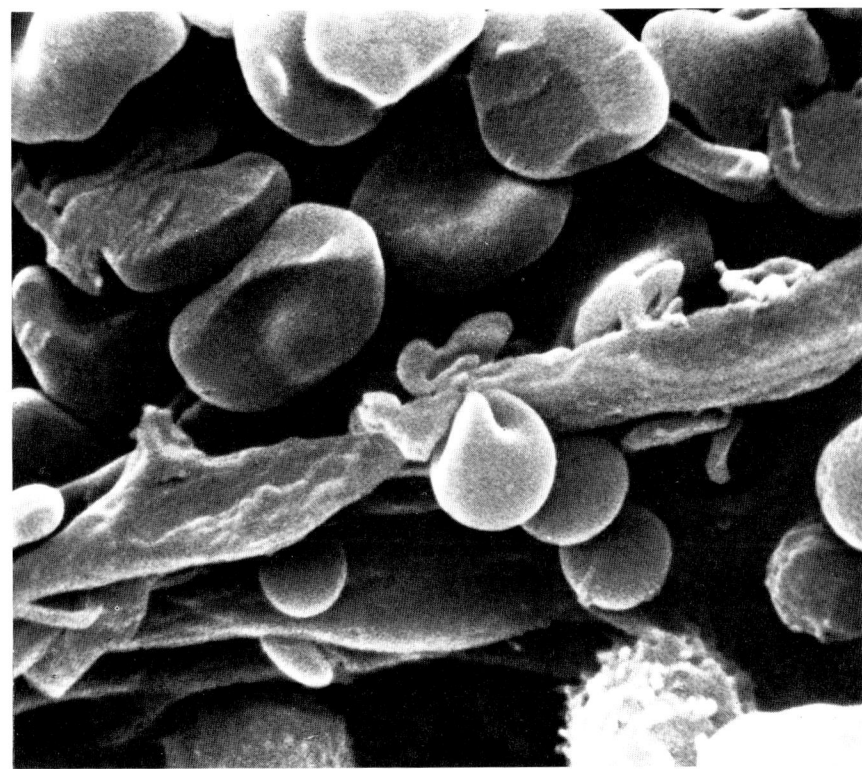

m

Part 2 ABNORMALITIES OF RED CELL PRODUCTION

1. APLASTIC MYELOPATHIES

A detailed description of these hematopoietic disorders involving marrow stem cells is given in Chapter 5.

2. ABNORMALITIES OF DNA SYNTHESIS (MEGALOBLASTIC ANEMIAS)

The megaloblastic anemias are a heterogeneous group of disorders characterized by morphologic features which represent correlates of altered deoxyribonucleic acid (DNA) synthesis [123, 124].

Since the morphological abnormalities are due to selective or combined deficiencies of the coenzymes vitamin B_{12} and folic acid which are required for the synthesis of proteins and DNA precursors, most of the megaloblastic anemias arise as a consequence of the lack of one or both these factors.

Whatever is the cause for the defect (increased demand, competition for vitamin, defective absorption, lack of intrinsic factor) the hematologic manifestations are the same and thus cannot be used to distinguish among different disorders [125-127]. For this reason, pernicious anemia which constitutes a distinct clinical entity (genetically determined disorder with defective intrinsic factor, IF, secretion and autoimmune disturbance, see **Fig. 29**) and which may in fact be considered as a prototype of the megaloblastic anemias, has been commonly used in the past as a misleading synonym for all conditions characterized by vitamin B_{12} deficiency. However, since the morphological features of this disease provide a paradigm for other disorders of this group, they will be discussed in this section.

2.1. Megaloblastic erythropoiesis

Megaloblastic erythropoiesis affects to a varying extent most of the proliferating cells. As a rule, megaloblasts [128-130] are larger than the corresponding normal cells. They have a greater amount of cytoplasm and an increased nuclear size (**Fig. 26**). Moreover, there is a delay in chromatin condensation leading to an asynchronous pattern between nuclear and cytoplasmic maturation.

When the anemia is not severe, the megaloblastic changes do not affect all proliferating cells, but are usually limited to a fraction of polychromatophilic erythroblasts.

The kinetics of megaloblastic proliferation differs from normal normoblastic erythropoiesis as regards the relative number of cells at various stages of differentiation. There are fewer cells reaching the E_4 stage of maturation (see **Fig. 25** and refs. 131, 132). Therefore, there is a relative increase in basophilic erythroid precursors in the marrow of patients with untreated pernicious anemia (**Fig. 27**).

Mitotic activity is increased in megaloblastic cells (mainly at the proerythroblastic stage) [133-135]. The mitotic figures show slender or elongated chromosomes [136], which are subject to fragmentation [137, 138]. There is severe disturbance in nucleoprotein synthesis leading to ineffective mitosis (**Fig. 28**). However, to establish the etiology of the megaloblastosis, specific biochemical assays are required [139, 140] in addition to recognition of the morphologic features (**Fig. 32**).

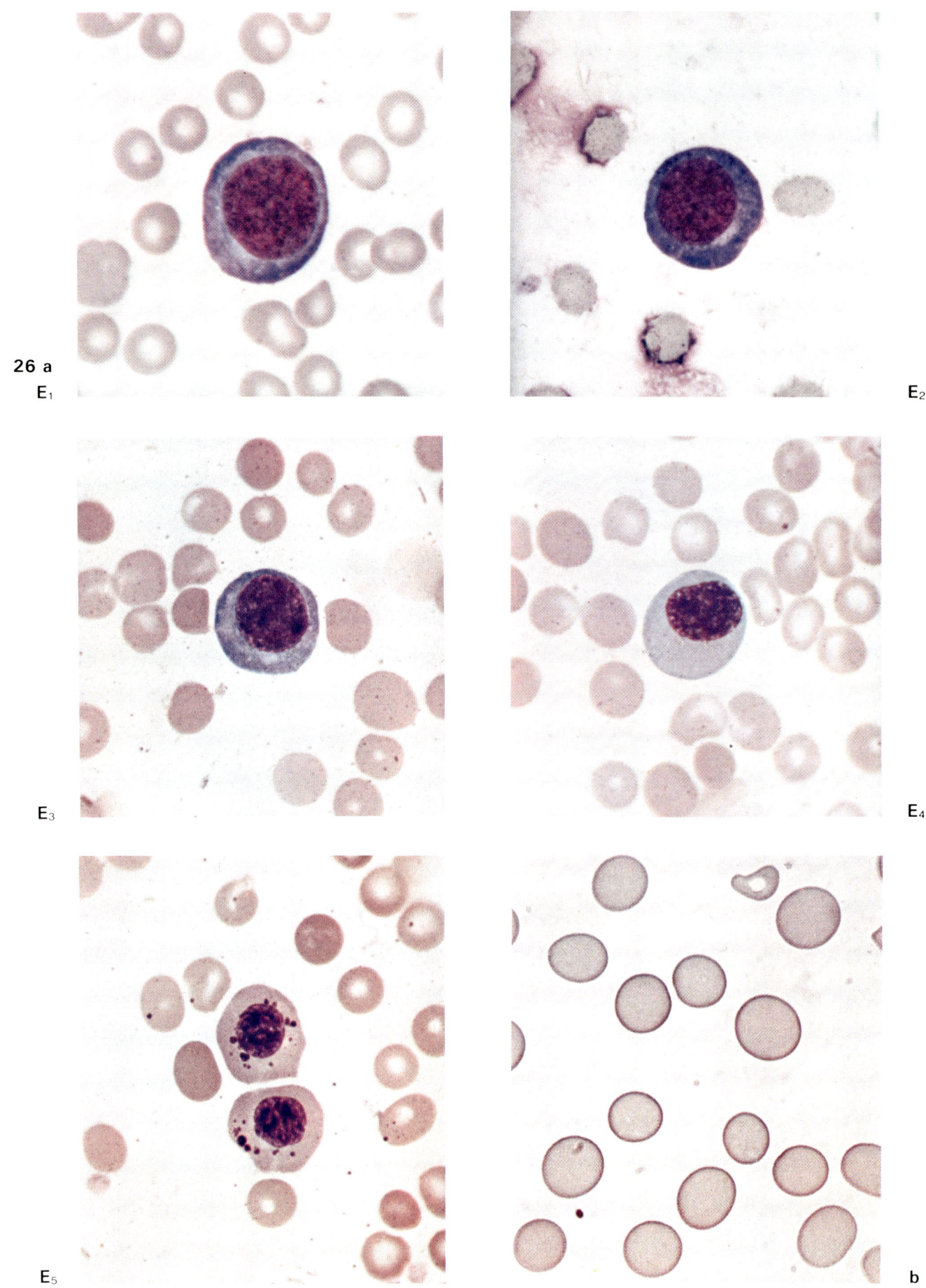

3 ERYTHROCYTES

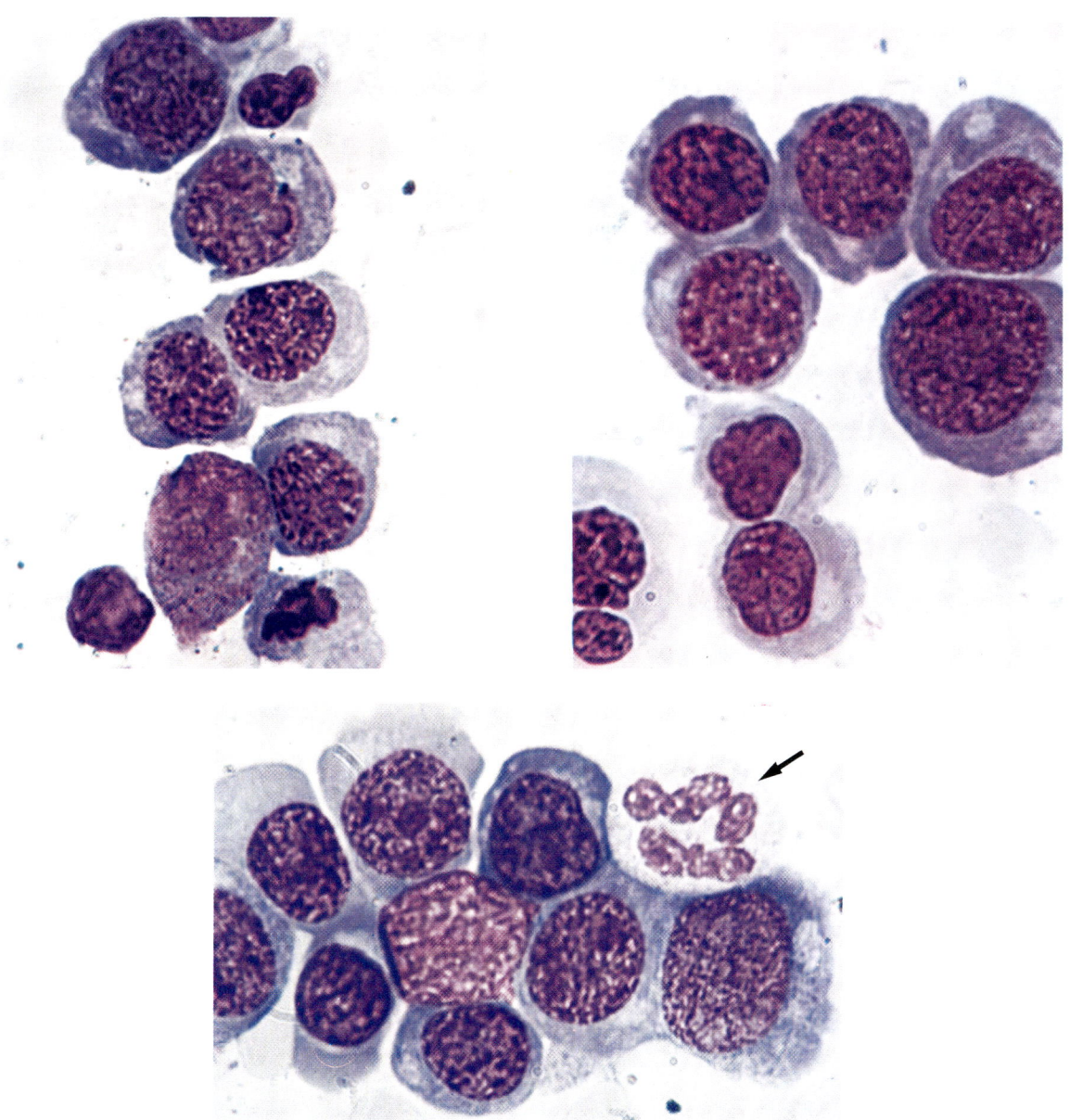

Fig. 27 Megaloblastic cells in the bone marrow of a patient with fully developed clinical features of pernicious anemia. Maturation beyond the basophilic erythroblast is rarely seen. Also note neutrophil with a hypersegmented nucleus (**arrow**).

Fig. 26 a) Differentiation sequence from the promegaloblast to the late polychromatophilic megaloblast ($E_1 \longrightarrow E_5$) in Giemsa-stained preparations.

Promegaloblast (E_1): This cell measures 10-30 μm in diameter and is characterized by a loosely arranged chromatin, by the presence of several nucleoli, and abundant basophilic cytoplasm.

Basophilic megaloblasts (E_2-E_3): These are cells (14-20 μm of diameter) with deeply basophilic cytoplasm. Their nuclei still present dispersed chromatin pattern. Nucleoli have almost disappeared.

Polychromatophilic megaloblasts (E_4-E_5): The size of these cells is quite variable, but is usually larger than normal. The "nucleo-cytoplasmic dissociation" is a striking feature of these cells, which retain finely dispersed chromatin, whereas the cytoplasm shows the beginning of hemoglobin synthesis. In the most severe forms, nuclear fragmentation and multiple Howell-Jolly bodies are seen. The reticulocyte stage is often omitted in the passage from the late polychromatophilic to the megalocyte.

b) Megalocytes (blood smear from a patient with pernicious anemia). Most of the cells display macro-ovalocytic features. A considerable degree of aniso- and poikilocytosis is also noted.

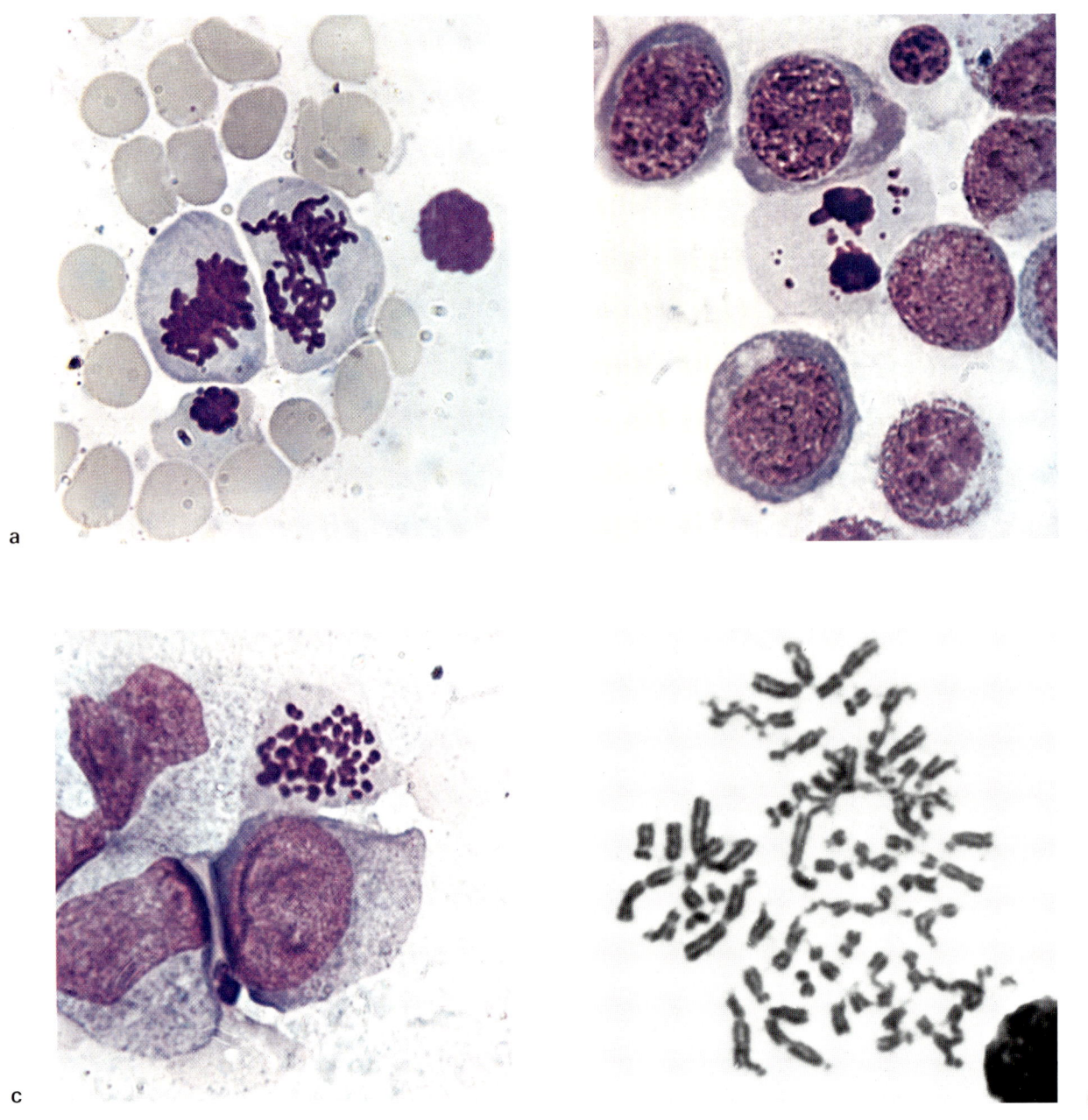

Fig. 28 a) Mitotic figures in megaloblastic cells. Chromosomes appear particularly elongated and irregularly distributed.
b) Abnormal mitotic figures in megaloblastic cells: anaphase with several chromosome fragments dispersed throughout the cytoplasm.
c) Clumping of chromosomes which appear as round-shaped chromatin masses.
d) Metaphase plate obtained by direct preparation from the bone marrow of a patient with pernicious anemia prior to any treatment. Multiple fragmentations of the chromosomes and interchanges are seen.
From Castoldi et al., ref. 137.

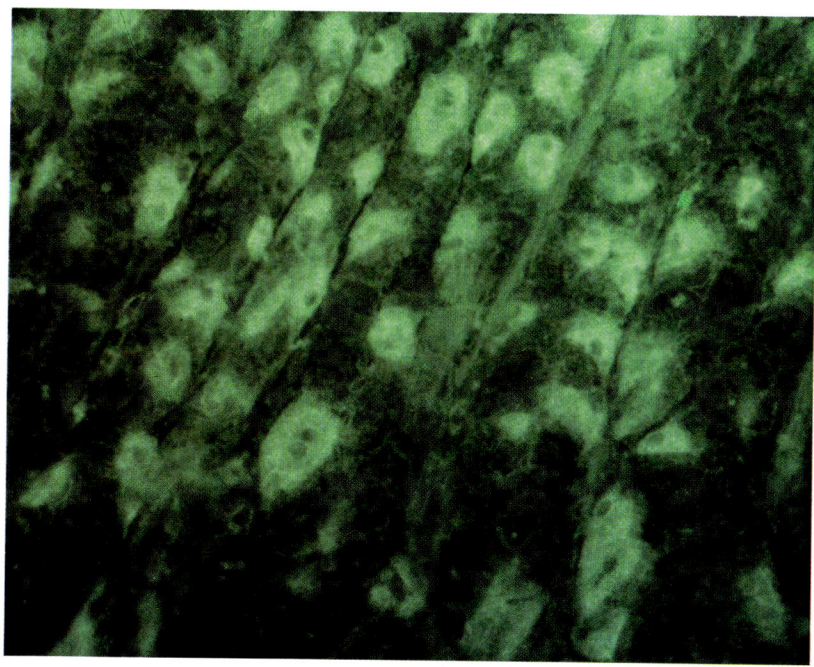

Fig. 29 *Patients with pernicious anemia may have antibodies to gastric parietal cells as well as to intrinsic factor, the glycoprotein which binds vitamin B_{12} before it can be absorbed. The indirect immunofluorescence technique was used to detect antibodies adsorbed onto gastric parietal cells.*
Courtesy of Prof. A.M. Marmont, S. Martino's Hospital, Genova.

Thus the use of a terminology mainly related to the definition of small morphological deviations from the classical megaloblastic erythropoiesis and implying a more or less defined reference to specific or prevailing factors, is avoided.

In fact, terms such as *macroblast* and *macroblastic anemia* were commonly used to characterize megaloblastic anemias mainly related to nutritional deficiencies [141] and whose morphological features were milder than those observed in pernicious anemia (**Fig. 30**). Likewise, the terms *transitional megaloblasts* [142] and *intermediate megaloblasts* have been used with different purposes, either for the elements appearing in the course of inadequately treated patients [143] or as a consequence of multiple metabolic disturbances as is the case of iron deficiency complicating vitamin B_{12} or folic acid deficiencies [144]. All these definitions lend support to the concept that megaloblastic anemia should be considered as a basic picture implying some different degrees of morphological expression [123].

Since the structural alterations of the cells reflect impaired DNA synthesis, they are readily observed in other cells or tissues with rapid turnover rates such as the granulocytic cells [145] (**Fig. 31**), gastric and oral mucosa and the genito-urinary tract (**Fig. 32**).

2.1.1. Cytochemical and ultrastructural features

The PAS (Periodic Acid-Schiff) reaction is negative in megaloblastic cells [149] and only a moderate increase in siderotic granules has been detected with the Perls' acid ferrocyanide reaction. There is an increase in the activity of the Embden-Meyerhof pathway, pentose phosphate shunt and tricarboxylic acid cycle [150].
Moreover, increased α-naphthyl-acetate esterase activity is detected similarly to some dyserythropoietic anemias [151, 152].

A positive benzidine reaction confirms the presence of hemoglobin in large cells with immature nuclear chromatin pattern.

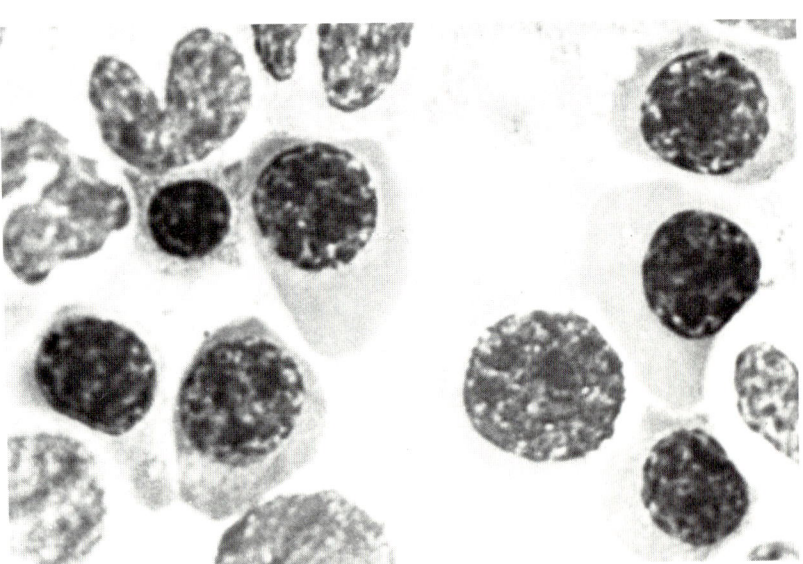

Fig. 30 *Megaloblastic changes limited to the more mature cells in a case of malabsorption syndrome.*

Ultrastructural analysis of megaloblastic erythropoiesis has shown a variety of abnormalities which are mainly expressed in more mature cells: reduced amount of heterochromatin, clefts, intranuclear inclusions, partial loss of the nuclear membrane, long strands of endoplasmic reticulum, autophagic vacuoles, increased number of free ferritin molecules, large siderosomes, degenerated mitochondria. Most of these alterations have been interpreted as degenerative changes leading to the death of the affected cells and to their phagocytosis by marrow macrophages [153-155].

Fig. 32 *It is still uncertain how the principal features of megaloblastic proliferation, i.e. abnormal size of the cells and asynchronous maturation of the nuclear and cytoplasmic components are related to the metabolic disturbances of these cells. While the nucleo-cytoplasmic dissociation has been attributed to delayed condensation of the chromatin in the maturing erythroblasts [134], the enlarged diameter of the cells indicates a normal rate of RNA and protein synthesis [146, 148] in the presence of blocked DNA replication and cell division. Impaired DNA synthesis is due to defective conversion of deoxyuridilate by thymidilate synthetase. However thymidilate synthesis may be affected only indirectly by vitamin B_{12} and folate deficiency, since these factors do not appear to be actively involved in any step of the DNA synthesis. Possibly vitamin B_{12} deficiency causes a failure of homocysteine methylation to methionine leading to reduced conversion of 5-methylene-tetrahydrofolate to tetrahydrofolate (THF). Thus, since most of the folate is trapped as methyl-THF, in the cells there is a decrease of the 5,10-methylene-THF, a folate coenzyme required for methylation of deoxyuridine in the synthesis of thymidilate.*

dUMP, deoxyuridine monophosphate; **dTMP**, deoxythymidine monophosphate; **dTTP**, deoxythymidine triphosphate; **dCTP**, deoxycytidine triphosphate; **dGTP**, deoxyguanosine triphosphate; **dATP**, deoxyadenosine triphosphate.

3 ERYTHROCYTES 81

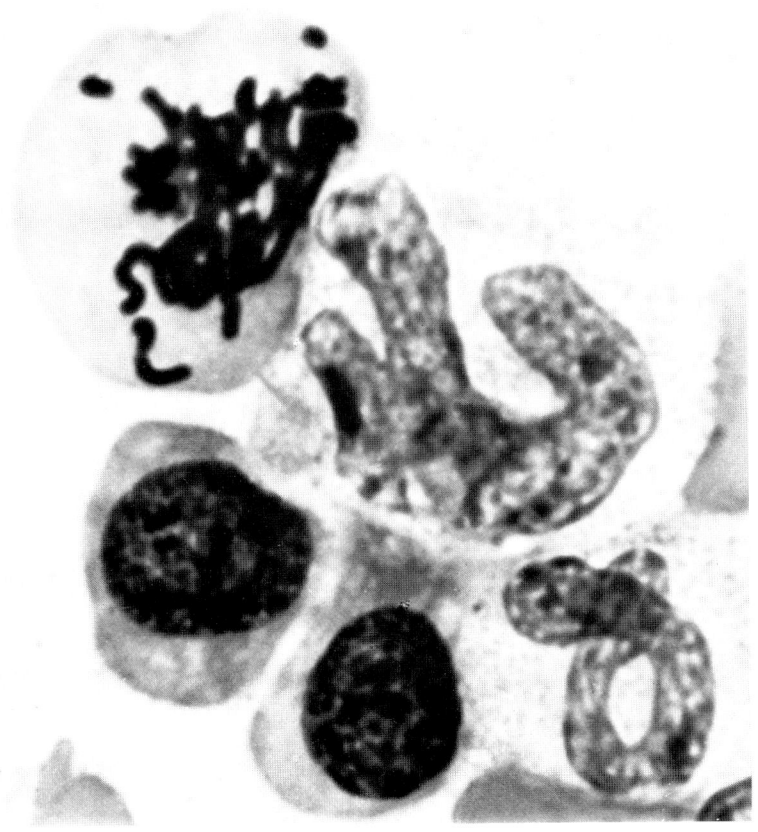

Fig. 31 Giant metamyelocytes with ribbon-like nuclei.

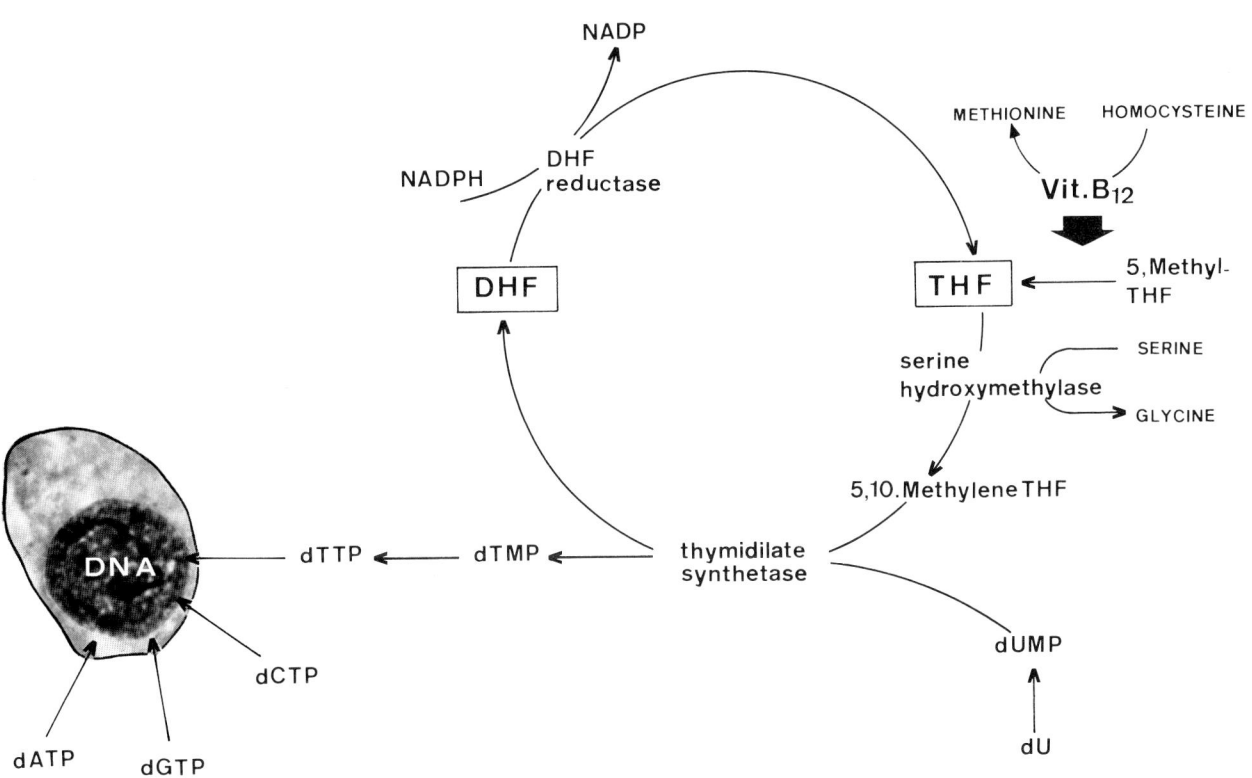

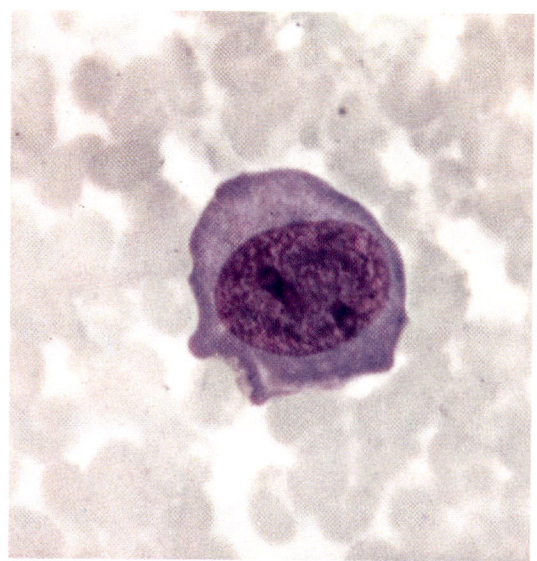
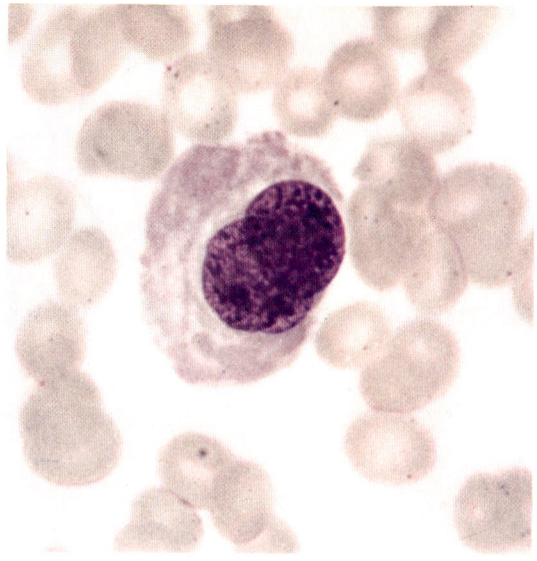
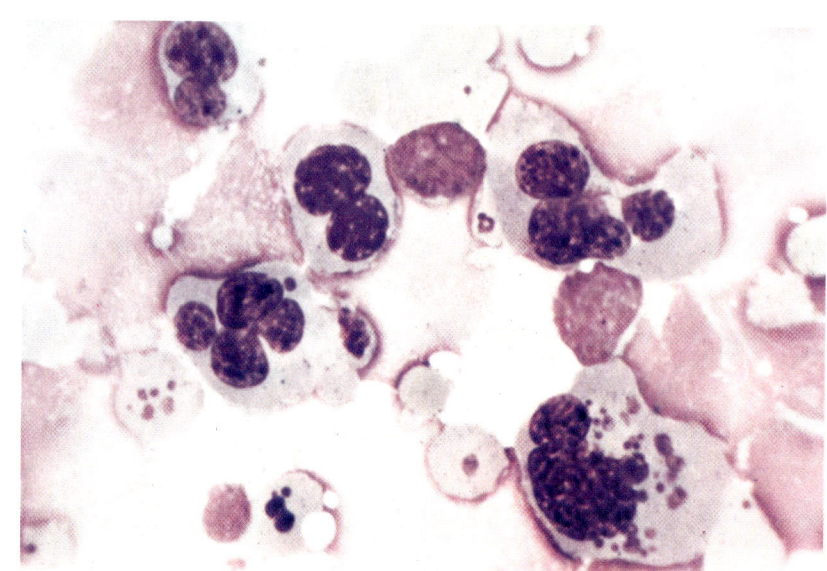

Fig. 33 a) Giant erythroblasts (polychromatophilic stage) in the bone marrow of a patient treated with 5-fluorouracil. Cytoplasm of some cells is characteristically "frayed" (**b**).
c) Giant multinucleated erythroblasts in a patient with acute lymphoblastic leukemia after prolonged treatment with 6-mercaptopurine and methotrexate.

2.2. Drug-induced megaloblastic changes

Megaloblastic changes may also be observed as a consequence of some medications which either impair intestinal absorption of vitamin B_{12} or folic acid or their utilization (e.g. anticonvulsants, oral contraceptives, antitubercular drugs) or act, as in the case of antimetabolite drugs, with predictable toxic effects (particularly methotrexate, 5-fluorouracil, arabinosyl-cytosine, 6-mercaptopurine). In all these instances, but particularly when cytotoxic drugs are administered, large cells with marked alteration of nuclear shape, karyorrhexis, and sometimes highly abnormal polyploid elements, are observed [156, 157] (**Fig. 33**).

Characteristically, most of these cells are polychromatophilic (*giant ortochromatic erythroblasts, binucleate polyploid oxyphil megalocytes*) [158]. Gian cells arising after therapy with cytotoxic drugs may represent cells which have been arrested after a synthetic period or in which DNA synthesis occurs at a very slow rate [148].

3 ERYTHROCYTES

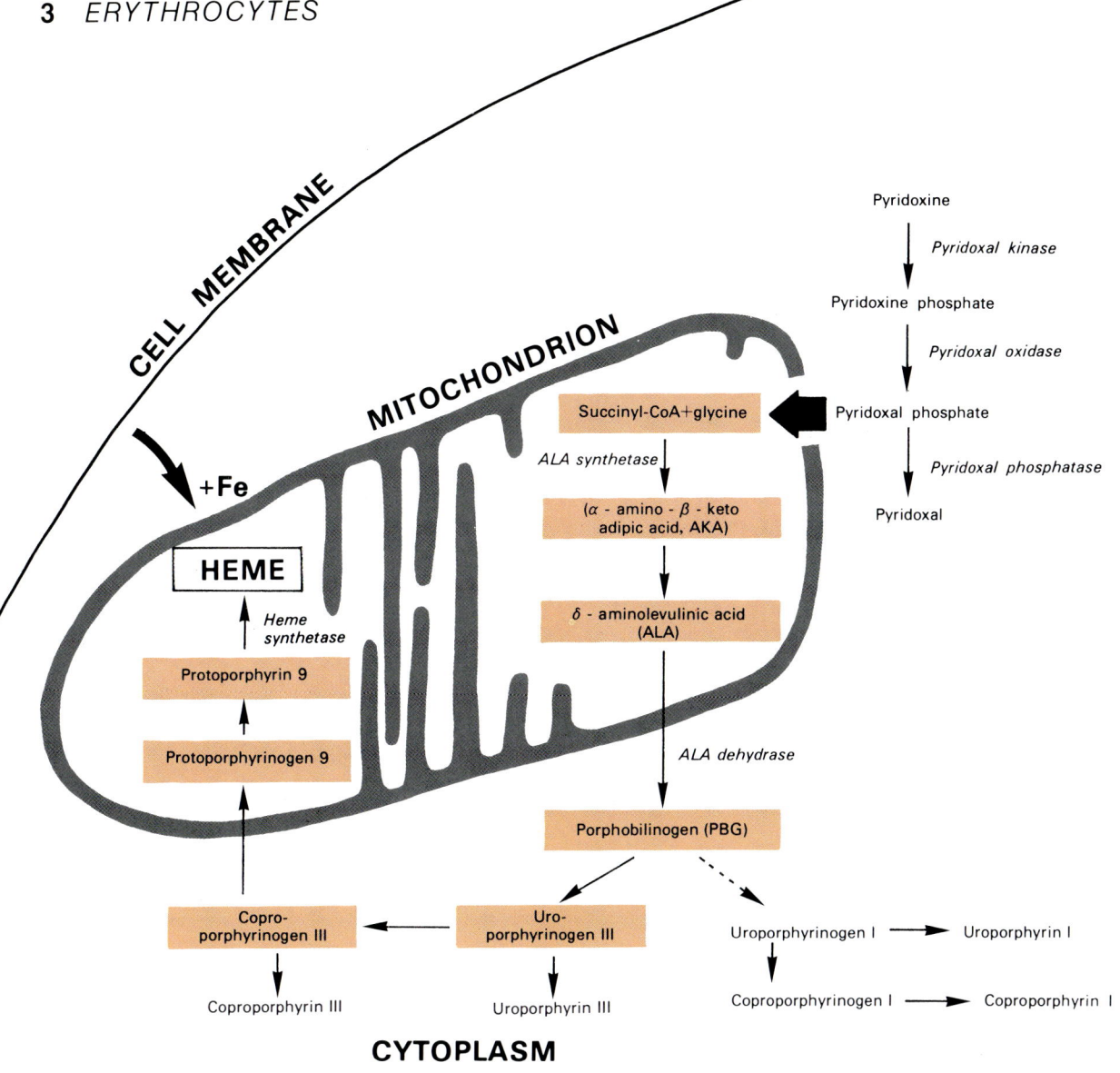

Fig. 34 *Schematic representation of the metabolic steps (intramitochondrial and cytoplasmic) leading to heme synthesis.*

3. DISORDERS RELATED TO DISTURBANCES OF HEMOGLOBIN SYNTHESIS

3.1. Dyserythropoiesis and dyserythropoietic anemias

The term *dyserythropoietic anemia* [159, 160] is sometimes employed as a useful albeit all-encompassing term that may refer to any kind of disturbed erythropoietic pattern, both congenital and acquired. It may be manifested by almost any quantitative, functional, morphological or biochemical abnormality of red cell precursors in blood or bone marrow [161, 162]. Under this large "umbrella", the manifestations of such well defined disorders as megaloblastic anemia, iron deficiency anemia, porphyria, thalassemia and hemoglobinopathy would be included as well as a large variety of syndromes of unknown etiology. However, once the reason for disorderly erythropoiesis has been established, the term dyserythropoietic anemia is replaced by a more specific terminology (see below). The retention of the term "dyserythropoietic anemia" in the case of the congenital variants reflects our ignorance in this area (see p. 92).

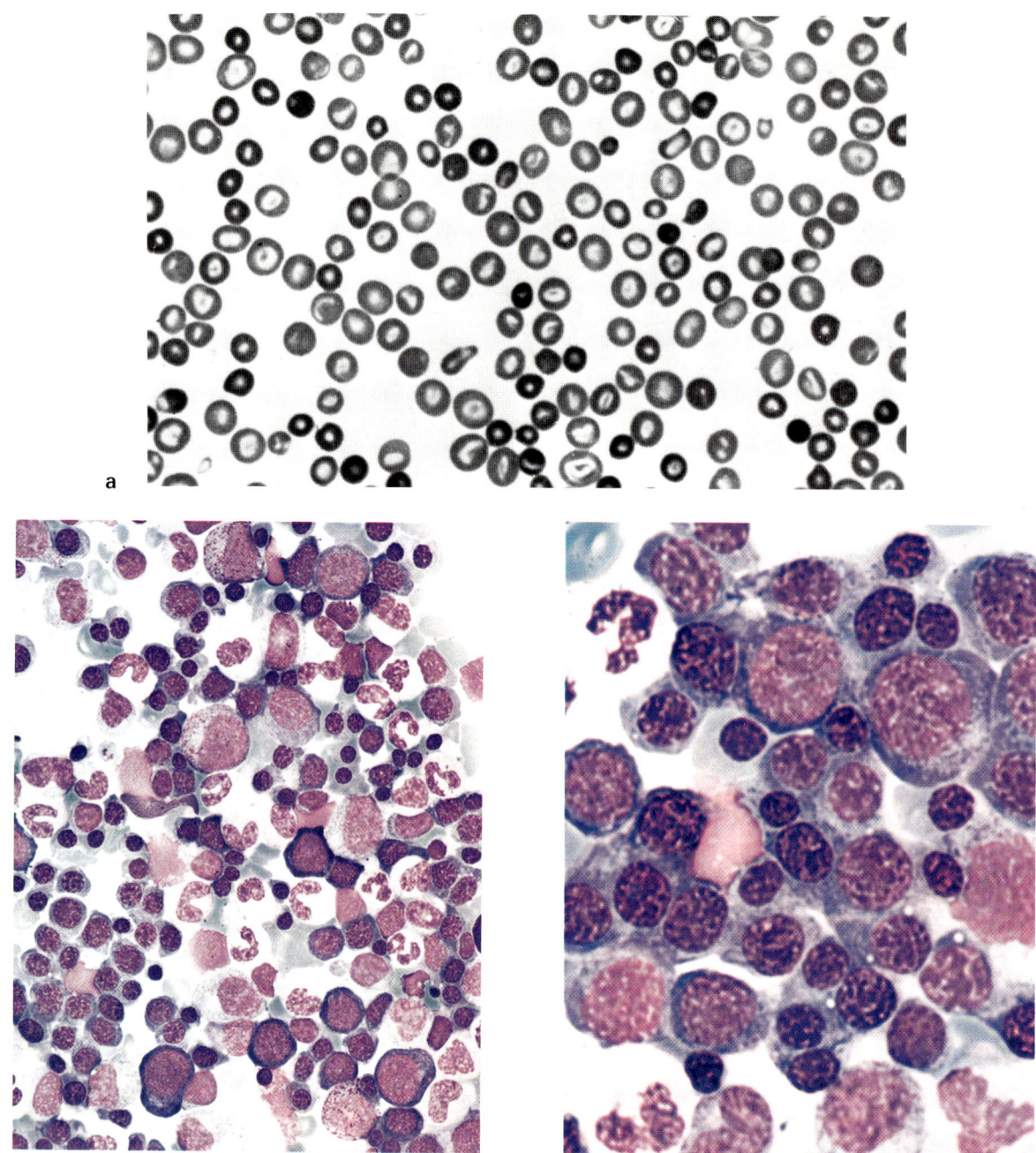

Fig. 35 a) Aniso- and poikilocytosis of the erythrocytes in a patient with primary acquired sideroblastic anemia. b) Hypercellular bone marrow in primary acquired sideroblastic anemia. c) At higher magnification, the macronormoblastic features of some erythroid cells are clearly shown.

3.2. Sideroblastic anemias

This group of disorders is characterized by disturbed erythroid proliferation leading to impaired hemoglobinization and abnormal iron deposition giving rise to "sideroblasts".
The biochemical defects underlying many of these conditions are not understood, but the basic abnormality relates to the inability of the erythroblasts to synthesize heme (**Fig. 34**). Most of these disorders, therefore, have features in common such as low hemoglobin, depressed reticulocyte count, hyperplastic marrow and increased plasma iron as a consequence of defective utilization. The conditions are also referred to as *sideroachrestic* [163, 164] or *refractory anemias* [165-168]. Colloquially, these anemias are said to have a full marrow with an empty blood. A still provisional classification of these disorders includes: a) *hereditary sideroblastic anemia* (X-linked or autosomal); b) *primary acquired sideroblastic anemia* either responsive or refractory to pyridoxine; c) *secondary*

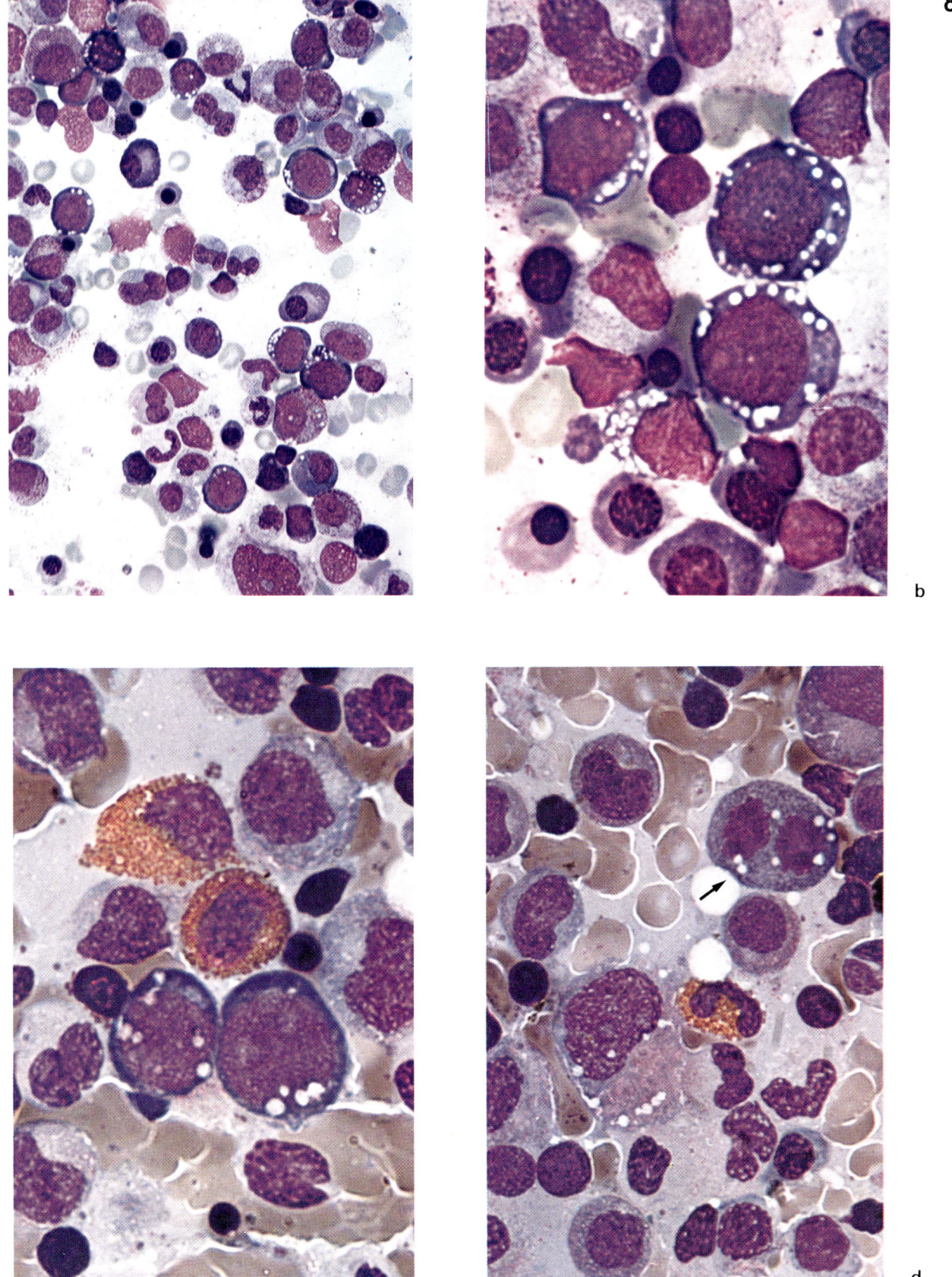

Fig. 36 a, b) Secondary acquired sideroblastic anemia (alcoholism). Prominent vacuolization of the basophilic erythroblasts is observable.
c) Chloramphenicol toxicity. Patient developed anemia and leukopenia. Vacuolization is seen in the cytoplasm of a pronormoblast and the cytoplasm and nucleus of a basophilic normoblast.
d) Vacuolization of an erythroid precursor in mitosis (**arrow**) as well as in a promyelocyte.
c, d) Courtesy of Dr. Zucker-Franklin, Department of Medicine, New York University.

Fig. 37 a) *Prussian blue stain showing free iron granules distributed throughout the cytoplasm of most of the erythroblasts either as confluent clumped masses or arranged as a ring around the nuclei ("ringed sideroblasts").*

b) *Combined staining for α-naphthyl-acetate esterase and Perls' reaction, showing heavy prussian blue precipitates and a strong enzymatic reaction in the red cell precursors.*

acquired sideroblastic anemia either specific due to malabsorption, alcohol, antitubercular drugs, lead, chloramphenicol, or non specific associated with leukemia and other myeloproliferative disorders [169-170].

The morphological patterns associated with sideroblastic anemias are illustrated in **Figures 35-41**.

Whilst in the hereditary forms a dimorphic population of hypochromic and normochromic red cells is present in the blood, in the acquired idiopathic forms a normochromic or even a macrocytic anemia may be observed. In all of these patients there is a marked anisocytosis and poikilocytosis (**Fig. 35 a**).
The marrow is hypercellular with an increased proportion of erythroid cells. As a rule, the cells are micronormoblastic in the hereditary sideroblastic anemias, whereas in the primary acquired forms a fraction of the erythroid population is macronormoblastic (**Figs. 35 b** and **c**). Poor hemoglobinization leads to a "ragged" appearance of the cytoplasm particularly of the polychromatophilic erythroblasts; furthermore, the cytoplasm of nucleated red cell precursors in patients with alcohol or chloramphenicol toxicity is often vacuolated (**Figs. 36 a, b, c**, etc).

As far as the iron content of the erythroblasts is concerned, two types of sideroblasts may be distinguished. One type is characterized by an increase of both the number and the size of siderotic granules scattered throughout the cytoplasm. This is common in disorders associated with increased transferrin saturation without significantly impaired hemoglobin synthesis (hemolytic disorders, megaloblastic anemias).
A second type, which is quite distinctive for the sideroblastic anemias is characterized by the presence of large, coarse granules clustered around the nucleus (*ringed sideroblast* [173]; *pathologic sideroblast* [174]) (**Fig. 37**).

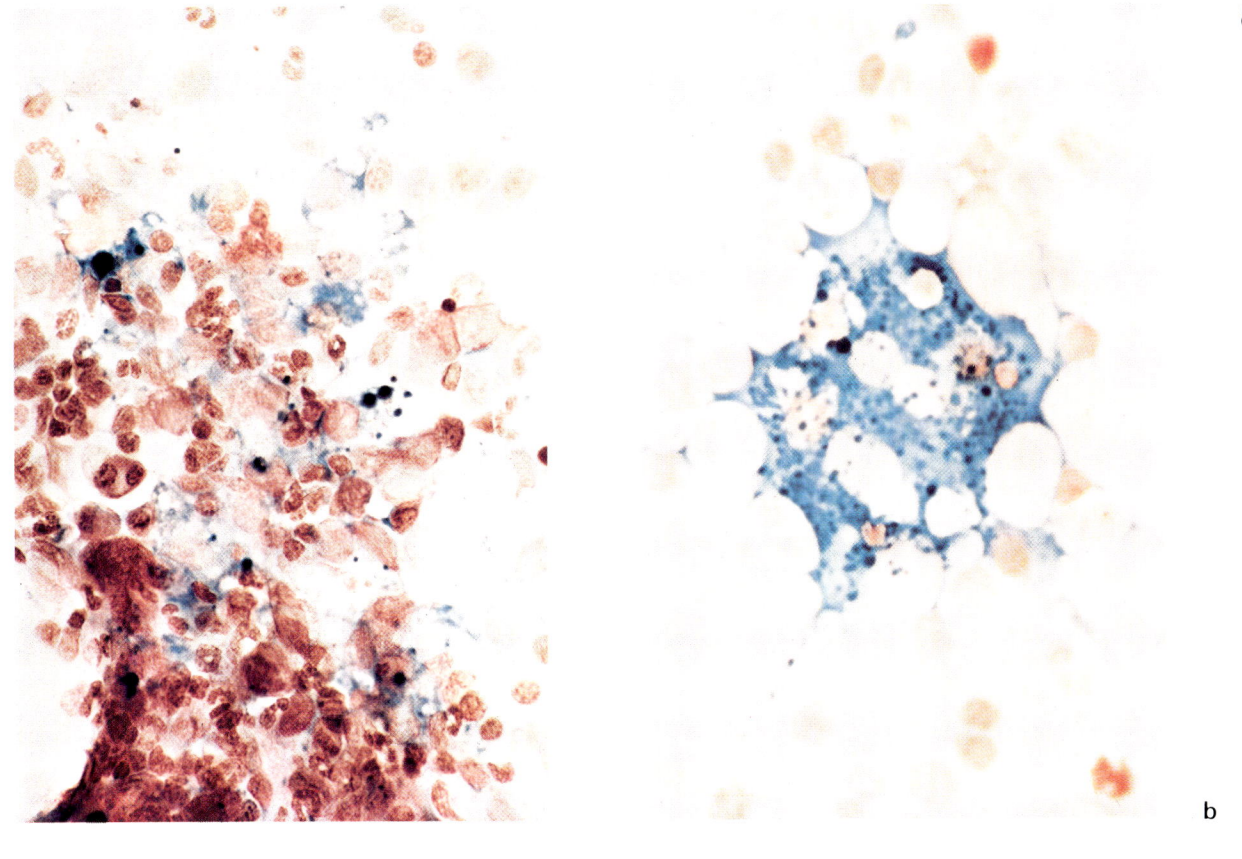

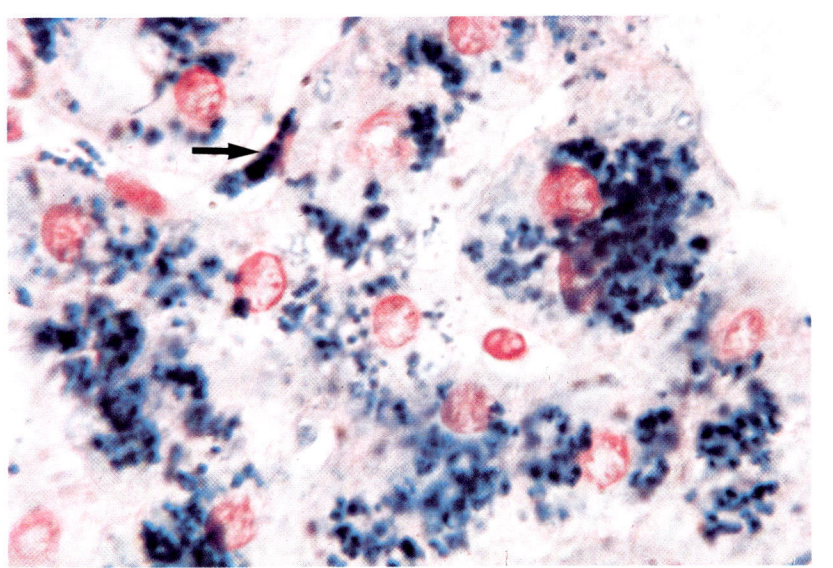

Fig. 38 a) *Patchy area from the marrow exhibiting increased iron stores in acquired idiopathic sideroblastic anemia.*
b) *Bone marrow macrophage exhibiting heavy Prussian blue precipitates.*
c) *Section from a liver biopsy with prominent iron deposits; a Kupffer cell is indicated by the* **arrow**.
In all of the preparations, iron is demonstrated by Prussian blue staining.

In patients with acquired sideroblastic anemia, iron may accumulate even in the immature basophilic erythroblasts where it may appear in vacuoles [175].

Reticulum cells are heavily laden with ferruginous micelles and show a homogeneous intense staining reaction with the Prussian blue (**Figs. 38 a** and **b**). Iron deposits may also be observed in other tissues, particularly in the liver (**Fig. 38 c**).

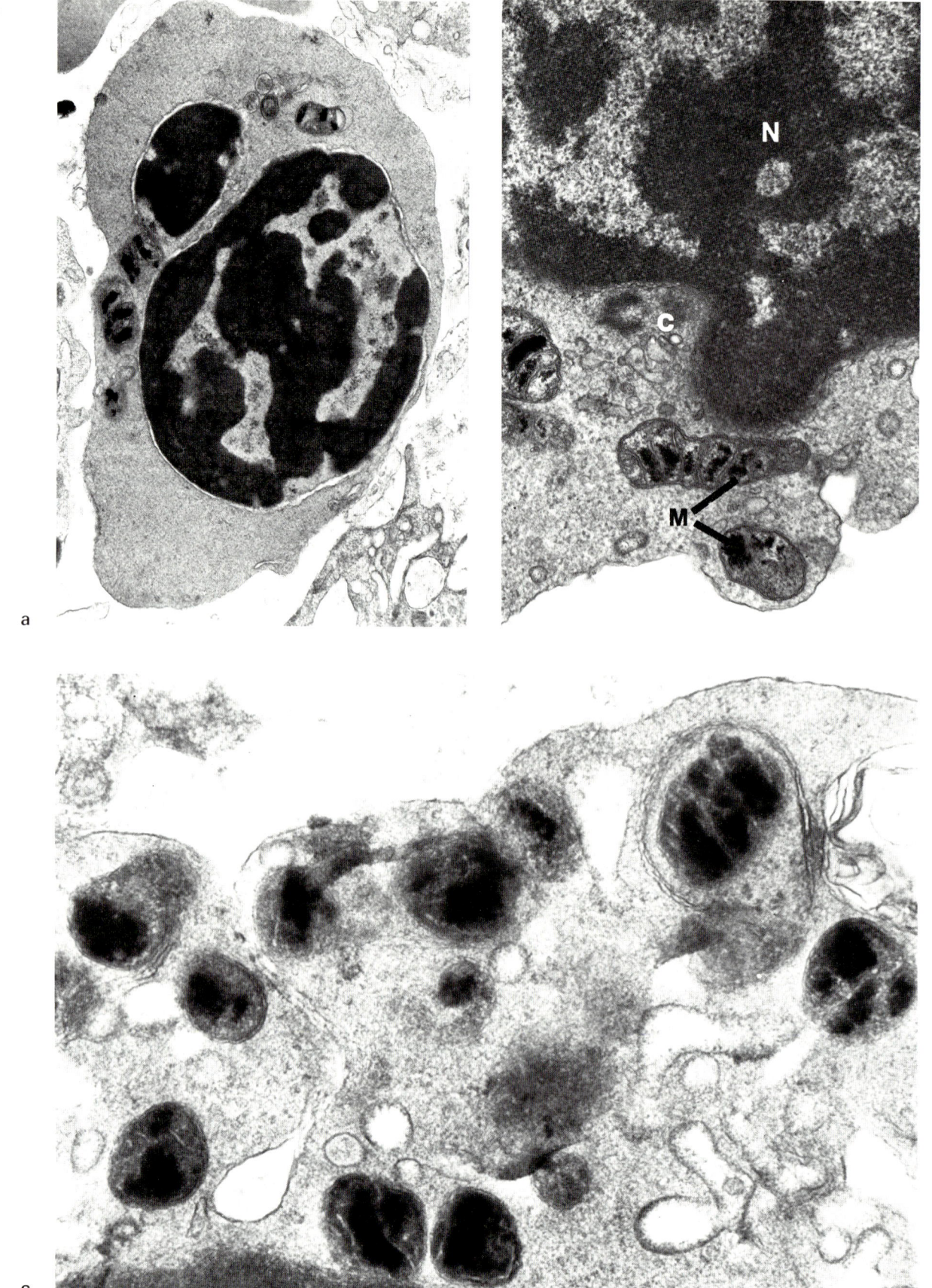

Fig. 39 a) Acquired idiopathic sideroblastic anemia showing erythroblasts with heavy iron deposition within the mitochondria. Rupture or separation of the cristae may arise from excessive iron accumulation. Perinuclear distribution of the structurally abnormal mitochondria accounts for the appearance of "ringed sideroblasts" ($\times$ 3,500).

b) Detail of an erythroblast obtained from the bone marrow of a patient with sideroblastic anemia illustrates "ferrugenous" deposits in mitochondria (**M**). Nucleus (**N**), centrioles (**C**) ($\times$ 31,000).
Courtesy of Dr. D. Zucker-Franklin, Department of Medicine, New York University.

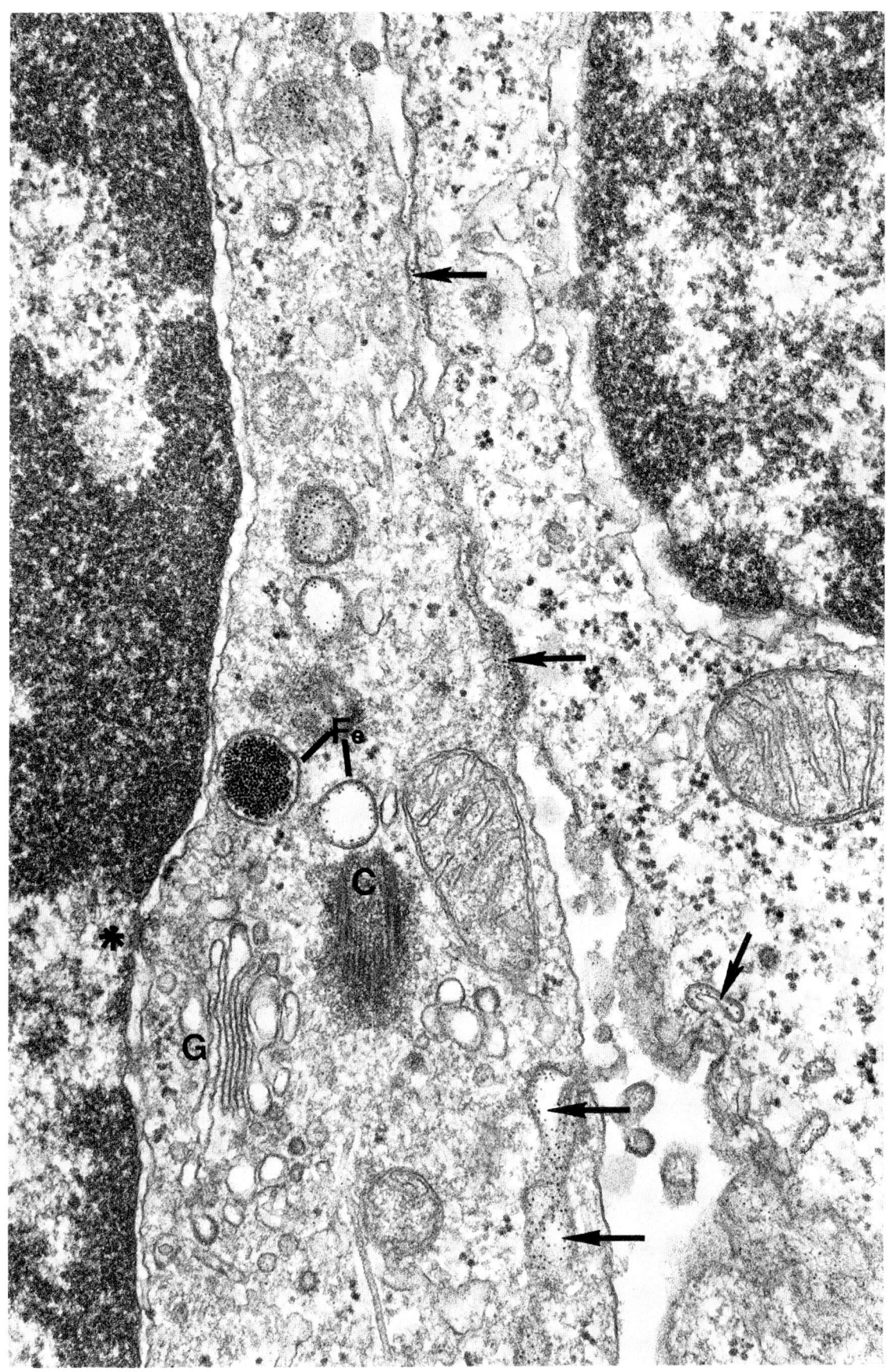

Fig. 39 c) Several swollen mitochondria with marked iron accumulation in the cytoplasm of an erythroblast (× 35,000).

d) Two adjacent erythroblasts from the bone marrow of a patient with increased iron storage. Note ferritin particles located on the plasma membrane of both cells and in invaginations of the surface membrane (**arrows**). Within the cell, ferritin has accumulated in membrane-bound structures (**Fe**). Golgi zone (**G**), centriole (**C**); asterisk indicates nuclear pore (× 57,000).
Courtesy of Dr. D. Zucker-Franklin, Department of Medicine, New York University.

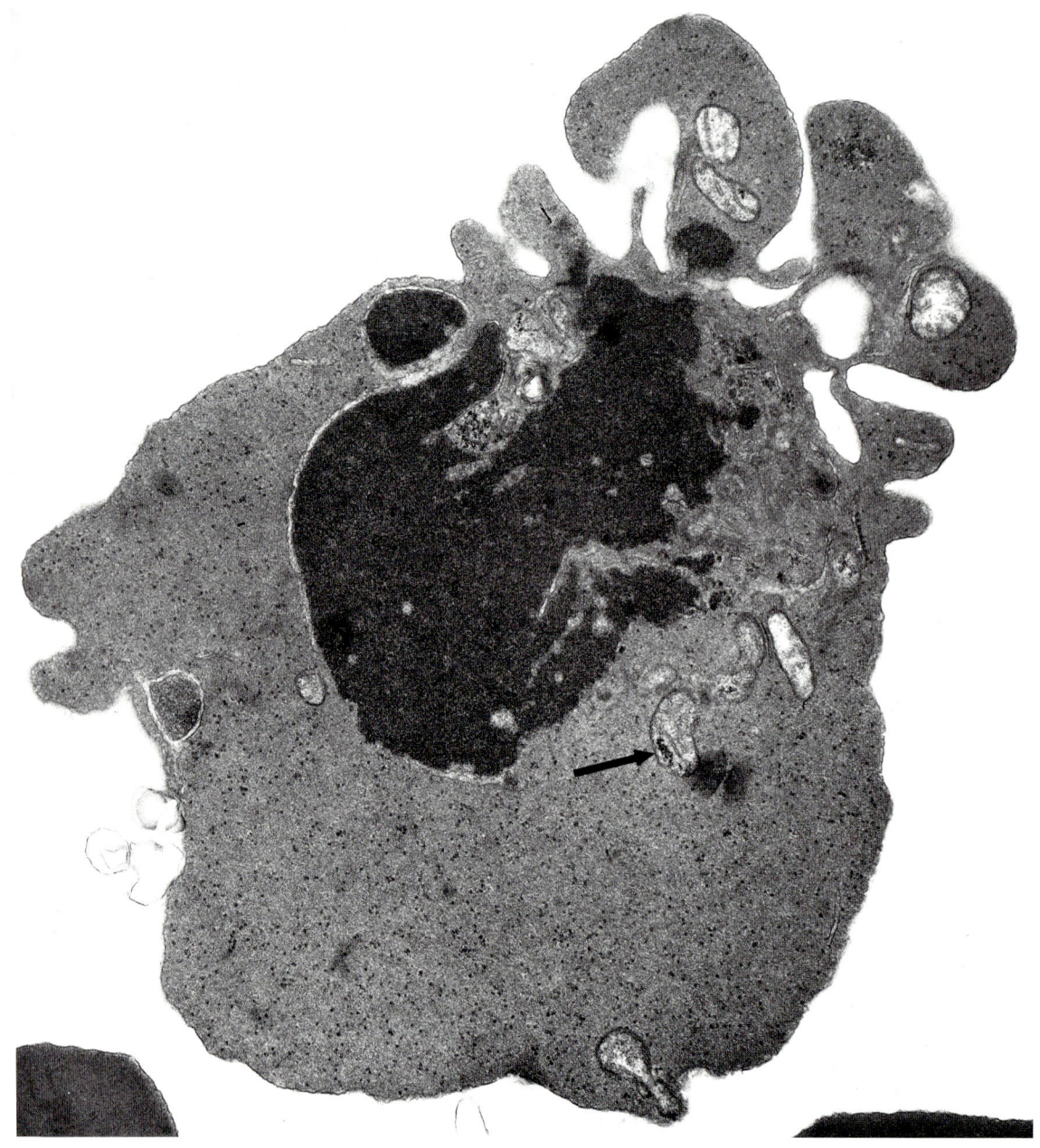

Fig. 40 a) Erythroblast obtained from the marrow of a patient with sideroblastic anemia associated with chronic myelogenous leukemia. The nucleus is probably in telophase of the final cell division. Its partial fragmentation reflects dyserythropoiesis. The contour of the cell resembles that of a reticulocyte. Fragments of the nucleus may already have been extruded. **Arrow** indicates mitochondrion containing ferrugenous micelles ($\times$ 26,000).
Courtesy of Dr. D. Zucker-Franklin, Department of Medicine, New York University.

3 ERYTHROCYTES

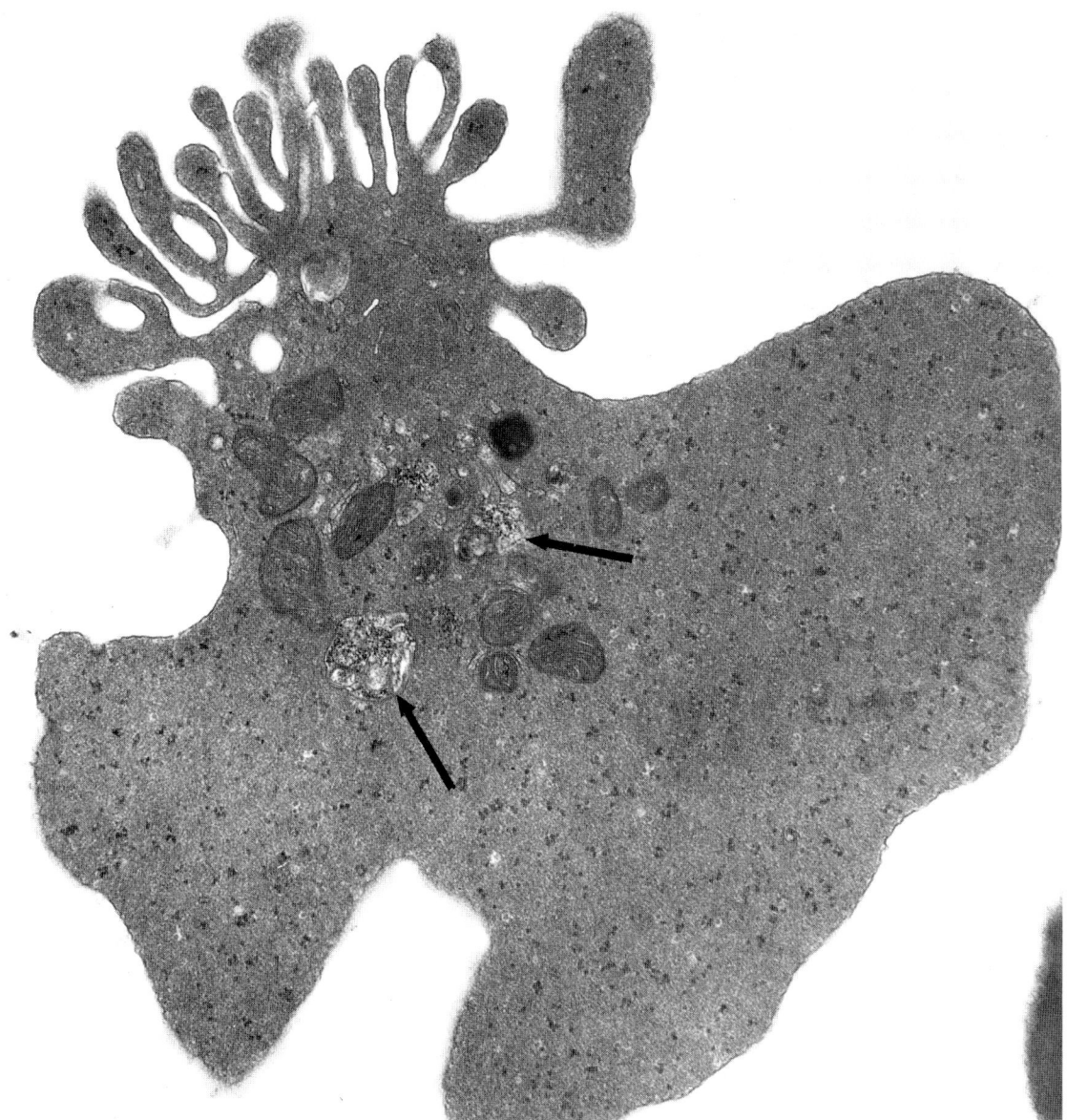

Fig. 40 b) *Reticulocyte from the marrow of a patient with ineffective erythropoiesis associated with chronic myelogenous leukemia. Note the excessive accumulation of ferritin (arrows) ($\times$ 29,000). Courtesy of Dr. D. Zucker-Franklin, Department of Medicine, New York University.*

With respect to other cytochemical features, PAS staining has been reported to be normal in the majority of cases [176], while α-naphthyl-acetate esterase activity has been found to be increased in most erythroblasts. On electron microscopy an abnormal accumulation of iron in the mitochondria is seen in most sideroblastic anemias.
Iron is deposited in between the cristae in the form of a finely granular electron-dense material. Accumulation of iron leads to degenerative processes of the affected organelles with disruption of the mitochondrial structure (**Fig. 39 a-d**) [177]. All these features are common to both the inherited and acquired conditions, including those associated with preleukemic states (refractory anemias with excess of myeloblasts, RAEM) [171].
Nuclear clefts and blebs are common features of hemopoietic dysplasia [178] (see p. 118); the overall features are reminiscent of those observed in acute leukemias (**Fig. 40 a, b**).

3.2.1. **Synartesis**, a peculiar morphological abnormality seen in some refractory anemias refers to a kind of junction which links one erythroblast to another and which may disturb the release of the cells from the bone marrow resulting in ineffective erythropoiesis (**Fig. 41**).

Originally "*synartesis*" [179, 180] (sunartésis = junction) was described as a feature in anemia due to membrane abnormalities, but it is probably a non specific feature seen in dyserythropoietic syndromes to a variable extent [181, 182]. In most instances, there is transverse alignement of the ferritin molecules which occupy the space between closely adjacent erythroblasts [183] and which give the appearance of intercellular junctions (septate-like junctions).

3.3. Congenital dyserythropoietic anemias

The congenital dyserythropoietic anemias (CDA) constitute a group of rare hereditary diseases characterized by ineffective erythropoiesis and bizarre nuclear abnormalities in the red cell precursors of the bone marrow. Three types of CDA have been distinguished [160, 161, 185-188] (Table 2).

3.3.1. **CDA type I** is extremely rare [184, 189-192] (**Figs. 42 and 45 a, b**). The basic pathogenetic mechanisms responsible for the erythroblastic abnormalities are unknown. Cytokinetic studies [193] as well as spectrophotometric analyses [194] have suggested an underlying disturbance in nucleoprotein synthesis which leads to abnormal mitotic divisions.

3.3.2. **CDA type II.** Some descriptions of this disorder had been reported in the literature [195-197] before the definition by Crookston *et al.* (1960) under the label of HEMPAS ("Hereditary Erythroblastic Multinuclearity with Positive Acidified Serum lysis test") (**Figs. 43 and 45 c**).

The condition is characterized by the presence of a positive acidified serum lysis test and by increased agglutinability of erythrocytes by anti-i antiserum. The defect has been attributed to the lack of sialoglycoproteins (glycophorin) which would in turn allow increased exposure of antigenic determinants (i sites) on the surface of the red cell membrane.

Abnormal mitotic divisions of erythroblasts may be responsible for the "marginal cisterna", a peculiar linear structure which runs along the inside of the red cell membrane and which may interfere with nuclear division or extrusion (see **Fig. 45**) [198].

3.3.3. **CDA type III** (**Fig. 44**) has been described in the past under different names such as *familial erythroid multinuclearity* [199] or *hereditary benign erythroreticulosis* [200]. The features observed in CDA type III are reminiscent of those observed in erythremic myelosis. Even morphologically the cells appear to be quite similar. The multinucleated erythroblasts appear to arise either as a consequence of multipolar mitoses or of acytokinesis [201]. On the other hand the polyploid uninucleated erythroblasts may reflect an underlying defect in DNA synthesis leading to endomitotic DNA replication or to a fusion of telophasic nuclei [202, 203].

Classification of CDA into three main types is empirical since there is considerable morphological overlap [204, 205].
Recently a series of variants have been described [206, 207], sometimes in association with other disorders such as thalassemia trait [208] or with mucopolysaccharidosis [209, 210].

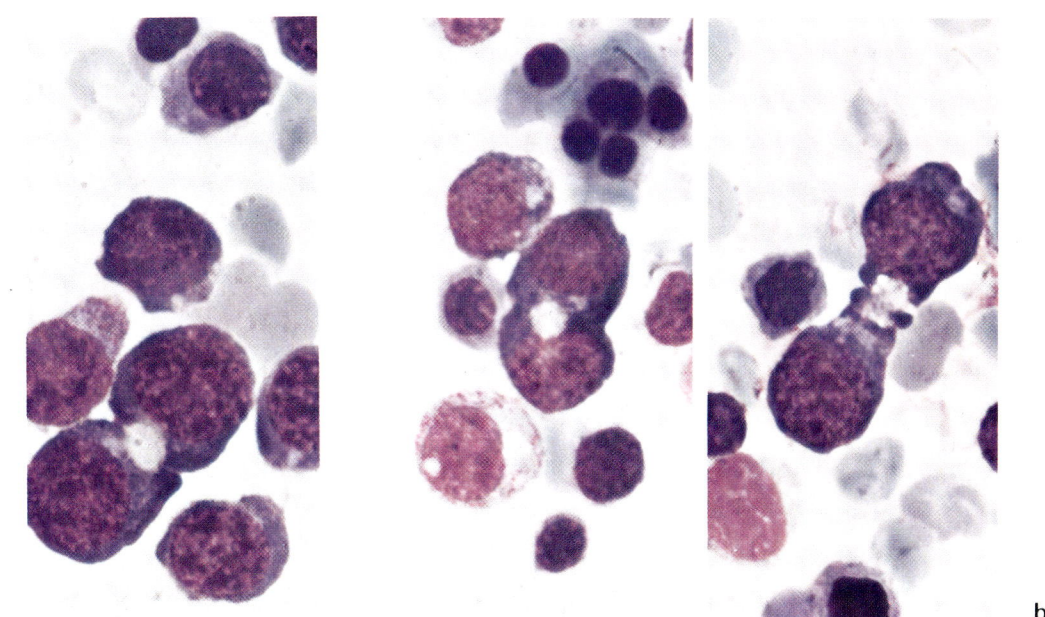

Fig. 41 Different features of erythroblastic "synartesis" (refractory anemia).
a) Clumping of basophilic erythroblasts. The cells seem to be tightly connected with each other as in a syncytial tissue.
b) Several erythroblasts are linked by junctions which delimit non basophilic clear zones.
Courtesy of Prof. A.M. Marmont, S. Martino's Hospital, Genova.

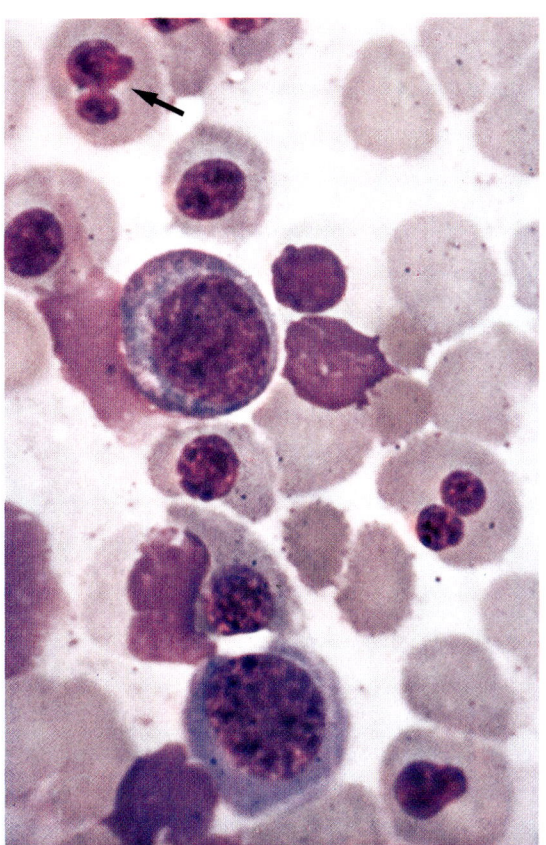
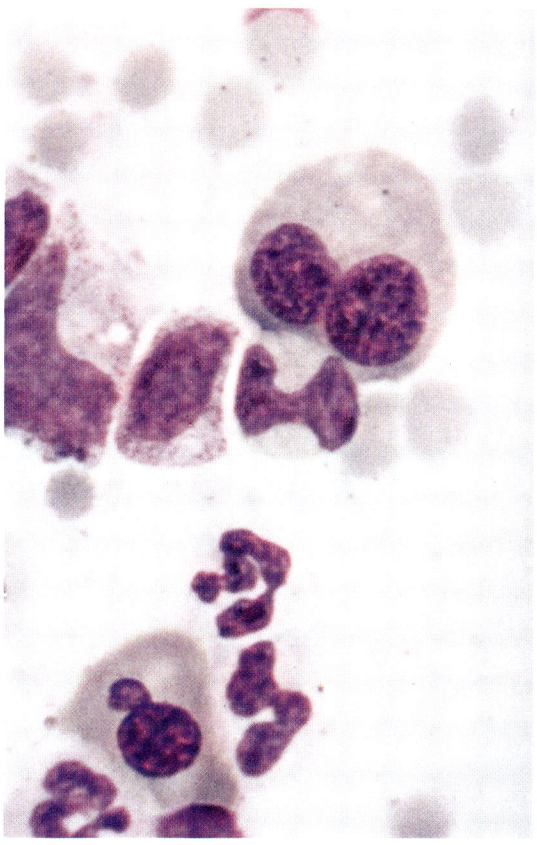

Fig. 42 a, b) CDA type I: Giant (megaloblastic) erythroblasts and erythroblastic internuclear chromatin bridges (**arrow**). Binucleated erythroblasts are readily observed.

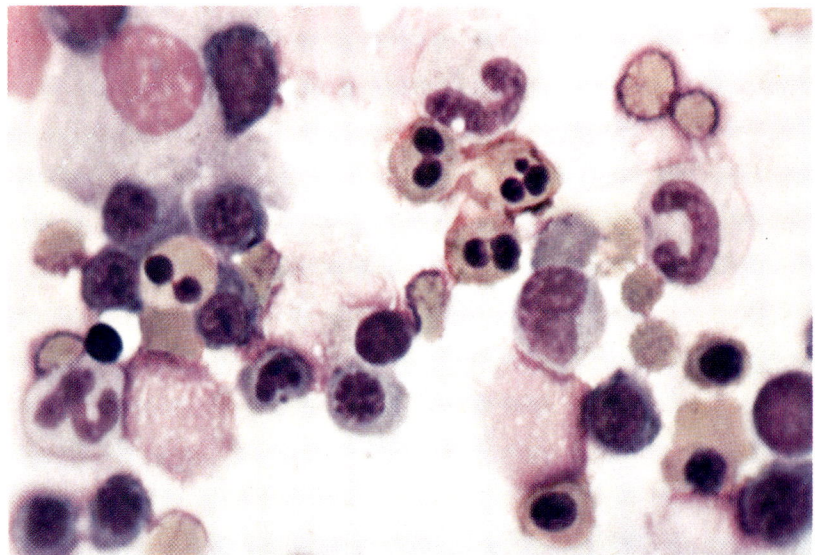

Fig. 43 CDA type II: Normoblastic hyperplasia, binucleation of most of the erythroblasts, karyorrhexis of some nuclei.

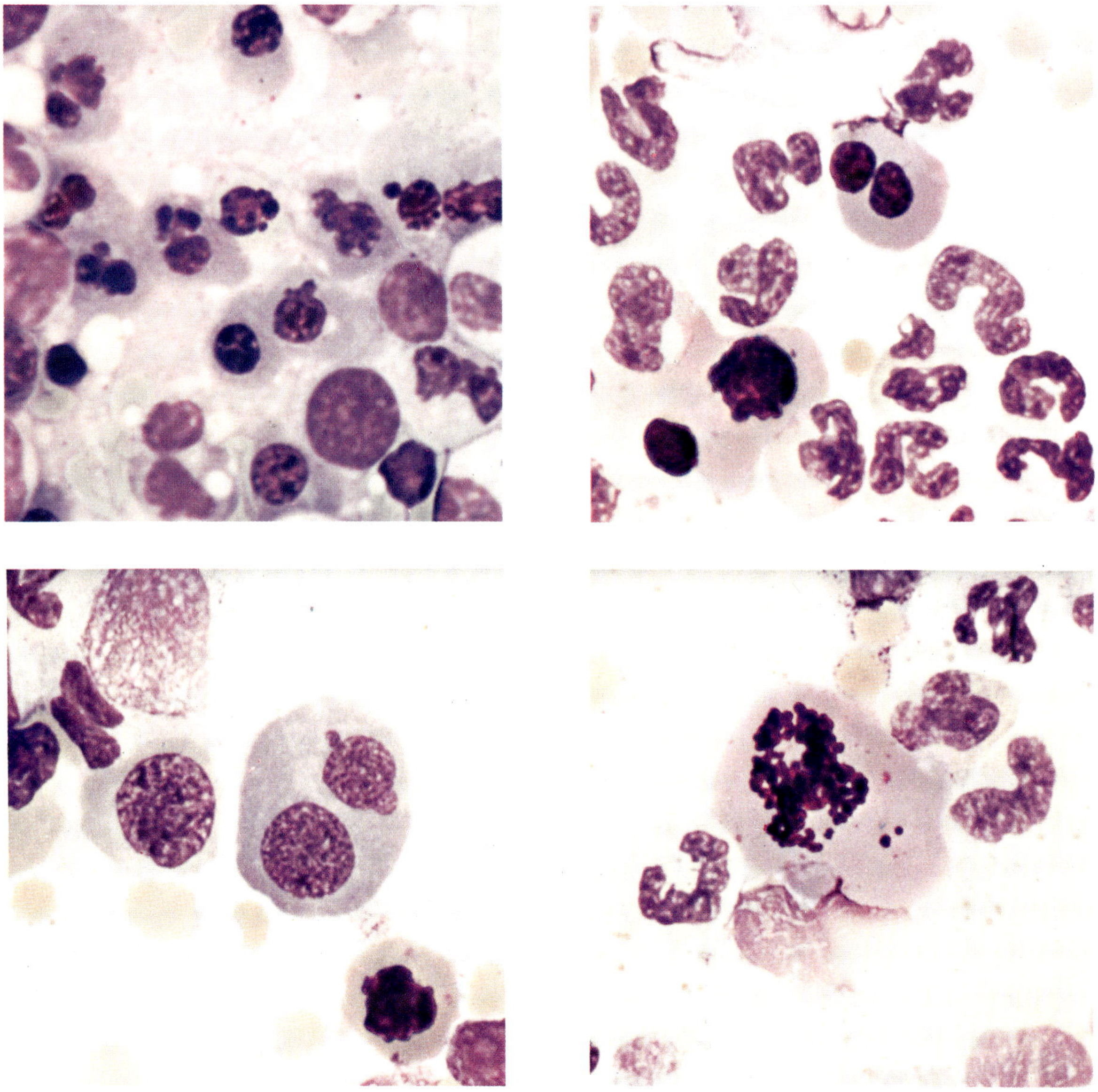

Fig. 44 a, b, c, d) CDA type III: Several erythroblasts with lobulated nuclei and karyorrhexis (**a, b, c**). Giant multinucleated erythroblasts (**c**), sometimes exhibiting abnormal mitotic figures (**d**).

3 ERYTHROCYTES

Table 2 PRINCIPAL FEATURES OF CONGENITAL DYSERYTHROPOIETIC ANEMIAS

	CDA I	CDA II	CDA III
Inheritance	Autosomal recessive	Autosomal recessive	Dominant
Blood	Macrocytic anisopoikilocytosis	Normocytic anisopoikilocytosis	Macrocytic anisopoikilocytosis
Marrow	Binucleated erythroblasts, megaloblastic features, intranuclear chromatin bridges, normal mitotic figures, cytoplasmic connections between cells, enlarged nuclear pores with partial loss of nuclear envelope and cytoplasmic portions invaginating into the nuclear area	High incidence of binucleated erythroblasts (10-40%), few multinucleated erythroblasts (up to 4 nuclei), pluripolar mitoses, karyorrhexis	Giant multinucleated erythroblasts, karyorrhexis, nuclear blebs
Excessive iron storage	+	−	+
Acidified serum test	−	+	−
Anti-i test	−	+	−

ULTRASTRUCTURAL FINDINGS IN CONGENITAL DYSERYTHROPOIETIC ANEMIAS

	CDA I	CDA II	CDA III
Nuclear:			
Enlargement of nuclear pores with partial loss of nuclear envelope	+	−	−
Vacuolization of the heterochromatin ("spongy structure")	+	−	−
Internuclear chromatin bridges	+	−	−
Clefts and blebs	+	−	+
Invagination of cytoplasmic portions into the nuclear area	+	−	+
Cytoplasmic:			
Myelin figures and autolytic areas	+	−	+
Iron-filled mitochondria	+	−	+
Cytoplasmic bridges	+	−	−
Presence of "marginal cisternae"	−	+	−

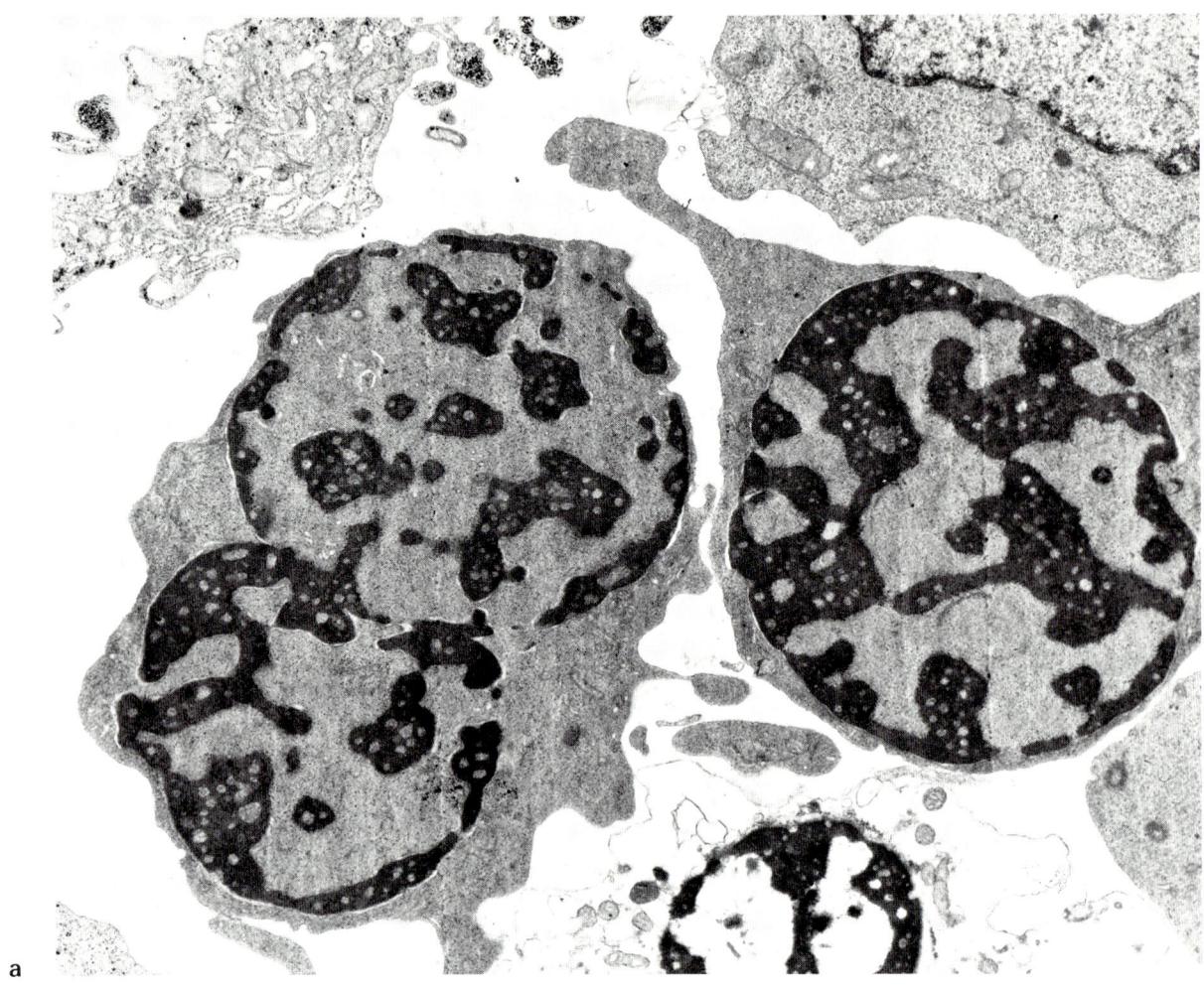

Fig. 45 a) CDA I. Two polychromatophilic normoblasts. One cell shows incomplete division of nuclei ($\times$ 8,500).
b) Normoblast in CDA I. Spongy remnants of nuclear chromatin. Nucleolus is reduced to a thin shell. Myelin figures and cytoplasmic organelles in the nuclear area. Mytochondria with iron deposits ($\times$ 16,500).
c) CDA II. Double membrane enclosing a cisterna at a distance of 40-60 nm from the inside of the plasma membrane ($\times$ 32,000).
Courtesy of Dr. J. Fortezza-Vila and Prof. H. Heimpel, Division of Hematology, University of Ulm.

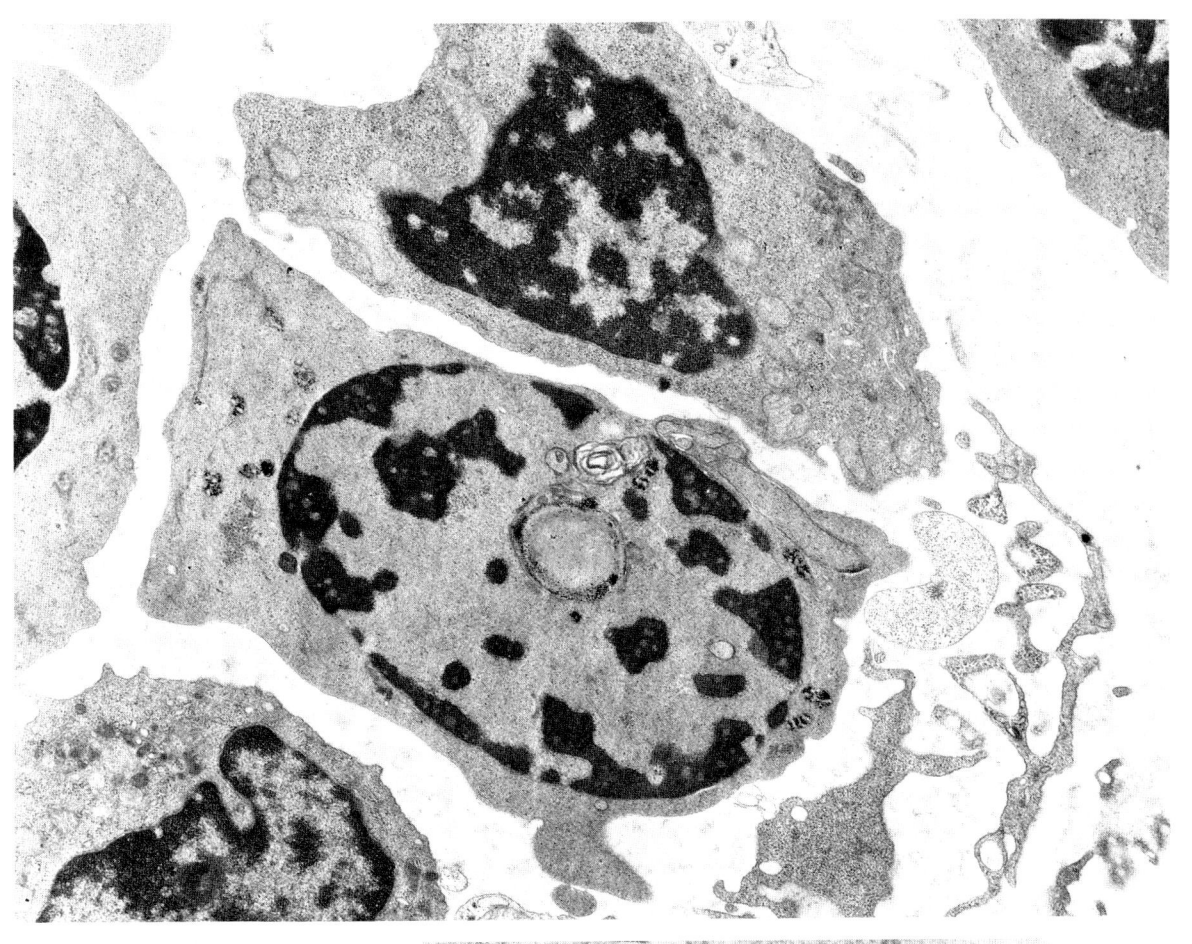

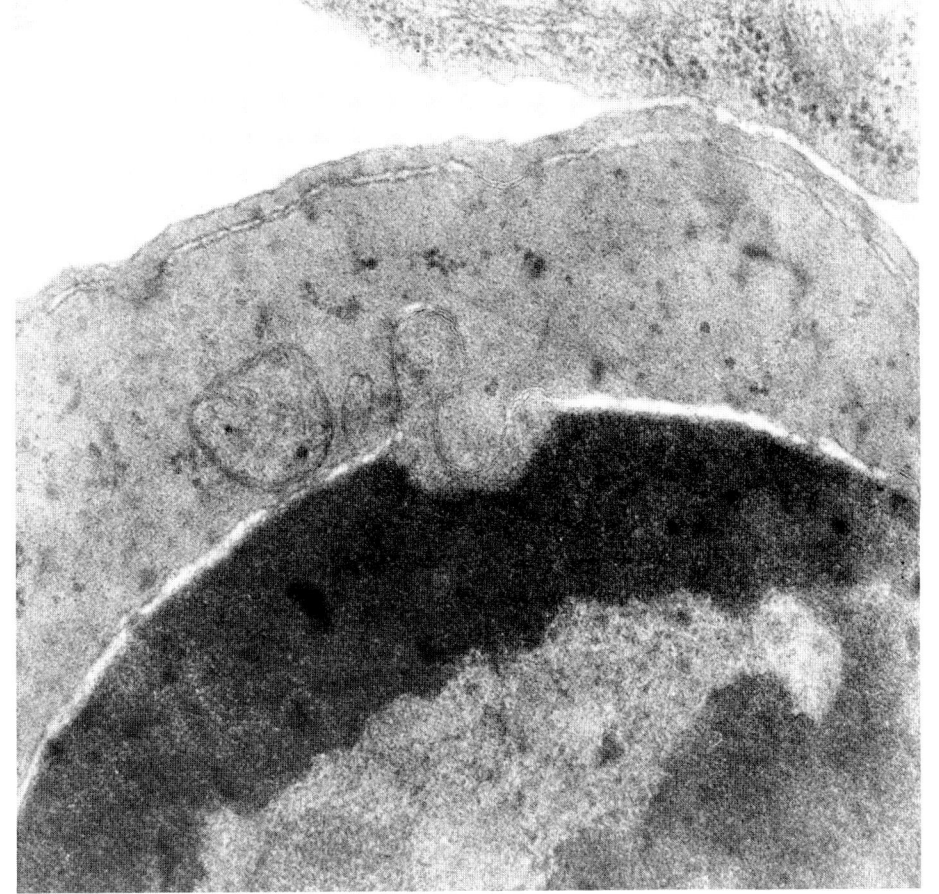

BLOOD CELLS

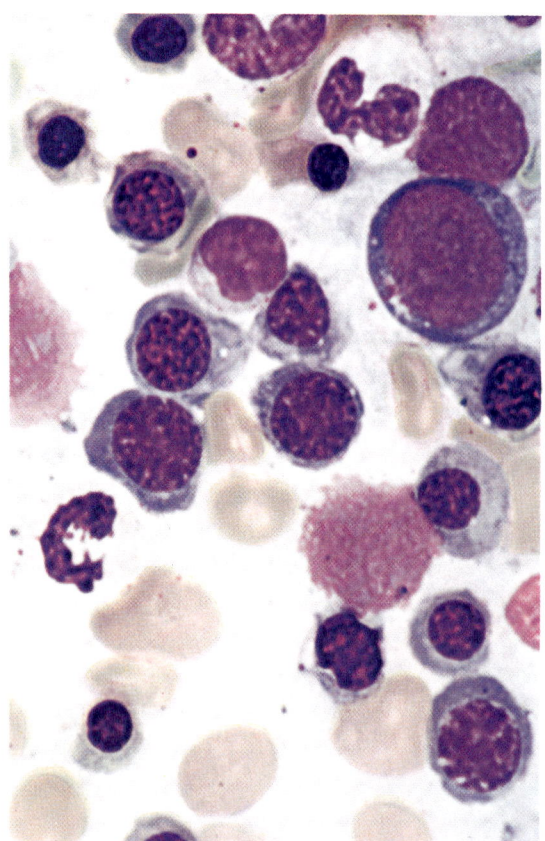

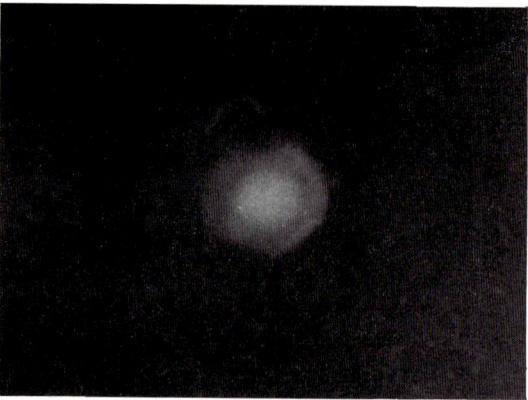

47 a

46   47 b

Fig. 46 *Erythroid hyperplasia with megaloblastic features in some bone marrow cells from a case of erythropoietic porphyria. Some mature erytroblasts show a "ragged cytoplasm".*

Fig. 47 a) *Red fluorescence (reproduced in white) of an erythroblastic nucleus (erythropoietic porphyria; unstained bone marrow smear).*
b) *Rod-like inclusion in an erythroblastic cell (fluorescence observation).*

3.4. Porphyrias

The porphyrias constitute a group of disorders which are classified on the basis of the principal site where the metabolic abnormalities occur into *erythropoietic* and *hepatic* forms [211-213]. The former group includes the congenital erythropoietic porphyria (Gunther's disease), the milder condition of erythropoietic (erythrohepatic) protoporphyria and the erythropoietic coproporphyria. Among the hepatic porphyrias the chronic cutaneous hepatic variant associated with alcoholism represents the most frequent disorder; other varieties (acute intermittent, variegate porphyria, and hereditary coproporphyria) are less frequently observed.
Congenital erythropoietic porphyria is most likely to have hematologic manifestations. The anemia is usually normochromic and associated with an increased number of reticulocytes and circulating erythroblasts. Microcytosis and hypochromia are sometimes observed.

The bone marrow shows erythroblastic hyperplasia, often with a dimorphic population, normoblastic and with pathological features respectively (mainly represented by porphyrin-laden erythroblasts). Not infrequently macroerythroblastosis is observed, which is possibly related to hemolysis and folate consumption (**Fig. 46**). The pathological population of erythroblasts exhibits abnormalities of nuclear shape, with lobulation and separation of chromatin masses. Nuclei may contain central inclusions of porphyrins or, according to some authors [211, 214], structures containing hemoglobin, since they stain deeply with benzidine.

Cytoplasmic abnormalities include irregular distribution of basophilia (*ragged erythroblasts*), vacuolization, basophilic stippling, iron granules and, less frequently, structures which have been referred to as porphyrin crystals [215].

A double population of erythroid precursors is easily detected by examination of unstained bone marrow smears with a fluorescence microscope. While most of the erythroblasts exhibit a red porphyrin fluorescence either inside or at the surface of the nucleus, some cells fail to fluoresce (**Fig. 47**). Only a fraction of the reticulocytes exhibit red fluorescence.

There is no clear explanation for the existence of a double population of cells. It may be related to a differential renewal rate. It is possible that cells which mature rapidly are more ready to produce the isomer type I of porphyrins because of deficient PBG-deaminase-uroporphyrogen isomerase production.

3.4.1. Erythropoietic protoporphyria.
This disorder is clinically characterized by photosensitivity, moderate anemia and frequent liver involvement (cirrhosis with cholestasis). The primary defect is diminished activity of ferrochelatase. Thus, protoporphyrin accumulates in erythrocytes and may be progressively deposited in the liver.

3.4.2. Symptomatic porphyrinopathies.
Most of the disorders that are associated with increased excretion of porphyrins are symptomatic since they are accompanied by alterations in heme synthesis or abnormal porphyrin excretion.

Symptomatic porphyrinopathies may be divided into protoporphyrinemias (from lead intoxication, iron deficiency, sideroblastic anemia, alcoholism) and coproporphyrinurias (from liver disorders, heavy metal intoxications, infectious diseases, or associated with some blood disorders such as thalassemia, aplastic anemia, leukemia, pernicious anemia). The underlying biochemical alterations in many of these conditions are still unknown. A disturbance in ferrochelatase activity has been claimed for most of the symptomatic protoporphyrinemias [216].

3.5. Iron deficiency anemia

Iron deficiency results in reduced hemoglobin concentration in the red cells manifested by hypochromia.

Thus *hypochromic anemia* has become a commonly used equivalent term for iron deficiency anemia. However, this term is incorrect [217], since a lowered hemoglobin concentration (associated with "hypochromasia") may occur in a variety of different clinical conditions. It is due either to failure of heme synthesis (as in sideroblastic anemia) or to reduced hemoglobin synthesis (as in thalassemic syndromes).

Furthermore, iron deficiency may exist before becoming evident on the blood smear [218]. In the early phases [219] which are principally characterized by the loss of iron storage (phase of *iron depletion*), hypochromia and microcytosis are usually lacking [217]. In this situation anemia is often normochromic and normocytic and a correct diagnosis can be made only by evaluating iron stores (*iron deficiency without anemia*) [220].

However aniso-poikilocytosis may be present in some patients without patent hypochromia making the differential diagnosis more difficult since it may also be seen in other conditions such as heterozygous β-thalassemia.

Determination of red cell indices (MCV, MCH and MCHC) are important in differentiating iron deficiency from other conditions [221] (**Fig. 48 b**). In advanced iron deficiency (Hb less than 8 gr %) the morphological diagnosis is easily made on the basis of poor hemoglobinization (presence of "annulocytes" in blood smears) and of the invariably associated aniso-poikilocytosis (*iron deficiency anemia*) (**Figs. 48 a, c, d**).

The iron deficient bone marrow shows an absolute increase in normoblasts. Erythropoiesis is orderly, but the impaired hemoglobinization leads to relative accumulation of basophilic precursors (**Fig. 49**). Morphological alterations are seen only in the late erythroblasts which present an irregularly stained

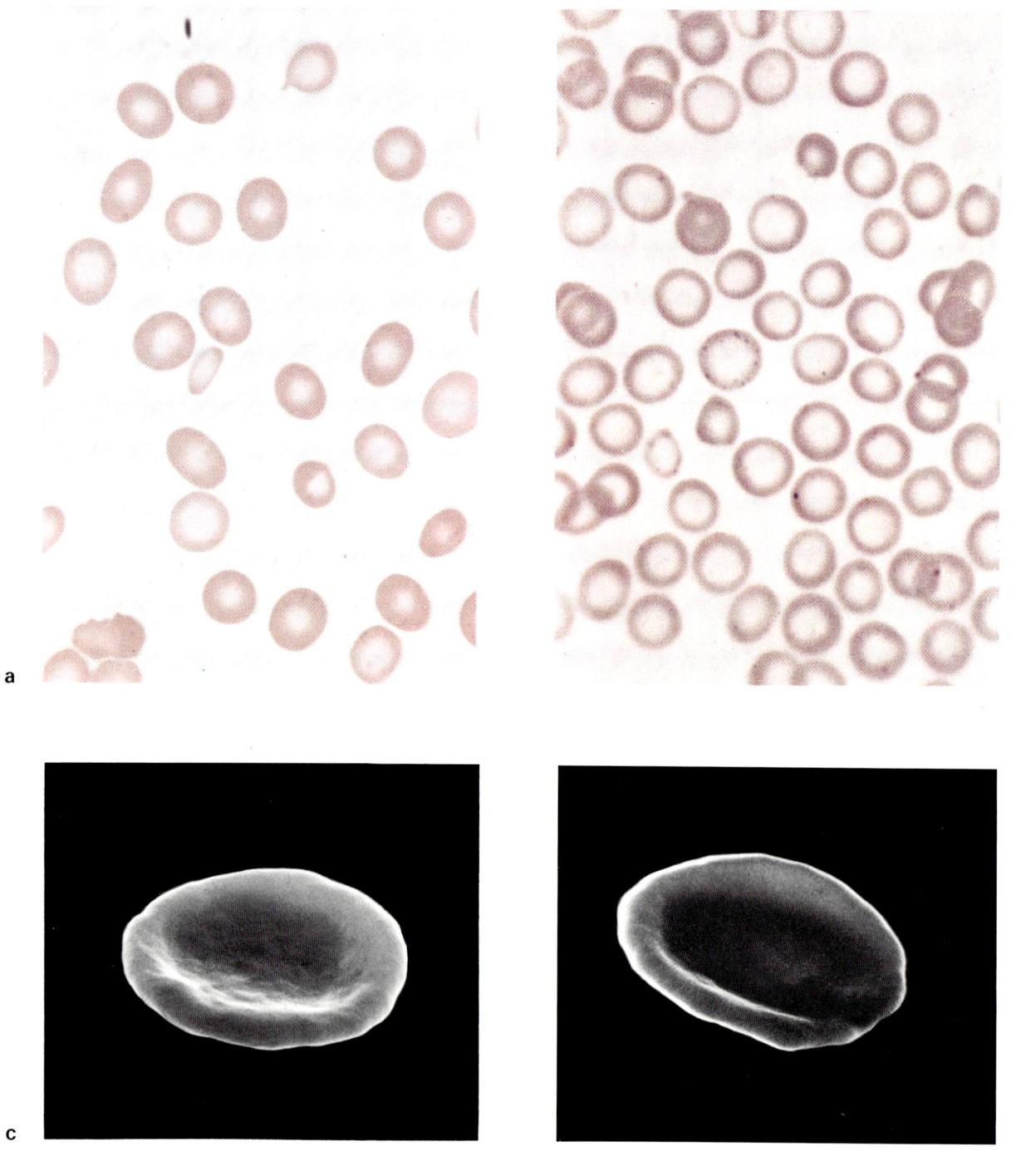

Fig. 48 a) Peripheral blood in severe iron deficiency anemia is characterized by the presence of hypochromic and microcytic erythrocytes. Poor hemoglobinization of the cells leads to the appearance of a thin rim of pigment at the inner side of the erythrocyte membrane ("annulocytes"). Poikilocytosis is also a common feature; target cells, cigar-shaped, tear drop elements and many other bizarre erythrocytic forms are frequently observed.

b) A picture of hypochromic microcytic anemia in thalassemia trait is shown for comparison. Although the determination of red cell indices is mandatory for a differential diagnosis from iron deficiency anemia (MCV reduced and MCHC near normal), an accurate smear interpretation may detect some important morphological features. The red cells in these patients are extremely thin and near normal in diameter giving only rise to moderate degree of anisocytosis.

c, d) Micro-leptocytes (SEM observation) ($\times$ 5,200).

3 ERYTHROCYTES

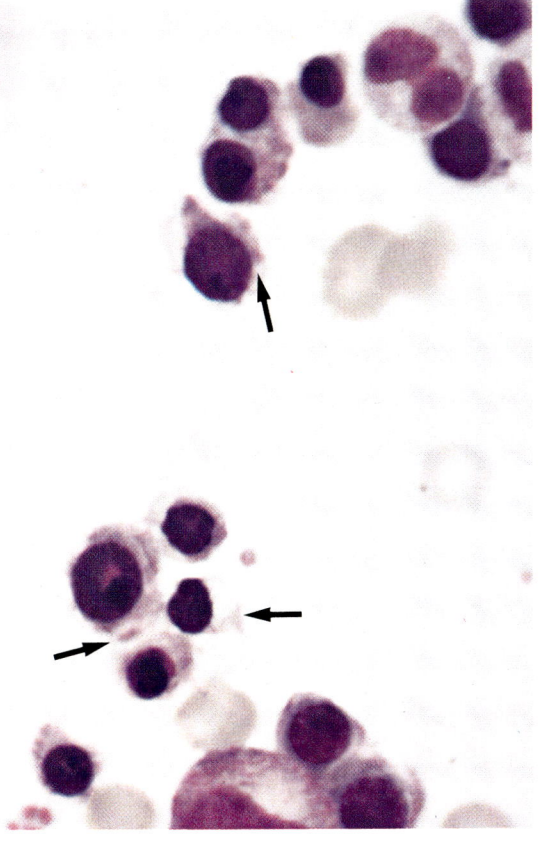
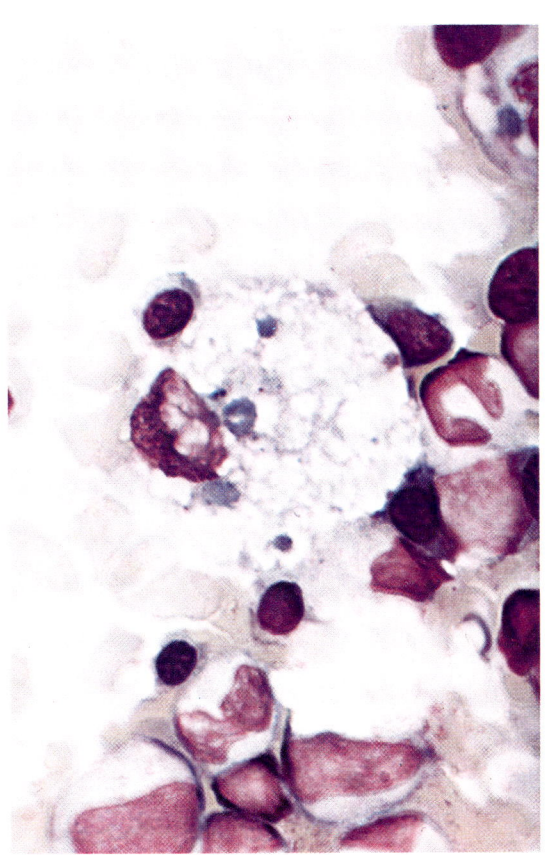

Fig. 49 The bone marrow of a patient with severe iron deficiency anemia. Erythropoiesis is normoblastic, but the erythroid cells exhibit defective hemoglobinization ("ragged cytoplasm") (**arrows**) and pycnotic nuclei.

Fig. 50 Reticulum cell surrounded by a few erythroblasts in iron deficiency anemia. Most of these cells do not show any positive reaction to Prussian blue staining.

cytoplasm. Nuclear abnormalities, such as irregularity in shape, karyorrhexis and occasional binucleation may also be seen.

There may be numerous reticulum cells in the marrow which do not show stainable iron within their cytoplasm (**Fig. 50**).

Analysis of stainable storage iron [222-224] as well as the evaluation of the number of sideroblasts in the marrow may further help to distinguish iron deficiency anemia from all other anemias. Although some discrepancies may arise from the evaluation of the Prussian blue reaction on histological sections of bone marrow, in comparison with cytological preparations [225], no stainable iron is present in the marrow of markedly iron deficient patients. Sideroblasts are significantly decreased in early stages of iron deficiency [226, 227] and they do not exceed 10% in the marrow (0 - 10%) of patients with overt iron deficiency anemia.

The picture of iron deficiency anemia may be further altered by the concomitance of other pathologic conditions (*complicated iron deficiency anemia*) [228] (hemolytic disorders, diseases associated with a decreased red cell formation such as infections and cancer).

3.6. Abnormalities of the globin synthesis

3.6.1. Thalassemia syndromes

The thalassemias constitute a group of inherited disorders characterized by a decreased rate of globin chain

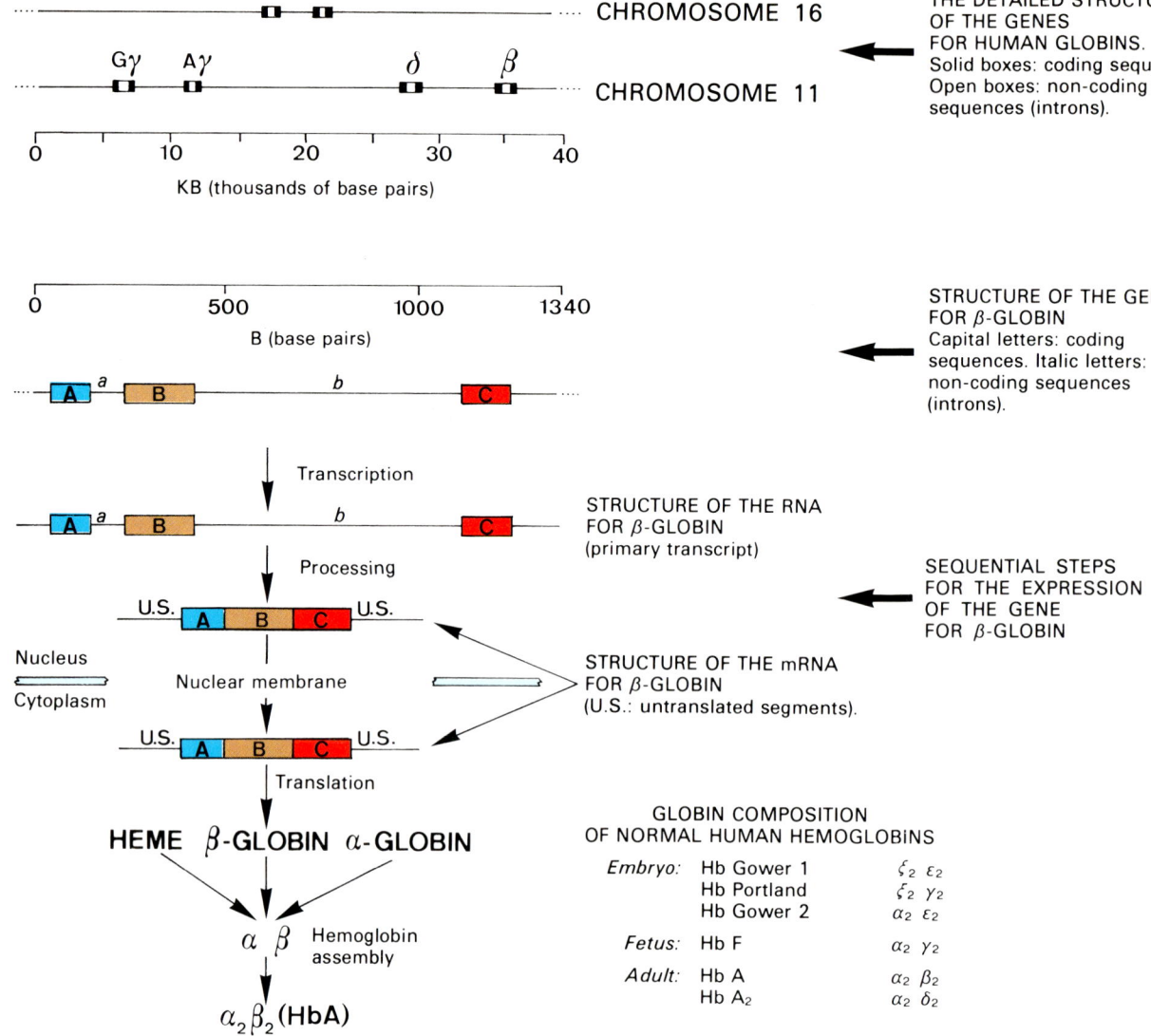

Fig. 51 Diagrammatic summary of current information on the structure, organization, and expression of the genes for human globins [229-233]. Advances in knowledge about the molecular defects recognize some distinct possible pathogenetic mechanisms of the thalassemic disorders, such as a deletion of genes for globin synthesis, a defective RNA transcription, a suppression of translation of mRNA (**arrows**). These mechanisms are known to be operative in some of the recognized forms of thalassemias. Courtesy of Prof. F. Conconi, Institute of Biochemistry, University of Ferrara.

production. The pathogenetic mechanisms are illustrated in **Figure 51**.

Since the rate of either α- or β-chain synthesis may be affected, two main types of thalassemia are recognized, α- and β-thalassemia respectively, with variants caused by distinct molecular defects [234-236] (**Fig. 52**).

The severity of the clinical expression of thalassemias will be defined here according to traditional terminology [246-249]. *Thalassemia major* is the most severe form which corresponds to the condition first reported by Cooley in 1925 and which includes most of the homozygous conditions. *Thalassemia minor* is a term applied to clinical states characterized by a milder degree of anemia and arising from a single gene involvement, as in heterozygotes. However, since there is a wide range of fluctuation in the clinical severity, the term of *thalassemia intermedia* has been introduced for those conditions which have manifestations that lie between the *major* and the *minor*

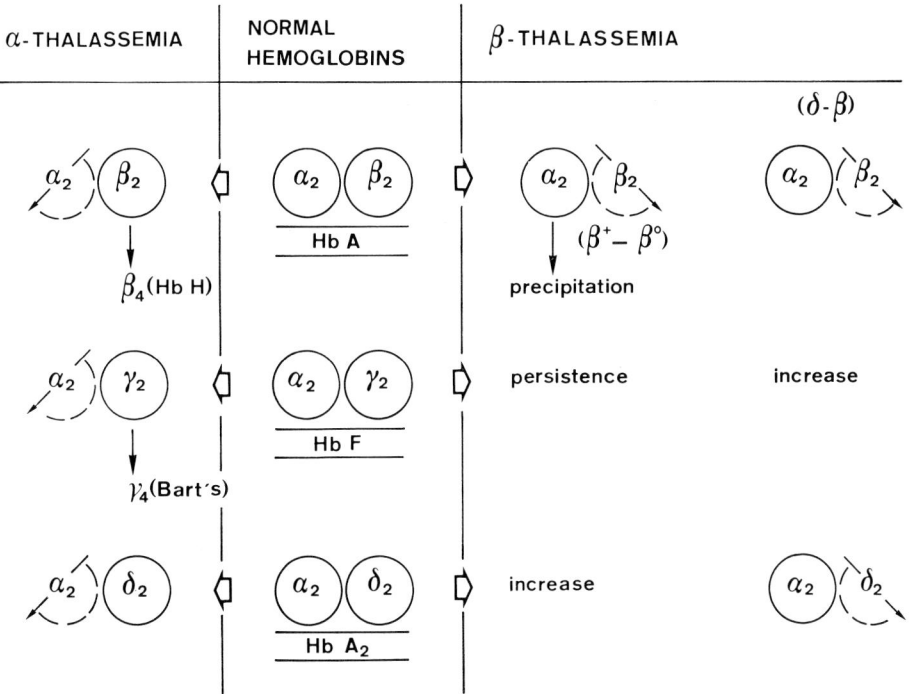

Fig. 52 β-thalassemias are characterized by a curtailed production of Hb A ($\beta_2\alpha_2$) and by an overwhelming production of α chains. Since γ and δ chain synthesis is not affected, there is an increased level of Hb F and Hb A_2 in thalassemia major and minor respectively. Advances in molecular biology have shown that the β-chain production may be totally absent or significantly reduced, allowing the identification of two principal varieties of β-thalassemia major, the β° and the β⁺ respectively. These variants are not due to the deletion of β-genes, but possibly to absent or reduced β-chain mRNA, with a few exceptions, as in thalassemia Ferrara [237] in which a defective translation of mRNA for β-globin is operative.
Another group of β-thalassemias is characterized by a reduced synthesis of β and δ chains (δ-β-thalassemia); this variant probably recognizes a gene deletion [238]. Furthermore some β-thalassemic disorders may arise from insufficiently synthesized abnormal globin chains (fusion variants of δ-β chains) known as Lepore hemoglobins [239, 240]. All these groups show several subvariants.
Involvement of the α-genes, in α-thalassemias, affects the synthesis of all of the normal hemoglobins (Hb A, Hb F, Hb A_2). Thus the presence of a reduced amount of α-chains allows the formation of tetramers of γ-chains (γ_4-Hb Bart's) in children and β-chains in the adults (β_4-Hb H). The amount of these hemoglobins depends on the degree of the α-chain defect [241-243].
Available data suggest the existence of four α-chain genes whose variable loss of function is responsible for the different types of α-thalassemias [244]. Deletion of α-genes results into a lethal condition ("Hydrops fetalis") characterized by the absence of α-chain synthesis and the presence of Bart's hemoglobin. The presence of 2 of 4 α-chain genes is associated with a mild clinical condition, the α-thalassemia trait (hypochromia and microcytosis without anemia), whereas no hematologic abnormalities are seen in the "silent carrier state" in which the presence of three active α-genes is suggested. The presence of only one active α-chain gene leads to hemoglobin H disease, a condition characterized by an increased amount of β_4 tetramers in adults (Hb H). However some cases of hemoglobin H disease appear to arise from heterozygous conditions between α-thalassemia and hemoglobin Constant Springs [245] which represent a terminal mutation of the α-chain and is connected with a reduced α-chain output.

forms. Thalassemia intermedia encompasses a series of disorders which range from the homozygous β-thalassemia of mild variety (as in Africans), to the double heterozygous (e.g. β-and δ β-thalassemia, α- and β-thalassemia) and to the association of β-thalassemia with hemoglobin variants involving β-chains, or even to some acquired clinical conditions such as severe folate deficiency [244].

These clinical distinctive patterns also apply to the morphological patterns of blood and bone marrow which, to some extent, correlate with the severity of the disease.

Pathophysiology of the morphological features. The morphological features of the thalassemia syndromes correlate with the degree of the erythropoietic dysfunction (ineffective erythropoiesis).

Anemia is a consequence of a decreased hemoglobin content in individual red cells which in turn is due to a defect in the synthesis of globin chains.

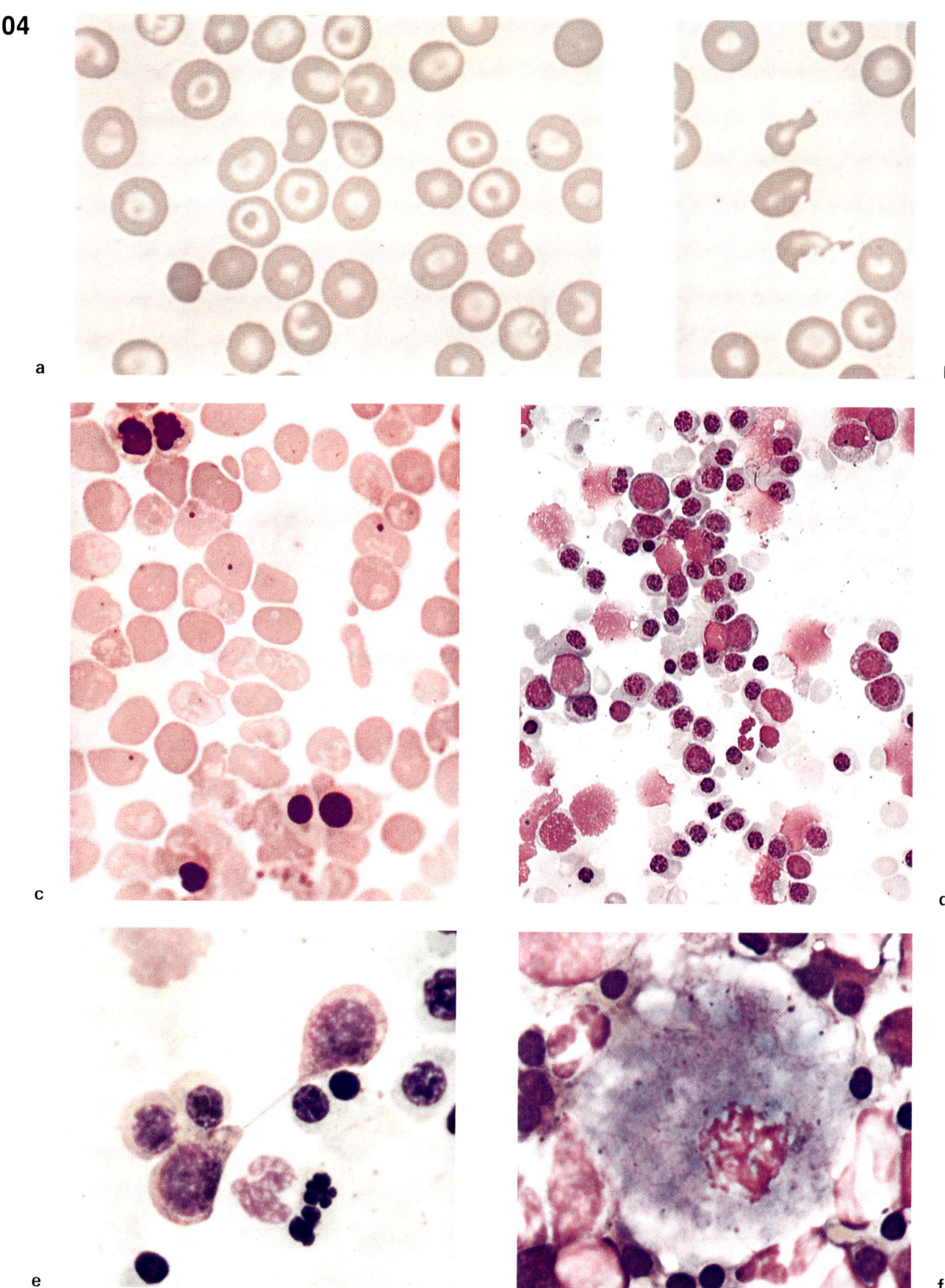

Fig. 53 a-f) Heterozygous β-thalassemia (thalassemia minor). There are many target cells and moderate anisopoikilocytosis (microcytes, tear-drop forms, schizocytes) (**a, b**). Nucleated red cells are observed after splenectomy, often in association with Howell-Jolly bodies (**c**) (see **Fig. 17**).
d, e, f) The bone marrow shows an erythroblastic hyperplasia (**d**) with orderly maturation. Some erythroid elements display filamentous connections as a consequence of fast regenerative processes (**e**). Reticulum cells may be numerous and contain several phagocytosed debris; they may exhibit a diffuse bluish cytoplasm (**f**).

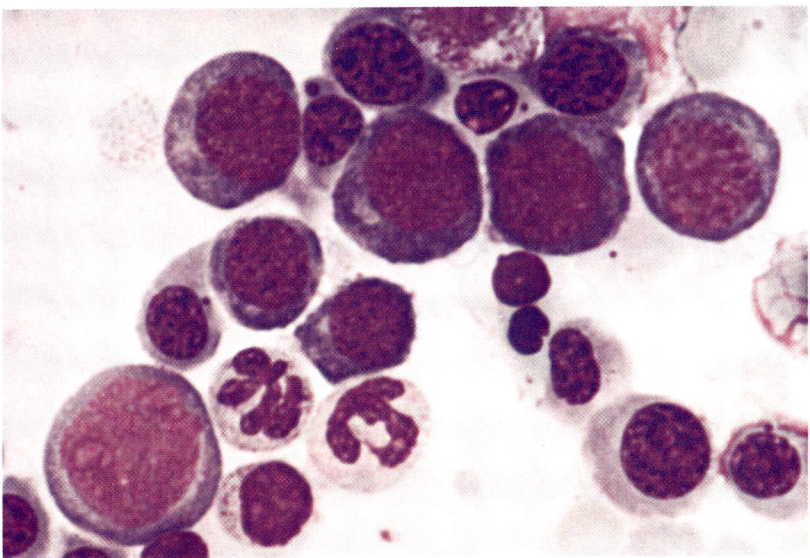

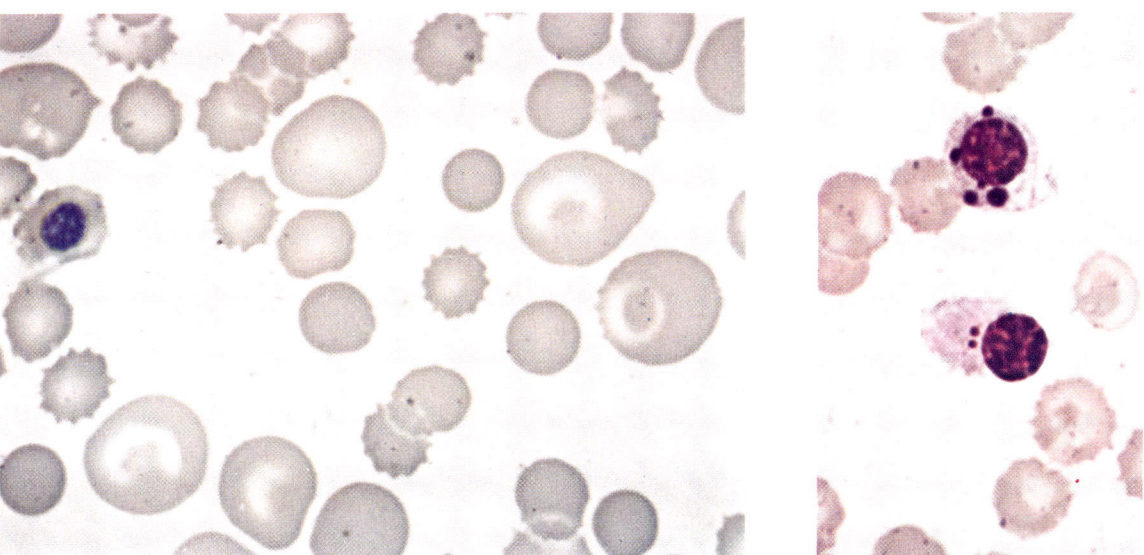

Fig. 54 a-c) *Heterozygous β-thalassemia associated with severe folic acid deficiency (thalassemia intermedia). In this case the morphological features are similar to those observed in β-thalassemia minor. However dyserythropoiesis is more frankly expressed and associated with megaloblastic changes in the marrow and in the blood (**a, b**). Nucleated red cell precursors are present in the circulation and often exhibit karyorrhexic nuclei (**c**).*

However, since there is imbalance in globin chain production, i.e. the unaffected globin chains continue to be synthesized at a normal rate, they accumulate and precipitate thereby damaging the cells and giving rise to the inclusions illustrated in **Figures 17-21**. Such inclusions are "pitted" by a healthy spleen leaving highly deformed cells (see **Figs. 24** and **25**). Such cells have a shortened lifespan aggravating the anemia. This in turn stimulates erythropoietin production which results in further marrow hyperplasia and metabolic disturbances, e.g. excessive folate consumption causing "megaloblastoid" changes, and excessive iron deposition from destroyed red cells (**Figs. 54 a-c**).

Morphological patterns. The most common morphological features of the thalassemic disorders are illustrated in **Figures 53-55** (for Hb H disease see **Fig. 21 c**). All these pictures may be significantly modified by the association with other disorders, such as hemoglobinopathies, or by some concomitant metabolic deficiencies (iron or folic acid).

Cytochemical studies have been conducted mainly on the cells of patients with β-thalassemia. A proportion of erythroblasts

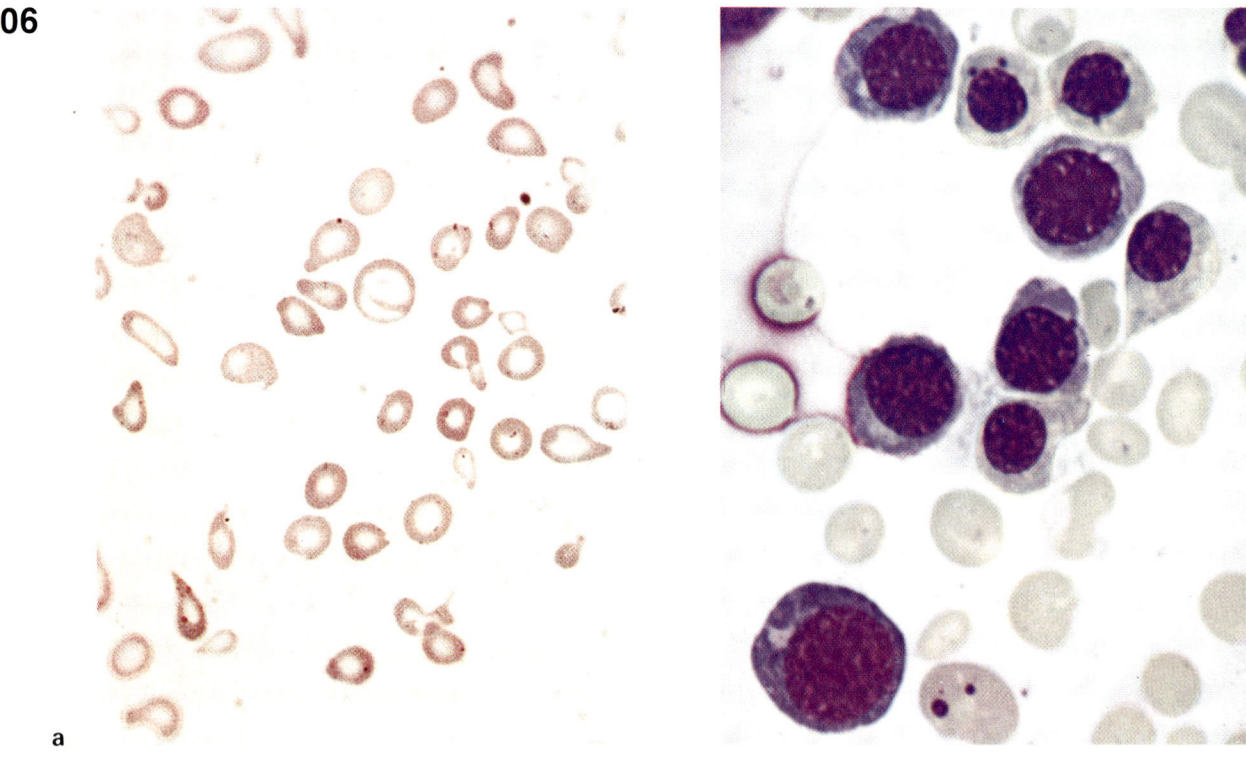

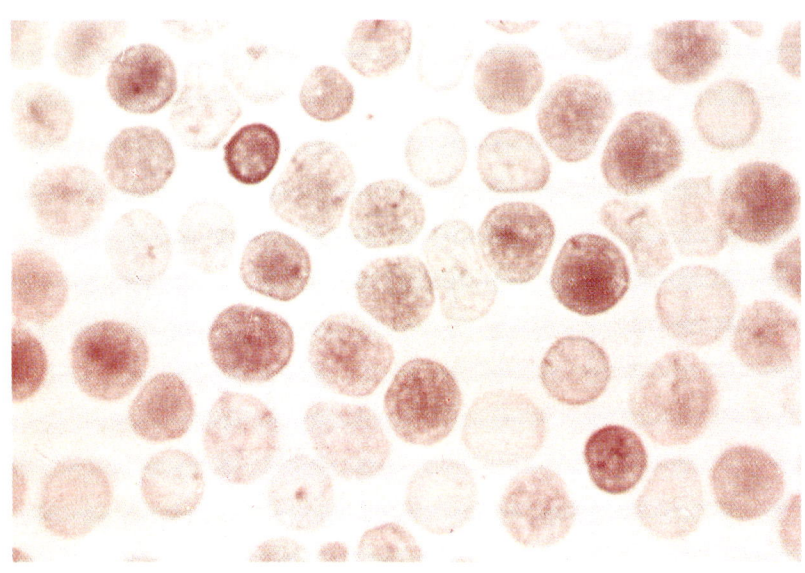

Fig. 55 a, b) Homozygous β-thalassemia (16 year old patient).

a) Anisopoikilocytosis (presence of microspherocytes, macrocytes, fragmented cells, and other bizarre shapes with cigar or tear-drop forms). Basophilic stippling is a common feature. Nucleated red cell precursors are present in the blood (mainly after splenectomy), and exhibit occasional mitotic figures.

b) The bone marrow exhibits gross erythroblastic hyperplasia; many cells show karyorrhexic nuclei and vacuolated cytoplasm. Megaloblastic changes are sometimes observed, as in this patient.

c) An increased level of fetal hemoglobin (Hb F) is characteristically present in homozygous β-thalassemia and may be detected in other thalassemia syndromes. Hb F is randomly distributed among the red cells, as demonstrated by the Kleihauer and Betke's acid elution test. Hb F containing cells ("Hb F cells") appear deeply stained. Thalassemic disorders should be distinguished from other clinical conditions characterized by the persistence of Hb F in adult life ("hereditary persistence of fetal hemoglobin", HPFH) [250] in which a homogeneous distribution of Hb F among the red cells occurs (Negro and Greek variants).

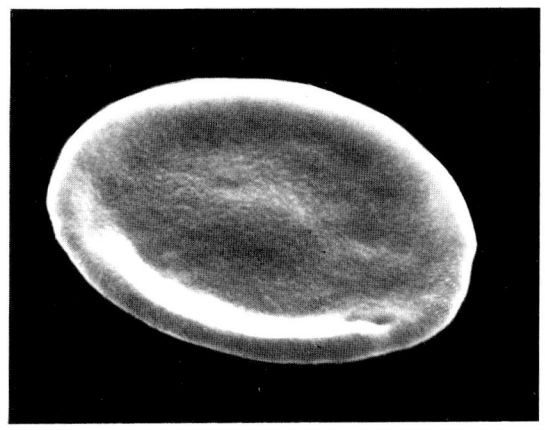
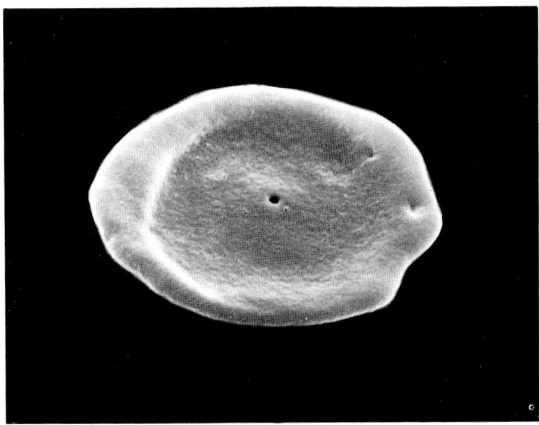
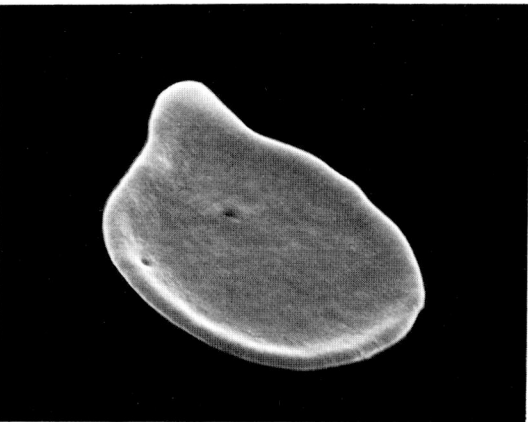

Fig. 56 a-d) Different features of the erythrocytes in patients with heterozygous β-thalassemia as viewed by scanning electron microscopy. Most of the cells are cup-shaped (codocytes) (× 5,200).

contain PAS-positive material [251, 252] which is probably glycogen.
The distribution of PAS-positive materials may be diffuse or in small dots, as revealed by the application of fluorescent Schiff reagents [253]. The number of positive cells increases with the maturity of the erythroblasts and is usually higher in thalassemia major in comparison with the other forms. There is an increased amount of stainable iron in the marrow.

Sideroblasts as well as hemosiderin laden macrophages are commonly seen.

Electron microscope studies of the erythroblasts and circulating red cells of patients with homozygous β-thalassemia have shown a series of abnormalities which are mostly related to reduced hemoglobin synthesis [254, 255]. The most distinctive features are cytoplasmic and intranuclear α-chain precipitates and the accumulation of iron either as free ferritin in the cytoplasm or as clusters within the mitochondria or in membrane bound vacuoles.
The red cells exhibit bizarre shapes with prominent indentations and elongated projections. In most cells, remnants of organelles (ferritin deposits, degenerated mitochondria, myelin figures) are still detectable (**Fig. 56**).

The fine structure of macrophages [256] in the bone marrow of thalassemic patients has been reviewed [257].

Figs. 56 e, f) Represent whole cells as seen by SEM.
g, h) Represent thin sections of similar cells.
Although SEM affords a better appreciation of the cell surface, TEM reveals cytoplasmic precipitates, remnants of organelles, and other inclusions (SEM, × 5,200; TEM, × 14,000).

3 ERYTHROCYTES

Figs. 56 i, j) *Ultrastructure of erythrocytes from a patient with homozygous β-thalassemia exhibits highly irregular contours, large vacuoles, degenerated organelles and siderosomes of different size (× 14,000).*

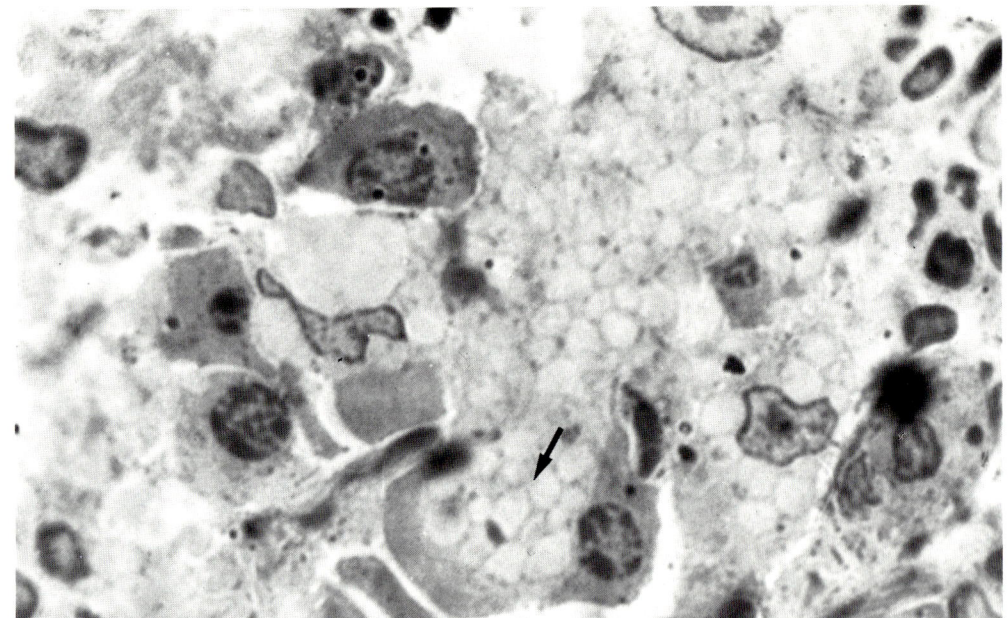

Fig. 57 a) Storage cell in the spleen of a thalassemic patient (homozygous β-thalassemia). **Arrow** indicates a cell in which the nucleus is displaced and the cytoplasm is filled with round-shaped bodies. (Semi-thin section stained with toluidine blue).

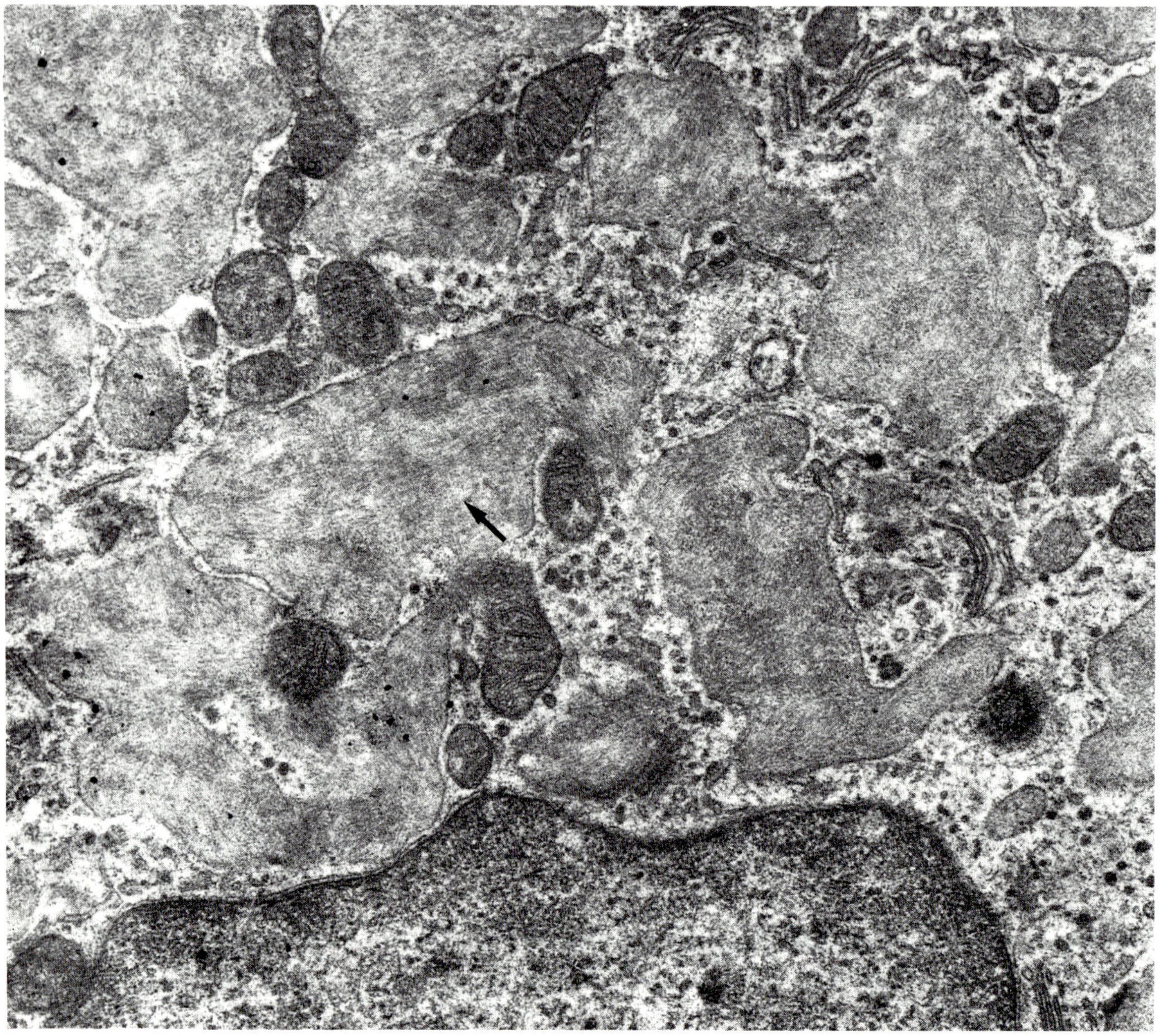

b) Ultrastructural features of a storage cell containing material with fibrillar structure (**arrow**). Mitochondria and rough endoplasmic reticulum are dispersed throughout the cytoplasm ($\times$ 5,000).
Courtesy of Prof. G. Fabris, University of Ferrara.

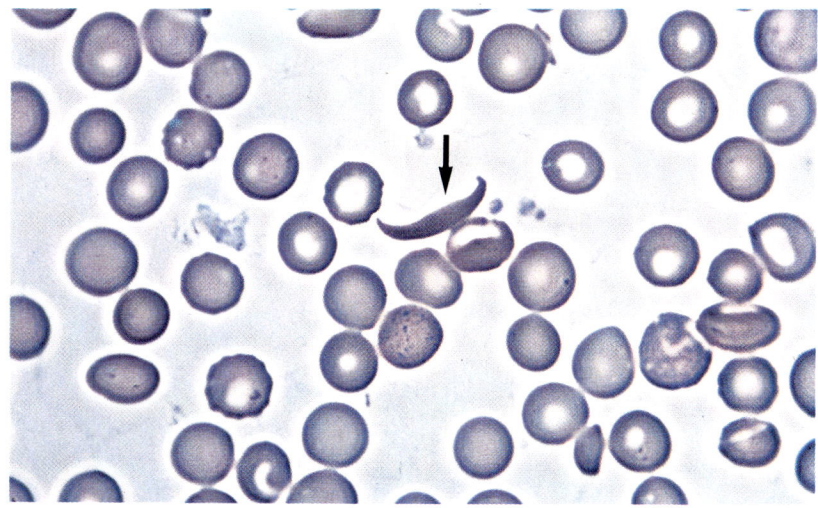

Fig. 58 *Elongated sickle-shaped red cell (**arrow**) observed in a blood smear (phase contrast). Courtesy of Prof. A.M. Marmont, S. Martino's Hospital, Genova.*

These cells appear to be located close to collagen fibers and to project some cytoplasmic processes into sinusoids where they appear to phagocytose portions of adjacent erythroblasts containing precipitated α-chains. By means of this mechanism precipitated α-chains may be eliminated from the erythroblasts, avoiding irreversible damage.

The splenic macrophages may look like foamy cells [258] as is the case in chronic myeloid leukemia or idiopathic thrombocytopenic purpura [259] or other conditions associated with excessive red cell destruction and incomplete digestion of erythrocytes [258] (see **Fig. 57**).

3.6.2. Abnormal hemoglobin: sickle cell anemia

Amino acid substitution in the hemoglobin molecule may alter its function and lead to aggregation of the pathological hemoglobin under a variety of conditions such as lowered oxygen tension or acidosis (sickling phenomenon) [260].
Sickle cell anemia (due to the replacement of glutamic acid by valine at position 6 at the N-terminal end of the β-chain [261, 262]), is the most common disorder among the aggregating hemoglobinopathies with clinical relevance (C, D, Hb S/thalassemia).
In sickle cell disease, anemia is usually severe with normocytic or even macrocytic features, associated with anisopoikilocytosis. Occasional sickle cells appear spontaneously in dry smears [263] (**Fig. 58**). The shape changes may be reversible after exposure to oxygen. However, once the deoxygenated Hb S has formed fibrils (see **Fig. 61**), the cells are probably irreversibly sickled.

This may be due to membrane alterations, e.g. loss of potassium in the early phase [264], increase in membrane Ca content in advanced stages [265, 266] or alterations in phosphorylation of the membrane constituents [267].

The sickling phenomenon is elicited by incubating red cells under lowered oxygen tension on a slide, under a sealed cover slip, or after addition of reducing substances which accelerate the precipitation of hemoglobin [268] (**Fig. 59**).

Irreversibly sickled cells are the principal cause for increased viscosity of the blood [269, 270]. Intravascular agglutination may be responsible for occlusion of small vessels in different organs. The clinical counterparts of such biophysical alteration of the red cell shape are manifested by leg ulcers, splenic, bone, and lung infarcts, renal dysfunction and abnormalities of the retinal vessels [271, 273] (**Fig. 60**).

The ultrastructural features of sickle cells are characterized by an arrangement of microtubular rods which are oriented in the long axes of the spicules (**Fig. 61**).

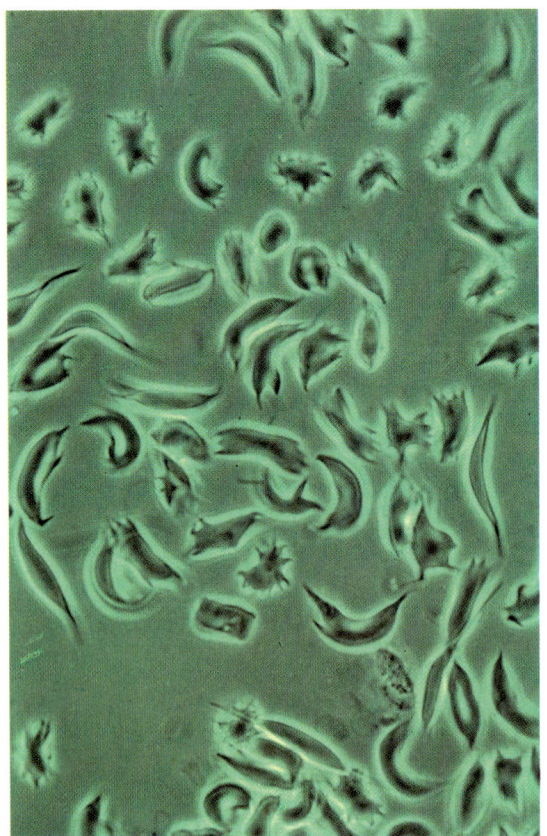 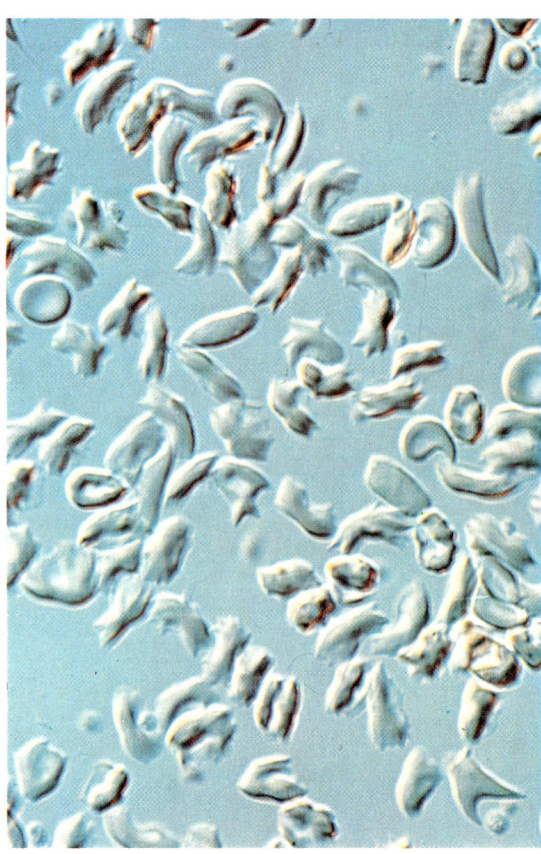

Fig. 59 Phase contrast (**a**) and interference microscopy (Nomarsky optics) (**b**) observations of sealed films of blood of the same patient. Holly-leaf sickling is seen.
Courtesy of Prof. A.M. Marmont, S. Martino's Hospital, Genova.

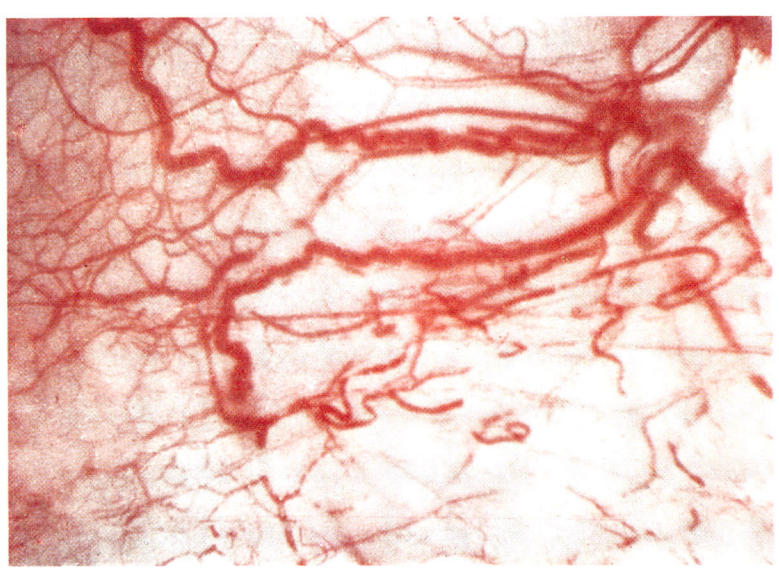

Fig. 60 Retinal vessels in sickle cell anemia showing segmentation believed to be due to sludging of clumped erythrocytes.
Courtesy of Prof. A.M. Marmont, S. Martino's Hospital, Genova.

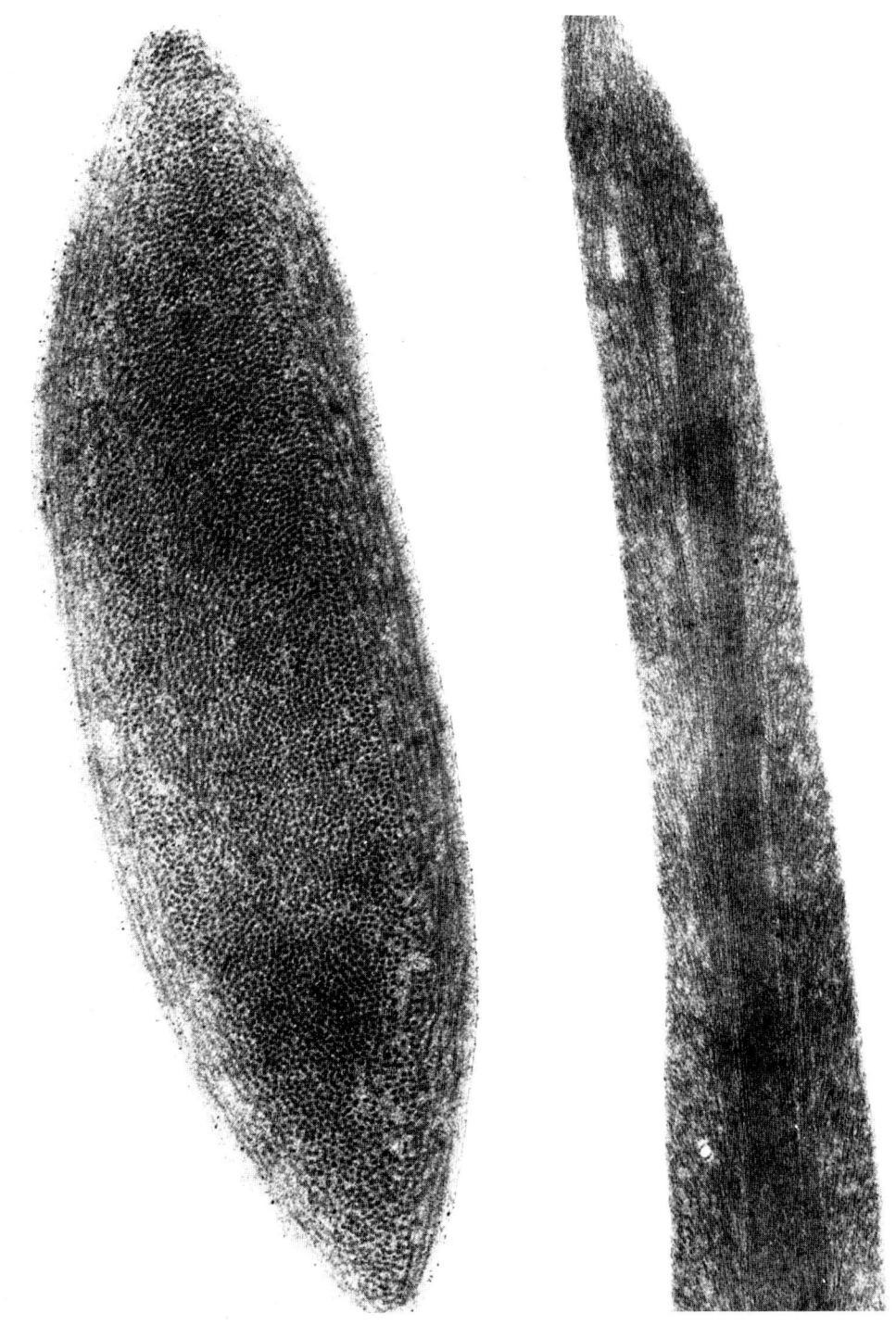

Fig. 61 Electron micrographs of sections of "irreversibly sickled" SS erythrocytes containing fibers composed of molecules of deoxygenated Hb S. As oxygenated "irreversibly sickled" cells do not contain fibers, they more properly should be referred to as "irreversibly deformed". Fibers are shown in cross section in **a** and, longitudinally in **b**. It should be noted that this regularity of parallel arrangement of fibers is usually confined to deoxygenated SS erythrocytes with an abnormal MCHC, whereas the fibers lie at random in deoxygenated SS cells with a normal MCHC (**a**, × 57,000; **b**, × 26,000).
Reproduced from Döbler, J. and Bertles, J.F., J. Exp. Med. 127: 711, 1968, with permission of the Authors and Publisher.

Rods are postulated to be formed by inter-twining in a helical structure of six filaments consisting of linearly polymerized molecules of deoxygenated hemoglobin [274]. The linear aggregation of sickle cell hemoglobin is not completely understood. It has been suggested that the valine-valine cyclization of the N-terminal end of the β-chain may lead to a key-like structure of the surface of the β-chain allowing a link with sites of the adjacent hemoglobin molecule [275].

3.6.3. Unstable hemoglobins

Maintenance of normal globin chain structure and, in particular, the area of the "pocket" containing the heme binding site appears to be of primary importance for the stability of the hemoglobin molecule. Substitution or deletions of amino acids in β- and α-chains at the site or in the proximity of heme binding is probably responsible for the instability of some hemoglobins to heating or oxidative stress [276-278].

Clinically overt hemolytic anemia is usually reflected on routine blood smears whereas milder abnormalities require special techniques for diagnosis. As in other hemolytic anemias microspherocytosis and polychromasia are the most common signs in the peripheral blood.

4. HYPERPROLIFERATIVE AND NEOPLASTIC ERYTHROPOIESIS

4.1. Acute erythremic myelosis and erythroleukemia

Autonomous proliferation of red cell precursors is seen in a series of related disorders: acute erythremic myelosis [279, 280], chronic erythremic myelosis [85, 86], acute erythroleukemia. These conditions have been collected under the name Di Guglielmo syndrome [281, 282]. Since these conditions are closely associated with the myeloproliferative syndromes in that the granulocytic and the megakaryocytic cell lines are usually also affected, the term "Di Guglielmo disease" is reserved for cases in which abnormal proliferation is manifested predominantly or exclusively in the erythroid line. It should be mentioned, however, that some morphologic overlap also exists between erythroleukemia and idiopathic sideroblastic anemia [283].

Morphologic features

A description of the pathology associated with erythremic myelosis will be limited to the red cell series in this chapter (**Figs. 62, 63**). The reader is referred to Chapters 4 and 10 for illustrations of granulocyte, megakaryocyte and platelet abnormalities in the myeloproliferative syndromes.

The marrow is often hypercellular with selective hyperplasia of the nucleated red cell precursors which recall aspects of megaloblastic anemia and exhibit nuclear and cytoplasmatic abnormalities [284-286].

Red cell morphology in the peripheral blood is not much affected, although some degree of macrocytosis may be observed. Nucleated red cells are almost invariably present, often exhibiting karyorrhexis.

Fig. 62 a-e) *Acute erythremic myelosis. The bone marrow is marked by a prominent erythroid hyperplasia (a). Basophilic proerythroblasts and erythroblasts are accumulating as a consequence of maturation arrest in the erythroid series. Some cells are large and highly polyploid and may present nuclear aberrations, including multinuclearity, irregular chromatin separation, persistence of nucleoli. Such abnormalities are mostly limited to basophilic erythroid elements, but they may be less frequently found, even in partially hemoglobinized cells (b, c). Chromosomes appear to form round-shaped masses of clumped chromatin (d, e). In a few instances erythroblastic or red cell phagocytosis has been seen.*

115

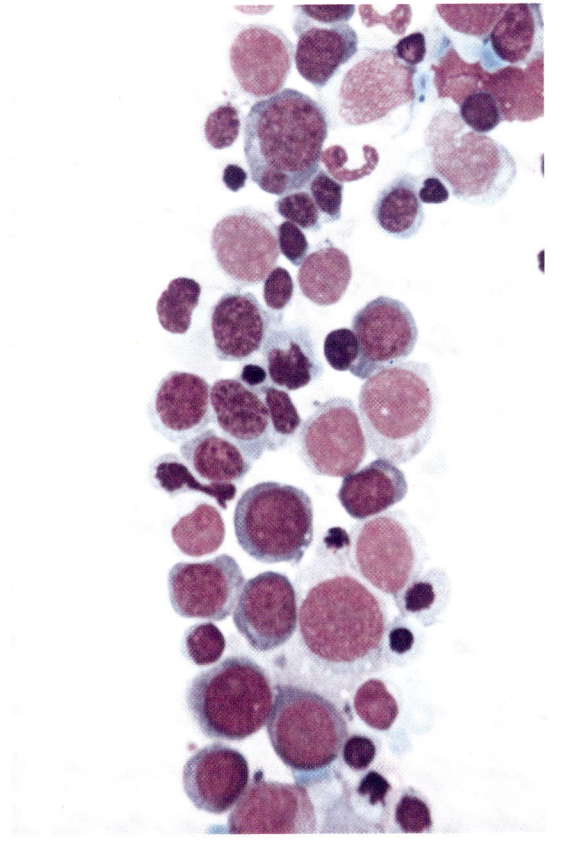

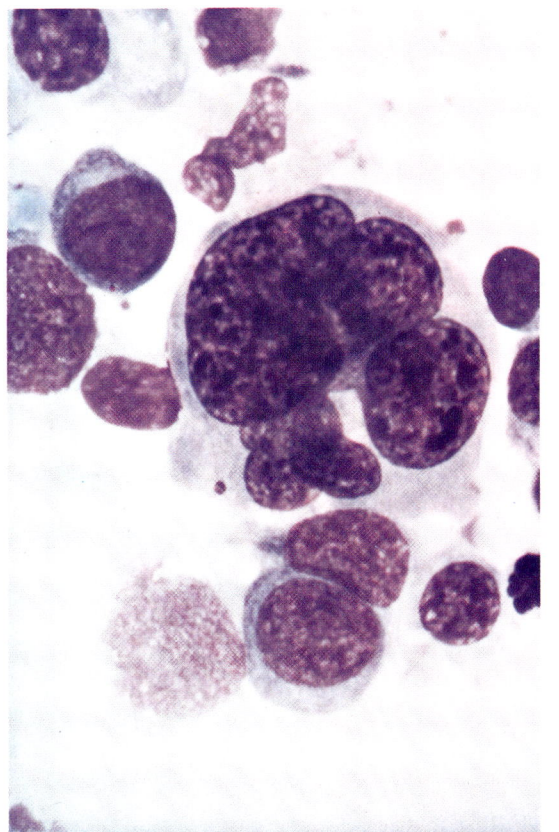

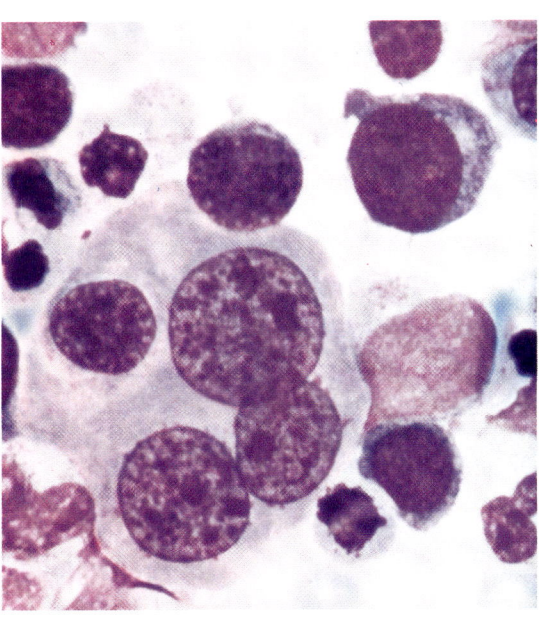

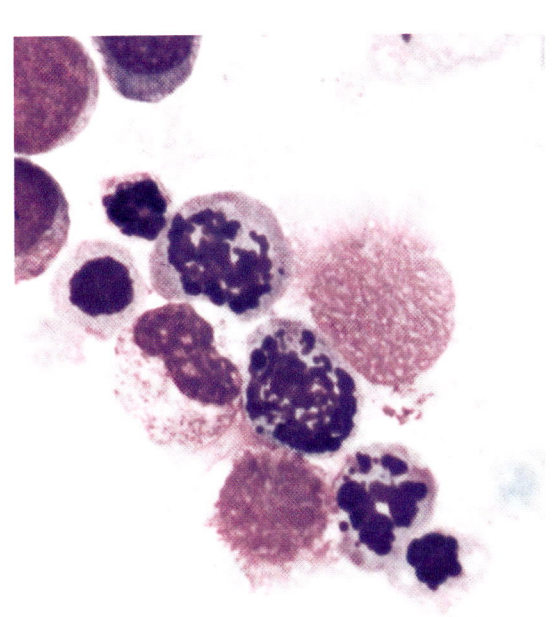

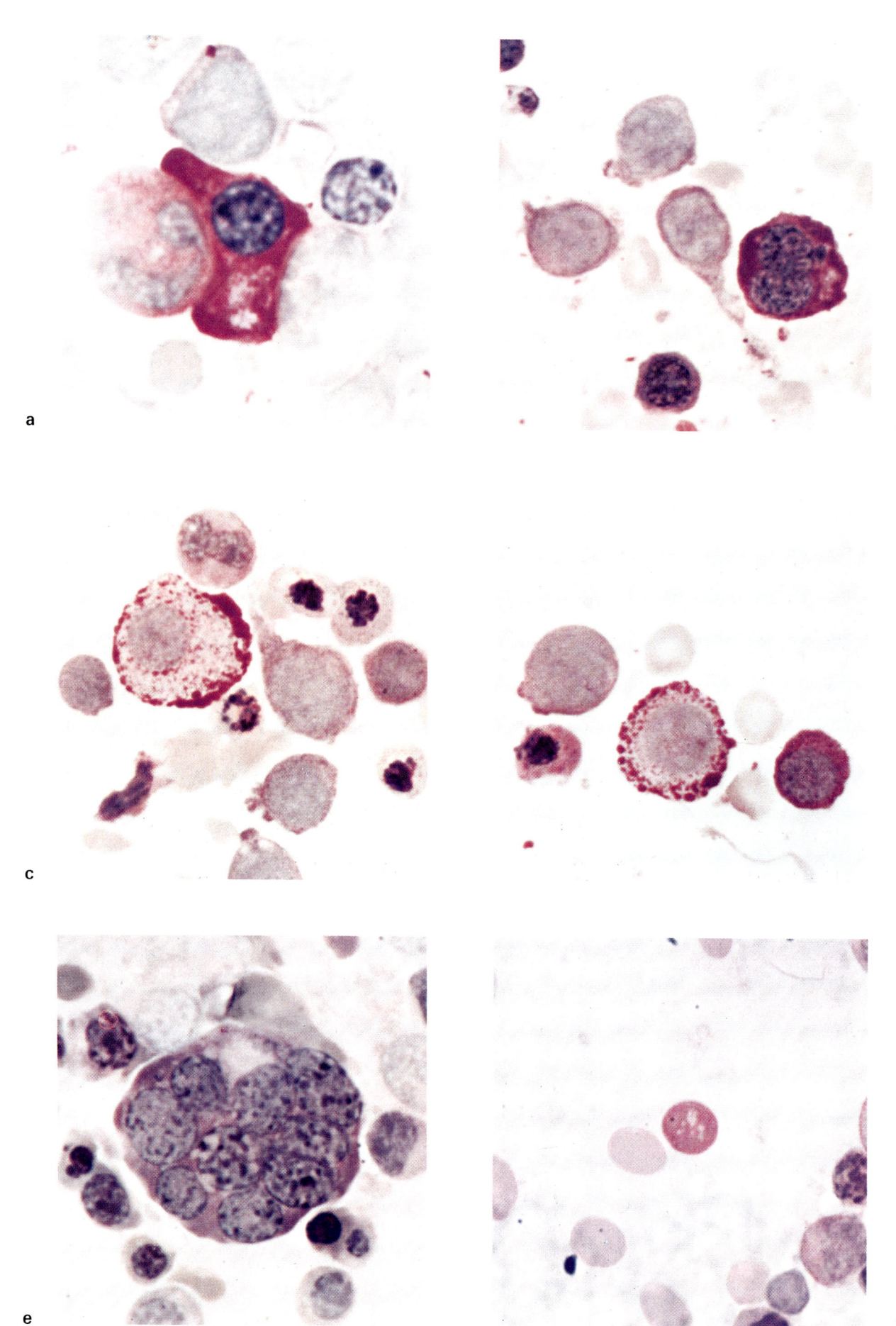

3 ERYTHROCYTES

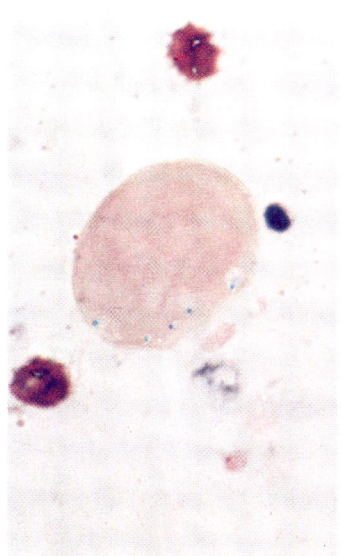
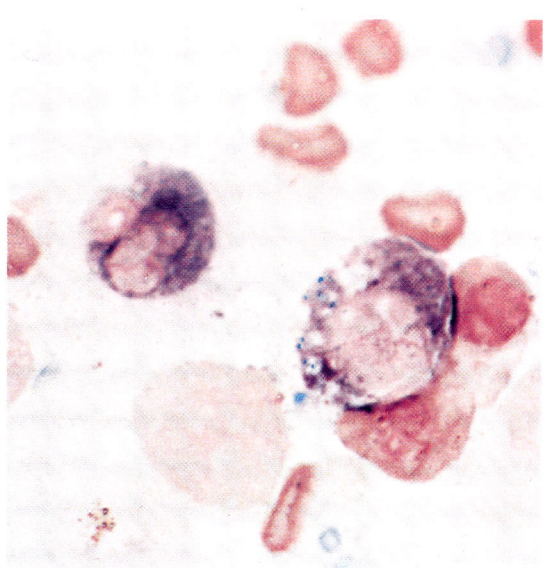

Fig. 64 Combined staining for AS-D-chloroacetate esterase and Prussian blue reaction on a bone marrow smear from a patient with acute erythremic myelosis.
a) Iron granules stained within vacuoles of the cytoplasm of a cell with negative reaction for specific esterase.
b) Iron granules with same distribution as in the former cell; the cytoplasm shows a positive reaction for specific esterase.

Most of the erythroid cells display an intense PAS reaction, with a variable pattern [287, 288]. A diffuse reaction is usually observed in more mature cells.

Since the intensity of PAS staining is weakened after amylase digestion, it has been suggested that the substance responsible for the staining is related to glycogen. However, other observations have suggested that PAS-positive material may be represented by glycoproteins [289] (**Fig. 63**).

As any other disorder characterized by the presence of dyserythropoietic features, erythremic myelosis presents sideroblastic cells, some with ringed features. Furthermore, a clearly increased perinuclear non specific esterase activity has been observed, mainly in mature erythroblasts, and a prominent acid phosphatase activity has been localized in a narrow zone near the nuclear membrane of the young erythroid cells.

Some erythroid precursors may demonstrate specific esterase activity (AS-D-chloroacetate esterase [290]). Since this enzyme is usually associated with cells of granulocytic origin, it has been suggested that the primitive erythroid precursors in erythremic myelosis may share some metabolic properties with the myeloid series. This suggestion has gained support by the simultaneous demonstration of prussian blue precipitates in cells which are positive for specific esterases (**Fig. 64**). Alternatively, some primitive erythroid-like cells may actually be elements of the monocytic series (promonocytes) which exhibit the capacity to phagocytose iron particles as in other hypersiderotic disorders [291, 292].

Fig. 63 a-d) Variable features of the distribution of the PAS reaction in the erythroblasts of erythremic myelosis.
a, b): Diffuse strongly positive reaction.
c, d): Intense granular positivity.
e) Giant multinucleated erythroblast showing a weakly positive PAS reaction.
f) Erythrocytes from peripheral blood exhibiting a diffuse intense positivity for the PAS reaction.

Table 3 MARKER STUDIES IN ERYTHROLEUKEMIA
(6 CASES)

Anti-cALL	—
Anti-granulocyte	—
Anti-T	—
Anti-p28,33 (HLA-DR)	—
Anti-Ig	—
Anti-glycophorin	+
Anti-spectrin	+
E (sheep) rosettes	—
TdT	—

Unpublished data of J. Robinson and M. Greaves, Imperial Cancer Research Fund, London.

See Part 2 of Chapter 8 for details of these membrane markers and TdT (Terminal deoxynucleotidyl Transferase).

These confusing abnormalities may be elucidated by means of membrane markers and enzyme analyses which may define the phenotype of various erythroleukemic cells more precisely [293]. Table 3 presents a list of such tests currently in use for this purpose.

The ultrastructural features of erythremic cells resemble those of the normal erythroid series [50, 285, 294, 295]. The immature red cell precursors are usually larger than the normal proerythroblasts and often show a vacuolated cytoplasm, an increased number of mitochondria and accumulation of glycogen. The nuclei of these cells are devoided of peripheral chromatin condensation and show large nucleoli.

With increasing maturity more nuclear-cytoplasmic asynchrony may develop. Mitochondria may still be present in large number and contain ferrugenous aggregates which resemble those seen in sideroblastic anemias. Late erythroid cells contain glycogen particles which may be dispersed throughout the cytoplasm or clumped together, paralleling the cytochemical distribution of the PAS-positivity.

4.2. Polycythemia vera

Polycythemia vera (PV) is a clonal hemopoietic stem cell disorder [296, 297] which may be included in the spectrum of myeloproliferative syndromes (**Fig. 65**). However some prominent features involving red cells, such as the absolute erythrocytosis, deserve consideration in this chapter.

Changes in red cell morphology parallel the different patterns of erythropoiesis during the course of the disease [298]. Erythropoiesis is orderly and usually confined to intramedullary sites in the early phases of the disease. In more advanced stages it involves extramedullary tissues [299-301]. Erythroid hyperplasia may be accompanied by some ultrastructural abnormalities which are common to most dyserythropoietic disorders (nuclear blebs and clefts, enlargement of nuclear pores) (**Fig. 65**). Red cell morphology is marked by aniso-poikilocytosis, ovalocytosis, elliptocytosis.

The appearance of morphologically abnormal cells with progression of the disease appears to go hand in hand with the emergence of a population of cells that are hypersensitive to erythropoietin and, therefore, have a growth advantage over normal cells [302].

Fig. 65 a) Low power view of a polycythemic bone marrow. All cell lines are shown but megakaryocytes are particularly prominent.
b) Ultrastructural features of the bone marrow in polycythemia vera (florid phase). Nucleated erythroid precursors are abundant and show orderly maturation. Cells indicated by **1**, **2**, **3** illustrate sequential maturation of erythroblasts (× 4,000).
Courtesy Dr. J. Thiele, Department of Medicine, University of Hannover.

3 ERYTHROCYTES 119

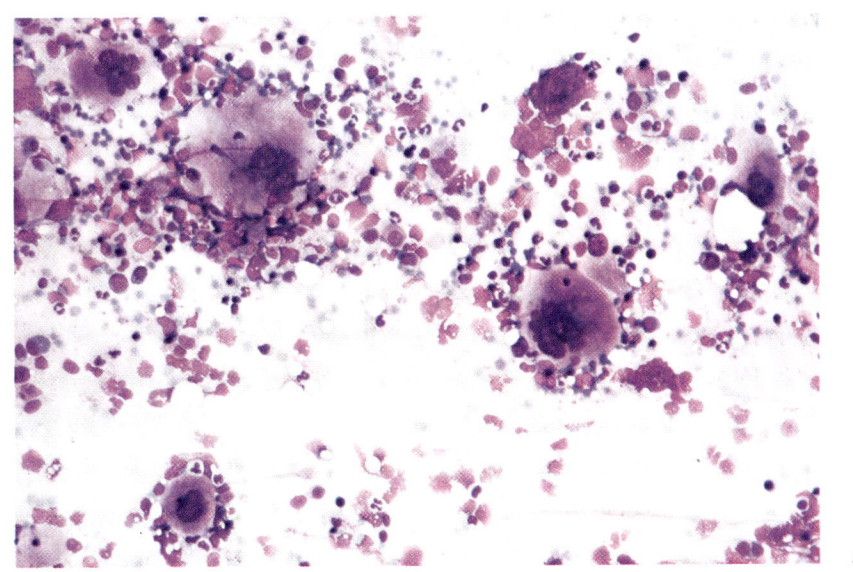

a

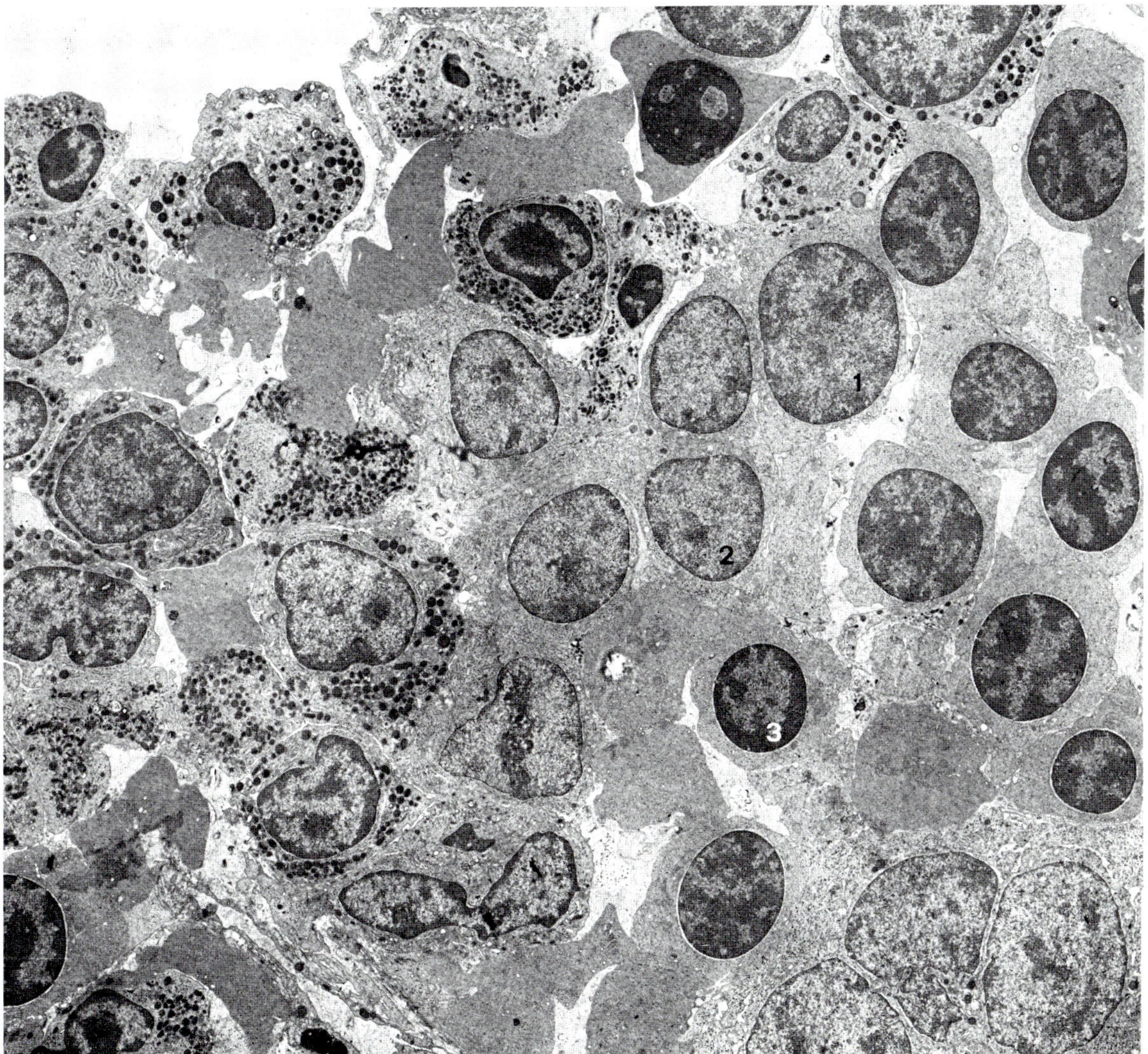

b

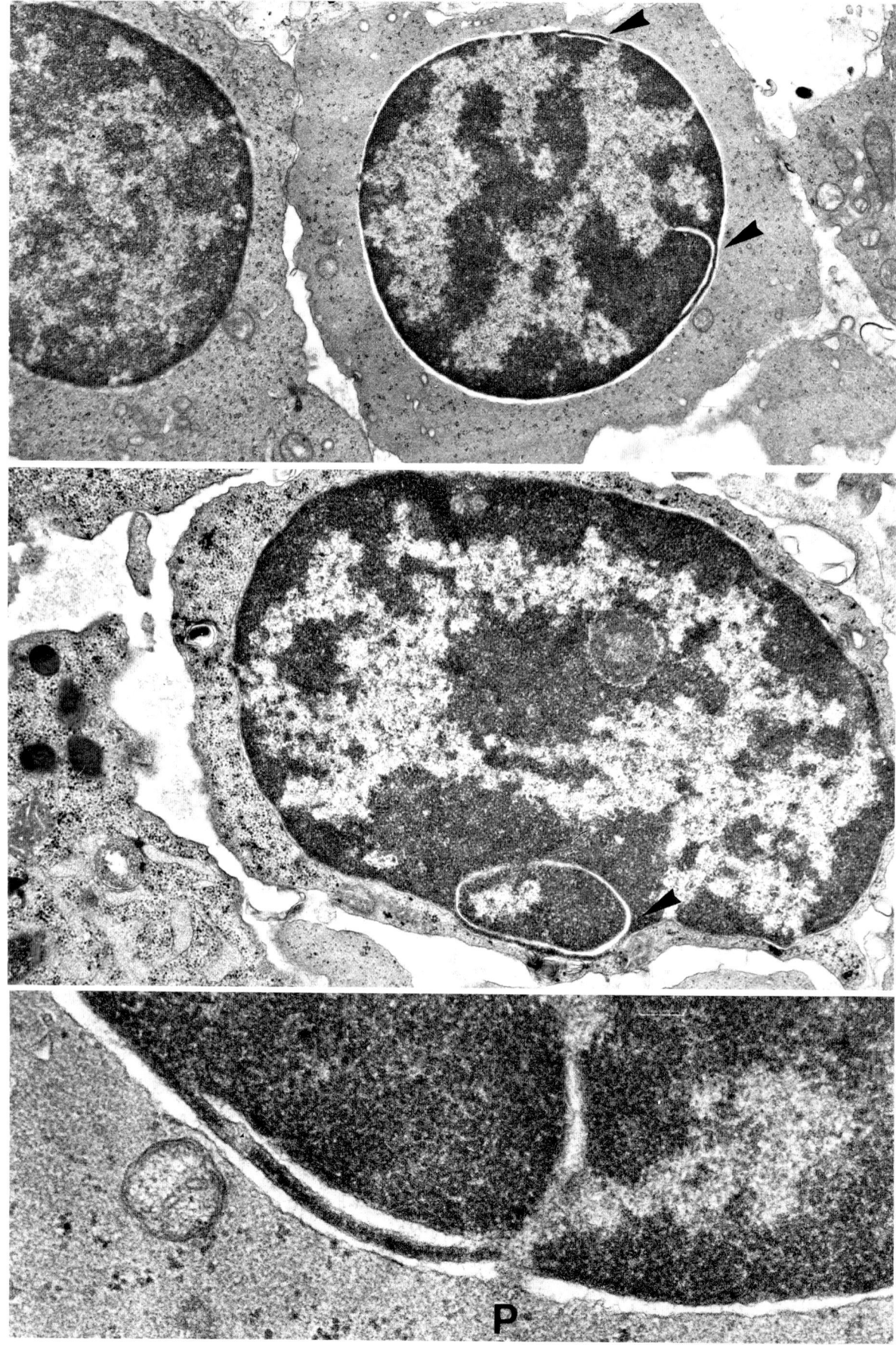

Fig. 65 c) Nuclear clefts (**arrowheads**) in erythroblasts of the marrow of a patient with polycythemia vera. A chromatin bridge is seen in association with a nuclear pore complex (**P**). Dyserythropoietic aspects are more commonly observed in the advanced stages of the disorder (**top**, × 13,000; **middle**, × 18,500; **bottom**, × 60,000). Courtesy of Dr. J. Thiele, Department of Medicine, University of Hannover.

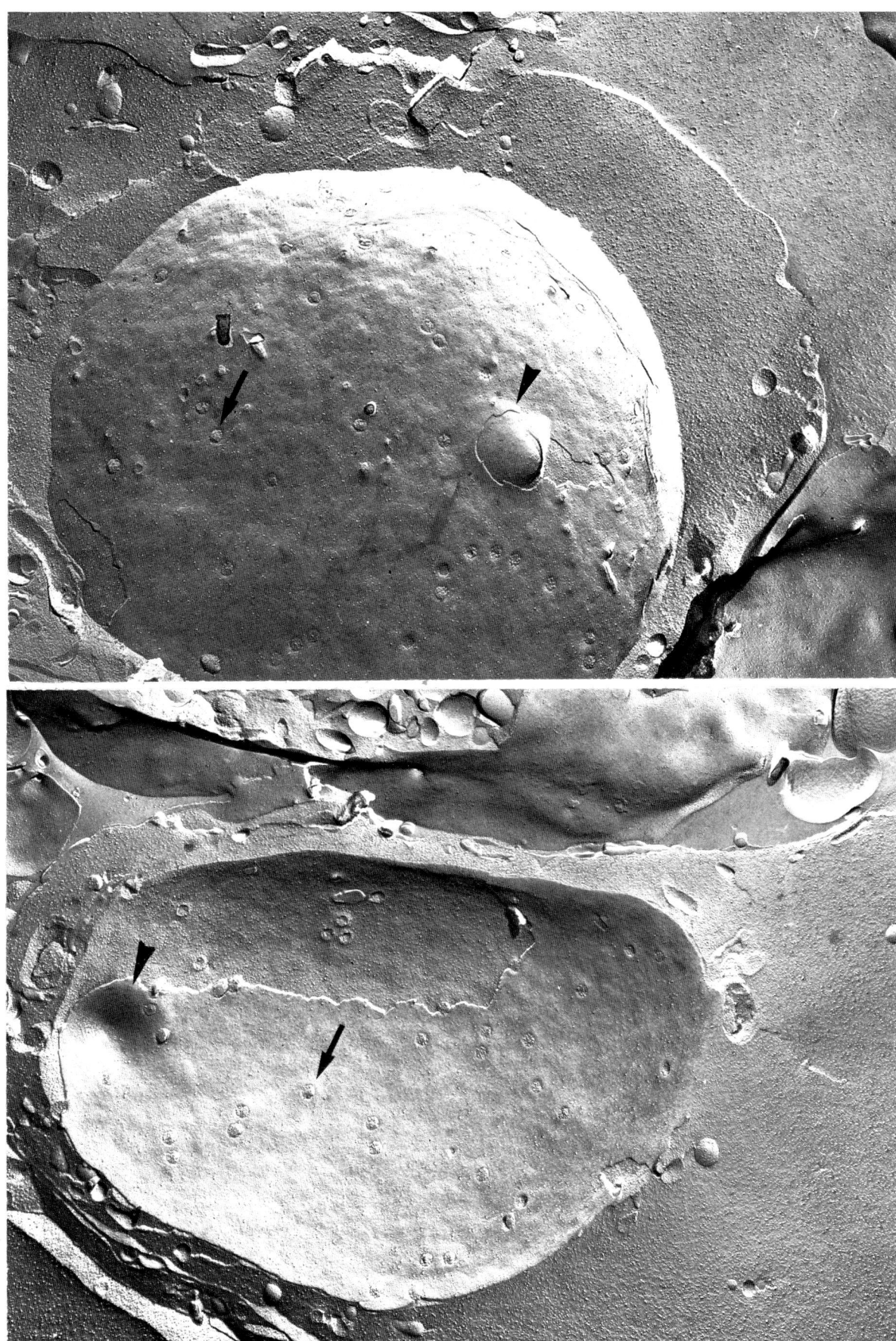

Fig. 65 d) Nuclei of erythroblasts in freeze-fracture replicas with localized bleb formation (**arrowheads**) seen from the outer leaflet (**top**) and from the inner leaflet (**bottom**). **Arrows** indicate nuclear pores ($\times$ 24,000). Courtesy of Dr. J. Thiele, Department of Medicine, University of Hannover.

Part 3   ABNORMALITIES OF RED CELL DESTRUCTION

1. HEREDITARY HEMOLYTIC ANEMIAS

1.1. Hereditary spherocytosis

Hereditary spherocytosis (HS) is an autosomal dominant trait in which a defect in the structure of the red cell membrane leads to premature destruction of erythrocytes in the spleen. That the condition is due to an intrinsic defect in the red cells is based on the observation that the cells have a markedly increased osmotic fragility *in vitro* and a shortened lifespan when they are transfused into normal individuals. The cells have an increased Na^+ influx stimulating the breakdown of ATP which in turn accelerates glycolysis [303-305].
This explains, in part, why the cells lyse more readily than normal cells on sterile incubation at 37 °C. *In vivo*, the resulting spherical shape of the erythrocytes renders the cells less able to traverse the sinuses of the spleen. The resulting erythrostasis aggravates the situation and may cause cells to assume a "hyperspheroidal" shape (**Fig. 66**). Additional abnormalities have been identified in the cytoskeletal proteins [306, 307] and the fatty acid composition of the membrane [308, 309]. These deserve further exploration.
On routine blood smears HS erythrocytes appear small, spheroidal (microspherocytes) and filled with hemoglobin. Spherocytes may be variable in number and their presence is better assessed by application of the osmotic fragility test or by the autohemolysis test. Anisocytosis is not usually as prominent as in other acquired hemolytic disorders. The bone marrow shows erythroid hyperplasia with occasional megaloblastic features as a consequence of excessive folate consumption due to chronic hemolysis.

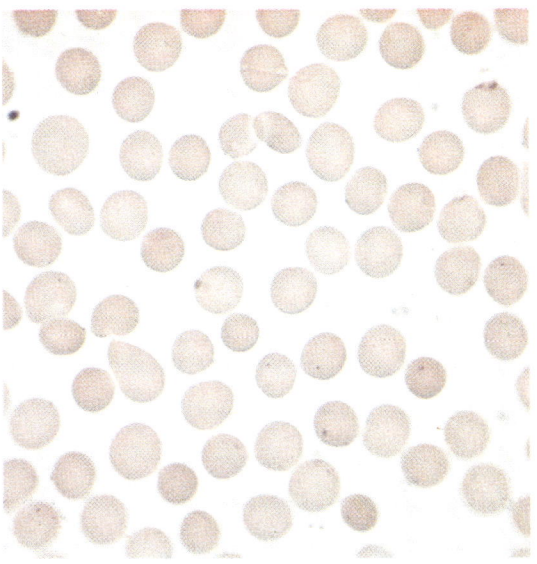
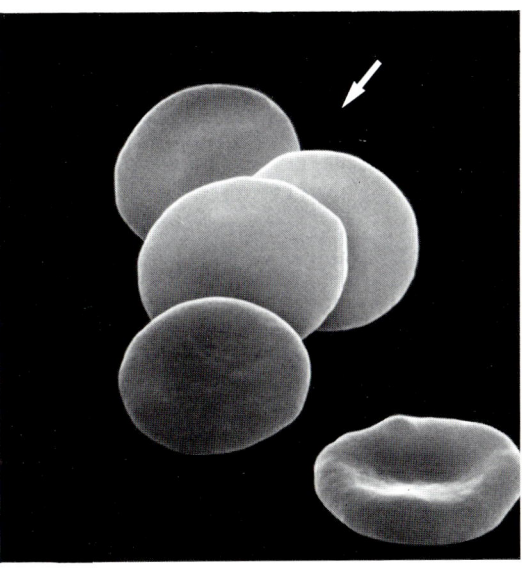

Fig. 66 *Hereditary spherocytosis.* **a)** *The blood smear is characterized by the presence of small round cells, with dense, uniformly staining hemoglobin ("spherocytes").* **b)** *A group of spherocytes (**arrow**) as seen by the scanning electron microscope ($\times$ 4,600).*

1.2. Elliptocytosis

This condition is reminiscent of red blood cells of several vertebrates [310].

Erythrocytes with oval or elliptic shape are seen in normal subjects (up to 15%); however, in hereditary elliptocytosis more than 25% of the red cells may consist of ellipotocytes. A continuous spectrum from circular to elongated elliptical cells is observed (**Fig. 67**). Some Authors have even attempted to classify the red cells of these patients [311, 312] according to the degree of elongation of their erythrocytes.

1.3. Acanthocytosis

This is a rare genetically determined disease resulting from defective synthesis of β-lipoproteins [313]. The disorder includes several clinical manifestations, such as progressive neurologic changes, steatorrhea, retinitis pigmentosa and a hematologic picture characterized by the occurrence of thorny red cells. These are normochromic and present irregularly spaced elongated projections (see **Fig. 24 a**). They should be distinguished from other spur cells observed in other conditions, e.g. in hepatocellular disorders ("burr cells") [314, 315] and uremia [316].

1.4. Enzyme deficiencies

Most erythrocyte enzyme deficiencies, whether involved in the hexose monophosphate shunt (e.g. glucose-6-phosphate dehydrogenase [317-322] and glutathione reductase) or related to the glycolytic pathway (e.g. pyruvate kinase [323-329]) result in various degrees of intermittent or chronic hemolytic anemia. The morphological abnormalities associated with these deficiencies do not exhibit specific diagnostic features and are characterized only by the structural changes seen in other hemolytic disorders (**Figs. 17-24**). For this reason, a detailed description of the genetic, biochemical and clinical aspects of these diseases is inappropriate within the confines of an Atlas. The reader is referred to excellent reviews on this subjects (e.g. Chapters 22 and 23 in Wintrobe's Clinical Hematology, pp. 769-793, 1974) [329].

2. PAROXYSMAL NOCTURNAL HEMOGLOBINURIA

Paroxysmal nocturnal hemoglobinuria (PNH) is a disorder clinically manifested by chronic intravascular hemolysis (increasing during sleep with overt hemoglobinuria) associated with persistent hemosideruria (Strübing-Marchiafava-Micheli's syndrome) [330].

There is good evidence that this disorder is due in part to the presence of a population of red cells (PNH cells) which are abnormally sensitive to the lytic action of serum complement (C_3) [331-333] (**Fig. 68**).

However, PNH may not be a separate disease entity, but rather a variant expression of a myeloproliferative disorder. This is suggested by the frequent association of PNH with aplastic anemia [334-340] or its termination in myelogenous leukemia. PNH cells may therefore be forerunners of a more fully developed syndrome.

The concept is in line with Dacie's suggestion [343] that the PNH defect is the result of a somatic mutation in a pluripotent stem cell of the marrow. This is confirmed by the observation of membrane abnormalities in cells belonging to the other lines (platelets and granulocytes) [344-346] and by the study of female patients heterozygous for glucose-6-phosphate dehydrogenase deficiency [347] or by the determination of the Hb F distribution in the red cell populations [348].
Analysis of the complement sensitive red cells has revealed at least three different populations (PNH I, PNH II, PNH III) with progressive sensitivity

3 ERYTHROCYTES

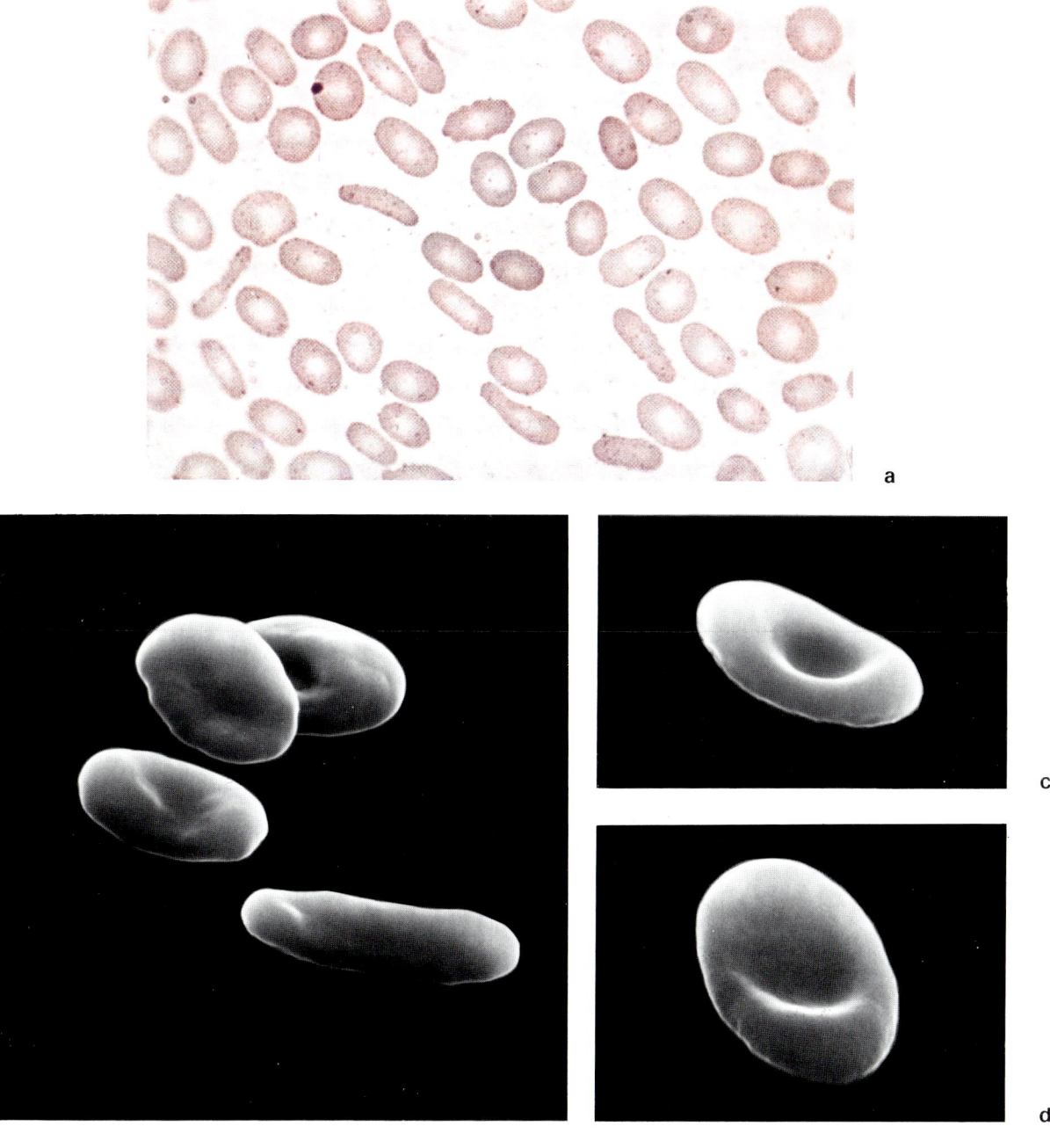

Fig. 67 a) Heterozygous elliptocytosis. Most of the cells are oval in shape; however some elongated forms ("cigar-shaped" cells) are observable.
b-d) Elliptocytes observed with the scanning electron microscope ($\times$ 5,200).

to lysis. The proportion of cells in each population is variable from patient to patient, but is usually stable for a long period of time [349-350].

The exact nature and the site of complement lysis remain largely unknown, and electron microscopic analyses have so far been inconclusive [351, 352].

Recognition of an abnormally low content of acetylcholinesterase in the cells [353] has led to many attempts to reproduce the red cell abnormality *in vitro* [354, 355]. Although these experiments have shed some light on the role of thiol groups in red cell lysis by complement, they have been unable to clarify the mechanism of complement fixation by PNH red cells.

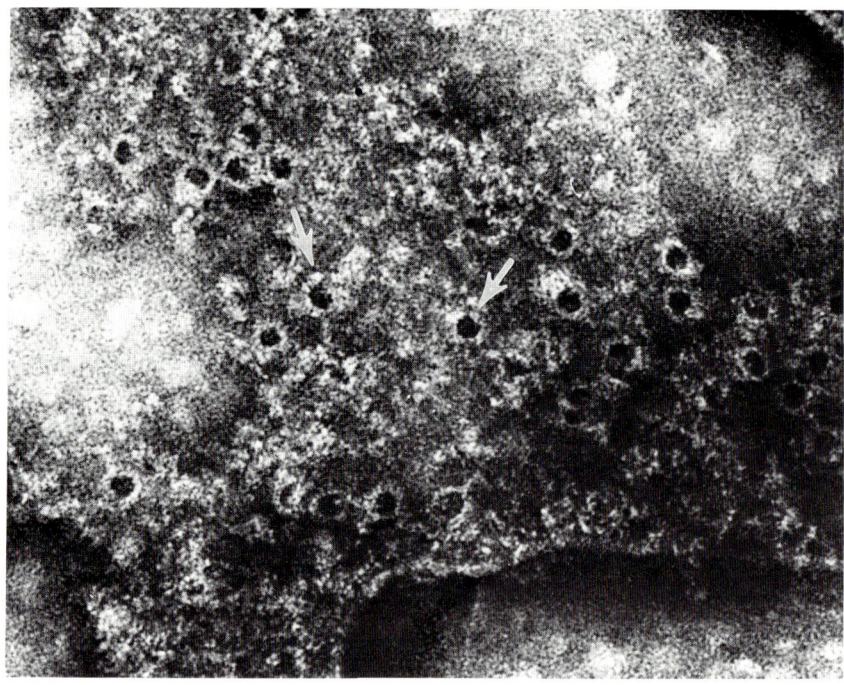

Fig. 68 *Fragment of sheep red cell membrane reacted with rabbit antibody and human complement. Stained with 2% sodium silicotungstate.* **Arrows** *indicate typical dimers of the C5b-q complex ($\times$ 318,750). Courtesy of Dr. Margaret J. Polley, Department of Medicine, Cornell University Medical Center.*

On routine smears PNH red cells show rather non-specific alterations. Due to chronic hemolysis there is a high percentage of young cells. Moreover, the almost constant and intermittently massive hemoglobinuria leads to iron deficiency manifested by depleted marrow stores and red cell morphology depicted in **Figure 48** on p. 100.
Also see **Figure 68** for mechanism of complement fixation and damage inflicted on the erythrocyte membrane.

3. ACQUIRED HEMOLYTIC DISORDERS

3.1. Anemia due to infection and infestation

Parasitic infestations may cause anemia by various mechanisms, e.g. direct damage to the red cell leading to its rapid destruction or indirectly by eliciting antibody formation which may lead to erythrocyte agglutination and sequestration by reticulo-endothelial cells. Several mechanisms may be operative simultaneously and influence the clinical course [359]. Only the most common infestations will be illustrated here (**Figs. 69-73**).

On a worldwide basis malaria is still the most prevalent parasite to cause anemia in man. Its most severe form is represented by *Plasmodium falciparum* (**Fig. 69**) which invades erythrocytes at all stages of maturation. A milder form of anemia is associated with infestations by *Plasmodium vivax* or *ovale* (**Fig. 70**) which appear to grow only in the younger cells of the erythroid population. Quartan malaria caused by *Plasmodium malariae* may not be associated with anemia since the organisms invade only relatively aged erythrocytes (**Fig. 71**). Because of the increased facility of international travel, it has become important for physicians to recognize these organisms in the blood smears of patients even in parts of the world where malaria has been eradicated.

3 ERYTHROCYTES

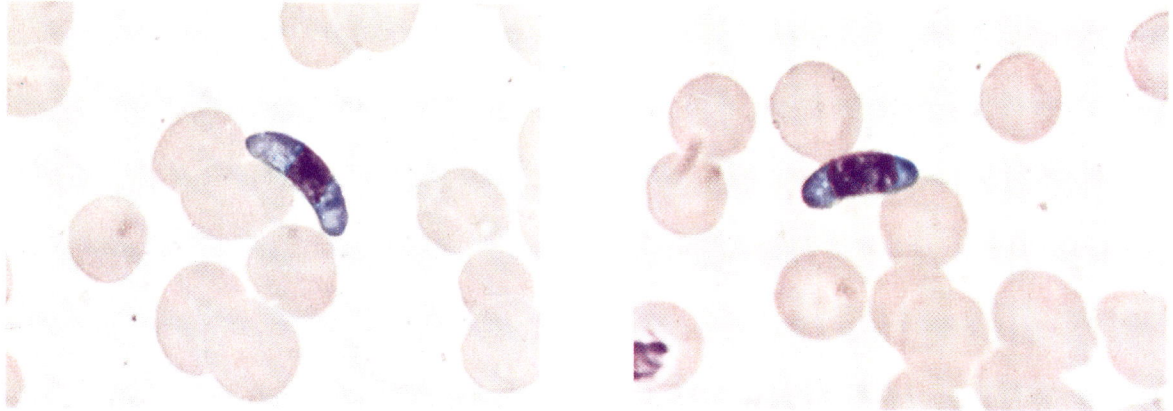

Fig. 69 Banana-shaped gametocytes from a patient with falciparum malaria (Plasmodium falciparum).

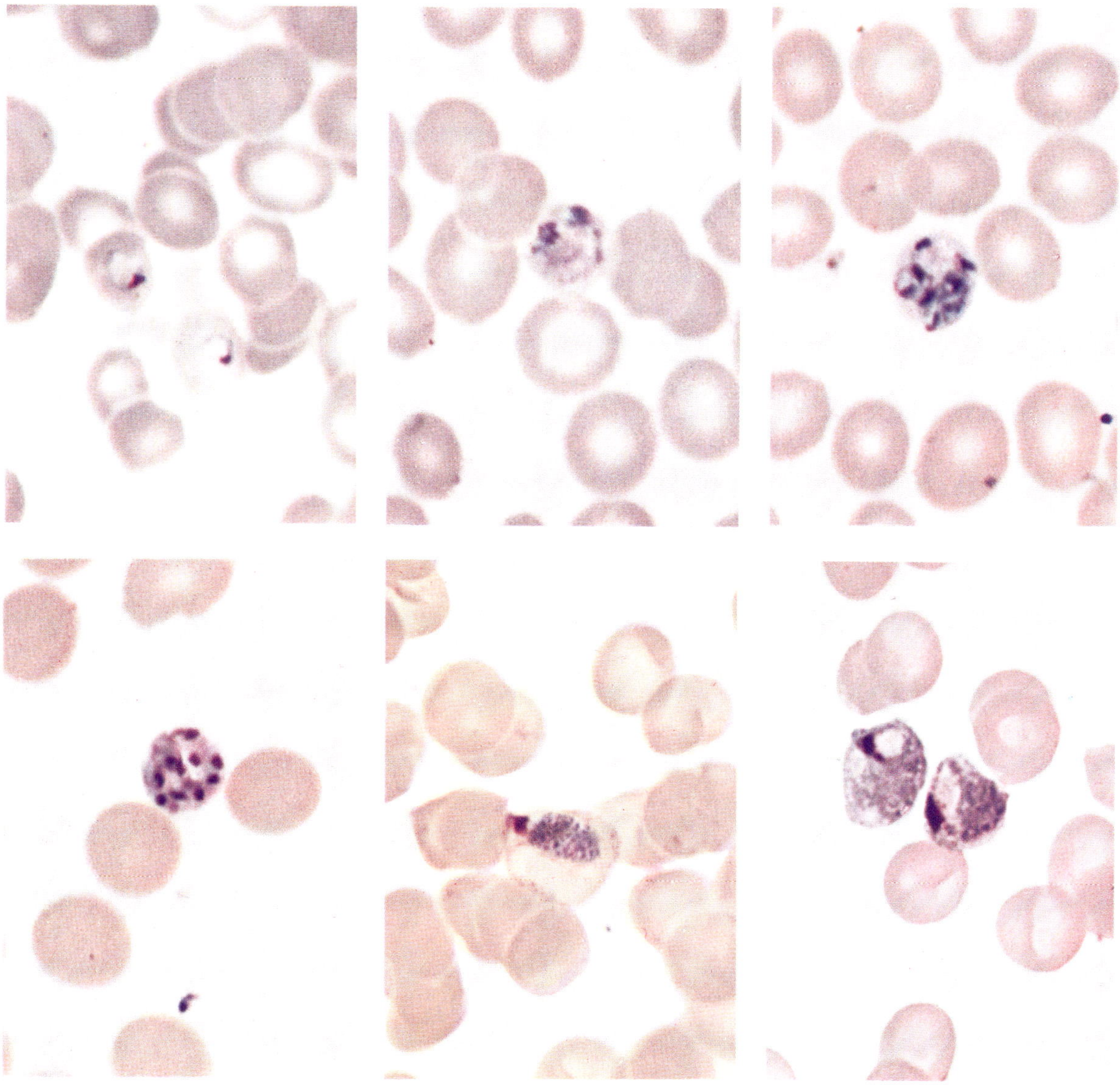

Fig. 70 Different forms of parasites in blood smears of tertian malaria (Plasmodium vivax).
a) Red cell containing trophozoites (anular schizonts). **b)** Late trophozoites (ameboid schizonts).
c, d) Red cells containing several merozoites. **e, f)** Gametocytes (female).

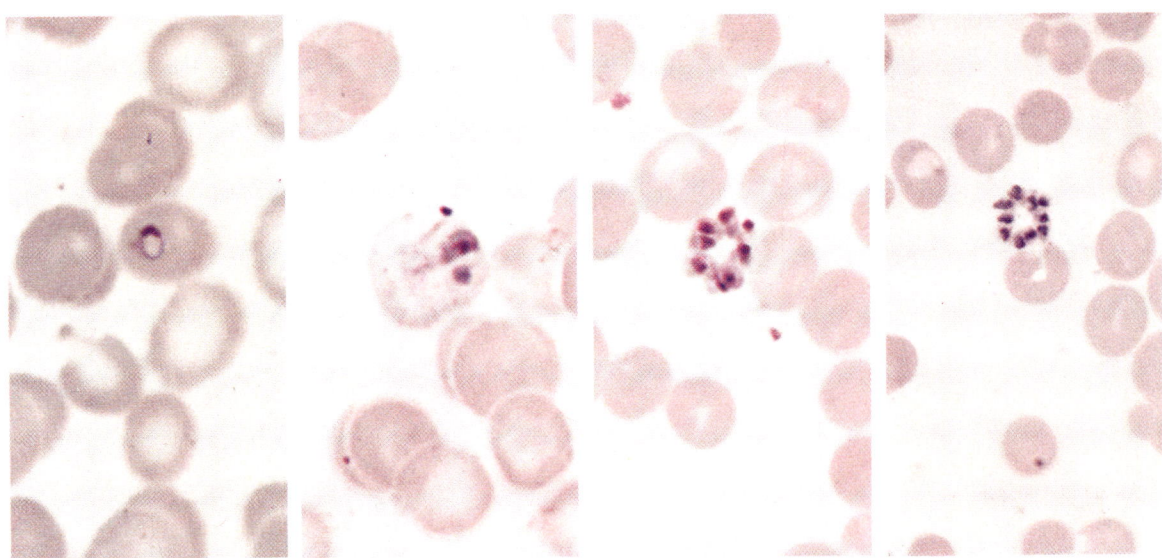

Fig. 71 Blood smears from a patient with quartan malaria (Plasmodium malariae). **a, b)** Trophozoites. **c, d)** Free merozoites.

The mechanisms by which the malarial parasite invades an erythrocyte has been elucidated by electron microscopy [360] (**Fig. 72**).

In addition to direct red cell damage [361], other mechanisms have also shown to be operative in causing anemia in malaria, e.g. transient depression of erythropoiesis and complement containing immune complexes which fix to the red cell surface [362]. The damaged red cells are partially or completely removed by the spleen.

A direct damage of the erythrocytes is observed in other infections such as human bartonellosis (Oroya fever) and in sepsis due to Clostridium welchii [363].

Bartonella bacilliformis is believed to adhere to the surface of the red cells, rather than penetrating into them. Damaged cells are removed by the liver and spleen.

Clostridium welchii causes hemolysis by producing a lecithinase (toxin) which releases highly active lysolecithins from the cell surface. A prominent microspherocytosis is seen under these conditions.

Babesiosis (Babesia microti) has been recognized recently as a cause of moderate to severe hemolytic anemia in man. Although well documented cases with overt parasitemia confirmed by blood smear (**Fig. 73**) are still limited in number, several epidemiologic studies related to patients with mild or subclinical infection, as suggested by serological data, have been reported in the past few years [364].

In other infectious disorders anemia may be related to hyperactivity of the reticulo-endothelial system, as in some chronic inflammatory diseases, or in *leishmaniasis* [365] (**Fig. 74**).

In the latter case the bone marrow and the spleen are infiltrated by parasitized reticulo-endothelial cells (Leishman-Donovan bodies). Although this process appears to represent a basic mechanism in the production of anemia, a complement mediated immune process has recently also been postulated for this infection [366].

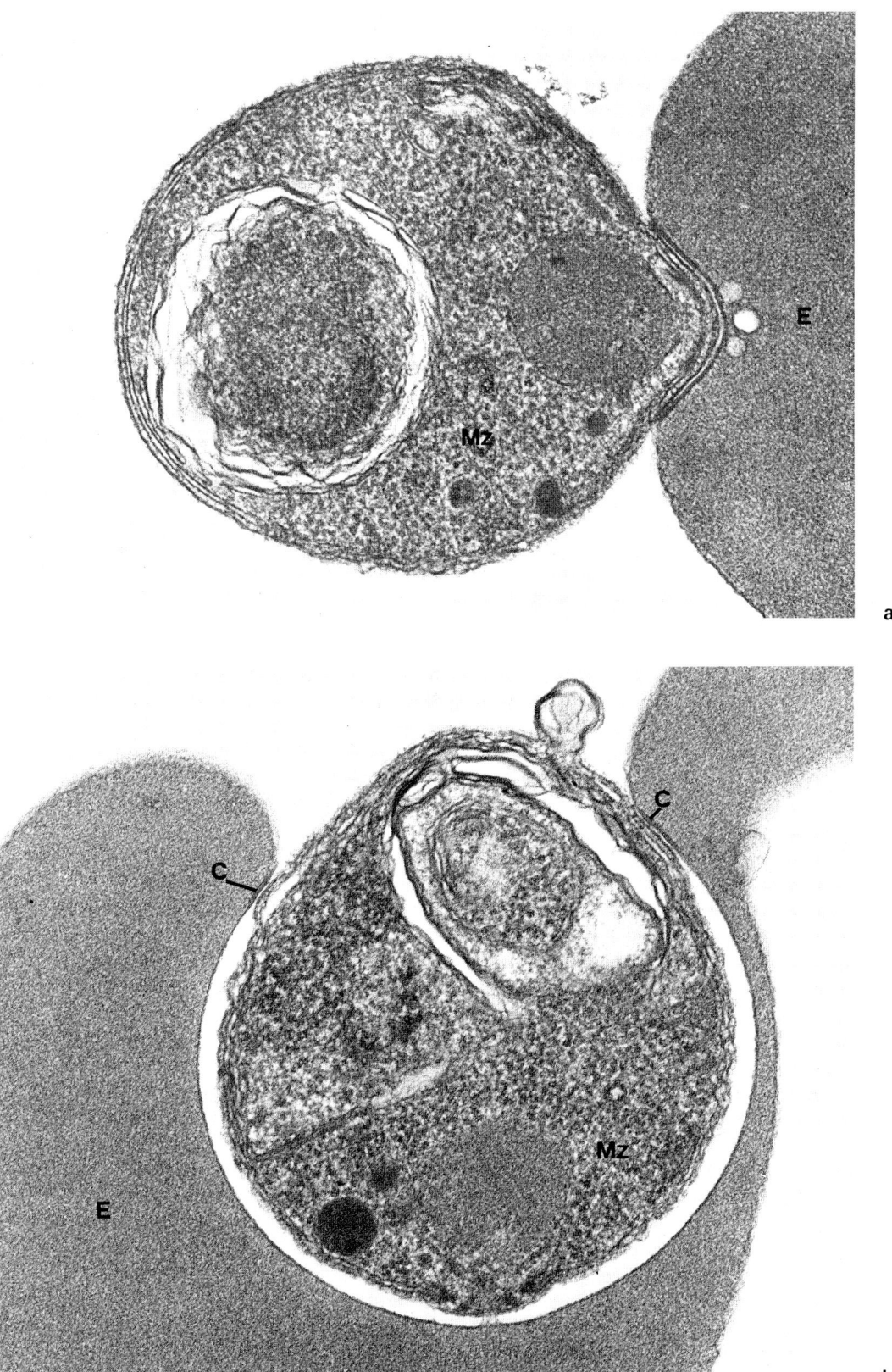

Fig. 72 Erythrocyte (E) is invaginated by merozoite (Mz); two different stages are illustrated: a) thickening of the erythrocyte membrane at the site of the attachment of the merozoite; b) the entry of the merozoite is almost completed. There is a firm attachmente (C) of the protozoan at the plasmalemma of the erythrocyte at each side of the entry orifice, following which the red cell invaginates to enclose the parasite ($\times$ 48,000). Courtesy of Prof. M. Aikawa, Case Western Reserve University, Cleveland, and the Publishers.

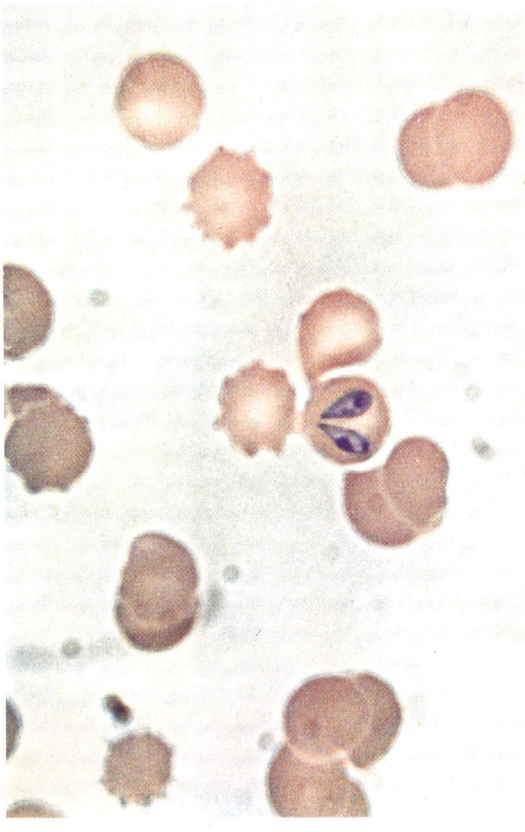
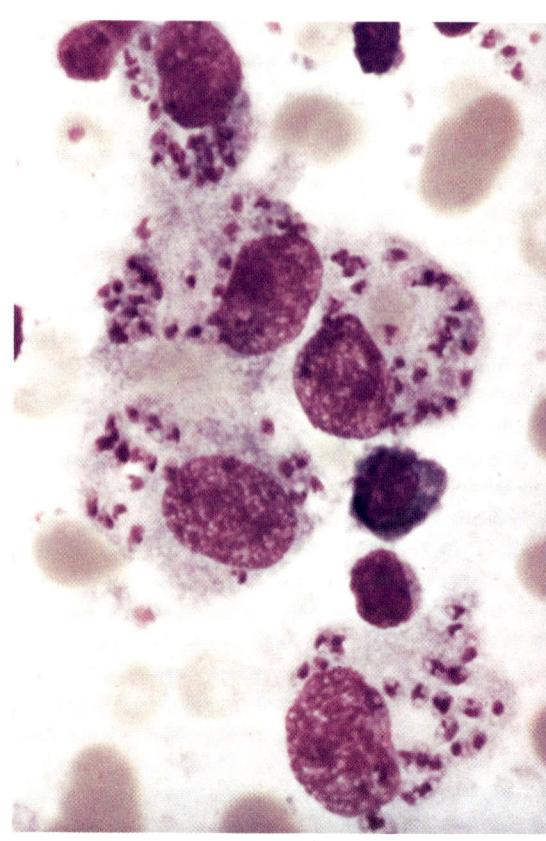

Fig. 73 *Babesiosis. The parasite, which is a thick-borne intraerythrocytic protozoan, exhibits a pyriform shape. Courtesy of Department of Zoology, University of Ferrara.*

Fig. 74 *Spleen imprint from a patient with leishmaniasis. Several histiocytes are filled with parasites.*

3.2. Chemical and drug-induced anemias

The morphological abnormalities seen in erythroid cells following administration of a variety of drugs are rather non-specific and may be reflected by functional rather than visible defects [367]. Furthermore, some effects appear to be dose-related, whereas in other instances the abnormalities are due to particular idiosyncrasies of patients such as an abnormal sensitivity of the stem cells or the inability to neutralize drug metabolites [368].

Some agents do not only damage hematopoietic cells, but also affect the interstitium and the microcirculation of the marrow [369-371].
Benzene poisoning is a good example of an agent causing dose-related damage [372] (**Fig. 75**). Other agents may impair the absorption of vitamin B_{12} or folate and thus be the cause of megaloblastic erythropoiesis.

Lead intoxication affects heme synthesis and may eventuate in acquired sideroblastic anemia. The resulting red cell abnormalities have been illustrated (see p. 84).

Drug-induced hemolytic anemias may also be mediated by immunologic mechanisms [373], e.g. *immune complex type* (as in the case of stibophen, phenacetin or quinine administration), b) *passive hemagglutination type* (mainly related to the use of penicillin and cephalosporins), c) *autoimmune type* (as reported for hydantoins, chlorpromazine and classically described for alpha-methyldopa which triggers the formation of antibodies against autologous determinants of the red cells).

3 ERYTHROCYTES

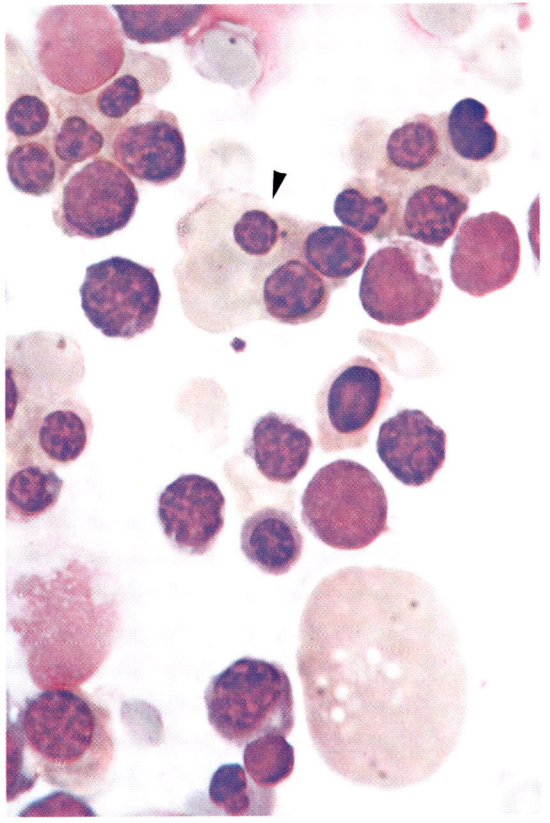 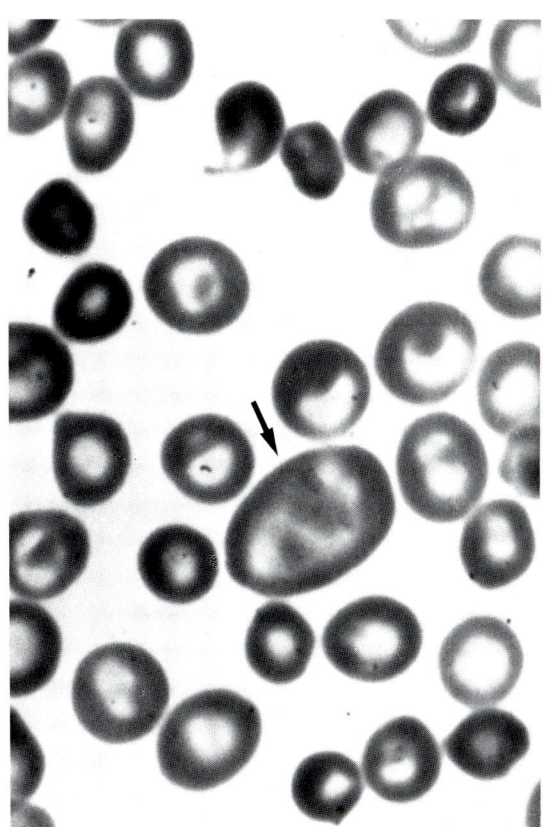

Fig. 75 a) Marked dyserythropoiesis (bone marrow) in a patient with benzene-induced anemia. Cells with two or three nuclei are also seen (**arrowhead**).
b) Large erythrocytes are observable even in the peripheral blood smears (**arrow**).

3.3. Autoimmune hemolytic anemias (AIHA)

These disorders, either idiopathic or secondary, are characterized by hemolytic states which do not depend on intrinsic defects of the red cells, but are mediated by antibodies or complement. Two major groups of AIHA are recognized, those with *warm-active autoantibodies* and those with *cold-active autoantibodies* respectively [374, 375].

The former are more common in older patients, often associated with lymphoreticular malignancies or systemic lupus erythematosus. In children they are usually related to viral infections or other acute diseases. Morphologically these conditions cannot be distinguished from other hemolytic states.

Serologic tests are mandatory to establish the diagnosis.

During active hemolysis there is marked aniso-poikilocytosis, spherocytosis, erythrocyte fragmentation and normoblastemia (**Fig. 76 a**).
A positive direct antiglobulin test may be helpful in differentiating AIHA from hereditary spherocytosis. Blood monocytes may occasionally show phagocytosed erythrocytes.

AIHA with cold-active autoantibodies is associated with several clinical disorders, such as cold agglutinin disease and paroxysmal cold hemoglobinuria.

Cold agglutinin disease (usually IgM antibodies with anti-I specificity) may occur as an acute condition accompanying *Mycoplasma pneumoniae* or infectious mononucleosis. Polychromasia,

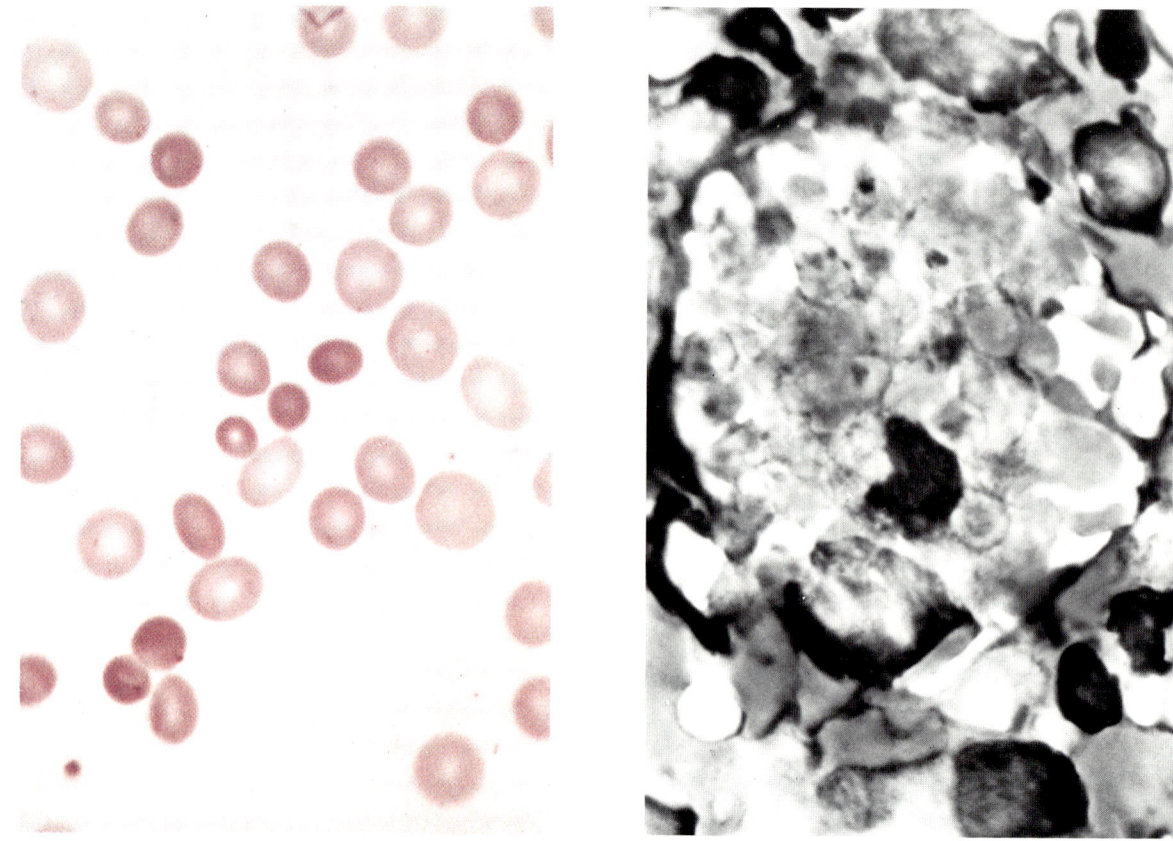

Fig. 76 a) *Auto-immune hemolytic anemia. There is a marked anisocytosis and spherocytosis.*
b) *Erythrophagocytic features in spleen imprints from a patient with lymphoma associated with cold agglutinin disease.*

spherocytosis, erythrophagocytosis and autoagglutination are observed. Chronic forms of cold agglutinin disease occur mainly in elderly patients with subclinical or fully developed. lymphoreticular tumors. Microspherocytosis, autoagglutination and erythrophagocytosis, mainly in the spleen, are prominent features (**Fig. 76 b**) [376].

4. THE ERYTHROCYTE FRAGMENTATION SYNDROMES

Although evidence of red cell fragmentation is found in a great number of hemolytic disorders, true erythroclasia occurs only in conditions that inflict direct mechanical damage to the cells. These include circulatory abnormalities brought about by diseased or prosthetic heart valves, small vessel aberrations as seen in thrombotic thrombocytopenic purpura (TTP), the infantile hemolytic uremic syndrome, malignant hypertension and large hemangiomata. The condition is usually referred to as microangiopathic hemolytic anemia [377, 378] and described in greater detail elsewhere (see **Fig. 77 c**) [379]. On the smear, all types of schistocytes are seen including so-called helmet or triangular cells, contracted cells and other distortions (**Fig. 77**) [378]. A more specific term for the crescent cell is keratocyte introduced by Bessis [97] to indicate an erythrocyte that has lost the central clear zone having successfully resealed its membrane after having been fragmented. This results in a double-horned appearance (see **Fig. 24 f** on p. 68). The final stage of acquired schistocytosis is an extremely small spherocyte (see **Fig. 77 a**).

3 ERYTHROCYTES

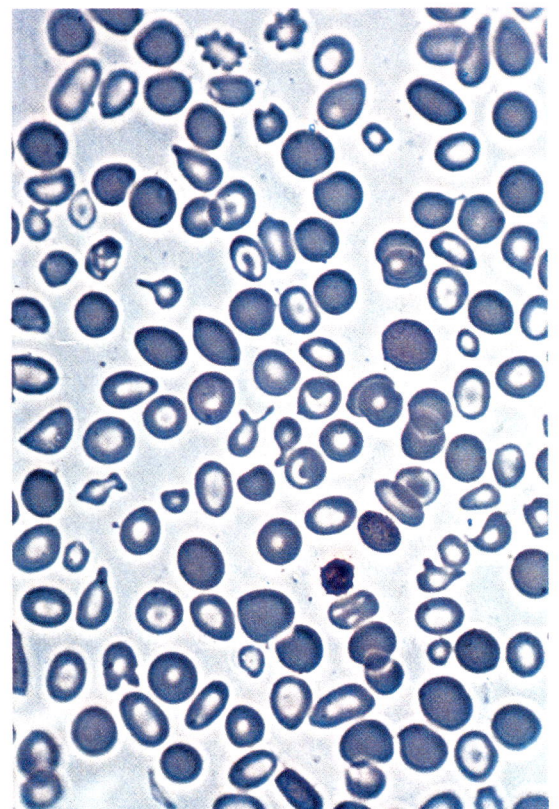

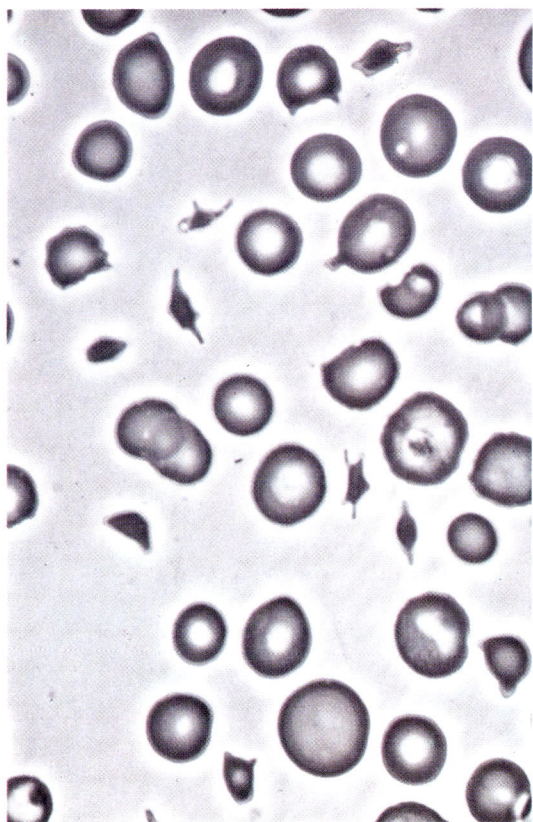

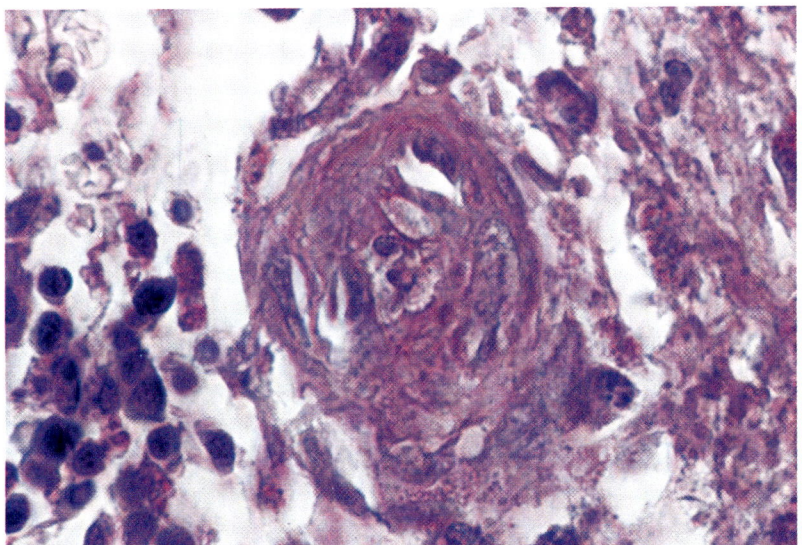

Fig. 77 a) Blood smear from a patient with TTP, showing prominent anisopoikilocytosis. Helmet, triangular and contracted cells are represented. Some spherocytes and target cells are also seen.

b) Typical erythrocyte fragmentation on a smear (TTP). All types of fragmented cells can be recognized. The larger cells could be identified as reticulocytes (phase contrast microscopy).

c) A capillary thrombosis in a bone marrow section. No inflammatory reaction can be seen.
Courtesy of Prof. A.M. Marmont, S. Martino's Hospital, Genova.

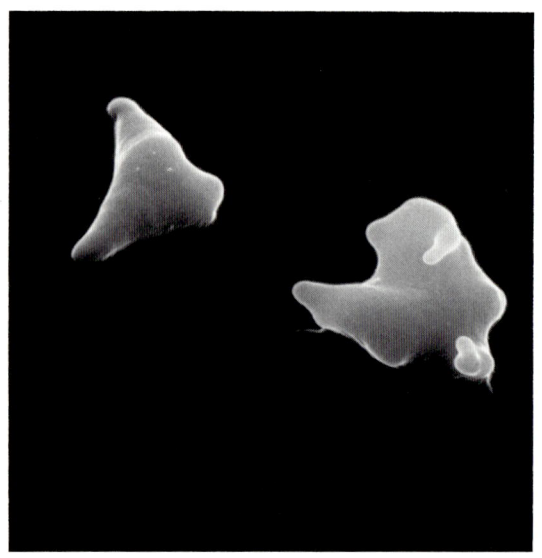 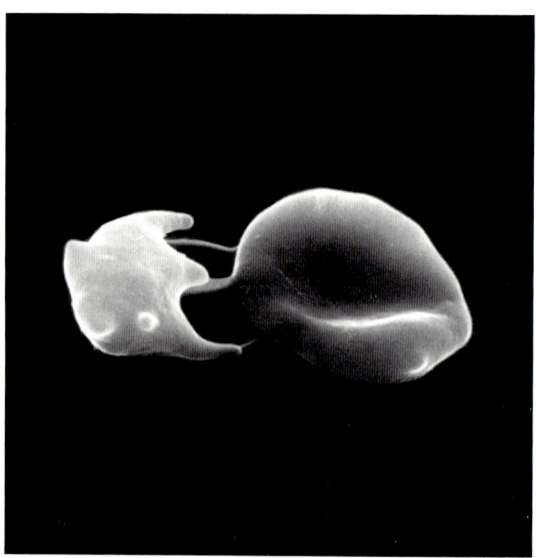

Fig. 77 d-e) Highly deformed cells, as seen by SEM, in a case of uremic hemolytic syndrome (× 5,200).

5. MYELOPHTHISIC ANEMIAS

The term "myelophthisic anemia" is used to describe a condition of the marrow which is a consequence of infiltration with abnormal cells (*space occupying lesions*) [386].

Solid metastatic tumors are often responsible for the infiltration of the marrow but, not infrequently, systemic hematologic proliferations (plasmocytic, lymphomatous or granulomatous) may cause myelophtisis.

Aspiration of the marrow, even if successful, often shows non-specific changes or normal morphology since the infiltration by metastatic cells is focally distributed.

The finding of clumped abnormal cells may be diagnostic (**Figs. 78 a-g**). The presence of osteoblasts and osteoclasts in such marrow can be misleading (**Figs. 78 h, i**) [387].

Diagnosis may be established by bone biopsy and examination of serial histologic sections [388] (**Figs. 78 j, k**).

The peripheral blood shows a moderate normochromic or even hypochromic anemia. Sometimes there is a prominent poikilocytosis due to fragmentation of the erythrocytes circulating through the occluded vessels (burr cells) [389]. Moderate increase of nucleated red cell precursors may be observed in association with an increased leukocyte count and the presence of toxic granulations within the polymorphonuclear leukocytes is common [390-393].

The pathogenesis of these features is still unclear. Several factors have been claimed to play a role, such as local stimulation, alterations in the sinusoidal barrier which controls the release of cells [392] and, possibly, production of "granulopoietic stimulating factors" by the neoplastic cells [393].

3 ERYTHROCYTES

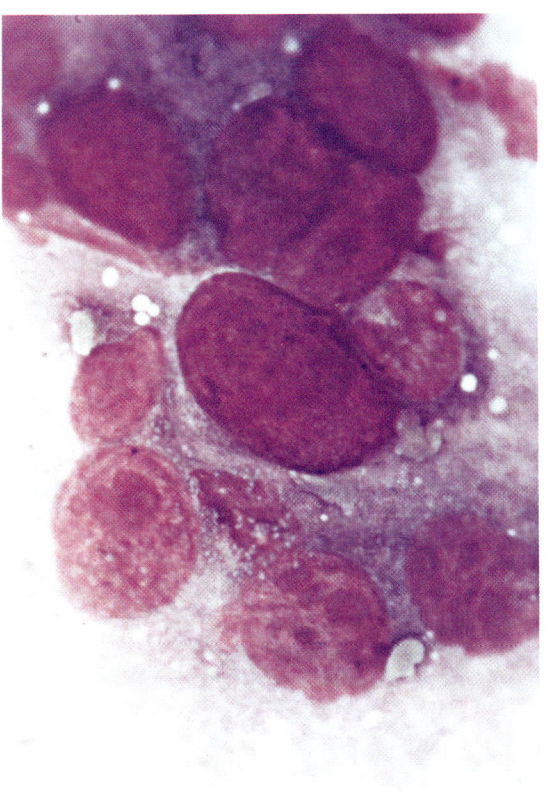

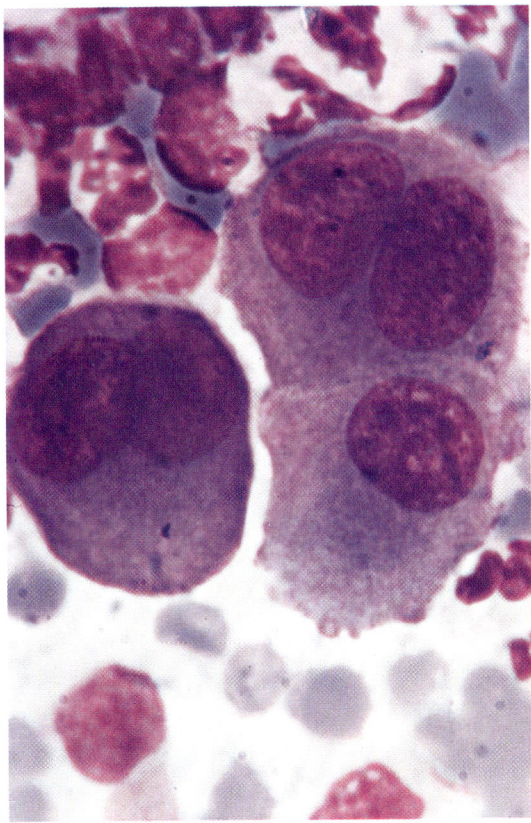

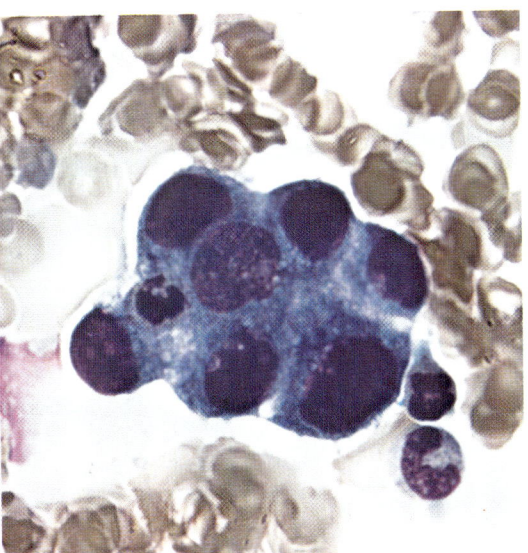

Fig. 78 a) Metastatic marrow in patient with prostatic carcinoma. Clumping of neoplastic cells is observed.
b) Cells from testicular carcinoma in bone marrow aspirate.
c) Marrow aspirates should be scanned for tumor cells at low magnification. They are often found separated from the marrow cells "in the dilute part of the smear". This clump is seen at higher magnification in **d**.
d) This clump of tumor cells found at low magnification (**c**) photographed with 100 × oil immersion.
Specimen obtained from a patient with carcinoma of the colon and myelophthisic anemia. In most instances, the origin of the tumor cannot be identified.
b, c, d) Courtesy of Dr. D. Zucker-Franklin, Department of Medicine, New York University.

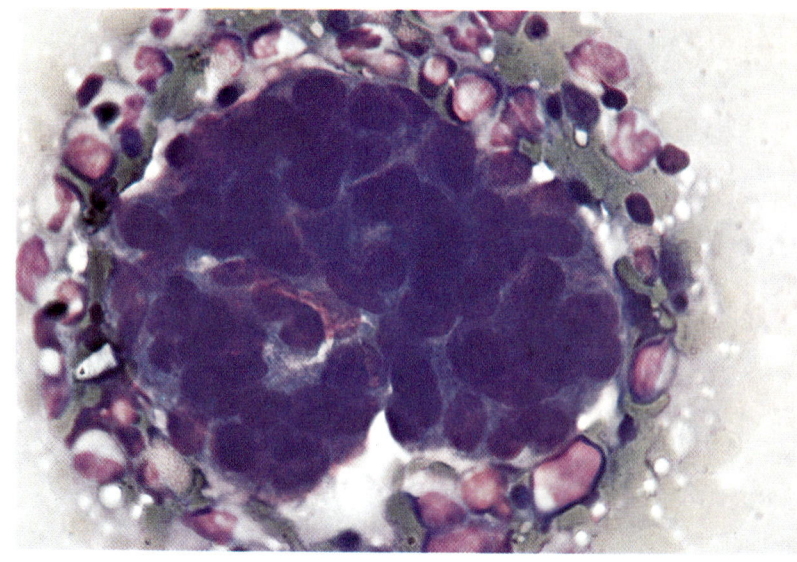

Fig. 78 e) Large clump of tumor cells in bone marrow aspirate showing displacement of normal hematopoietic tissue. The monotony of the cells within the clump makes distinction from marrow cells quite easy.
Courtesy of Dr. D. Zucker-Franklin, Department of Medicine, New York University.

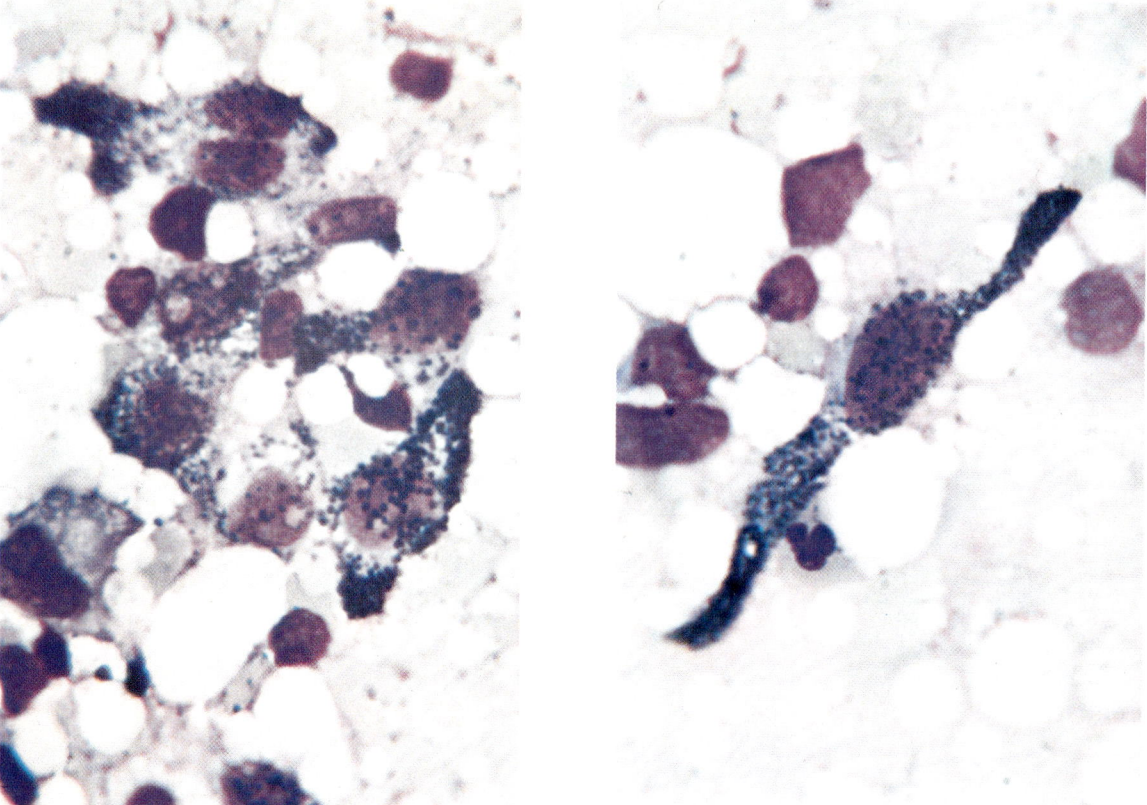

Figs. 78 f, g) Bone marrow smear showing massive infiltration with metastatic cells from melanosarcoma. Note the heavily pigmented cytoplasm of the neoplastic cells.

3 ERYTHROCYTES

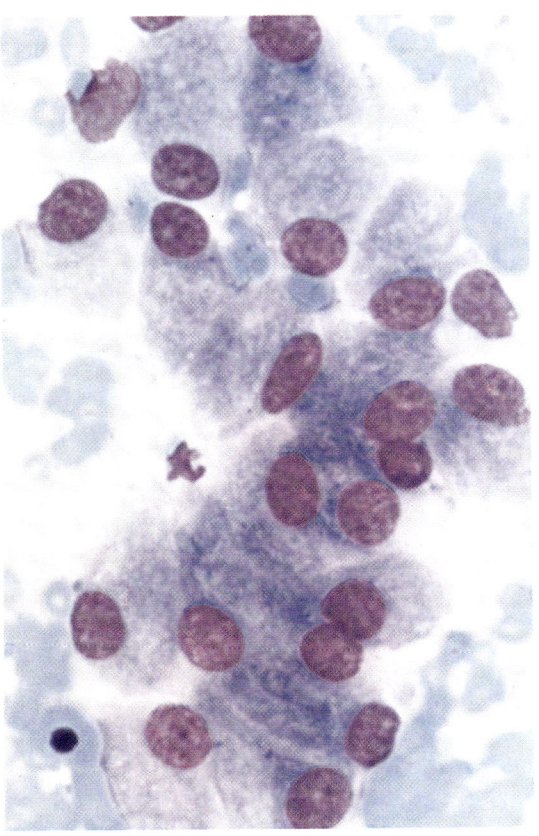
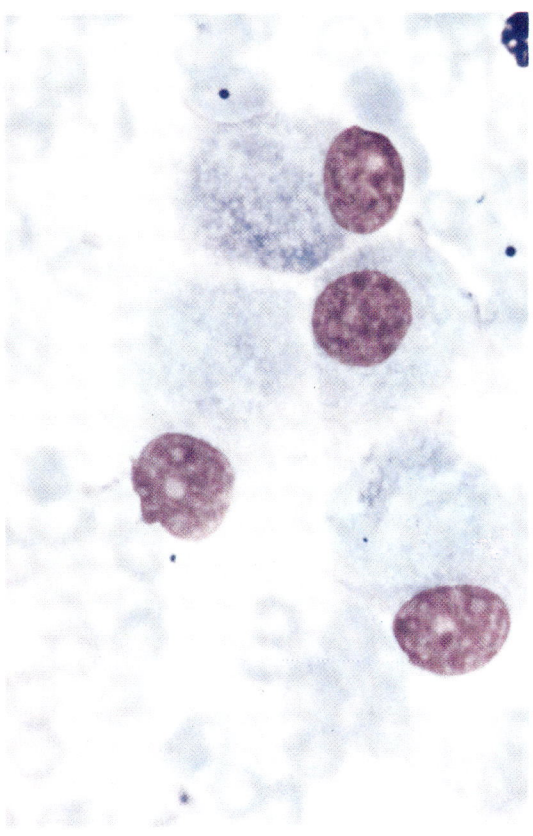

Figs. 78 h, i) *Group of osteoblasts in a bone marrow smear. At higher magnification (i) these cells appear to display abundant basophilic cytoplasm containing a large pale area separated from the perinuclear zone. The nucleus, eccentrically placed, exhibits one or two nucleoli, and a fine reticular chromatin pattern.*

REFERENCES

1. Boycott A.E.: *The blood as a tissue: hypertrophy and atrophy of the red corpuscles*. Proc. Roy. Soc. Med., 23, 15, 1929.
2. Schofield R., Lajtha L.G.: *Cellular kinetics of erythropoiesis*. In: Congenital Disorders of Erythropoiesis. Ciba Foundation Symposium, Elsevier North Holland, 37, 3, 1976.
3. Bessis M., Mize C., Prenant M.: *Erythropoiesis: Comparison of in vivo and vitro amplification*. Blood Cells, 4, 155, 1978.
4. Lajtha L.G.: *Discussion on the meaning of the term amplification*. Blood Cells, 4, 171, 1978.
5. Kelemen E., Calvo W., Fliedner T.M.: *Atlas of human hemopoietic development*. Springer, Heidelberg, 1979.
6. Gilmour J.R.: *Normal haemopoiesis in intrauterine and neonatal life*. J. Path. Bact., 52, 25, 1941.
7. Bloom W., Bartelmez G.W.: *Hemopoiesis in young human embryos*. Amer. J. Anat., 67, 21, 1940.
8. Thomas D.B., Yoffey J.M.: *Human foetal haematopoiesis. II. Hepatic haematopoiesis in the human foetus*. Brit. J. Haemat., 10, 193, 1964.
9. Quattrin N., Dini E., De Rosa L.: *Dyserythropoietic features of human erythropoiesis and their clinical significance*. In: Metcalf D., Condorelli M., Peschle C. (Eds.): Leukemia and aplastic anemia. Pensiero Sci. Ed., Rome, p. 281, 1976.
10. Kalpaktsoglou P.K., Emery J.L.: *Human bone marrow during the last three months of intrauterine life. A histological study*. Acta haemat. (Basel), 34, 228, 1965.
11. Marks J., Gairdner D., Roscoe J.D.: *Blood formation in infancy. III. Cord blood*. Arch. Dis. Child., 30, 117, 1955.
12. Alpen E.L., Cranmore D.: *Observations on the regulation of erythropoiesis and on cellular dynamics by Fe^{59} autoradiography*. In: The Kinetics of Cellular Proliferation. Stohlman F. Jr. ed., Grune & Stratton, New York and London, 1959.
13. Jacobson L.O., Goldwasser E., Gurney C.W.: *Transfusion-induced polycythaemia as a model for studying factors influencing erythropoiesis*. In: Ciba Symposium on Haematopoiesis. Wolstenholme G.E.W. and O'Connor M. eds., Churchill, London, 1960.
14. Till J.E., McCulloch E.A.: *A direct measurement of the radiation sensitivity of normal mouse bone marrow cells*. Radiat. Res., 14, 213, 1961.
15. Adamson J.W., Torok-Storb B., Lin N.: *Analysis of erythropoiesis by erythroid colony formation in culture*. Blood Cells, 4, 89, 1978.
16. Stephenson J.R., Axelrad A.A., McLeod D.L., Shreeve M.M.: *Induction of colonies of hemoglobin-synthesizing cells by erythropoietin in vitro*. Proc. Natl. Acad. Sci., U.S.A., 68, 1542, 1971.
17. Lajtha L.G.: *Kinetics of haemopoietic stem cells*. Haematologia, 5, 359, 1971.
18. Gregory C.J., McCulloch E.A., Till J.E.: *Erythropoietic progenitors capable of colony formation in culture. State of differentiation*. J. Cell. Physiol., 81, 411, 1973.
18. Peschle C.: *Erythropoiesis*. Ann. Rev. Med., 31, 303, 1980.
19. Axelrad A.A., McLeod D.L., Shreeve M.M., Heath D.S.: *Properties of cells that produce erythrocytic colonies in vitro*. In: Proceedings of the Second International Workshop on Hemopoiesis in Culture. Robinson W.A. ed., HEW (NIH) Publ. 74-205, 226, 1973.

20. Gregory C.J., Eaves A.C.: *Human marrow cells capable of erythropoietic differentiation in vitro. Definition of three erythroid colony responses.* Blood, *49*, 855, 1977.
21. Gregory C.J., Eaves A.C.: *Three stages of erythropoietic progenitor cell differentiation distinguished by a number of physical and biologic properties.* Blood, *51*, 527, 1978.
22. Lord B.I., Mori K.J., Wright E.G., Lajtha L.G.: *Proliferation regulators in haemopoietic cell populations.* Blood Cells, *3*, 451, 1977.
23. Cline M.J., Golde D.W.: *Cellular interactions in haemopoiesis.* Nature, *277*, 177, 1979.
24. Goldwasser E., Kung C.K.H.: *Purification of erythropoietin.* Proc. Natl., Acad. Sci. (U.S.A.), *68*, 697, 1971.
25. Gordon A.S., Cooper G.W., Zanjani E.D.: *The kidney and erythropoiesis.* Semin. Hemat., *4*, 337, 1967.
26. Miller M.E.: *The interaction between the regulation of acid-base and erythropoietin production.* Blood Cells, *1*, 449, 1975.
27. Krantz S.B., Jacobson L.O.: *Erythropoietin and the regulation of erythropoiesis.* University of Chicago Press, 1970.
28. Peschle C., Condorelli M.: *Regulation of fetal and adult erythropoiesis.* In: Congenital Disorders of Erythropoiesis. Ciba Foundation Symposium, Excerpta Medica, Elsevier, North Holland, 37, 25, 1976.
29. Lucarelli G., Porcellini A., Carnevali C., Carmena A., Stohlman F.: *Fetal and neonatal erythropoiesis.* Ann. N.Y. Acad. Sci., *149*, 544, 1968.
30. Gordon A.S., Condorelli M., Peschle C.: *Regulation of erythropoiesis.* Il Ponte, Milano, 1971.
31. Peschle C.: *Regulation of erythropoiesis and its defects.* Brit. J. Haemat., *3 i* (Suppl.), 69, 1975.
32. Rifkind R.A., Marks P.A.: *The regulation of erythropoiesis.* Blood Cells, *1*, 417, 1975.
33. Harrison P.R.: *Analysis of erythropoiesis at the molecular level.* Nature, *262*, 353, 1976.
34. Iscove N.N., Sieber F.: *Erythroid progenitors in mouse bone marrow detected by macroscopic colony formation in culture.* Exp. Hematol., *3*, 32, 1975.
35. Goldwasser E.: *Some molecular aspects of red cell differentiation.* In: Gordon A., Condorelli M., Peschle C.: Regulation of erythropoiesis. 1st Intern. Conf. on Hematopoiesis, Publ. House « Il Ponte », pp. 227-233, 1971.
36. Chamberlain J.K., Leblond P.F.: Weed R.I.: *Reduction of adventitial cell cover. An early direct effect of erythropoietin on bone marrow ultrastructure.* Blood Cells, *1*, 635, 1975.
37. Wickramasinghe S.N.: *Human bone marrow.* Blackwell Sci. Publ., Oxford, London, 1975.
38. Lessin L.J., Bessis M.: *Morphology of the erythron.* In: Hematology, Williams W.J., Beutler E., Erslev A.J., Rundles R.W. eds., McGraw-Hill Book Co., New York, p. 103, 1977.
39. Bond V.P., Fliedner T.M., Cronkite E.P., Rubini J.R., Robertson J.S.: *Cell turnover in blood and blood-forming tissues studied with tritiated thymidine.* In: The kinetics of cellular proliferation, F. Stohlman Jr. ed., Grune & Stratton, New York and London, 1959.
40. Bessis M., Breton-Gorius J.: *Diapedèse des reticulocytes et des erythroblastes.* Compt. Rend. Acad. Sci., *251*, 465, 1960.
41. Tavassoli M., Crosby W.H.: *Fate of the nucleus of the marrow erythroblast.* Science, *179*, 912, 1973.
42. Chamberlain J.K., Lichtman M.A.: *Marrow cell egress: specificity of the site of penetration into the sinus.* Blood, *52*, 959, 1978.
43. Tavassoli M.: *The marrow-blood barrier* (Annotation). Brit. J. Haemat., *41*, 297, 1979.
44. Tavassoli M., Shaklai M.: *Absence of tight junctions in endothelium of marrow sinuses: possible significance for marrow cell egress.* Brit. J. Haemat., *41*, 303, 1979.
45. Thorell B.: *Studies on the formation of cellular substances during blood cell production.* Acta Med. Scand., Suppl. 200, 1947.
46. Storti E., Mauri C., Quaglino D.: *Cytochemistry in normal and pathological hemopoiesis: biological and diagnostic implications.* Proc. 6th Intern. Congr. Clinical Pathology, C.E.P.I., Roma, pp. 415-433, 1966.
47. Grasso J.A., Woodard J.W., Swift H.: *Cytochemical studies of nucleic acids and proteins in erythrocytic development.* Proc. Natl. Acad. Sci. (U.S.A.), *50*, 134, 1963.
48. Bessis M.: *Living blood cells and their ultrastructure.* Springer, Berlin, New York, 1973.
49. Tanaka Y., Goodman J.R.: *Electron microscopy of human blood cells.* Harper & Row, New York, 1972.
50. Cawley J.C., Hayhoe F.G.J.: *Ultrastructure of haemic cells.* W.B. Saunders Co., London, 1973.
51. Bessis M., Breton-Gorius J.: *Iron metabolism in the bone marrow as seen by electron microscopy: a critical review.* Blood, *19*, 635, 1962.
52. Tanaka Y., Brecher G., Bull B.: *Ferritin localization on the erythroblast cell membrane and rhopheocytosis in hypersiderotic human bone marrow.* Blood, *28*, 758, 1966.
53. Jandl J.H., Inman J.K., Simmons R.L., Allen D.W.: *Transfer of iron from serum iron binding protein to human reticulocytes.* J. Clin. Invest., *38*, 161, 1959.
54. Sullivan A.L., Grasso J.A., Weintraub L.R.: *Micropinocytosis of transferrin by developing red cells: an electron-microscopic study utilizing ferritin-coniugated transferrin and ferritin-conjugated antibodies to transferrin.* Blood, *47*, 133, 1976.
55. Perls M.: *Nachweis von Eisenoxyd in gewissen Pigmenten.* Virchow's Arch. Path. Anat., *39*, 42, 1867.
56. Lajtha L.G., Oliver R.: *Studies on the kinetics of erythropoiesis: a model of the erythron.* In: Ciba Foundation Symposium on Haemopoiesis, Wolstenholme G.E.W. and O'Connor M. eds., Churchill, London, 1960.
57. Stohlman F.: *Humoral regulation of erythropoiesis. XIV. A model for abnormal erythropoiesis in thalassemia.* Ann. N.Y. Acad. Sci., *119*, 578, 1964.
58. Yataganas X., Gahrton G., Thorell B.: *DNA, RNA and hemoglobin during erythroblast maturation. A cytophotometric study.* Exp. Cell Res., *62*, 254, 1970.
59. Bessis M., Bricka M.: *Aspect dynamique des cellules du sang. Son étude par microcinématographie en contraste de phase.* Rév. Hémat., *7*, 407, 1952.
60. Bessis M., Breton-Gorius J., Thiery J.P.: *Rôle possible de l'hémoglobine accompagnant le noyeau des érythroblastes dans l'origine de la stercobiline eliminée précocement.* C.R. Acad. Sci. (Paris), *252*, 2300, 1961.
61. Heilmeyer L., Westhäuser R.: *Reifungstadien überlebenden Reticulozyten in vitro und ihre Bedeutung für die Schätzung der Hämoglobinproduktion in vivo.* Z. Klin. Med., *121*, 361, 1932.
62. Mel H.C., Prenant M., Mahandas N.: *Reticulocyte motility and form: studies on maturation and classification.* Blood, *49*, 1001, 1977.
63. Bessis M., Breton-Gorius J.: *Le reticulocyte. Colorations vitales et microscopie électronique.* Nouv. Rév. Franç. Hémat., *4*, 77, 1964.
64. Marmont A.: *Acridine orange fluorescence microscopy in hematology.* Proc. 7th Congr. Europ. Soc. Hematol., Part 2, *36 i*, 1960.
65. Schiffer L.M.: *Fluorescence microscopy with acridine orange: a study of hemopoietic cells in fixed preparations.* Blood, *19*, 200, 1962.
66. Thaer A., Becker H.: *Microscope fluorometric investigations on the reticulocytic maturation distribution as diagnostic criterion of disordered erythropoiesis.* Blut, *39*, 339, 1972.
67. Castoldi G.L., Yam L.T., Mitus W.J.: *Cytochemical demonstration of dihydro-orotic acid dehydrogenase in blood and bone marrow cells.* Acta haemat. (Basel), *39*, 203, 1968.
68. Branemark P.I., Bagge U.: *Intravascular rheology of erythrocytes in man.* Blood Cells, *3*, 11, 1977.
69. Lacelle P.L., Evans E.A., Hochmuth R.M.: *Erythrocyte membrane elasticity, fragmentation and lysis.* Blood Cells, *3*, 335, 1977.
70. Singer S.J., Nicolson G.L.: *The fluid mosaic model of the structure of cell membranes.* Science, *175*, 720, 1972.
71. Greenwalt T.J.: *The human red cell in vitro.* Grune & Stratton, New York, 1973.

72. Shohet S.B., Ness P.M.: *Hemolytic anemias. Failure of the red cell membrane*. Med. Clin. North Am., *60*, 913, 1976.
73. Marchesi V.T., Furthmayr H., Tomita M.: *The red cell membrane*. Ann. Rev. Biochem., *45*, 667, 1976.
74. Finean J.B., Coleman R., Michell R.H.: *Membranes and their cellular functions*. 2nd ed., Blackwell Sci. Publ., Oxford, 1978.
75. Fairbanks G., Steck T.L., Wallach D.F.H.: *Electrophoretic analysis of the major polypeptides of the human erythrocyte membrane*. Biochemistry, *10*, 2606, 1971.
76. Steck T.L.: *The organization of proteins in the human red blood cell membrane*. J. Cell Biol., *62*, 1, 1974.
77. Anselstetter V.: *Gel electrophoresis of the human erythrocyte membrane proteins: aberrant patterns in hematological and non hematological diseases*. Blut, *36*, 135, 1978.
78. Bennett V., Stenbuck P.J.: *The membrane attachment protein for spectrin is associated with band 3 in human erythrocyte membranes*. Nature, *280*, 468, 1979.
79. Tilney L.G., Detmers P.: *Actin in erythrocyte ghosts and its association with spectrin*. J. Cell Biol., *66*, 508, 1975.
80. Brewer G.J. (ed.): *Erythrocyte structure and function*. Liss, New York, 1975.
81. Yunis J.J., Yunis E.: *Cell antigens and cell specialization. I. A study of blood group antigens on normoblasts*. Blood, *22*, 53, 1963.
82. Mazumdar P.M.H.: *Agglutination of normoblasts with anti-D*. Vox Sang., *11*, 90, 1966.
83. Gahmberg C.G., Jakinen M., Andersson L.C.: *Expression of the major sialoglycoprotein (glycophorin) on erythroid cells in human bone marrow*. Blood, *52*, 379, 1978.
84. Bessis M.: *L'îlot érythroblastique, unité fonctionnelle de la moelle osseuse*. Rev. Hémat., *13*, 8, 1958.
85. Di Guglielmo G., Quattrin N.: *Mielosi eritremica cronica*. Haematologica (Pavia), *24*, 1, 1942.
86. Heilmeyer L., Schoener W.: *Die chronische reine Erythroblastose des Erwachsenen als leukämie-paralleler Prozess des erythrozytären Systems*. Dtsch. Arch. Klin. Med., *187*, 225, 1941.
87. Marmont A.: *Transplantation hemopoiesis. Morphological bone marrow studies after allogeneic marrow transplantation in man for severe aplastic anemia and acute leukemia*. Nouv. Rév. Franç. Hémat., *21*, 133, 1979.
88. Policard A., Bessis M.: *Micropinocytosis and rhopheocytosis*. Nature, *194*, 110, 1962.
89. Bessis M., Breton-Gorius J.: *Iron metabolism in the bone marrow as seen by electron microscopy. A critical review*. Blood, *19*, 635, 1962.
90. Le Charpentier Y., Prenant M.: *Isolement de l'îlot érythroblastique. Etude en microscopie optique et électronique à balayage*. Nouv. Rév. Franç. Hémat., *15*, 119, 1975.
91. Castoldi G.L.: *I fenomeni rigenerativi midollari dopo antimitotici*. Min. Med., *57*, 1102, 1965.
92. Jolly J.: *Recherches sur la formation des globules rouges des mammiferes*. Arch. Anat. Microsc., *9*, 133, 1907.
93. Discombe G.: *L'origine des corps de Howell-Jolly et des anneaux de Cabot*. Sangre, *29*, 262, 1948.
94. Rondanelli E.G., Trenta A., Magliulo E., Vannini V., Gerna G.: *Morphogénèse des micronoyaux supplementaires (pseudo-corps de Jolly) dans les cellules érythropoietiques irradiées*. Acta Haemat. (Basel), *35*, 232, 1966.
95. Koyama S.: *Studies on Howell-Jolly bodies*. Acta Hematol. Jap., *23*, 20, 1960.
96. van Oye E.: *L'origine des anneaux de Cabot*. Rev. Haematol., *9*, 173, 1954.
97. Bessis M.: *Réinterpretation des frottis sanguins*. Masson-Springer, Paris-Berlin, 1976.
98. Jensen W.N., Moreno G.D., Bessis M.: *An electron microscopic description of basophilic stippling in red cells*. Blood, *25*, 933, 1965.
99. Pappenheimer A.M., Thompson W.P., Parker D.D., Smith K.E.: *Anemia associated with unidentified erythrocytic inclusions*. Q.J. Med. Sci., *14*, 75, 1945.
100. Crosby W.H.: *Siderocytes and the spleen*. Blood, *12*, 165, 1957.
101. Rifkind R.A., Danon D.: *Heinz body anemia: an ultrastructural study. Heinz body formation*. Blood, *25*, 885, 1965.
102. Jacob H.S.: *Mechanism of Heinz body formation and attachment to the red cell membrane*. Semin. Hemat., *7*, 341, 1970.
103. Sears D.A., Friemnan J., White D.R.: *Binding of intracellular protein to the erythrocyte membrane during incubation: the production of Heinz bodies*. J. Lab. Clin. Med., *86*, 722, 1975.
104. Gabuzda T.G.: *Hemoglobin H and the red cell*. Blood, *27*, 568, 1966.
105. Carrell R.W., Lehmann H.: *The unstable hemoglobin hemolytic anemias*. Semin. Hemat., *6*, 116, 1969.
106. Ballas S.K., Burka E.R.: *Protease activity in the human erythrocyte: localization to the cell membrane*. Blood, *53*, 875, 1979.
107. Rifkind R.A.: *Heinz body anemia: an ultrastructural study. II. Red cell sequestration and destruction*. Blood, *26*, 433, 1965.
108. Brecher G., Bessis M.: *Present status of spiculed red cells and their relationship to the discocyte-echinocyte transformation. A critical review*. Blood, *40*, 333, 1972.
109. Weed R.I., Bessis M.: *The discocyte-stomatocyte equilibrium of normal and pathologic red cells*. Blood, *41*, 471, 1973.
110. Ponder E.: *Hemolysis and related phenomena*. Grune & Stratton, New York, p. 10, 1948.
111. Lock S.P., Smith R.S., Hardisty R.M.: *Stomatocytosis: a hereditary red cell anomaly associated with haemolytic anaemia*. Brit. J. Haemat., *7*, 303, 1961.
112. Davidson R.J., How J., Lessels S.: *Acquired stomatocytosis. Its prevalence and significance in routine hematology*. Scand. J. Haemat., *19*, 47, 1977.
113. Bessis M.: *Corpuscles. Atlas of red blood cell shapes*. Springer, Berlin, New York, 1974.
114. Weed R.I., Chailley B.: *Calcium-pH interactions in the production of shape change in erythrocytes*. Nouv. Rév. Franç. Hémat., *12*, 777, 1972.
115. Palek J., Liu S.C., Snyder L.M.: *Metabolic dependence of protein arrangement in human erythrocyte membranes. I. Analysis of spectrin-rich complexes in ATP-depleted red cells*. Blood, *51*, 385, 1978.
116. Bessis M., Brecher G.: *Action du plasma conservé sur la forme des globules rouges*. Nouv. Rév. Franç. Hémat., *11*, 305, 1971.
117. Longster G.H., Tovey L.A.D.: *The effects of certain blood-grouping sera on the red cell surface as seen by the scanning electron microscope*. Brit. J. Haemat., *23*, 635, 1972.
118. Lambertenghi-Deliliers G., Pozzoli E., Praga C.: *Le cellule del sangue al microscopio a scansione*. Farmitalia, Milano, 1976.
119. Preston F.E., Lee D.: *The effects of phenothiazines on human erythrocytes: an ultrastructural study*. Brit. J. Haemat., *20*, 563, 1971.
120. Lambertenghi G., Ferrone S., Sirchia G.: *Surface ultramicroscopy of paroxysmal nocturnal hemoglobinuria erythrocytes*. Acta Haemat. (Basel), *44*, 257, 1970.
121. Dacie J.V., Lewis S.M.: *Practical haematology*. Fifth ed., Churchill-Livingstone, Edinburgh, pp. 84-119, 1975.
122. Bessis M., Weed R., Leblond P. (eds.): *Red cell shape: physiology, pathology, ultrastructure*. Springer, New York, 1973.
123. Chanarin I.: *The megaloblastic anemias*. Blackwell Scientific Publications, Oxford and Edinburgh, pp. 339-377, 1969.
124. Beck W.S.: *Erythrocyte disorders – Anemias related to disturbance of DNA synthesis (megaloblastic anemias)*. In Hematology. Williams W.J., Beutler E., Erslev A.J. and Rundles R.W. eds., McGraw-Hill Book Co., New York, 1977.
125. Bloch M.: *Megaloblastic anemias*. Chapter 10 in *Mechanism of anemia*. Weinstein J. and Beutler E. eds., McGraw-Hill Book Co., New York, 1962.
126. Treiff R.R.: *Folic acid deficiency anemias*. Semin. Hemat., *7*, 23, 1970.

127. Magnus E.M.: *Folate studies. Folate and vitamin B_{12} values in relation to bone marrow pattern.* Scand. J. Haemat., Suppl. No. 24, Munksgaard, Copenhagen, pp. 100-104, 1975.
128. Ehrlich P.: *Farbenanalytische Untersuchungen zur Histologie und Klinik des Blutes.* Hirschwald, Berlin, 1891.
129. Jones O.P.: *The origin of megaloblasts and normoblasts in biopsied human marrow and the difference between the two series.* Anat. Rec. (Suppl.), 58, 23, 1934.
130. Fieschi A., Astaldi G.: *La coltura in vitro del midollo osseo. Problemi di fisiopatologia ematologica studiati con la tecnica della coltura dei tessuti.* Tipografia del Libro, Pavia, 1946.
131. Messner H., Fliedner T.M., Cronkite E.P.: *Kinetics of erythropoietic cell proliferation in pernicious anemia.* Series Haemat., II/4, 44, 1969.
132. Wickramasinghe S.N., Chalmers D.G., Cooper E.H.: *Arrest of cell proliferation and protein synthesis in megaloblasts of pernicious anemia.* Acta Haemat. (Basel), 41, 65, 1969.
133. Rondanelli E.G., Gorini P., Magliulo E., Fiori G.P.: *Differences in proliferative activity between normoblasts and pernicious anemia megaloblasts.* Blood, 34, 542, 1964.
134. Killmann S.A.: *Cell classification and kinetic aspects of normoblastic and megaloblastic erythropoiesis.* Cell Tissue Kinet., 3, 217, 1970.
135. Boll I.T.M., Koenigs H.P.: *The kinetics of the normal, the megaloblastic and the sideroachrestic erythropoiesis estimated by colchicine blocking* in vitro. Blood, 37, 204, 1971.
136. Polli E.: *Il problema dell'origine del megaloblasto e dei rapporti di esso con il sistema mieloide differenziato. Ricerche sulla struttura nucleare.* Arch. Sci. Med., 82, 426, 1946.
137. Castoldi G.L., Scapoli G.L., Dallapiccola B., Spanedda R.: *Analyse des anomalies chromosomiques dans l'anémie pernicieuse.* Nouv. Rév. Franç. Hémat., 9, 769, 1969.
138. Lawler S.D., Roberts P.D., Hoffbrand A.V.: *Chromosome studies in megaloblastic anemia before and after treatment.* Scand. J. Haemat., 8, 309, 1971.
139. Goldberg L.S., Fudenberg H.H.: *The autoimmune aspects of pernicious anemia.* Am. J. Med., 46, 489, 1969.
140. Hoffbrand A.V.: *Vitamin B_{12} and folate metabolism: the megaloblastic anemias and related disorders.* In: Blood and its disorders. R.M. Hardisty, D.J. Weatherall eds., Blackwell Sci. Publications, Oxford-London, pp. 392-472, 1974.
141. Schartum-Hansen H.: *Zur Morphologie des Sternalpunktates bei perniziöser Anämie und makroblastischen Anämien.* Folia Haemat. (Lpz.), 58, 145-159, 1937.
142. Dawson D.W.: *The bone marrow picture of folic acid deficiency in pregnancy.* J. Obstet. Gynec., 69, 38-46, 1962.
143. Downey H.: *The megaloblast-normoblast problem.* J. Lab. Clin. Med., 39, 837, 1952.
144. Fudenberg H.H., Estren S.: *Non-Addisonian megaloblastic anemia. The intermediate megaloblast in the differential diagnosis of pernicious and related anemias.* Am. J. Med., 25, 198, 1958.
145. White J.C., Leslie I., Davidson J.N.: *Nucleic acids of bone marrow cells, with special reference to pernicious anemia.* J. Path. Bact., 66, 291, 1953.
145. Lindenbaum J., Nath B.J.: *Megaloblastic anaemia and neutrophil hypersegmentation.* Brit. J. Haemat., 44, 511, 1980.
146. Glazer H.S., Mueller .F., Jarrold T., Sakurai K., Will J.J., Vilter R.R.: *Effect of vitamin B_{12} and folic acid on nucleic acid composition of the bone marrow of patients with megaloblastic anemia.* J. Lab. Clin. Med., 43, 905, 1954.
147. Beck W.S.: *The metabolic basis of megaloblastic erythropoiesis.* Medicine (Baltimore), 43, 715, 1964.
148. Wickramasinghe S.N., Cooper E.H., Chalmers D.C.: *A study of erythropoiesis by combined morphologic, quantitative, cytochemical and autoradiographic methods. Normal human bone marrow, vitamin B_{12} deficiency and iron deficiency.* Blood, 31, 304, 1968.
149. Quaglino D., Hayhoe F.G.J.: *Periodic-acid Schiff positivity in erythroblasts with special reference to Di Guglielmo's disease.* Brit. J. Haemat., 6, 26, 1960.
150. Stuart J., Skowron P.N.: *A cytochemical study of marrow enzymes in megaloblastic anaemia.* Brit. J. Haemat., 15, 443, 1968.
151. Rozenszajin L., Leibovich M., Shoham D., Epstein J.: *The esterase activity in megaloblasts, leukaemic and normal haemopoietic cells.* Brit. J. Haemat., 14, 605, 1968.
152. Kass L., Peters C.L.: *Non-specific esterase activity in pernicious anemia and chronic erythremic myelosis.* Am. J. Clin. Path., 68, 273, 1977.
153. Ito K., Ito N., Sato S., Katsunuma H.: *Electron microscopic study on the megaloblasts in pernicious anemia.* Acta Hemat. Jap., 27, 436, 1964.
154. Goodman J.R., Wallerstein R.O., Hall S.G.: *The ultrastructure of the bone marrow histiocytes in megaloblastic anaemia and the anaemia of infection.* Brit. J. Haemat., 14, 471, 1968.
155. Wickramasinghe S.N., Bush V.: *Electron microscopic and high resolution autoradiographic studies of megaloblastic erythropoiesis.* Acta Haemat. (Basel), 57, 1, 1977.
156. Stebbins R., Scott J., Herbert V.: *Drug-induced megaloblastic anemias.* Semin. Hemat., 10, 235, 1973.
157. Baserga A., Castoldi G.L.: *Sex chromatin after cytostatic drugs.* Lancet, ii, 106, 1966.
158. Undritz E.: *Hämatologische Tafeln:.* Sandoz, Basel, 1952.
159. Berendson S., Lowman J., Sundberg D., Watson C.J.: *Idiopathic dyserythropoietic jaundice.* Blood, 24, 1, 1964.
160. Crookston J.A., Crookston M.C., Burnie K.L., Francombe W.H., Dacie J.V., Davis J.A., Lewis S.M.: *Hereditary erythroblastic multinuclearity with a positive acidified-serum test. A type of congenital dyserythropoietic anaemia.* Brit. J. Haemat., 17, 11, 1969.
161. Heimpel H., Wendt F.: *Congenital dyserythropoietic anemia with karyorrhexis and multinuclearity of erythroblasts.* Helv. Med. Acta, 34, 103, 1968.
162. Lewis S.M., Verwilghen R.L. (eds.): *Dyserythropoiesis.* Academic Press, London-New York-San Francisco, 1977.
163. Heilmeyer L., Keiderling W., Bilger R., Bernauer H.: *Ueber chronische refractäre Anämien mit sideroblastischen Knochenmark (Anemia refractoria sideroblastica).* Folia Haemat. (Frankfurt), 2, 49, 1958.
164. Heilmeyer L., Emmrich J., Hennemann H.H., Keiderling W., Lee M., Bilger R., Schubothe H.: *Ueber eine chronische hypochrome Anämie bei zwei Geschwistern auf der Grundlage einer Eisenverwertungstörung (Anemia hypochromica sideroachrestica hereditaria).* Folia Haemat. (Frankfurt), 2, 61, 1958.
165. Björkman S.E.: *Chronic refractory anemia with sideroblastic bone marrow: a study of four cases.* Blood, 11, 250, 1956.
166. Dacie J.V., Smith M.D., White J.C., Mollin D.L.: *Refractory normoblastic anaemia: a clinical and haematologic study of seven cases.* Brit. J. Haemat., 5, 56, 1959.
167. Mollin D.L.: *Sideroblasts and sideroblastic anaemia.* Brit. J. Hemat., 11, 41, 1965.
168. Bernard J., Lortholary P., Levy J.P., Boiron M., Najean Y., Tanzer J.: *Les anémies normochromes sidéroblastiques primitives.* Nouv. Rév. Franç. Hémat., 3, 723, 1963.
169. Tura S., Baccarani M., Ricci P., Zaccaria A., Muller-Berat N.: *Anemia diseritropoietica idiopatica acquisita.* Atti XXIV Congr. Naz. Soc. It. Ematologia, Pavia, pp. 65-144, 1973.
170. Linman J.W., Bagby G.C. Jr.: *The preleukemic syndrome: clinical and laboratory features, natural course and management.* Blood Cells, 2, 11, 1976.
171. Dreyfus B.: *Preleukemic states. I. Definition and classification. II. Refractory anemia with excess of myeloblasts in the bone marrow (Smoldering acute leukemia).* Blood Cells, 2, 33, 1976.
172. Yunis A.A.: *Chloramphenicol toxicity.* In: Blood disorders due to drugs and other agents. Girwood R.H. ed., Excerpta Medica, Amsterdam, p. 107, 1973.

173. Bowmann W.D.: *Abnormal ("ringed") sideroblasts in various hematologic and non hematologic disorders.* Blood, *18*, 662, 1961.
174. Bessis M., Jensen W.N.: *Sideroblastic anaemia, mitochondria and erythroblastic iron.* Brit. J. Haemat., *11*, 49, 1965.
175. Larizza P., Orlandi F.: *Electron microscopic observations on bone marrow and liver tissue in hereditary refractory sideroblastic anemia.* Acta haemat. (Basel), *31*, 9, 1964.
176. Kuschner J.P., Lee G.R., Wintrobe M.M., Cartwright G.E.: *Idiopathic refractory sideroblastic anemia: clinical and laboratory investigation of 17 patients and review of the literature.* Medicine, *50*, 139, 1971.
177. Bessis M., Breton-Gorius J.: *Ferritin and ferruginous micelles in normal erythroblasts and hypochromic hypersideremic anemias.* Blood, *14*, 423, 1959.
178. Maldonado J.E., Maigne J., Lecoq D.: *Comparative electron-microscopic study in the erythrocytic line in refractory anemia (Preleukemia) and myelo-monocytic leukemia.* Blood Cells, *3*, 167, 1976.
179. Breton-Gorius J., Flandrin G., Daniel M.Th., Brouet J.C.: *Septate-like junctions acquired by erythroblasts in a case of refractory anemia.* Scand. J. Haemat., *10*, 219-224, 1973.
180. Flandrin G., Daniel M.Th., Breton-Gorius J., Brouet J.C., Bernard J.: *Ilot érythroblastique anormal dû au développement de jonctions intercellulaires (Synartèse érythroblastique). Un nouveau mécanisme d'anémie. Problèmes posés par le diagnostic.* Nouv. Rév. Franç. Hémat., *14*, 161-180, 1974.
181. Frisch B., Lewis S.M., Swan M.: *Intercellular contacts between erythroid precursors in the bone marrow in dyserythropoiesis.* Brit. J. Haemat., *33*, 469-475, 1976.
182. Wickramasinghe S.N., Bush V.: *An electron microscope study of the intercellular contacts between the erythroblasts of patients with hypersiderotic bone marrows.* Scand. J. Haemat., *19*, 25-32, 1977.
183. Tanaka Y., Brecher G., Bull B.: *Ferritin localization on the erythroblast cell membrane and rhopheocytosis in hypersiderotic human bone marrows.* Blood, *28*, 758-769, 1966.
184. Wendt F., Heimpel H.: *Kongenitale dyserythropoietische Anämie bei einem zweieiigen Zwillingpaar.* Med. Klin., *62*, 172, 1967.
185. Breton-Gorius J., Daniel M., Clauvel J., Dreyfus B.: *Anomalies ultrastructurales des érythroblastes et des érythrocytes dans six cas de dysérythropoèse congénitale.* Nouv. Rév. Franç. Hémat., *12*, 653, 1972.
186. Lewis S.M., Nelson D.A., Pitcher C.S.: *Clinical and ultrastructural aspects of congenital dyserythropoietic anaemia type I.* Brit. J. Haemat., *23*, 113, 1972.
187. Wong K.Y., Hug G., Lampkin B.C.: *Congenital dyserythropoietic anemia type II: ultrastructural and radioautographic studies of blood and bone marrow.* Blood, *39*, 23, 1972.
188. Björksten B., Holmgren G., Roos G., Stenling R.: *Congenital dyserythropoietic anaemia type III: an electron microscopic study.* Brit. J. Haemat., *38*, 17, 1978.
189. Meuret G., Boll I., Graf Keyserlingk D., Heissmeyer H.: *Morphologische und kinetische Befunde bei einer kongenitalen dyserythropoietischen Anämie.* Blut, *21*, 341, 1970.
190. Clauvel J.P., Cosson A., Breton-Gorius J., Flandrin G., Faille A., Bonnet-Gajdos M., Turpin F., Bernard J.: *Dysérythropoèse congénitale.* Nouv. Rév. Franc. Hémat., *12*, 653, 1972.
191. Bianchini E., Ferrari L., Tentoni M.: *Le anemie diseritropoietiche. Inquadramento della diseritropoiesi e descrizione di un caso di CDA tipo I e di casi di diseritropoiesi acquisita.* Atti XXIV Congr. Naz. Soc. It. Ematologia, Pavia, pp. 31-54, 1973.
192. Maldonado J.E., Taswell H.F.: *Type I dyserythropoietic anemia in an elderly patient.* Blood, *44*, 495, 1974.
193. Queisser W., Spiertz E., Jost E., Heimpel H.: *Proliferation disturbances of erythroblasts in congenital dyserythropoietic anemia type I and II.* Acta Haemat. (Basel), *45*, 65, 1971.
194. Meuret G., Tschan P., Schlüter G., Graf Keyserlingk D., Boll I.: *DNA-, histone-, RNA-, hemoglobin-content and DNA-synthesis in erythroblasts in a case of congenital dyserythropoietic anemia type I.* Blut, *24*, 32, 1972.
195. De Lozzio C.B., Valencia J.I., Accame F.: *Chromosomal study in erythroblastic endopolyploidy.* Lancet, *i*, 1004, 1962.
196. Roberts P.D., Wallis P.G., Jackson A.D.: *Hemolytic anemia with multinucleated erythroblasts in the marrow.* Lancet, *i*, 1186, 1962.
197. Schärer K., Marti H.R., Baumann Th.: *Konstitutionelle Anämie mit Kernteilungsstörungen der Erythroblasten.* Schweiz. Med. Wschr., *95*, 1511, 1965.
198. Verwilghen R.L., Tan P., De Wolf-Peeters C., Broeckaert-Vanorshoven A., Louwagie A.C.: *Cell membrane anomaly impeding cell division.* Experientia, *27*, 1467, 1971.
199. Wolff J.A., von Hofe F.: *Familial erythroid multinuclearity.* Blood, *6*, 1274, 1951.
200. Bergström I., Jacobsson L.: *Hereditarity benign erythroreticulosis.* Blood, *19*, 296, 1962.
201. Goudsmit R., Beckers D., de Bruijne J.I.D., Engelfriet C.P., James J., Morselt A.F.W., Reynierse E.: *Congenital dyserythropoietic anaemia type III.* Brit. J. Haemat., *23*, 97, 1972.
202. Wickramasinghe S.N., Goudsmit R.: *Some aspects of the biology of multinucleate and giant mononucleate erythroblasts in a patient with CDA, type III.* Brit. J. Haemat., *41*, 485, 1979.
203. Wickramasinghe S.N., Chalmers D.D., Cooper E.H.: *A study of ineffective erythropoiesis in sideroblastic anemia and erythremic myelosis.* Cell Tissue Kinet., *1*, 43, 1968.
204. Heimpel H.: *Kongenitale dyserythropoietische Anämien.* Blut, *31*, 261, 1975.
205. Schuppler J., Cornu P., Krey G., Gudat F., Speck B.: *Congenital dyserythropoietic anemia with ultrastructural features of type I and type II.* Blut, *31*, 271, 1975.
206. Mc Bride J.A., Wilson W.E.C., Baille N.: *Congenital dyserythropoietic anemia type IV.* Am. Soc. Hemat., San Francisco. Blood, *38*, 837, 1971.
207. Sansone G.: *A new type of congenital dyserythropoietic anaemia.* Brit. J. Haemat., *39*, 537, 1978.
208. Weatherall D.J., Clegg J.B., Knox-Macauley H.H.M., Bunch C., Hopkins C.R., Temperley I.J.: *A genetically determined disorder with features both of thalassaemia and congenital dyserythropoietic anaemia.* Brit. J. Haemat., *24*, 681, 1973.
209. Quattrin N.: *Una nuova malattia tesaurismotica: mucopolisaccaridosi genotipica diseritropoietica.* Min. Pediat., *23*, 672, 1971.
210. Quattrin N.: *Dyserythropoietische Anämien.* Schweiz. Med. Wschr., *105*, 65, 1975.
211. Schmid R., Schwartz S., Watson C.J.: *Porphyrin content of bone marrow and liver in the various forms of porphyria.* Arch. Int. Med., *93*, 167, 1954.
212. Elder G.H., Gray C.H., Nicholson D.C.: *The porphyrias: a review.* J. Clin. Path., *25*, 1013, 1972.
213. Waldenström J.G.: *The porphyrias.* In: *Hematology.* Williams W.J., Beutler E., Erslev A.J., Rundles R.W. eds., McGraw-Hill Book Co., New York, p. 551, 1977.
214. Larizza P.: *The problem of erythropoietic porphyria in the light of the latest advances in biochemistry and morphology.* Panminerva Med., *4*, 315, 1962.
215. Varadi S.: *Haematological aspects in a case of erythropoietic porphyria.* Brit. J. Haemat., *4*, 270, 1958.
216. Doss M.: *Hematological disturbances of porphyrin metabolism.* In: *Strategies in clinical hematology.* Gross R., Hellriegel K.P. eds., Rec. Results in Cancer Research (69), Springer, Berlin-Heidelberg-New York, pp. 97-109, 1979.
217. Fairbanks V.F., Fahey J.L., Beutler E.: *Clinical disorders of iron metabolism.* Grune & Stratton, New York and London, pp. 128-228, 1971.
218. Fairbanks V.F., Beutler E.: *Iron deficiency.* In: *Hematology.* Williams W.J., Beutler E., Erslev A.J., Rundles R.W. eds., McGraw-Hill Book Co., New York, p. 363, 1977.
219. Finch C.A., Beutler E., Brown E.B., Crosby W.H.,

Hegsted M., Moore C.V., Pritchard J.A., Sturgeon P., Wintrobe M.M.: *Iron deficiency in the United States.* J.A.M.A., *203*, 407, 1968.
220. Jacobs A., Worwood M. (eds.): *Iron in Biochemistry and Medicine.* Academic Press, London and New York, 1974.
221. Wintrobe M.M.: *Clinical hematology.* Lea & Febiger, Philadelphia, pp. 621-670, 1974.
221. England J.M., Fraser P.: *Discrimination between iron-deficiency and heterozygous-thalassemia syndromes in differential diagnosis of microcytosis.* Lancet, *i*, 145, 1979.
222. Rath C.E., Finch C.A.: *Sternal marrow hemosiderin: a method for the determination of available iron stores in man.* J. Lab. Clin. Med., *33*, 81, 1948.
223. Beutler E.: *Clinical evaluation of iron stores.* New Engl. J. Med., *256*, 692, 1957.
224. Wallerstein R.O.: *Marrow iron.* J.A.M.A., *238*, 1661, 1977.
225. Fong T.P., Okafor L.A., Thomas W., Westerman M.P.: *Stainable iron in aspirated and needle-biopsy specimens of marrow: a source of error.* Am. J. Hemat., *2*, 47, 1977.
226. Hansen H.A., Weinfeld A.: *Hemosiderin estimations and sideroblast counts in the differential diagnosis of iron deficiency and other anemias.* Acta Med. Scand., *165*, 333, 1959.
227. Bainton D.F., Finch C.A.: *The diagnosis of iron deficiency anemia.* Am. J. Med., *37*, 62, 1964.
228. Block M.H.: *Text-Atlas of hematology.* Lea & Febiger, Philadelphia, p. 74, 1976.
229. Fritsch E.F., Lawn R.M., Maniatis T.: *Characterization of deletions which affect the expression of fetal globin genes in man.* Nature, *279*, 598, 1979.
230. Weatherhall D.J., Clegg J.B.: *Recent developments in the molecular genetics of human hemoglobin.* Cell, *16*, 467, 1979.
231. Flavell R.A., Kooler J.M., Deboer E., Little P.F.R., Williamson R.: *Analysis of the β- δ-globin gene loci in normal and Hb Lepore DNA: direct determination of gene linkage and intergene distance.* Cell, *15*, 25, 1978.
232. Mears J.G., Ramirez F., Leibowitz D., Bank A.: *Organization of human δ- and β-globin genes in cellular DNA and the presence of intragenic inserts.* Cell, *15*, 15, 1978.
233. Little P.F.R., Flavell R.A., Kooler J.M., Annison G., Williamson R.: *The structure of the human fetal globin gene locus.* Nature, *278*, 227, 1979.
234. Ingram V.M., Stretton A.O.W.: *Genetic basis of the thalassemia diseases.* Nature, *184*, 1903, 1959.
235. Weatherhall D.J., Clegg J.B.: *The thalassemia syndromes.* 2nd ed., Blackwell, Oxford, 1972.
236. Bank A.: *The thalassemia syndromes.* Blood, *51*, 369, 1978.
237. Conconi F., Rowley P.T., Del Senno L., Pontremoli S., Volpato S.: *Induction of β-globin synthesis in the β-thalassemia of Ferrara.* Nature, *238*, 83, 1972.
238. Ottolenghi S., Comi P., Giglioni R., Tolstoshev P., Panyon W.G., Mitchell G.J., Williamson R., Russo G., Musumeci S., Schiliro G., Tsistrakis G.A., Charache S., Wood W.G., Clegg J.B., Weatherhall D.J.: *δ-β-thalassemia is due to a gene deletion.* Cell, *9*, 71, 1978.
239. Gerald P.S., Diamond I.K.: *The diagnosis of thalassemia trait by starch block electrophoresis of the hemoglobin.* Blood, *13*, 61, 1958.
240. Baglioni C.: *The fusion of two peptide chains in hemoglobin Lepore and its interpretation as a genetic deletion.* Proc. Natl. Acad. Sci. (U.S.A.), *48*, 1880, 1962.
241. Hunt J.A., Lehmann H.: *Abnormal human hemoglobins: hemoglobin "Bart's": a fetal hemoglobin without alpha-chains.* Nature, *184*, 872, 1959.
242. Rigas D.A., Koler R.D., Osgood E.E.: *New hemoglobin possessing a higher electrophoretic mobility than normal adult hemoglobin.* Science, *171*, 372, 1955.
243. Gouttas A., Fessas Ph., Tsevrenis H., Xefteri E.: *Description d'une nouvelle varieté d'anémie hémolitique congénitale (Etude hématologique, électrophorétique et génétique).* Sang, *26*, 911, 1955.
244. Weatherhall D.J.: *The thalassemias.* In: *Hematology.* Williams W.J., Beutler E., Erslev A.J., Rundles R.W. eds., McGraw-Hill Book Co., New York, p. 391, 1977.
244. Adams J.G., Steinberg M.H.: *Alpha-thalassemia.* Am. J. Hemat., *2*, 317, 1977.
245. Weatherhall D.J., Clegg J.B.: *The α-chain termination mutants and their relationship to the α-thalassemias.* Phil. Trans. Roy. Soc., *271*, 411, 1975.
246. Cooley T.B., Lee P.: *A series of cases of splenomegaly in children with anemia and peculiar bone changes.* Trans. Am. Pediatr. Soc., *37*, 29, 1925.
247. Rietti F.: *Hemolytic anemias with increased osmotic resistance of the erythrocytes.* Acta Med. Scand., *125*, 451, 1946.
248. Silvestroni E., Bianco I.: *Le emoglobine umane.* Ed. Istituto "Gregorio Mendel", Roma, 1963.
249. Baserga A., Barrai I., Coppo M., Bonomo L., Carcassi U., Castaldi G., Tentori L.: *Aspetti internistici della talassemia minor.* Relaz. LXXXI Congr. Naz. Soc. It. Medicina Interna, Roma, 1980.
250. Huisman T.H.J., Schroeder W.A., Efremov G.D., Duma H., Mladenovsky B., Hyman C.B., Rachmilewitz E.A., Bower N., Miller A., Brodie A., Shelton J.R., Shelton J.B., Apell G.: *The present status of the heterogeneity of fetal hemoglobin in β-thalassemia. An attempt to unify some observations in thalassemia and related conditions.* Ann. N.Y. Acad. Sci., *232*, 107, 1974.
251. Astaldi G., Rondanelli E.G., Bernardelli E., Strosselli E.: *An abnormal substance present in the erythroblasts of thalassemia major. Cytochemical investigations.* Acta haemat. (Basel), *12*, 145, 1954.
252. Fessas Ph., Papayannopoulou T.: *Cytochemical observations on β-thalassemia.* Acta haemat. (Basel), *34*, 1, 1965.
253. Yataganas X., Gahrton G., Fessas Ph., Kesse-Elias M., Thorell B.: *Proliferative activity and glycogen accumulation of erythroblasts in β-thalassaemia.* Brit. J. Haemat., *24*, 651, 1973.
254. Polliack A., Rachmilewitz E.A.: *Ultrastructural studies in β-thalassaemia major.* Brit. J. Haemat., *24*, 319, 1973.
255. Wickramasinghe S.N., Bush V.: *Observations on the ultrastructure of erythropoietic cells and reticulum cells in the bone marrow of patients with homozygous β-thalassaemia.* Brit. J. Haemat., *30*, 395, 1975.
256. Zaino E.C., Rossi M.B., Pham T.D., Azar H.A.: *Gaucher's cells in thalassemia.* Blood, *38*, 457, 1971.
257. Wickramasinghe S.N., Hughes M.: *Some features of bone marrow macrophages in patients with homozygous β-thalassaemia.* Brit. J. Haemat., *38*, 23, 1978.
258. Beltrami C.A., Bearzi I., Fabris G.: *Storage cells of spleen and bone marrow in thalassemia: an ultrastructural study.* Blood, *41*, 901, 1973.
259. Quattrin N.: *Sea-blue histiocytosis.* Haematologica (Pavia), *62*, 320, 1977.
260. Lehmann H., Huntsman R.G.: *Man's hemoglobin.* J.B. Lippincott Co., Philadelphia, 1966.
261. Pauling L., Itano H.A., Singer S.J., Wells I.C.: *Sickle cell anemia, a molecular disease.* Science, *110*, 543, 1949.
262. Ingram V.M.: *Gene mutation in human hemoglobin. The chemical difference between normal and sickle cell hemoglobin.* Nature, *180*, 326, 1957.
263. Herrick J.B.: *Peculiar elongated and sickle-shaped red corpuscles in a case of severe anemia.* Arch. Int. Med., *6*, 517, 1910.
264. Tosteson D.C., Carlssen E., Dunham E.T.: *The effects of sickling on iron transport. I. Effect of sickling on potassium.* J. Gen. Physiol., *39*, 31, 1955.
265. Jensen M., Shohet S.B., Nathan D.G.: *The role of red cell energy metabolism in the generation of irreversible sickled cells in vitro.* Blood, *42*, 835, 1973.
266. Eaton J.W., Skelton T.D., Swofford H.S., Kolpin C.E., Jacob H.S.: *Elevated erythrocyte calcium in sickle cell disease.* Nature, *246*, 105, 1973.
267. Hosey M.M., Tao M.: *Altered erythrocyte membrane phosphorylation in sickle cell disease.* Nature, *263*, 424, 1976.
268. Daland G.A., Castle W.B.: *A simple and rapid method for demonstrating sickling of the red blood cells:*

the use of reducing agents. J. Lab. Clin. Med., 33, 1085, 1948.
269. Klug P.P., Lessin S.: *Microvascular blood flow of sickled erythrocytes. A dynamic morphologic study.* Blood Cells, 3, 263, 1977.
270. Chien S.: *Rheology of sickle cells and erythrocyte content.* Blood Cells, 3, 283, 1977.
271. Comer P.B., Fred H.L.: *Diagnosis of sickle cell disease by ophtalmoscopic inspection of the conjunctiva.* New Engl. J. Med., 271, 344, 1964.
272. Paton D.: *Conjunctival sign of sickle cell disease.* Am. J. Ophtalmol., 68, 627, 1962.
273. Condon P.L., Serjeant G.R.: *Ocular findings in homozygous sickle-cell anemia in Jamaica.* Am. J. Ophtalmol., 73, 533, 1972.
274. Perutz M.F.: *Hemoglobin: genetic abnormalities.* New Scientist & Science Journal, 50, 757, 1971.
275. Murayama M.: *Molecular mechanisms of red cell "sickling".* Science, 153, 145, 1966.
276. White J.M.: *The unstable hemoglobins.* Brit. Med. Bull., 32, 219, 1976.
277. Sansone G.: *Acquisizioni moderne in tema di emoglobinopatie.* La Ricerca Clin. Lab., 1, 259, 1971.
278. Lehmann H., Huntsman R.G.: *Man's hemoglobins.* J.B. Lippincott Co., Philadelphia, 1977.
279. Di Guglielmo G.: *Ricerche di ematologia. I. Un caso di eritroleucemia.* Folia Med., 13, 386, 1917.
280. Di Guglielmo G.: *Eritremie acute.* Boll. Soc. Med. Chir. Pavia, 40, 665, 1926.
281. Dameshek W., Baldini M.: *The Di Guglielmo syndrome.* Blood 13, 192, 1958.
282. Dameshek W.: *The Di Guglielmo syndrome revisited.* Blood, 34, 567, 1969.
283. Hayhoe F.G.J., Quaglino D.: *Refractory sideroblastic anemia and erythremic myelosis: possible relationship and cytochemical observations.* Brit. J. Haemat., 6, 381, 1960.
284. Castoldi G.L., Yam L.T., Mitus W.J., Crosby W.H.: *Chromosomal studies in erythroleukemia and in chronic erythremic myelosis.* Blood, 31, 202, 1968.
285. Di Guglielmo G.: *Le malattie eritremiche ed eritroleucemiche.* Ed. Pensiero Sci., Roma, 1962.
286. Sondergaard-Pedersen H.: *Erythrophagocytosis by pathological erythroblasts in the Di Guglielmo syndrome.* Scand. J. Haemat., 13, 260, 1974.
287. Quaglino D., Hayhoe F.G.J.: *Periodic acid Schiff positivity in erythroblasts with special reference to Di Guglielmo's syndrome.* Brit. J. Haemat., 6, 26, 1960.
288. Hayhoe F.G.J., Quaglino D., Doll R.: *The cytology and cytochemistry of acute leukemias.* Her Majesty's Stationary Office, London, 1964.
289. Astaldi G., Strosselli E., Sauli S.: *Histochemical research on erythroblast PAS-positivity under various pathological conditions.* Proc. 9th Congr. Europ. Soc. Hematology, Lisbon, Basel, Karger, p. 86, 1963.
289. Spremolla G., Di Stasio L., Mirenda P., Saba P.: *Mielosi eritremiche, eritroleucemiche e megacariocitemiche.* Omnia med. terap., 1, 68, 1972.
290. Kass L.: *Cytochemical abnormalities of atypical erythroblasts in acute erythremic myelosis.* Acta haemat. (Basel), 54, 321, 1975.
290. Kass L.: *Esterase activity in erythroleukemia.* Am. J. Clin. Path., 67, 368, 1977.
291. Yam L.T., Li C.Y., Crosby W.H.: *Cytochemical identification of monocytes and granulocytes.* Am. J. Clin. Path., 55, 283, 1971.
292. Yam L.T., Finkel H.E., Weintraub L.R., Crosby W.H.: *Circulating iron-containing macrophages in hemocromatosis.* New Engl. J. Med., 279, 512, 1968.
293. Hoffbrand A.V., Ganeshaguru K., Llewelin P., Janossy G.: *Biochemical markers in leukemia and lymphoma.* In: Gross R., Hellriegel K.P.: *Strategies in Clinical Hematology.* Rec. Res. Cancer Res., 69, Springer, Berlin-New York, pp. 25-39, 1979.
294. Bessis M., Thiery J.P.: *Electron microscopy of human white blood cells and their stem cells.* Int. Rev. Cytol., 12, 199, 1961.
295. Huhn D., Kuboth W., Schmalzl F.: *Di Guglielmo syndrome.* Dtsch. Med. Wschr., 98, 355, 1973.
296. Adamson J.W., Fialkow P.J., Murphy S., Prchal J.F., Steinemann L.: *Polycythemia vera. Stem-cell and probable clonal origin of the disease.* New Engl. J. Med., 295, 913, 1976.
297. Bunch C., Wood W.G., Weatherhall D.J., Adamson J.W.: *Cellular origins of the fetal-hemoglobin-containing cells of normal adults.* Lancet, i, 1163, 1979.
298. Pollycove M., Winchell H.S., Lawrence J.H.: *Classification and evolution of patterns of erythropoiesis in polycythemia vera as studied by iron kinetics.* Blood, 28, 807, 1966.
299. Block M.H.: *Text-Atlas of hematology.* Lea & Febiger, Philadelphia, pp. 277-298, 1976.
300. Roberts B.E., Miles D.W., Woods C.G.: *Polycythemia vera and myelosclerosis: a bone marrow study.* Brit. J. Haemat., 16, 75, 1969.
301. Wassermann L.R.: *Polycythemia vera – its course and treatment. Relation to myeloid metaplasia and leukemia.* Bull. N.Y. Acad. Med., 3, 343, 1954.
302. Eaves C.J., Eaves A.C.: *Erythropoietin (Ep) dose-response curves for three classes of erythroid progenitors in normal human marrow and in patients with polycythemia vera.* Blood, 52, 1196, 1978.
303. Mohler D.N.: *Adenosine triphosphate metabolism in hereditary spherocytosis.* J. Clin. Invest., 44, 1417, 1968.
304. Jacob H.S.: *The defective red cell in hereditary spherocytosis.* Annual Review of Medicine, 20, 41, 1969.
305. Wiley J.S.: *Coordonated increase of sodium leak and sodium pump in hereditary spherocytosis.* Brit. J. Haemat., 22, 529, 1972.
306. Jacob H.S., Ruby A., Overland E.S., Mazia D.: *Abnormal membrane protein of red blood cells in hereditary spherocytosis.* J. Clin. Invest., 50, 1800, 1971.
307. Engelhard R.: *Impaired reassemblance of red blood cell membrane components in hereditary spherocytosis.* In: *Membrane in Disease.* Bolis L., Hoffman J.F., Leaf A. eds., Raven Press, New York, p. 75, 1976.
308. Kuiper P.J.C., Livni A.: *Differences in fatty acid composition between normal erythrocytes and hereditary spherocytosis affected cells.* Biochem. Biophys. Acta, 260, 755, 1972.
309. Zail S.S.: *The erythrocyte membrane abnormality of hereditary spherocytosis (Annotation).* Brit. J. Haemat., 37, 305, 1977.
310. Dresbach M.: *Elliptical human red corpuscles.* Science, 19, 469, 1904.
311. Lipton E.: *Elliptocytosis with hemolytic anemia: the effect of splenectomy.* Pediatrics, 15, 67, 1955.
312. Proietti-Orlandi F., De Ferrari A., Marotti F., Rossi-Mori A., Paleani-Vettori P.G., Torlontano G.: *Determinazione automatica del grado di deformazione ellittica dei globuli rossi.* LAB, J. Res. Lab. Med., 4, 383, 1978.
313. Baasen F.A., Kornzweig A.L.: *Malformation of the erythrocytes in a case of atypical retinitis pigmentosa.* Blood, 5, 381, 1950.
314. Smith J.A., Lonergan E.T., Sterling K.: *Spur-cell anemia. Hemolytic anemia with red cells resembling acanthocytes in alcoholic cyrrhosis.* New Engl. J. Med., 271, 396, 1964.
315. Cooper R.A., Diloy-Puray M., Lando P., Greenberg M.S.: *An analysis of lipoproteins, bile acids and red cell membranes associated with target cells and spur cells in patients with liver disease.* J. Clin. Invest., 51, 3182, 1972.
316. Cooper R.A.: *Pathogenesis of burr cells in uremia.* J. Clin. Invest., 49, 22, 1974.
317. Carcassi U.: *Eritroenzimopatie ed anemie emolitiche.* Ed. Omnia Med., Pisa, 1959.
318. Larizza P., Brunetti P., Grignani F.: *Anemie emolitiche enzimopeniche.* Arch. Hemat., 45, 1, 1960.
319. Luzzatto L., Allan N.C.: *Different properties of glucose-6-phosphate dehydrogenase from human erythrocytes with normal and abnormal levels.* Biochem. & Biophys. Res. Commun., 21, 547, 1965.
320. Beutler E.: *Glucose-6-phosphate dehydrogenase deficiency.* In: *Hematology*, 2nd ed. Williams W.J., Beutler E., Erslev A.J., Rundles R.W. eds., McGraw-Hill Book Co., New York, pp. 466-479, 1977.

321. Yoshida A., Beutler E.: *Human glucose-6-phosphate dehydrogenase variants: a supplementary tabulation.* Ann. Hum. Genet., *41*, 437, 1978.
322. Johnson G.J., Allen D.W., Cadman S., Fairbanks V.F., White J.G., Lampkin B.C., Kaplan M.E.: *Red-cell-membrane polypeptide aggregates in glucose-6-phosphate dehydrogenase mutants with chronic hemolytic disease.* New Engl. J. Med., *301*, 522, 1979.
323. Tanaka K.R., Paglia D.E.: *Pyruvate kinase deficiency.* Semin. Hemat., *8*, 367, 1971.
324. Kahn A., Marie J., Galand C., Boivin P.: *Chronic hemolytic anemia in two patients heterozygous for erythrocyte pyruvate kinase deficiency. Electrofocusing and immunological studies of erythrocyte and liver pyruvate kinase.* Scand. J. Haemat., *16*, 250, 1976.
325. Zanella A., Rebulla P., Vullo C., Izzo C., Tedesco F., Sirchia G.: *Hereditary pyruvate kinase deficiency: role of the abnormal enzyme in red cell pathophysiology.* Brit. J. Haemat., *40*, 551, 1978.
326. Oski F.A., Nathan D.G., Sidel V.W., Diamond L.K.: *Extreme hemolysis and red-cell distortion in erythrocyte pyruvate kinase deficiency. I. Morphology, erythrokinetics and family enzyme studies.* New Engl. J. Med., *270*, 1023, 1964.
327. Keitt A.S.: *Pyruvate kinase deficiency and related disorders of red cell glycolysis.* Amer. J. Med., *41*, 762, 1966.
328. Nathan D.G., Oski F.A., Sidel V.W., Gardner F.H., Diamond L.K.: *Studies of erythrocyte spicule formation and hemolytic anaemia.* Brit. J. Haemat., *12*, 385, 1966.
329. Leblond P.F., Lyonnais J., Delage J.M.: *Erythrocyte populations in pyruvate kinase deficiency anaemia following splenectomy. I. Cell morphology.* Brit. J. Haemat., *39*, 55, 1978.
329. Beutler E.: *Red cell enzyme defects as nondiseases and as diseases.* Blood, *54*, 1, 1979.
329. Valentine W.N.: *Hemolytic anemia and inborn errors of metabolism.* Blood, *54*, 549, 1979.
330. Crosby W.H.: *Paroxysmal nocturnal hemoglobinuria: a classic description by Paul Strübing in 1882 and a bibliography of the disease.* Blood, *6*, 270, 1951.
331. Crosby W.H.: *Paroxysmal nocturnal hemoglobinuria. Plasma factors of the hemolytic system.* Blood, *8*, 444, 1953.
332. Rosse W.F., Logue G.L., Adams J., Crookston J.H.: *Mechanisms of immune lysis of the red cells in hereditary erythroblastic multinuclearity with a positive acidified serum test and paroxysmal nocturnal hemoglobinuria.* J. Clin. Invest., *53*, 31, 1974.
333. Götze O., Muller-Eberhard H.J.: *Lysis of erythrocytes by complement in the absence of antibody.* J. Exp. Med., *132*, 898, 1970.
333. Biesecker G., Podack E.R., Halverson C.A., Müller-Eberhard H.J.: *C5b-q Dimer: isolation from complement lysed cells and ultrastructural identification with complement-dependent membrane lesions.* J. Exp. Med., *149*, 448-458, 1979.
333. Dourmashkin R.R.: *The structural events associated with the attachment of complement components to cell membrane in reactive lysis.* Immunology, *35*, 205-212, 1978.
333. Boros T., Douramshkin R.R., Humphrey J.H.: *Lesions in erythrocyte membranes caused by immune hemolysis.* Nature, *202*, 251, 1964.
334. Jenkins D.E. Jr., Hartmann R.C.: *Paroxysmal nocturnal hemoglobinuria terminating in acute myeloblastic leukemia.* Blood, *33*, 274, 1969.
335. Holden D., Lichtman H.: *Paroxysmal nocturnal hemoglobinuria with acute leukemia.* Blood, *33*, 283, 1969.
336. Kaufmann R.W., Schechter G.P., Mc Farland W.: *Paroxysmal nocturnal hemoglobinuria terminating in acute granulocytic leukemia.* Blood, *33*, 287, 1969.
337. Carmel R., Coltman C.A., Yatteau R.F., Costanzi J.J.: *Association of paroxysmal nocturnal hemoglobinuria with erythroleukemia.* New Engl. J. Med., *283*, 1329, 1970.
338. Tso S.C., Chan T.K.: *Paroxysmal nocturnal haemoglobinuria and chronic myeloid leukemia in the same patient.* Scand. J. Haemat., *10*, 384, 1973.
339. Crosby W.H.: *Paroxysmal nocturnal hemoglobinuria. Report of a case complicated by an aregenerative (aplastic) crisis.* Ann. Int. Med., *39*, 1107, 1953.
340. Hirsch J., Ungar B., Robinson J.S.: *Paroxysmal nocturnal hemoglobinuria: an acquired dyshemopoiesis.* Aust. Ann. Med., *13*, 24, 1964.
341. Dameshek W.: *Paroxysmal nocturnal hemoglobinuria. A "candidate myeloproliferative disorder".* Blood, *33*, 263, 1969.
342. Luzzatto L., Familusi J.B., Williams C.K.O., Junaid T.A., Rotoli B., Alfinito F.: *The PNH abnormality in myeloproliferative disorders: associations of PNH and acute erythremic myelosis in two children?* Haematologica (Pavia), *64*, 13, 1979.
343. Dacie J.V.: *The hemolytic anemias.* Part. IV, Grune & Stratton, New York, 1967.
344. Aster R.V., Enright S.E.: *A platelet and granulocyte defect in paroxysmal nocturnal hemoglobinuria: usefulness for detecting platelet antibodies.* J. Clin. Invest., *48*, 1199, 1968.
345. Craddock P.R., Fehr J., Jacop H.S.: *Complement-mediated granulocyte dysfunction in paroxysmal nocturnal hemoglobinuria.* Blood, *47*, 931, 1976.
346. Lewis S.M., Dacie J.V.: *Neutrophil (leucocyte) alkaline phosphatase in paroxysmal nocturnal haemoglobinuria.* Brit. J. Haemat., *11*, 549, 1965.
347. Oni S.B., Osunkoya B.O., Luzzatto L.: *Paroxysmal nocturnal hemoglobinuria. Evidence for monoclonal origin of abnormal red cells.* Blood, *36*, 145, 1970.
348. Papayannopoulou T., Rosse W., Stomatoyannopoulou G., Chen P., Adams J.: *Fetal-hemoglobin in paroxysmal nocturnal hemoglobinuria (PNH): evidence for derivation of Hb F-containing erythrocytes (F cells) from the PNH clone as well as from normal hemopoietic stem cell lines.* Blood, *52*, 740, 1978.
349. Rosse W.F., Adams J.P., Thorpe A.M.: *The population of cells in paroxysmal nocturnal haemoglobinuria of intermediate sensitivity to complement lysis. Significance and mechanisms of increased immune lysis.* Brit. J. Haemat., *28*, 181, 1974.
350. Rosse W.F.: *Variations in the red cells in paroxysmal nocturnal haemoglobinuria.* Brit. J. Haemat., *24*, 327, 1973.
351. Lewis S.M., Danon D., Marikovsky Y.: *Electron microscope studies of the red cells in paroxysmal nocturnal haemoglobinuria.* Brit. J. Haemat., *11*, 689, 1965.
352. Lambertenghi-Deliliers G., Ferrone S., Ranzi T.: *L'eritrocita umano in condizioni normali e patologiche al microscopio elettronico a scansione.* Gazz. San., *42*, 15, 1971.
353. De Sandre G., Ghiotto G.: *An enzymatic disorder in the erythrocytes of paroxysmal nocturnal haemoglobinuria. A deficiency in acetylcholinesterase activity.* Brit. J. Haemat., *6*, 39, 1960.
354. Sirchia G., Ferrone S., Mercuriali F.: *The action of two sulphydryl compounds on normal human red cells. Relationship to the red cells of paroxysmal nocturnal hemoglobinuria.* Blood, *25*, 502, 1965.
355. De Sandre G., Vettore L., Corrocher R., Cortesi S., Perona A.: *Ham-positive red cells induced in vitro by N-acetylcisteine or D-penicillamine.* Brit. J. Haemat., *15*, 437, 1968.
356. Goldstein B.C.: *Production of paroxysmal nocturnal hemoglobinuria-like red cells by reducing and oxidizing agents.* Brit. J. Haemat., *26*, 49, 1974.
357. Sirchia G., Ferrone S., Milani R., Mercuriali F.: *Observations on certain enzyme activities of normal human red cells treated with suhphydryl compounds.* Blood, *28*, 98, 1966.
358. Sirchia G., Mercuriali F., Ferrone S.: *Cephalotin-treated normal red cells: a new type of PNH-like cells.* Experientia, *24*, 495, 1968.
359. Conrad M.E.: *Hematologic manifestations of parasitic infections.* Semin. Hemat., *8*, 267, 1971.
359. Luzzatto L.: *Review: Genetics of red cells and susceptibility to malaria.* Blood, *54*, 961, 1979.
360. Aikawa M., Miller L.H., Johnson J., Rabbege J.: *Erythrocyte entry by malarial parasites. A moving junction between erythrocyte and parasite.* J. Cell Biol., *77*, 72, 1978.
361. Conrad M.E.: *Pathophysiology of malaria. Hematologic*

observations in human and animal studies.
Ann Int. Med., *70*, 134, 1969.
362. Woodruff A.W., Ansdell V.E., Pettitt I.E.: *Cause of anemia in malaria.* Lancet, *i*, 1055, 1979.
363. Dacie J.V.: *The hemolytic anemias.* 2nd ed., pt. 3, Grune & Stratton, New York, Chap. 15, pp. 908-922, 1967.
364. Anderson A.E., Cassaday P.B., Healy G.R.: *Babesiosis in man: sixth documented case.* Am. J. Clin. Path., *62*, 612, 1974.
364. Ruebush T.K., Juranek D.D., Chisholm E.S., Snow P.C., Healy G.R., Sulzer A.J.: *Human babesiosis on Nantucket island. Evidence for self-limited and subclinical infections.* N. Engl. J. Med., *297*, 825. 1977.
364. Healy G.R., Ruebush II T.K.: *Morphology of Babesia microti in human blood smears.* Am. J. Clin. Path., *73*, 107, 1980.
365. Martins J.M., de Alencar J.E., Magalhaes V.B.: *The anemia of kala-azar.* Rev. Inst. Med. Trop. S. Paulo, *7*, 47, 1965.
366. Woodruff A.W., Topley E., Knight R., Downie C.G.B.: *The anaemia of kala-azar.* Brit. J. Haemat., *23*, 319, 1972.
367. Castoldi G.L.: *Aspetti citologici generali e cromosomici nelle emopatie da farmaci.* Min. Pediat., *30*, 1439, 1978.
368. Girwood R.H.: *Blood disorders due to drugs and other agents.* Excerpta Medica, Amsterdam, 1973.
369. Knospe W.H., Crosby W.H.: *Aplastic anemia: a disorder of the bone marrow sinusoidal microcirculation rather than stem-cell failure?* Lancet, *i*, 20, 1971.
370. Fliedner T.M.: *Funktionelle Struktur der hämatopoietischen Stammzellenspeicher: Ihre Relevanz für das Problem der Knochemarkinsuffizienz.* In: Knochemarkinsuffizienz, Berichtstand des Deutsch-Osterreichischen Kongresses für Hämatologie, Wien. Lehmanns, München, p. 5, 1975.
371. Baserga A.: *Preleukemic states in the light of the leukemia cytokinetics.* Blood Cells, *2*, 285, 1976.
372. Rondanelli E., Gorini P.: *Effets du benzene sur la mitose érythroblastique.* Acta Haemat. (Basel), *26*, 281, 1961.
373. Miescher P.A., Pepper J.J.: *Drug-induced immunologic blood dyscrasias.* In: Textbook of Immunopathology. Miescher P.A., Müller-Eberhard H. eds., Grune & Stratton, New York, 1976.
374. Dacie J.V.: *The hemolytic anemias: congenital and acquired.* 3rd ed., Part II. "The Auto-immune Hemolytic Anemias", Grune & Stratton, New York, 1967.
375. Pirofsky B.: *Autoimmunization and the autoimmune hemolytic anemias.* The Williams & Wilkins Co., Baltimore, 1969.
376. Schubothe H.: *The cold hemagglutinin disease.* Semin. Hemat., *3*, 27, 1966.
377. Brain M.C., Dacie J.V., Hourihan D.O.B.: *Microangiopathic hemolytic anemia. The possible role of vascular lesions in pathogenesis.* Brit. J. Haemat., *8*, 358, 1962.
378. Dacie J.V.: *The hemolytic anemias, congenital and acquired. Part III. Secondary or symptomatic hemolytic anemia.* Churchill, London, 1967.
379. Wintrobe M.M.: *Clinical hematology.* Lea & Febiger, Philadelphia, 1974.
380. Venkatachalam M.A.: *Microangiopathic hemolytic anemia in rats with malignant hypertension.* Blood, *32*, 278, 1968.
381. Bull B.S., Rubenberg M.L., Dacie J.F., Brain M.C.: *Microangiopathic haemolytic anemia. Mechanisms of red cell fragmentation.* Brit. J. Haemat., *14*, 643, 1968.
382. Bull B.S., Kuhn I.N.: *The production of schistocytes by fibrin strands. A scanning electron microscope study.* Blood, *35*, 104, 1970.
383. Harker L.A., Slichter S.J.: *Platelets and fibrinogen consumption in man.* New Engl. J. Med., *287*, 999, 1972.
384. Marmont A.M., Damasio E.E., Rossi E., Spriano M.: *Thrombotic thrombocytopenic purpura successfully treated with a combination of dipyridamole and aspirin.* Haematologica (Pavia), *65*, 222, 1980.
385. Amorosi E.L., Karpaktin S.: *Antiplatelet treatment of thrombotic thrombocytopenic purpura.* Ann. Intern. Med., *86*, 102, 1977.
386. Vaughan J.M.: *Leuco-erythroblastic anemia.* J. Path. Bact., *42*, 541, 1936.
387. Emerson C.P., Finkel H.E.: *Problem of tumor cell identification in the bone marrow.* Cancer, *19*, 1527, 1966.
388. Contreras E., Ellis L.D., Lee R.E.: *Value of the bone marrow biopsy in the diagnosis of metastatic carcinoma.* Cancer, *29*, 778, 1972.
389. Forshaw J., Hardwood L.: *Poikilocytosis associated with carcinoma.* Arch. Intern. Med., *117*, 203, 1966.
390. Kremer W.B., Laszlo J.: *Hematologic effect of cancer.* In: Cancer Medicine. Holland J.F., Frei E. eds., Lea & Febiger, Philadelphia, p. 1085, 1973.
391. Weick J.K., Hagedorn A.B., Linman J.W.: *Leucoerythroblastosis. Diagnostic and prognostic significance.* Mayo Clin. Proc., *49*, 111, 1974.
392. Brittin G.M., Brecher G.: *Appearance of bone marrow smears with necrotic tumor cells.* Blood, *38*, 229, 1971.
393. Robinson W.A.: *Granulocytopoiesis in neoplasia.* In: Paraneoplastic syndromes. Hall T.C. ed., Ann. N.Y. Acad. Sci., *230*, 212, 1974.

Acknowledgement

This work was supported in part by grants from C.N.R. (Rome) n. 79.00613.96 and n. 80.01509.96. Technical assistance of the Electron Microscopy Center of the University of Ferrara is gratefully acknowledged.

4
Neutrophils

A.M. MARMONT and E. DAMASIO

Division of Hematology, S. Martino's Hospital, Genova, Italy

D. ZUCKER-FRANKLIN

Department of Medicine, New York University, New York, U.S.A.

Part 1 NORMAL STRUCTURE AND PHYSIOLOGY

1. DIFFERENTIATION AND MATURATION

Polymorphonuclear leukocytes (PMN's) develop in orderly progression, albeit with amplification, through a chain of identifiable precursors in the marrow to the mature endstage cells which enter circulating blood. Many different and increasingly sophisticated methods have been used to investigate the events that lead from the primitive pluripotent hemopoietic stem cell to the mature, circulating neutrophil (see Chapter 2). Such studies suggest that between the pluripotent stem cell and the recognizable granulocyte precursors there exist committed stem cells of lesser or greater restriction. One of these gives rise to granulocyte/monocyte colonies *in vitro* (CFU-GM) and is considered the immediate precursor of both the neutrophilic and monocytic lineages [1, 2]. This cell may well be the one which transforms and gives rise to the so-called "myelomonocytic" leukemias (see below).

To date, this assumption is still based on morphology as the surface antigens of granulocytic cells have been less extensively studied than those of lymphoid cells. However, specific granulocyte surface antigens [3] as well as distinct glycoproteins [4] have been described. Experiments utilizing the fluorescence activated cell sorter (see Chapter 1) revealed that CFU-GM may have HLA-DR (Ia-like) antigens on their surface [5]. Since Ia-like antigens are thought to be involved in cellular interactions in immune responses, these studies raise the intriguing possibility that HLA-DR molecules may also play a regulatory role in early hematopoiesis.

The earliest morphologically identifiable precursor in the bone marrow is the myeloblast (**Figs. 1** and **2**), although the term hemocytoblast is still retained in the French and Italian literature [7, 8, 9]. The cell measures 15-18 μm in diameter and has a large nucleus with finely dispersed chromatin and several nucleoli. The cytoplasm is scant, lightly basophilic and agranular [6]. Some investigators require the presence of at least a few azurophilic granules to establish granulocytic commitment [10]. Ultrastructurally (**Figs. 3, 4**) the nucleus of the myeloblast exhibits mostly euchromatin, synthetically "active" DNA and several small nucleoli. The cytoplasm is replete with ribosomes. There are a few profiles of rough endoplasmic reticulum accounting for the basophilia on light microscopy. Rare small granules are usually present. In a fraction of myeloblasts, peroxidase activity can be demonstrated in the perinuclear space before the appearance of the granules. Although this requires electron microscopy, the effort may be warranted in acute leukemias when the presence of peroxidase helps to distinguish myeloblasts from lymphoblasts [11] (see **Fig. 77**).

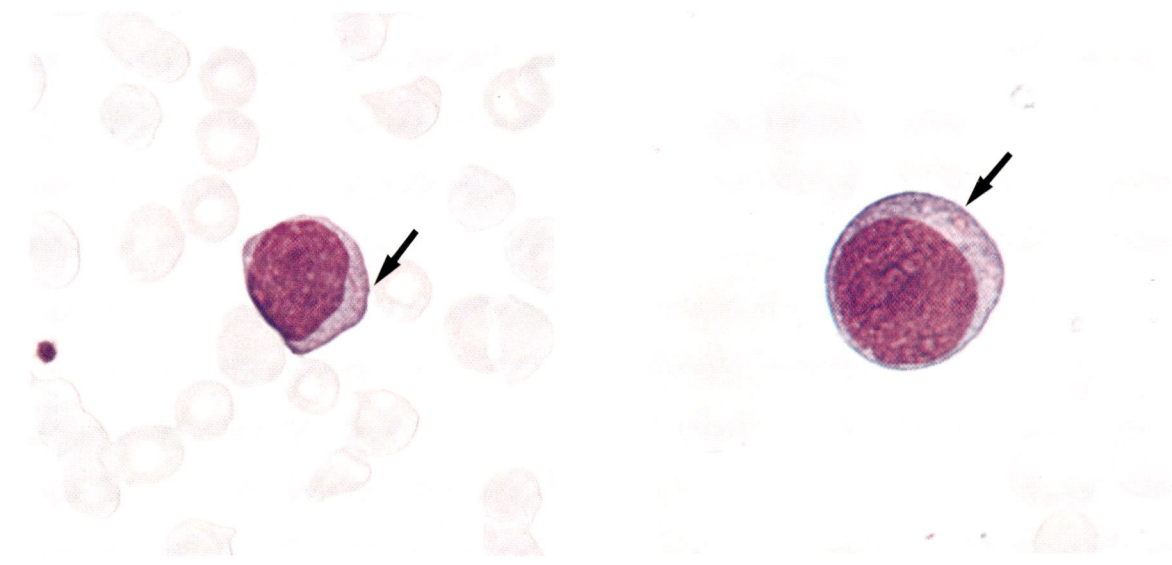

Fig. 1 Myeloblast, normal marrow. In this very immature cell, a few small azurophilic granules are indicated by an **arrow**.

Fig. 2 Myeloblast, normal marrow. Compared with the cell in **Fig. 1**. This myeloblast appears more mature. Azurophilic granules are indicated by an **arrow**.

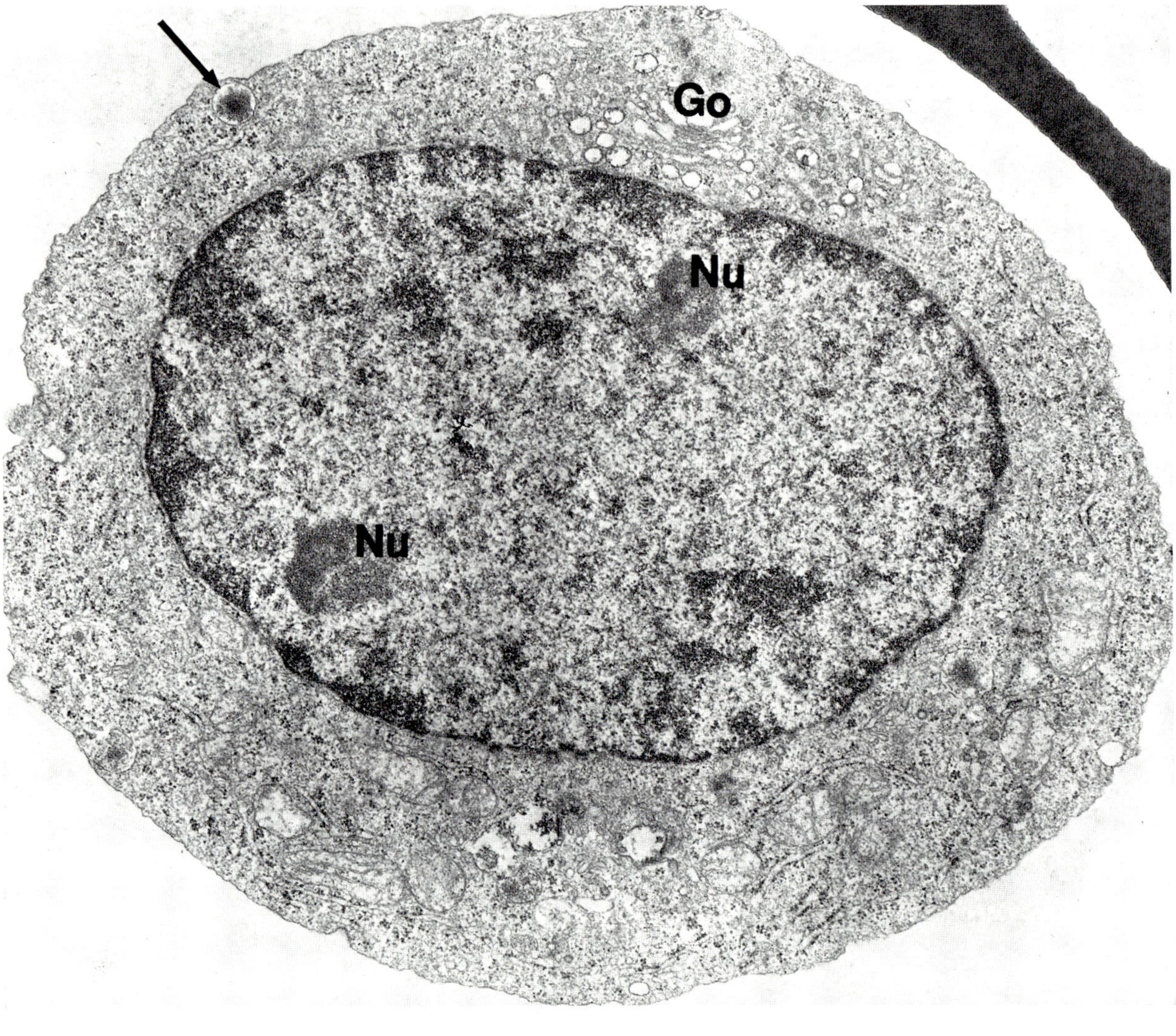

4 NEUTROPHILS

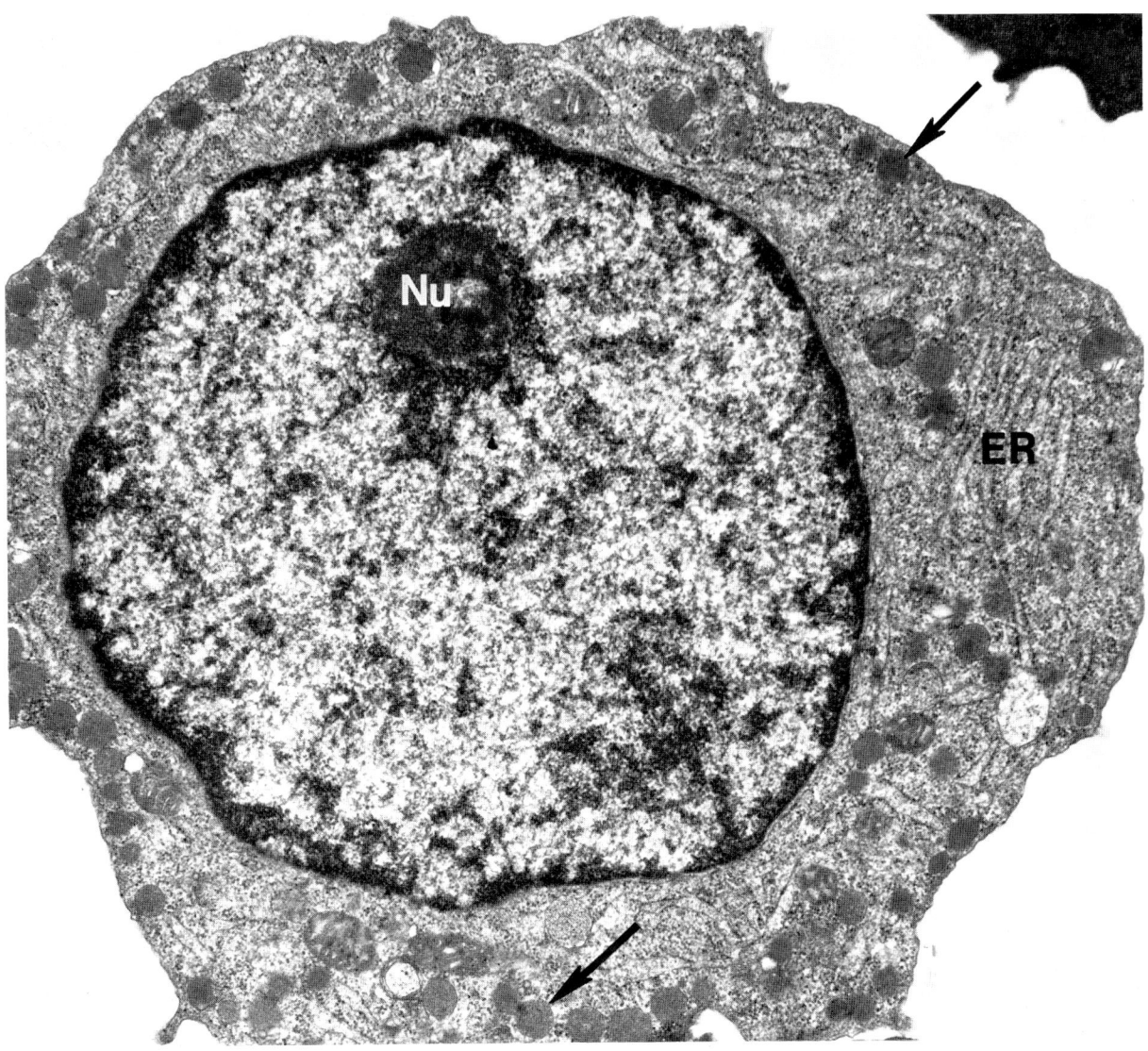

Fig. 4 Example of a cell which on light microscopy would be identified as a myeloblast because of the paucity of its granules (**arrows**), round nucleus with dispersed chromatin and relatively large nucleolus (**Nu**). It is obviously more differentiated than the cell depicted in **Figure 3**. Rough endoplasmic reticulum (**ER**) (× 19,000).

Fig. 3 Myeloblast, normal marrow. The nucleus is round, has finely dispersed chromatin and two small nucleoli (**Nu**). Leukemic myeloblasts usually show larger nucleoli. The Golgi zone is small (**Go**). There are few, if any, granules (**arrow**). The ones seen in this electron micrograph would probably not be noted on light microscopy. This cell might be difficult to distinguish from a lymphocyte. The cytoplasm is replete with ribosomes and a few profiles of rough endoplasmic reticulum are seen (× 19,000).

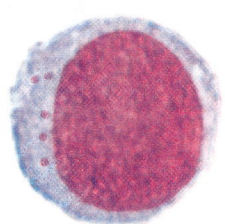 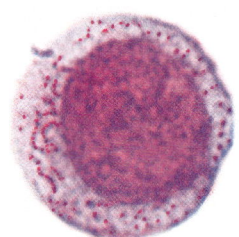

Fig. 5 *Early promyelocyte (I) with some azurophilic granules and basophilic cytoplasm.*

Fig. 6 *Late promyelocyte (II). Numerous azurophilic granules are dispersed in the acidophilic cytoplasm.*

Some degree of confusion exists as regards the next maturation stage, the promyelocyte. In the English literature, two closely related but morphologically distinguishable stages, that is a precursor with basophilic cytoplasm and relatively few azurophilic granules (**Fig. 5**) and a slightly later precursor with almost no cytoplasmic basophilia and an abundance of azurophilic granules (**Fig. 6**) (compare **Figs. 4, 5, 6, 7, 8**) are classified together.

Both are defined as promyelocytes and only rarely is a distinction made between early and late promyelocytes, corresponding to that made by Undritz [12] between promyelocyte I and II. Other authors who accept the term promyelocyte for cells with "fine" azurophilic granules, like Rohr [13], distinguish three cells, unripe, half-ripe and ripe myelocytes.

The first contains azurophilic granules only, the second a mixture of azurophilic and specific granules, and the third specific granules only. Rohr's classification is no longer tenable because it has been established that even mature neutrophils possess some primary granules. To avoid confusion, we must point out that the French and Italian literature still uses the term myeloblast for all cells with azurophilic granules and the term promyelocyte for cells possessing a mixture of azurophilic and specific granules with a preponderance of the first.

These definitions are of some importance because of their relevance to the classification of acute leukemias. The ultrastructural features of promyelocytes are illustrated in **Figures 7, 8 a** and **b**, and described in detail in the legends. It is now generally accepted that the bulk of the azurophilic (primary) granules are formed during the promyelocyte stage [14, 15] and that the myelocyte stage is marked by the appearance of the secondary, "specific" granules.

Although the distinction of only two types of granules is undoubtedly also an oversimplification [16], it has become of practical value not only in defining the stages of development, but also when evaluating cellular function in disease states [17-20]. Primary azurophilic granules are membrane-bound packets of enzymes, i.e. lysosomes. Most of them appear to bud from the inner, concave face of the Golgi apparatus [21] and have been shown to contain myeloperoxidase, elastase, lysozyme, cathepsin G, and many acid hydrolases [6, 22, 23].

The myelocyte stage (**Fig. 9**) begins with the formation of the secondary (specific) granules and ends when the cell has acquired a full complement of these structures. At this stage, synthesis of azurophilic granules ceases and their number decreases by dilution during

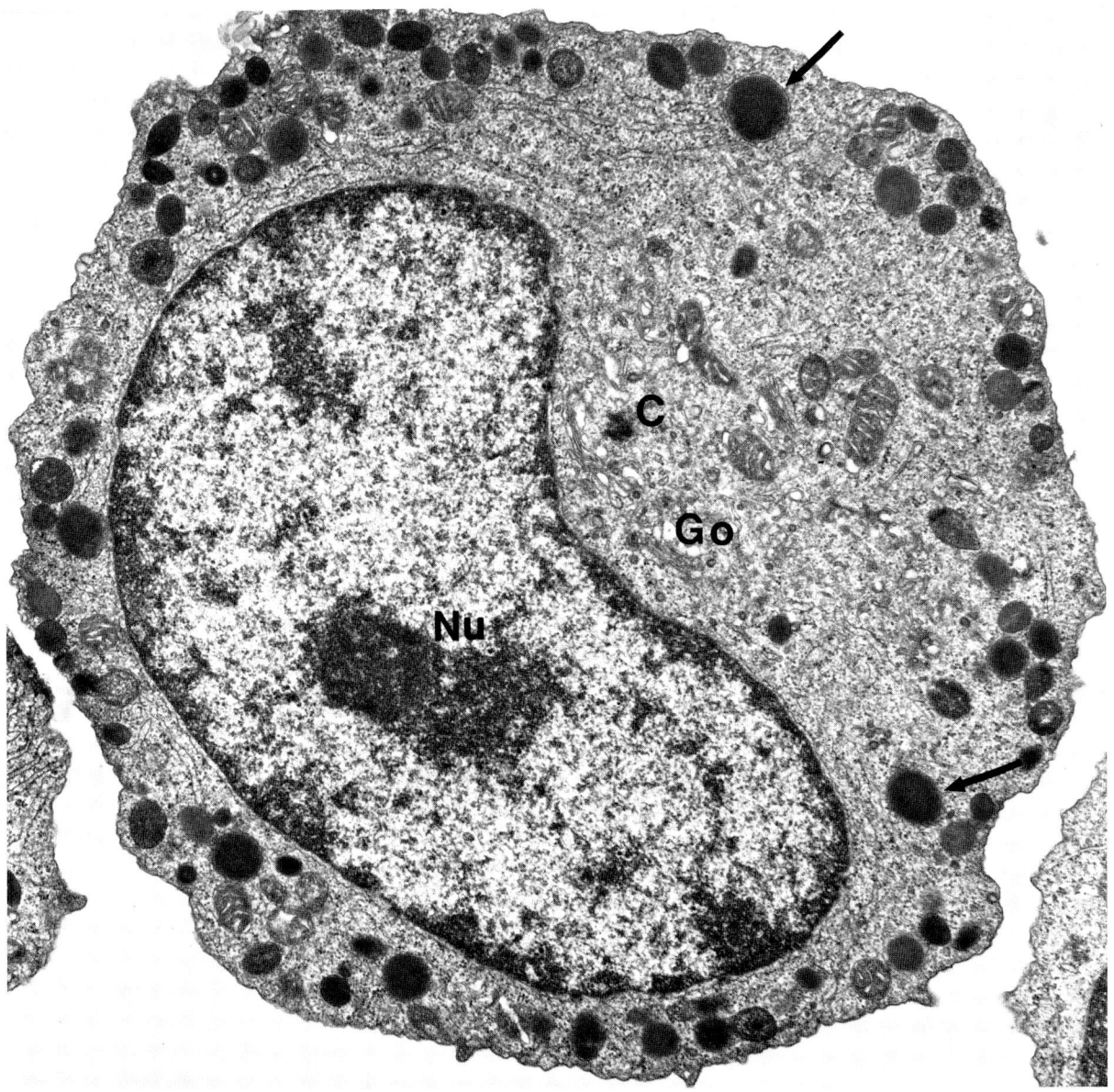

Fig. 7 Early promyelocyte. Its nuclear features resemble those of the myeloblast illustrated in **Figure 4**. However, there is a marked increase in the number and size of the granules and some (**arrows**) have the size and electron opacity of primary (azurophilic) granules. The Golgi zone (**Go**) is large. There are still numerous profiles of RER. **C**, centriole. This cell should be compared with the cells depicted in **Figures 4** and **8** ($\times$ 17,000).

subsequent mitotic divisions. Although the division between promyelocytes and myelocytes is somewhat arbitrary, immunofluorescent double staining techniques with fluorescein and rhodamine-conjugated antisera directed against different neutrophil enzymes have confirmed that primary and secondary granules are synthesized at different stages of granulocyte differentiation [24] (**Figs. 12 a-n**).

The secondary (specific, neutrophil) granules are smaller, more electron lucent (**Fig. 8**) and have been shown to contain lactoferrin and lysozyme. They are responsible for the characteristic color of neutrophils in Romanowsky-stained preparations. Alkaline phosphatase also appears during the myelocyte stage of differentiation but whether its localization is limited to the granules is not yet certain (**Fig. 12**).

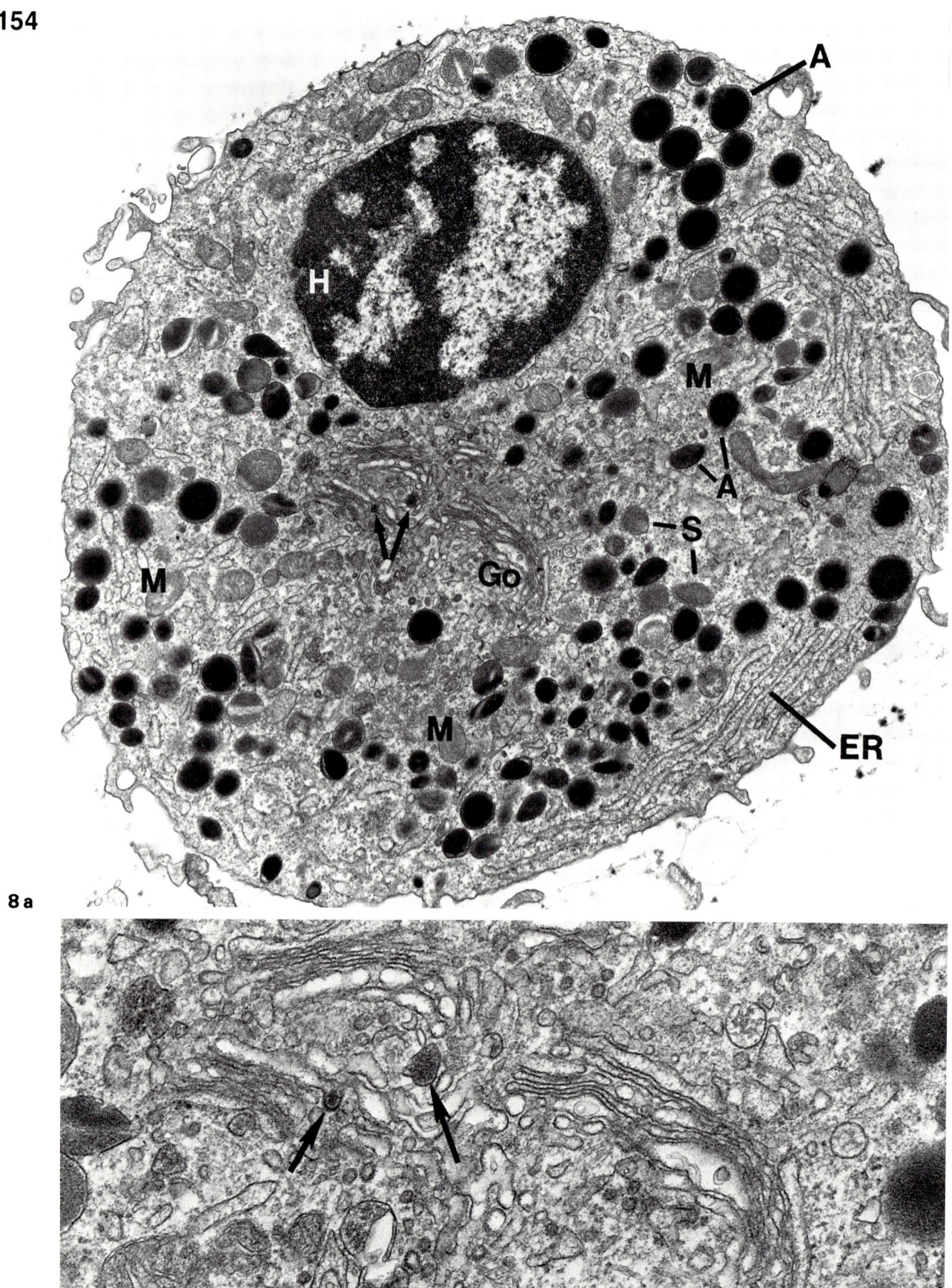

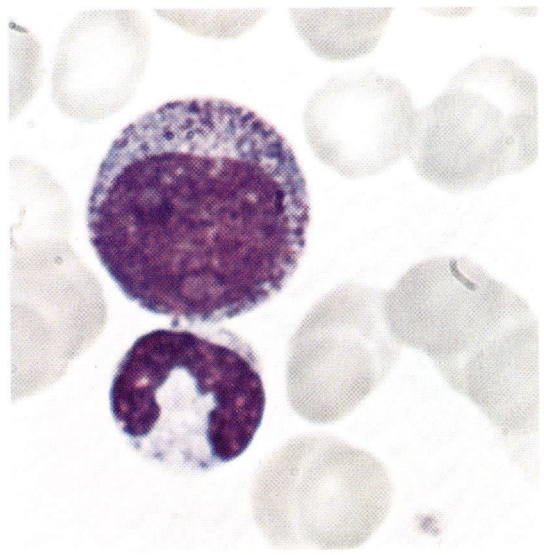

Fig. 9 A myelocyte (top) and a metamyelocyte (bottom).

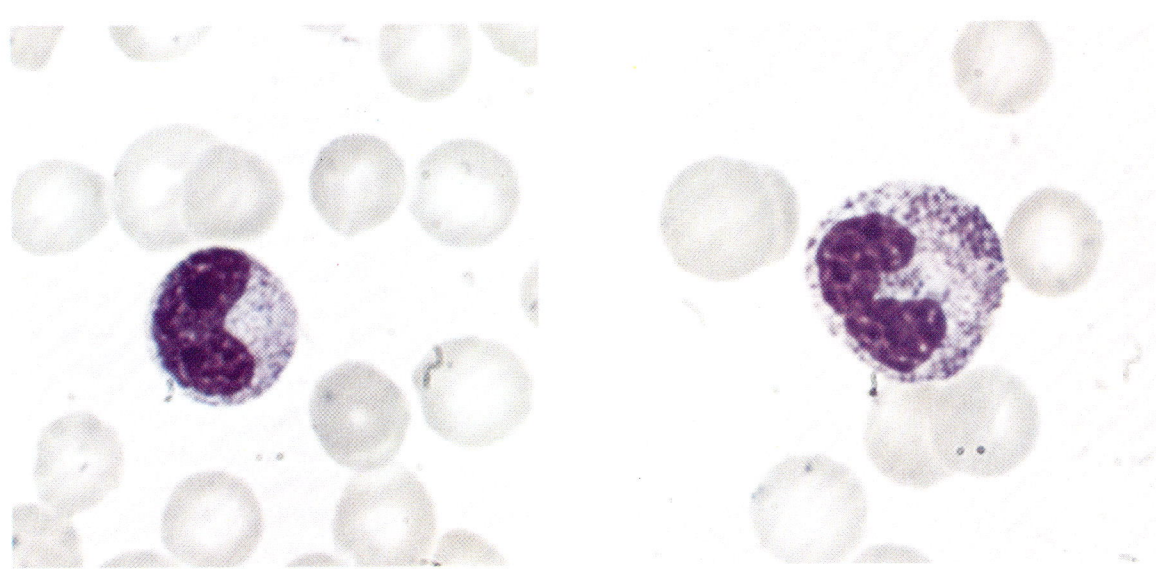

10   11

Figs. 10 and 11) Progressive maturation of metamyelocytes to "stab" form of nucleus.

The metamyelocyte is the immediate precursor of the mature neutrophil which is no longer capable of cell division (**Figs. 10-11** and **13-15**). It is easily recognized by its indented or horseshoe-shaped nucleus and full complement of neutrophilic granules. A "band" or "stab" form precedes true nucleus lobulation which is typical of circulating end stage cells (**Figs. 13-15**).

Mature neutrophils, their cytochemistry and ultrastructural features are illustrated in **Figures 16-18** and **25-30** and described in the accompanying legends.

Fig. 8 a) Late promyelocyte. Although only a small section of the nucleus is visible, the increase in condensed heterochromatin (**H**) is noteworthy. The majority of granules represent azurophilic (**A**) i.e. primarily lysosomes, but some less electron dense, smaller, specific granules (**S**) have already formed. There are still many profiles of rough endoplasmic reticulum (**ER**) and the large Golgi zone (**Go**) which is seen at higher magnification in **Figure 8 b** is still "packaging" new granules (**arrows**). **M**, mitochondria ($\times$ 17,000).

b) Higher resolution of the Golgi zone of the cell illustrated in **Figure 8 a** shows the "budding" of granules to better advantage (**arrow**). **A**, azurophilic or primary granule. **M**, mitochondria ($\times$ 44,000).

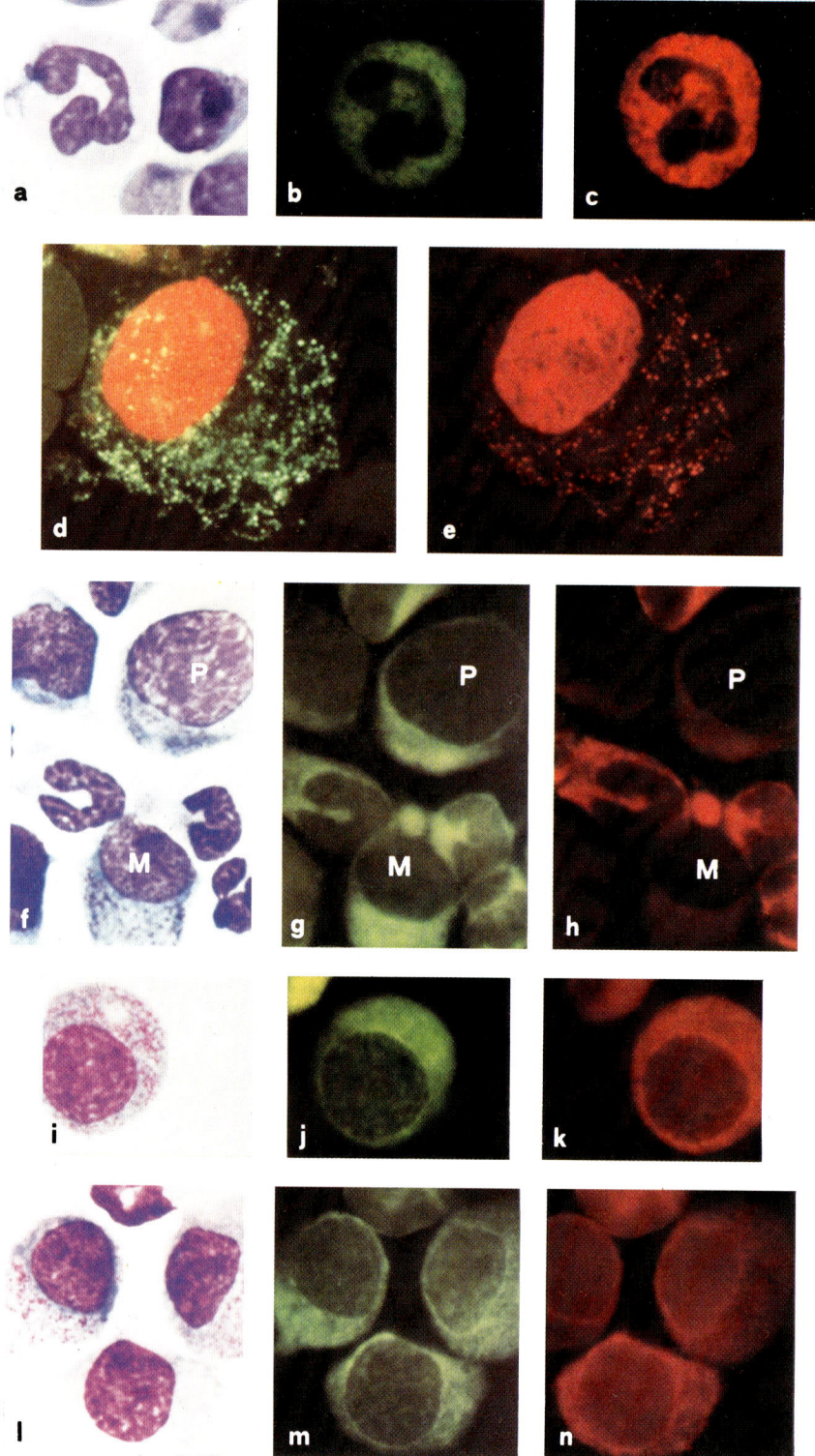

Fig. 12 Simultaneous immunofluorescent and Romanowsky stains of normal human bone marrow (a-c). Bone marrow neutrophil reacted with May Grünwald-Giemsa (a), fluorescein-labelled antimyeloperoxidase (b), and rhodamine-labelled antilactoferrin (c). Negative staining of other marrow elements by the conjugates demonstrates specificity. d, e) Promyelocyte stained with fluorescein-labelled antimyeloperoxidase (d), rhodamine-labelled antielastase (e) and counterstained with methyl green. Rupture of the cytoplasmic membrane allowed dispersion of the granules and emphasizes the conjoint binding of both markers in identical granules.
f-h) Promyelocyte (P) and myelocyte (M) stained with May Grünwald-Giemsa (f), fluorescein-labelled antimyeloperoxidase (g), and rhodamine-labeled antilactoferrin (h). Lactoferrin is not present in the promyelocyte but is strongly reactive in more mature cells in this field. Myeloperoxidase is present in all cells.
i-k) Myelocyte stained with May Grünwald-Giemsa (i), fluorescein-labelled anti-cathepsin G (j), and rhodamine-labelled antilactoferrin (k) showing the appearance of a specific granule marker in the cell.
l-n) Three myelocytes and one band form stained with May Grünwald-Giemsa (l), fluorescein-labelled anticathepsin G (m), and rhodamine-labelled antilysozyme (n). Lysozyme appears more intense in the more mature cells (top and bottom), while an azurophilic granule marker decreased or remained the same. Similar results were seen with lactoferrin. Courtesy of Dr. Pryzwansky (see ref. 24).

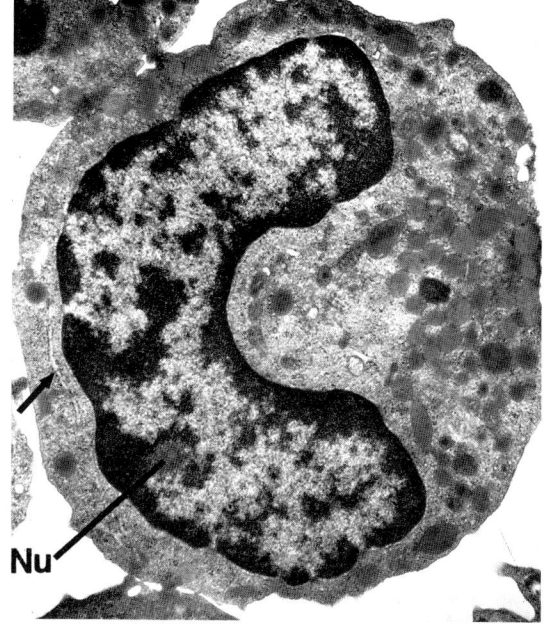

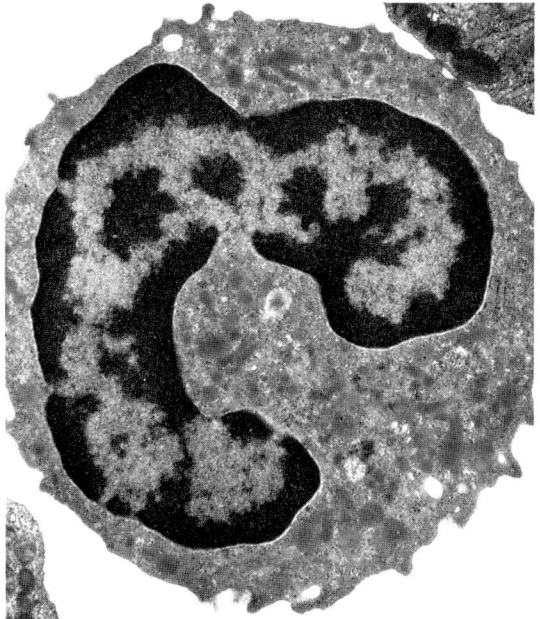

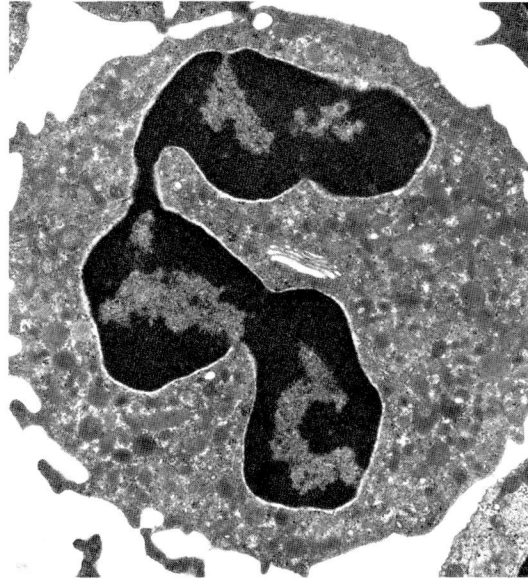

Figs. 13, 14, 15 Cells chosen to illustrate progressive maturation of the nucleus and cytoplasm from myelocyte via metamyelocyte to stab and mature neutrophil which takes place without further mitoses. Note particularly the progressive loss of euchromatin and increased peripheral distribution of heterochromatin (more electron opaque). The nucleolus (**Nu**) still visible in **Figure 13** (a cell, which on light microscopy might be identified as a myelocyte) is gradually lost as the nucleus becomes horseshoe-shaped, indented and finally multilobed. Profiles of RER (**arrow** in **Figure 13**), ribosomes and mitochondria are also gradually lost and the ratio of specific to primary granules increases (**Fig. 13**, × 11,500; **Fig. 14**, × 10,200; **Fig. 15**, × 11,500).

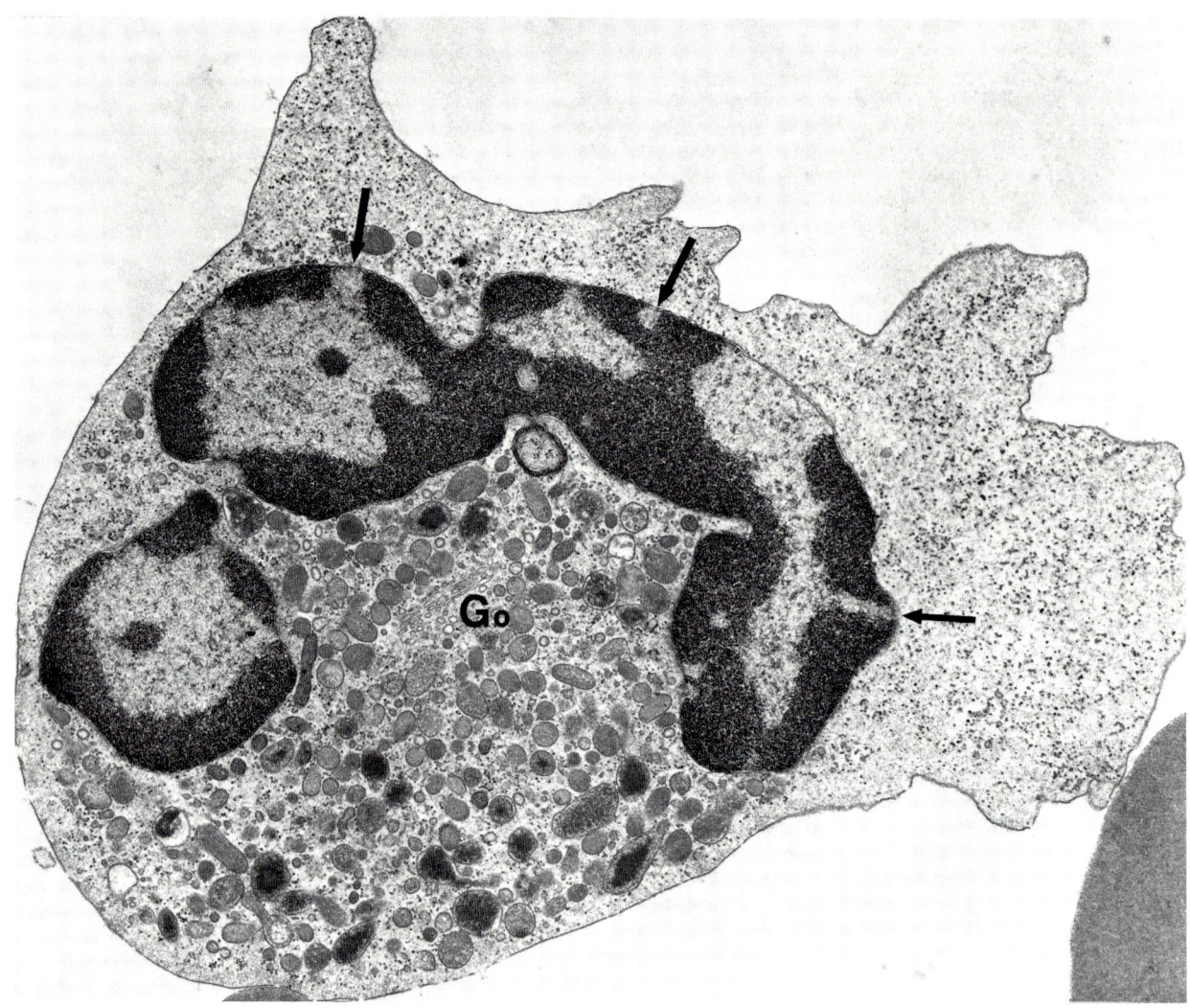

Fig. 16 Mature peripheral blood neutrophil. The nucleus is multilobed. The peripheral distribution of heterochromatin is only interrupted by channels of euchromatin where it is in continuity with nuclear pores (**arrows**). Note the heterogeneity of the granules and the fact that the primary granules (more electron dense) represent a minority population. There are few mitochondria, ribosomes and no RER. The Golgi zone is very small (**Go**). The black dots in the cytoplasm represent glycogen particles. The distance between the granules and the outer cell membrane ranges between 100-250 nm and is never less than 40 nm. A leading edge of cytoplasm or a pseudopod is always devoid of granules. Therefore, fusion of granule membranes with the surface membrane does not occur unless the cell is triggered (see text) ($\times$ 17,500).

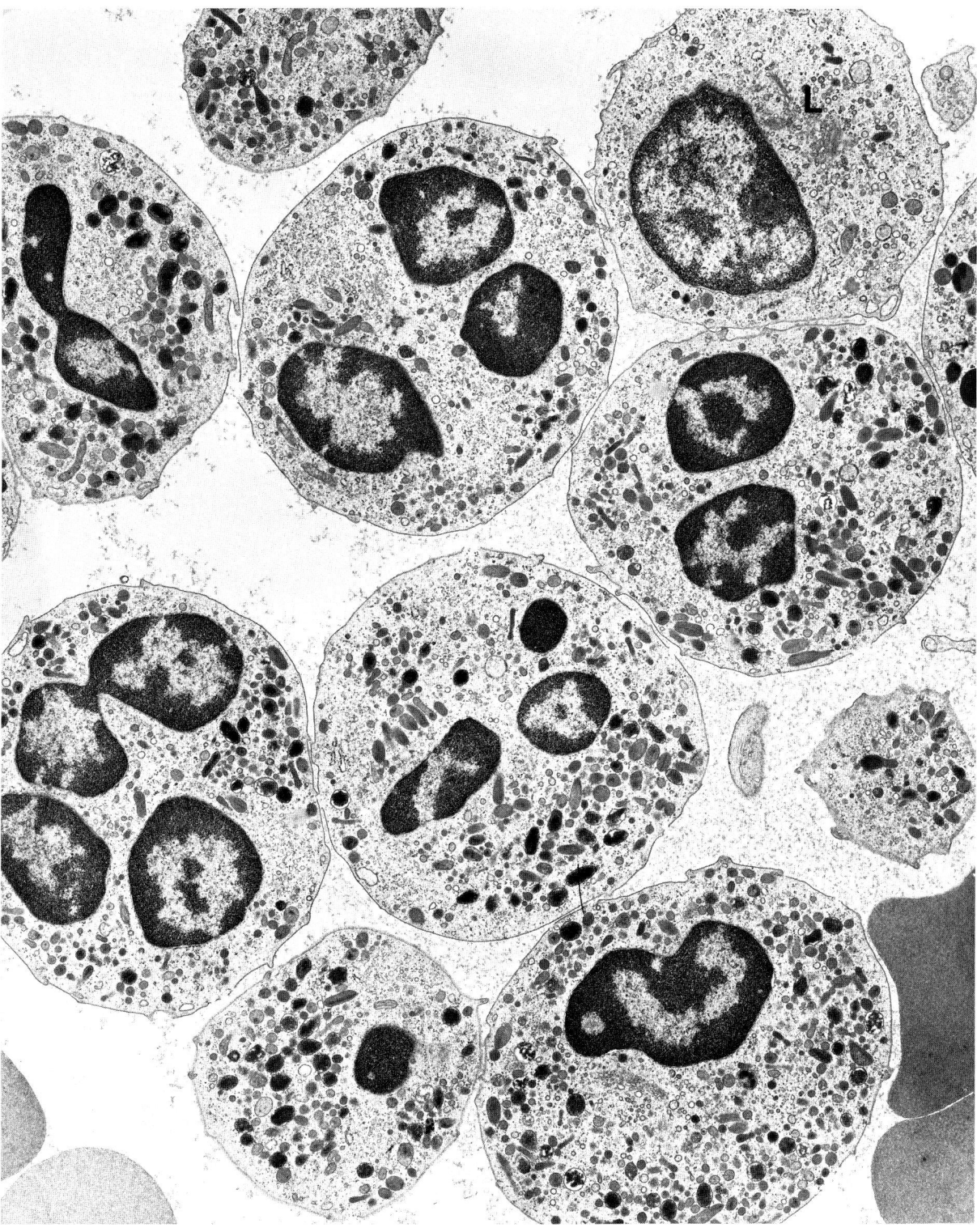

Fig. 17 Survey view of peripheral blood neutrophils obtained from a healthy individual illustrates the remarkable uniformity in the morphology of the cells. A lymphocyte (**L**) is seen in the right top corner of the illustration ($\times$ 8,500).

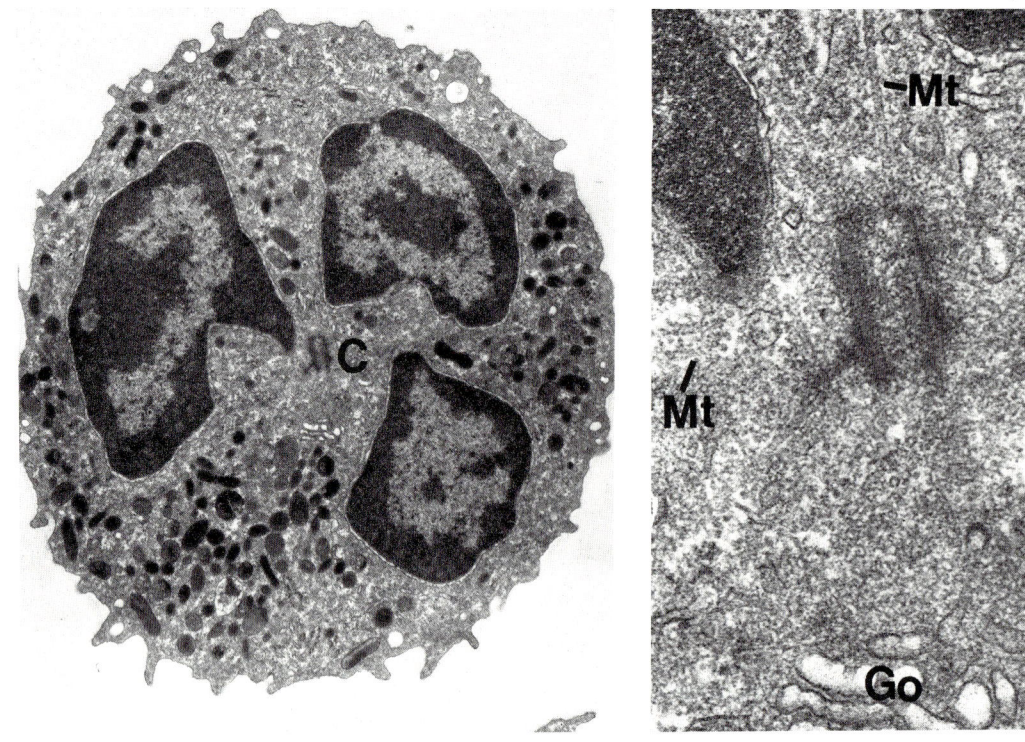

Fig. 18 a) Mature neutrophil sectioned through its centrosphere shows the location of the centriole (C) in a resting, circulating neutrophil. This area is illustrated at higher magnification in b (× 13,000).
b) Centriolar region of the cell shown in a at high resolution. Note microtubules (Mt) which emanate from this region. The atrophied Golgi zone (Go) is at bottom (× 66,000).

A few aspects deserve emphasis. Mature polymorphonuclear leukocytes (PMN's) (Fig. 19) are probably the only nucleated cells (perhaps with the exception of the acidophilic normoblasts) which do not possess well-delineated nucleoli, thus making it unlikely that the circulating neutrophil is still engaged in much protein synthesis. Although there are a few reports of de novo protein synthesis from amino acid precursors, this may be attributed to an admixture of less mature PMN's which are invariably present among isolated neutrophil preparations used for such analyses. Most of the chromatin appears as peripherally distributed, electron dense, "inactive" heterochromatin. Nuclear "inactivity" is also suggested by the cells' inability to incorporate ^{3}H-thymidine into DNA. It is noteworthy, however, that the nucleus still retains numerous nuclear pores which are in continuity with the remaining euchromatin (Fig. 16). The filamentous connections between nuclear lobes, seen by conventional microscopy, consist of extensions of heterochromatin delimited by membranes which are in continuity with the membranes surrounding the nuclear lobes [25] (Figs. 20 a, b). Since this continuity cannot be seen in every plane of section, some electron micrographs may show nuclear "rings" which seem to surround an area of cytoplasm (Fig. 20). Such "rings" are commonly found in thin sections of hypersegmented PMN's and have, at times, been mistaken for unusual forms of lysosomes. The significance of nuclear lobulation has remained unexplained, although the degree of lobulation may serve as a clue to some diseases (see p. 185). Osmotic swelling of the nucleus results in the disappearance of the filamentous connections between the lobes and "rounding-up" of the nucleus. Ultrastructurally the connections between the lobes also disappear but the lobes retain their identity within a common space [26] (Fig. 21).

4 NEUTROPHILS

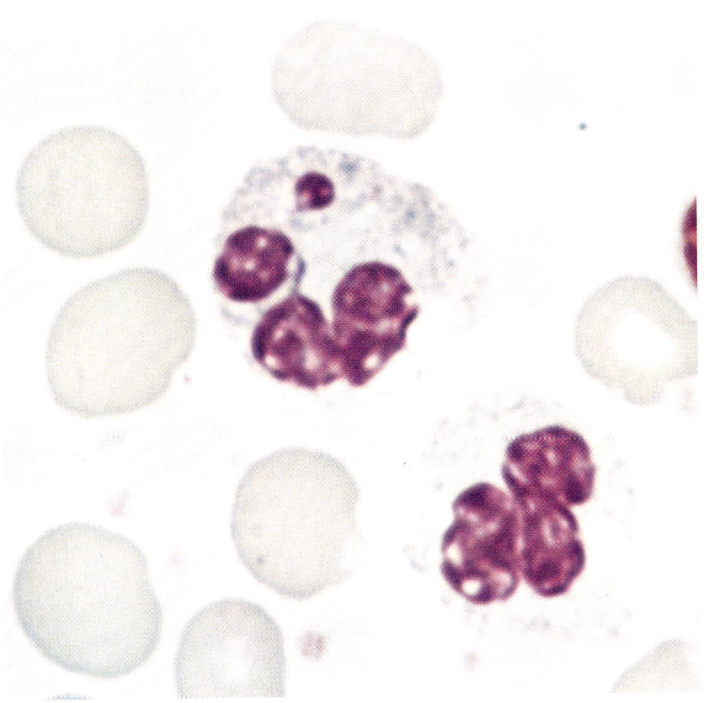

Fig. 19 Two mature neutrophils from the peripheral blood of a female subject. In one of the cells a "drumstick" is clearly discernible.

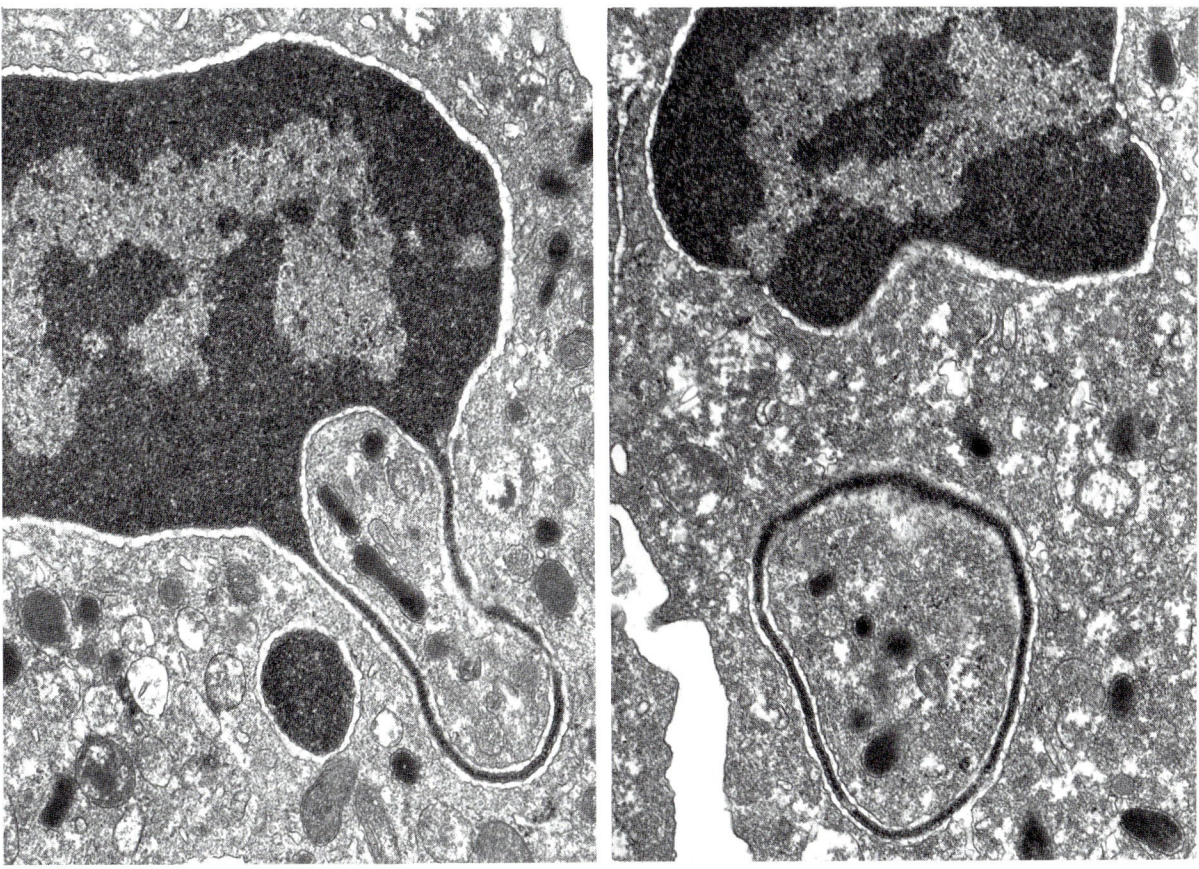

Fig. 20 a, b) Ultrastructure of "filaments" which connect the nuclear lobes. The word filament is a misnomer. In reality, the connections consist of nuclear heterochromatin delimited by the outer and inner nuclear membranes which are in continuity with those surrounding the nuclear lobes (see text) (× 28,000).

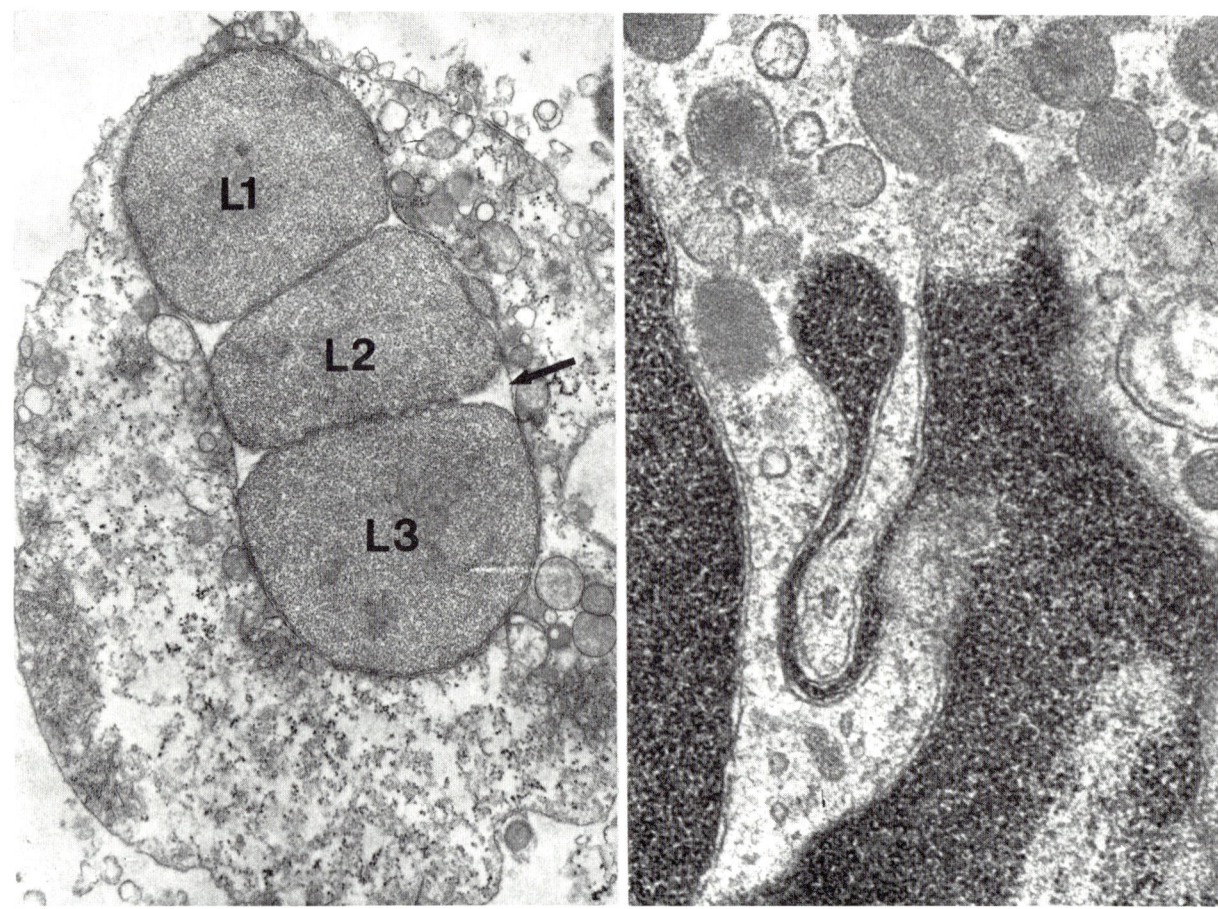

Fig. 21 *PMN exposed to streptolysin for 2 minutes. The separation of nuclear membranes by radiolucent material (**arrow**) seems to have forced the nuclear lobes (**L1, L2, L3**) into one space while each lobe has retained its identity by virtue of its own membrane ($\times$ 14,000).*
Reproduced from ref. 26 with permission of the publisher.

Fig. 22 *Ultrastructural appearance of nuclear appendage probably representing female sex chromatin ("drumstick") ($\times$ 52,000).*

2. SEX CHROMATINS

The nucleus of the mature neutrophil may serve to determine the genetic sex of an individual. The non-extended X chromosome of a normal XX female is present as a "drumstick" projecting from one of the nuclear lobes visible in about 2-3% of the adult neutrophil population [27]. The solid, round projections can be seen with almost any stain.
They are connected to a lobe of the nucleus by a very thin filament and should not be confused with other non-specific nuclear appendages (**Figs. 22, 23**). Drumsticks and/or nodules may be found in males with Klinefelter's syndrome (XXY), whereas they are absent in females with Turner's syndrome [28, 29].
With quinacrine-fluorescence, the presence of the "Y chromatin body" may be resolved in the circulating leukocytes of normal males [30-32]. In granulocytes fluorescent small clubs are particularly conspicuous (**Fig. 24**). Although more advanced techniques of karyotype analysis have superseded the identification of nuclear appendages (see Chapter 11) occasionally determination of sex chromatin on interphase cells, because they can be studied on routine blood smears, may be very useful. The interested reader is referred to ref. 33 for a more detailed description of the methods and pitfalls of these analyses.

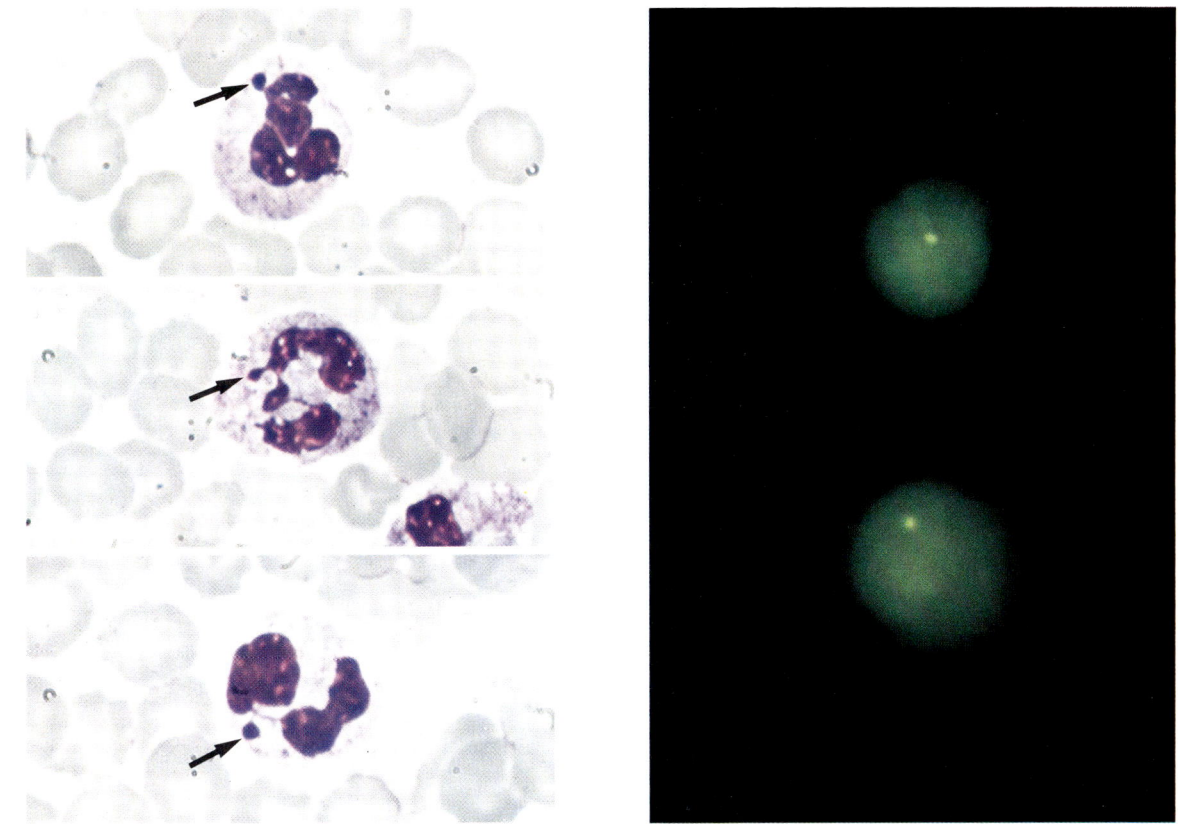

Fig. 23 a, b, c) Nuclear appendages identified as "drumsticks" (**arrows**) from the peripheral blood of normal females.

Fig. 24 Fluorescent "Y" bodies demonstrated by quinacrine fluorescence in bone marrow cells from a female patient transplanted with a male donor.

3. CYTOPLASM AND CYTOCHEMISTRY

The cytoplasm of the mature neutrophil contains about 200 granules of which roughly one-third are azurophilic and the rest are considered "specific" [6]. The morphologic heterogeneity of the granules is best appreciated on electron microscopy (**Figs. 16, 17**), but it is not yet known whether the morphologic heterogeneity is indicative of qualitative or quantitative differences of the enzymes contained in individual granules. At any rate, the strong peroxidase positivity of mature neutrophils (**Fig. 25**) as well as the ultrastructural localization of the enzyme seem to indicate that primary granules still remain present at this stage. The cells are also strongly positive when stained with the periodic acid Schiff (PAS) reagent (**Figs. 26 a, b**). This correlates with the abundance of glycogen particles seen on electron microscopy (**Fig. 16**). Indeed, the major source of energy for the cell is glycolysis even during the respiratory burst associated with phagocytosis [34]. Myeloblasts are PAS-negative. This distinguishes them from lymphoblasts which usually contain small to coarse PAS-positive granules. Neutrophil alkaline phosphatase (LAP) is a late enzyme which is contained in the secondary specific granules and is believed to participate in their protein and carbohydrate metabolism [35] (**Fig. 27**).

The alkaline phosphatase reaction is probably one of the most useful enzyme tests used clinically [36]. Inflammation and infections increase LAP positivity to the extent where this test is included in the routine workup of patients with a leukocytosis of unknown etiology. The LAP score is elevated in leukemoid reactions, polycythemia vera and some cases of myelofibrosis. It is low or absent

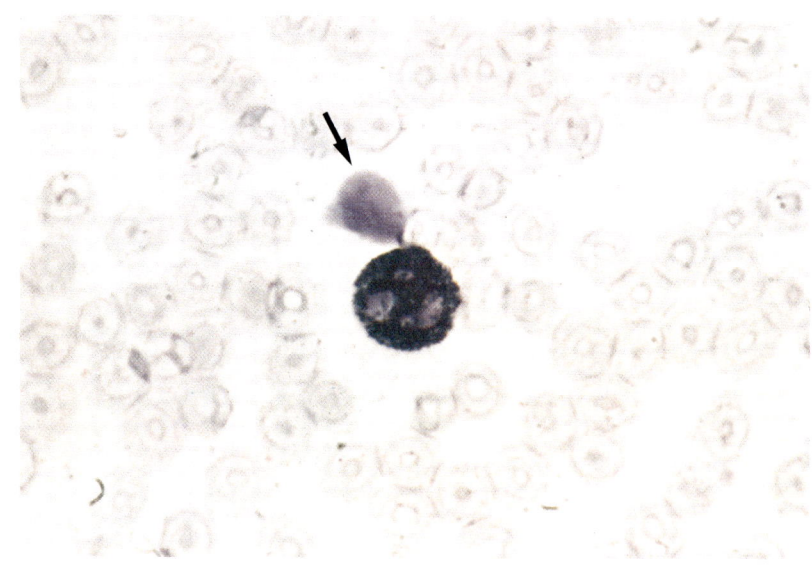

Fig. 25 Mature neutrophil with positive peroxidase reaction; nuclear counterstain with hematoxylin. **Arrow** indicates negative mononuclear cell. Monocytes are sometimes positive.

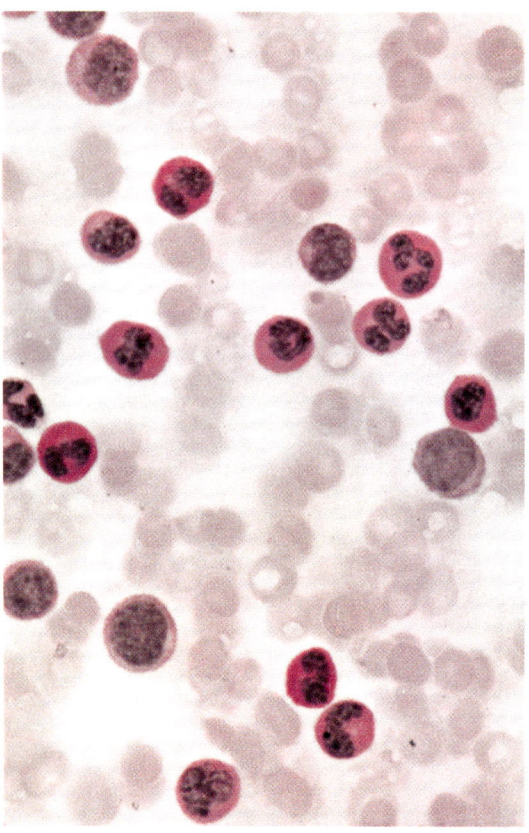

a

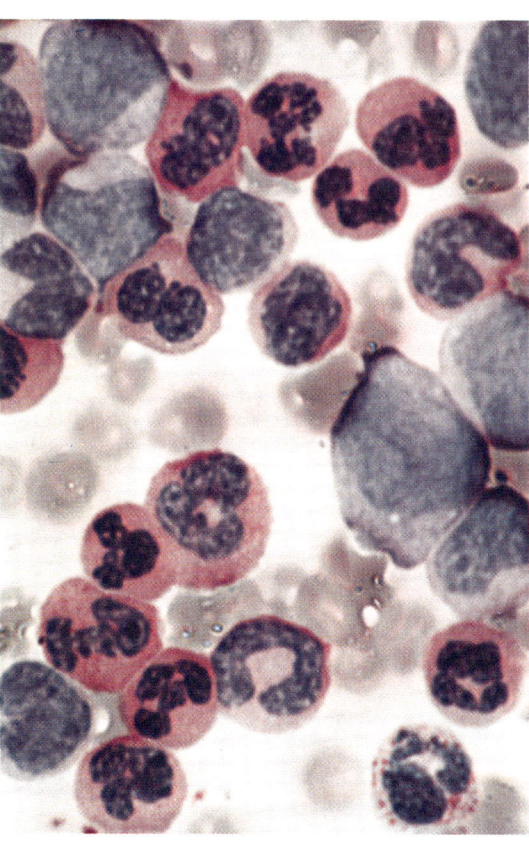

b

Fig. 26 a, b) PAS-reaction of peripheral blood (**a**) and bone marrow (**b**) illustrates increase in glycogen content (pink stain more intense) as neutrophils mature.

4 NEUTROPHILS

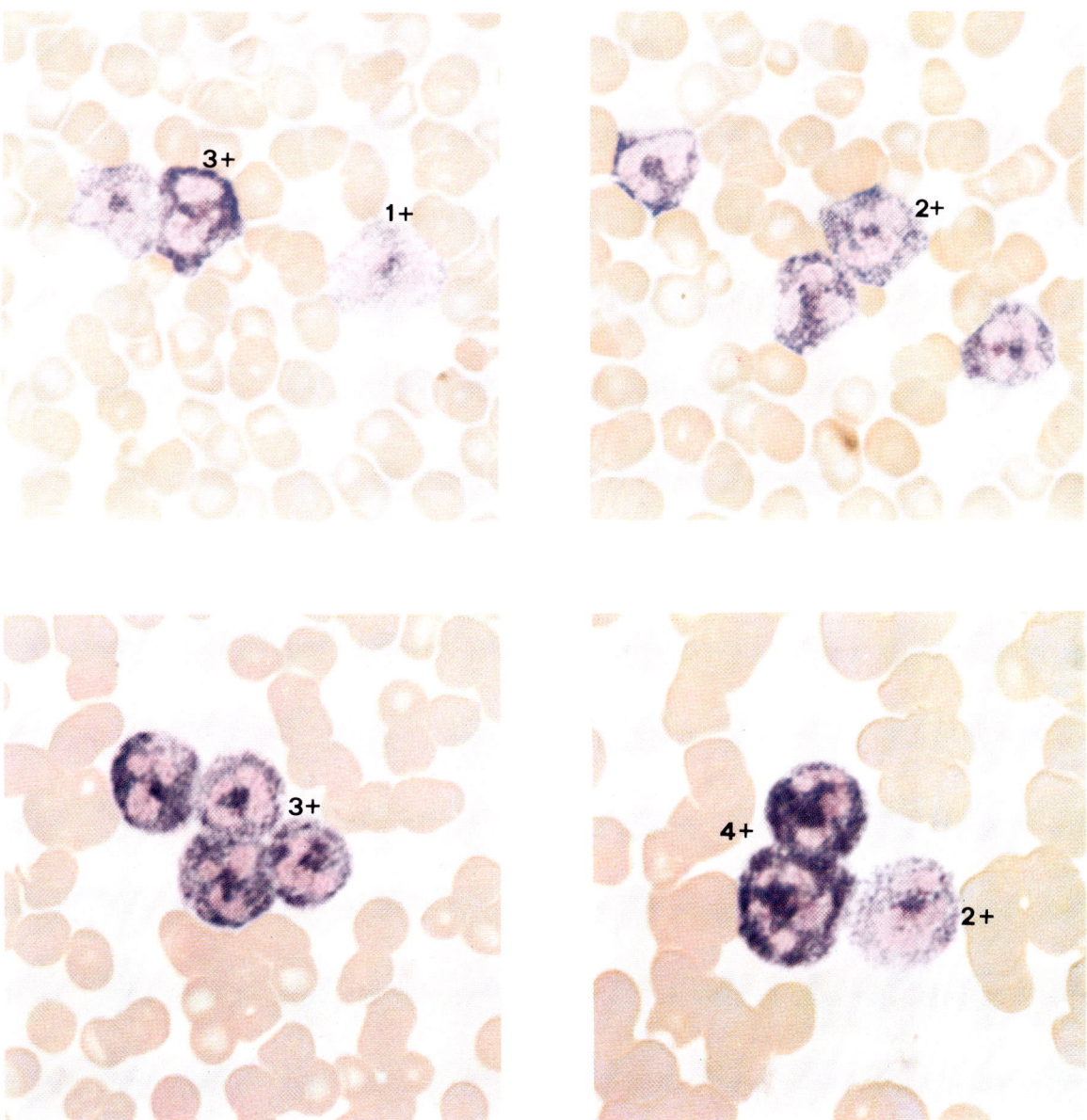

Fig. 27 Cytochemical localization of alkaline phosphatase in mature neutrophils. The cells show a different intensity of staining and are usually classified into stages 1+ to 4+ of Kaplow (see ref. 36). Although the evaluation of stain intensity is to some extent subjective, most observers arrive at some standard as indicated by the numbers 1+ to 4+ in the illustrations. The score is derived from the average obtained by counting a minimum of 100 cells.

in chronic myelogenous leukemia and in paroxysmal nocturnal hemoglobinuria [37]. The Sudan Black reaction, which is a rather non-specific stain for neutral fats and phospholipids, is also positive as it would be for any cell with many membrane-bound organelles (**Fig. 28**). Lymphoblasts are usually negative [37], probably because they have few, if any, membrane-bound organelles. In addition, a positive esterase reaction helps to distinguish the granulocytic from the monocytic series.

The naphthol-AS-D-chloroacetate esterase (NASDCA) reaction is a reliable cytochemical stain for the granulocytic series [38] (**Figs. 29 a, b**). Among the other non-specific esterases present in leukocytes, α-naphthyl-acetate esterase (ANA) and naphthol-AS-D-acetate esterase (NASDA) are contained in granulocytes as well as in monocytes. It is weaker in the former but in monocytes it is inhibited by NaF. The cytochemistry of leukemic neutrophils is discussed on pp. 201 and 212.

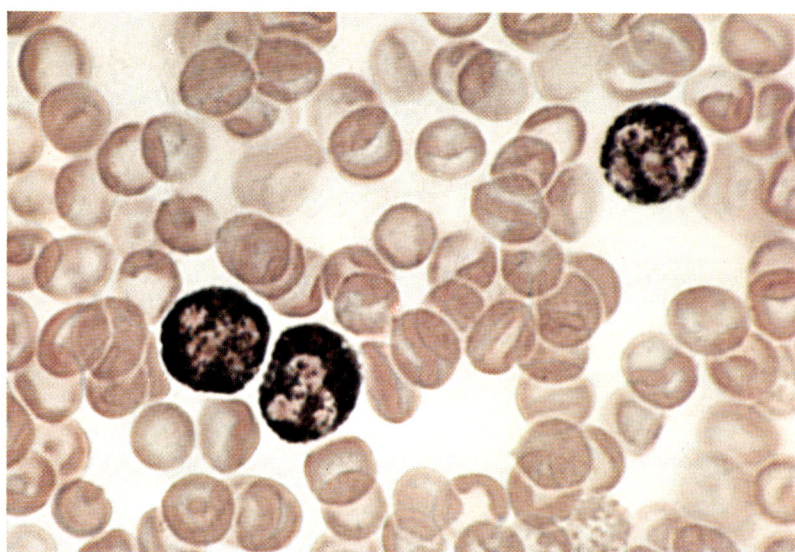

Fig. 28 Blood smear illustrating Sudan black reaction of mature neutrophils.

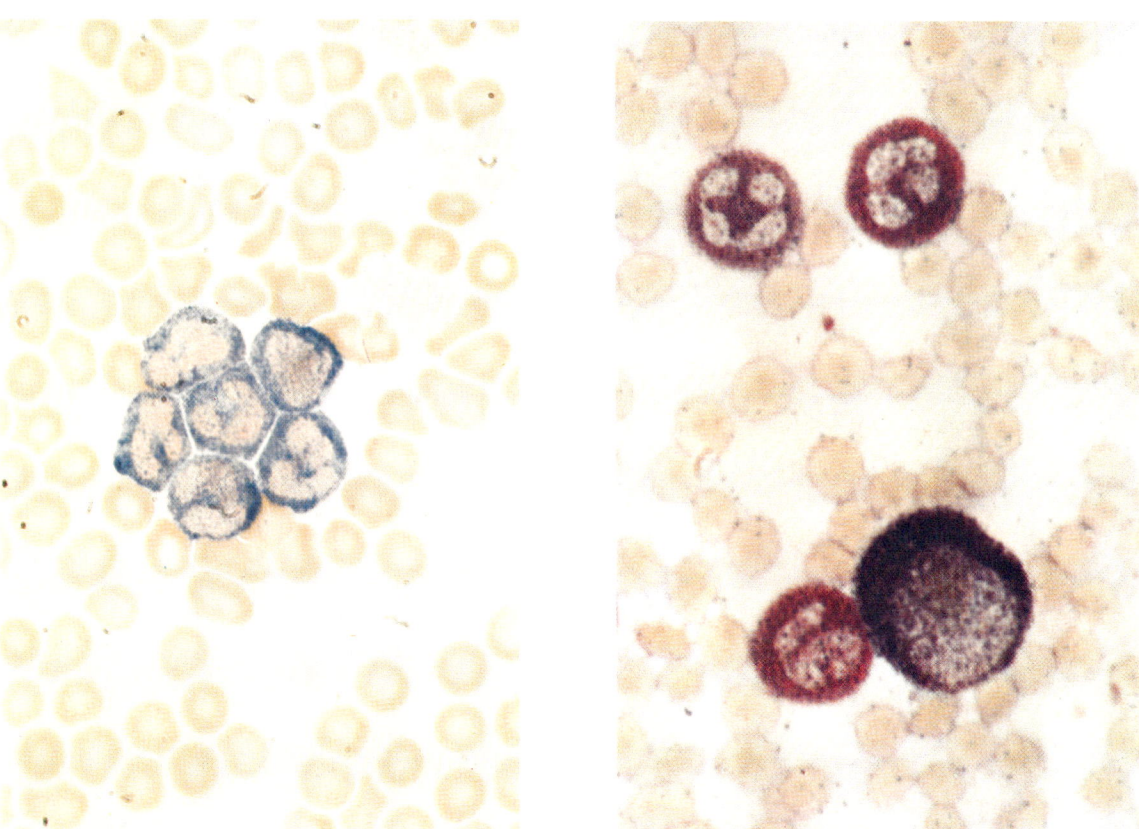

Fig. 29 a) A group of mature neutrophils shows strong positivity for naphthol AS-D-chloroacetate esterase.
b) Combined staining for naphthol AS-D-chloroacetate esterase and PAS. The esterase reaction is strongly positive in a promyelocyte and weak in three mature neutrophils which also show some PAS-positivity.
b) Courtesy of Dr. G.L. Castoldi, University of Ferrara.

4. KINETICS AND HUMORAL REGULATION OF GRANULOCYTES

Differentiation and maturation of myeloblasts to mature, circulating neutrophils takes about 7-11 days. Myelocytes constitute the largest population of dividing cells in the bone marrow and represent an efficient amplifying system. With a half-life of 6-7 hours, their turnover and production rate are prodigious (16.3×10^8, per kg, per 24 hrs) [6, 39, 144]. The circulating pool of granulocytes is in dynamic equilibrium with the marginated one which is about of the same size, or a little larger, and may be mobilized by stress, pyrogens and other factors. Studies utilizing leukocyte alkaline phosphatase seem to indicate that the passage from the circulating to the marginated pool is not random but selective [39]. Another important mobilizable pool is represented by mature neutrophils which are retained in the bone marrow (see ref. 144).

There are humoral factors that stimulate the mobilization of granulocytes from the post-mitotic pool in the bone marrow and others, chalones (for review see ref. 40), which inhibit mitosis. Currently, the most investigated of these are the colony stimulating factors (CSF) necessary for the growth of granulocyte-macrophage colonies *in vitro* (see Chapter 2). They appear to constitute a family of glycoproteins produced by mononuclear phagocytes [41]. Prostaglandins of the E series have been shown to inhibit granulocytopoiesis *in vitro* [42]. A central surveillance and effector role of macrophages has been conceived as a self-regulating medullary unit [41].

5. CHEMOTAXIS AND LOCOMOTION

Much of what has been learned about leukocyte physiology in recent years does not lend itself to visual documentation and will therefore only be summarized and referenced here. However, the structural concomitants of chemotaxis, locomotion, phagocytosis, and degranulation are now well understood. These have greatly helped in gaining insight into the cell's normal function and, in some instances, have clarified defects underlying disease. The motility of leukocytes has been studied for more than a century with increasing refinements in techniques of microscopy and cinemicrophotography. In the absence of stimuli, *in vitro* locomotion of the cells appears to be random, but always preceded by extension of a pseudopod at the leading end and the assumption of asymmetric shape leaving the nucleus towards the rear (**Fig. 30**). The stimuli which cause mature neutrophils to egress from the bone marrow [43, 44] or marginated neutrophils to diapedese from the circulation into tissues during normal homeostasis is not known. It is, however, clear that the cells pass between contiguous endothelial cells, first by inserting a pseudopod and subsequently by penetrating the basement membrane most often in areas where it is incomplete [45]. It is likely that inflammatory stimuli, such as histamine and serotonin, which induce contraction of endothelial cells, promote egress of neutrophils by virtue of newly formed inter-endothelial gaps [46]. Much more has been learned about directed locomotion, i.e. leukocyte chemotaxis, the mechanism whereby leukocytes are attracted by and migrate towards chemical stimuli. These studies have become possible with the development of *in vitro* methods, such as the Boyden chamber [47] and others [48]. The history and biochemical aspects of chemotaxis cannot be detailed here and have been excellently reviewed elsewhere [49-51]. In brief, chemotactic factors may be derived from the activation of the complement system (by the classical or alternative pathway), by the fibrinolytic and kinin-generating system, by products derived from cells (leukocytes and platelets), by products derived from bacteria (endotoxin), by prostaglandins, and by well-defined synthetic peptides, such as formyl-methionyl-leucyl-phenylalanine [52]. In each case, the chemoattractant must exist

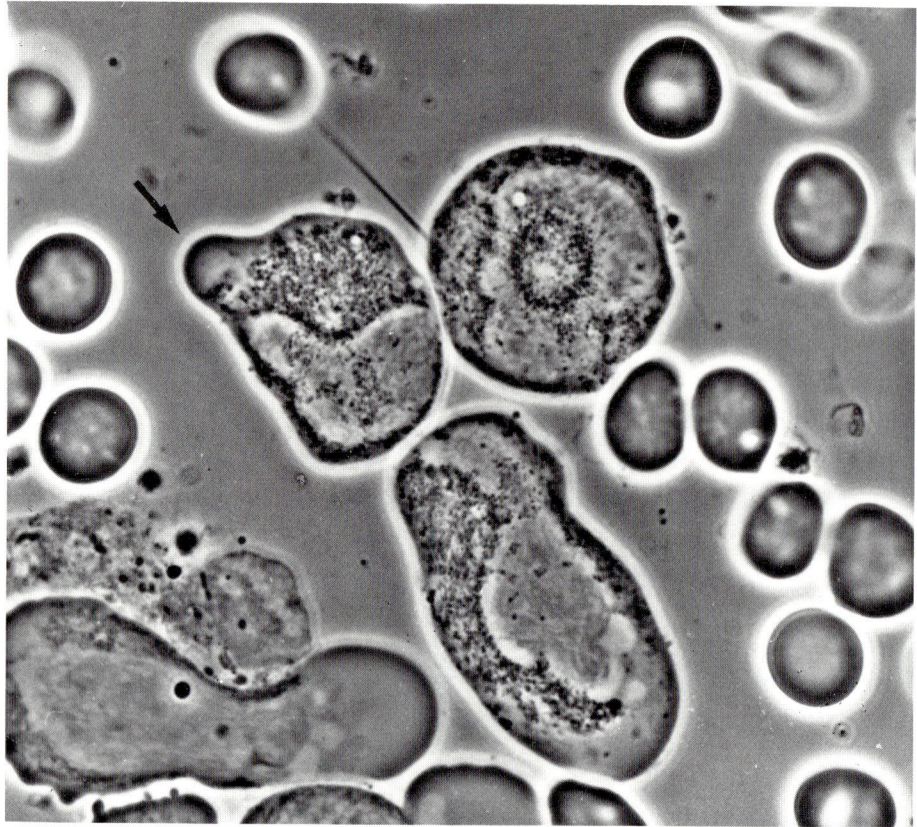

Fig. 30 *Phase photomicrograph of neutrophils. Agranular pseudopods are noteworthy (**arrow**). The nucleus stays in the rear of the cell during locomotion.*

as a gradient. This causes a predictable reorientation of the cell and its internal structures [53] which is illustrated in **Figures 31** and **32**.

Numerous inhibitors of chemotaxis have also been described. Some of these are present in serum, others are cell associated. In any case, the balance between stimulation of chemotaxis and inactivation of chemotactic factors plays an important role in modulation of the inflammatory response [54, 55]. Defects in this system have clinical consequences and are discussed on p. 196.

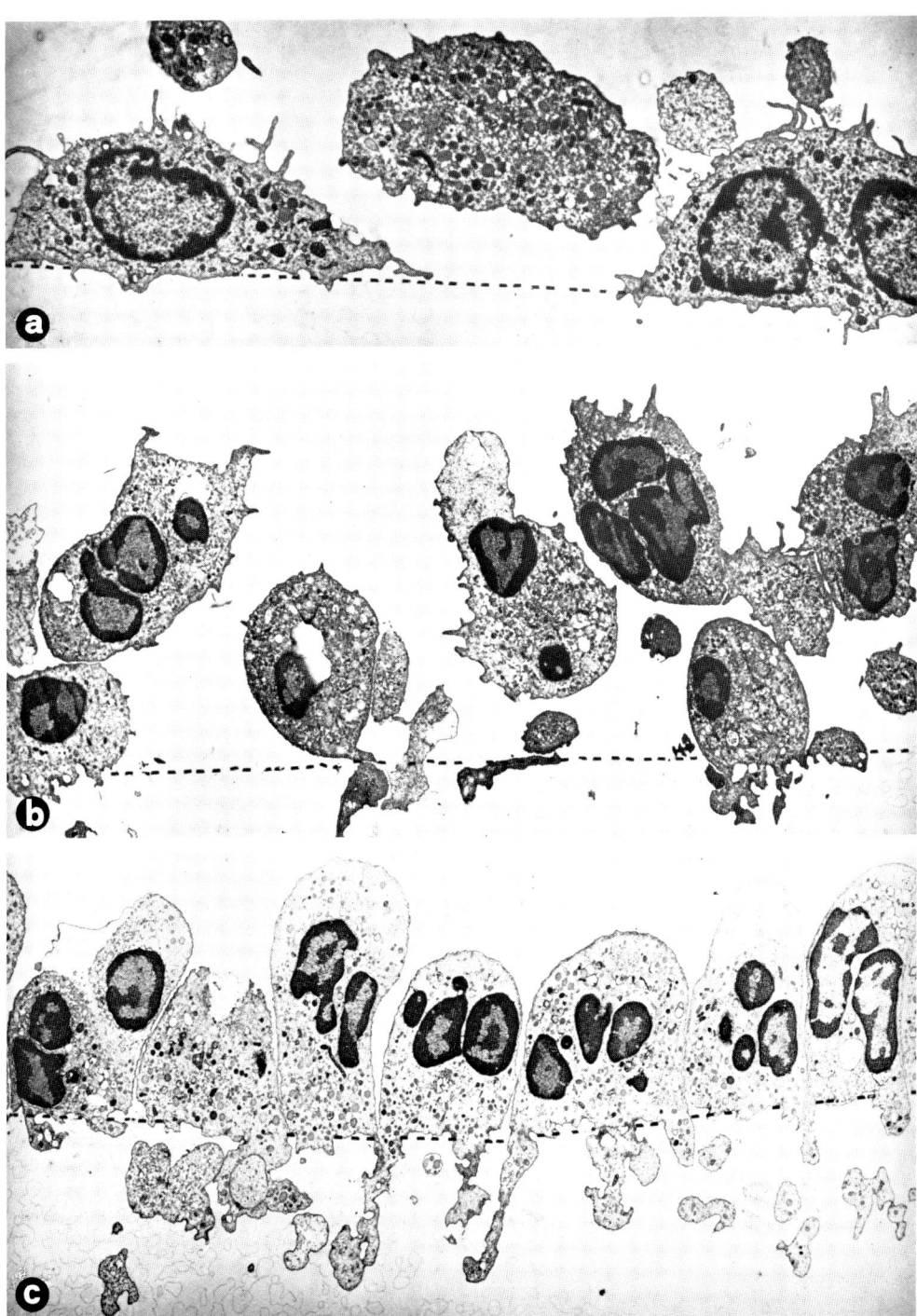

Fig. 31 Neutrophil chemotaxis examined in a modified Boyden chamber [47]. The chamber contains a micropore filter (stippled line) which separates the cell (top) from the chemoattractant below.
In a no chemotactic factor was present and the cells settled randomly on the filter ($\times$ 6,800).
In b a chemotactic factor was present at equal concentrations on both sides of the filter. This increased random movement and deformity of the cells ($\times$ 3,300).
In c chemotactic factor is present only below the filter. This caused marked polarization with all cells oriented in the same direction ($\times$ 3,450).
Courtesy of Dr. John Gallin, National Institute of Allergy & Infectious Diseases, reproduced from ref. 53 with permission of the publisher.

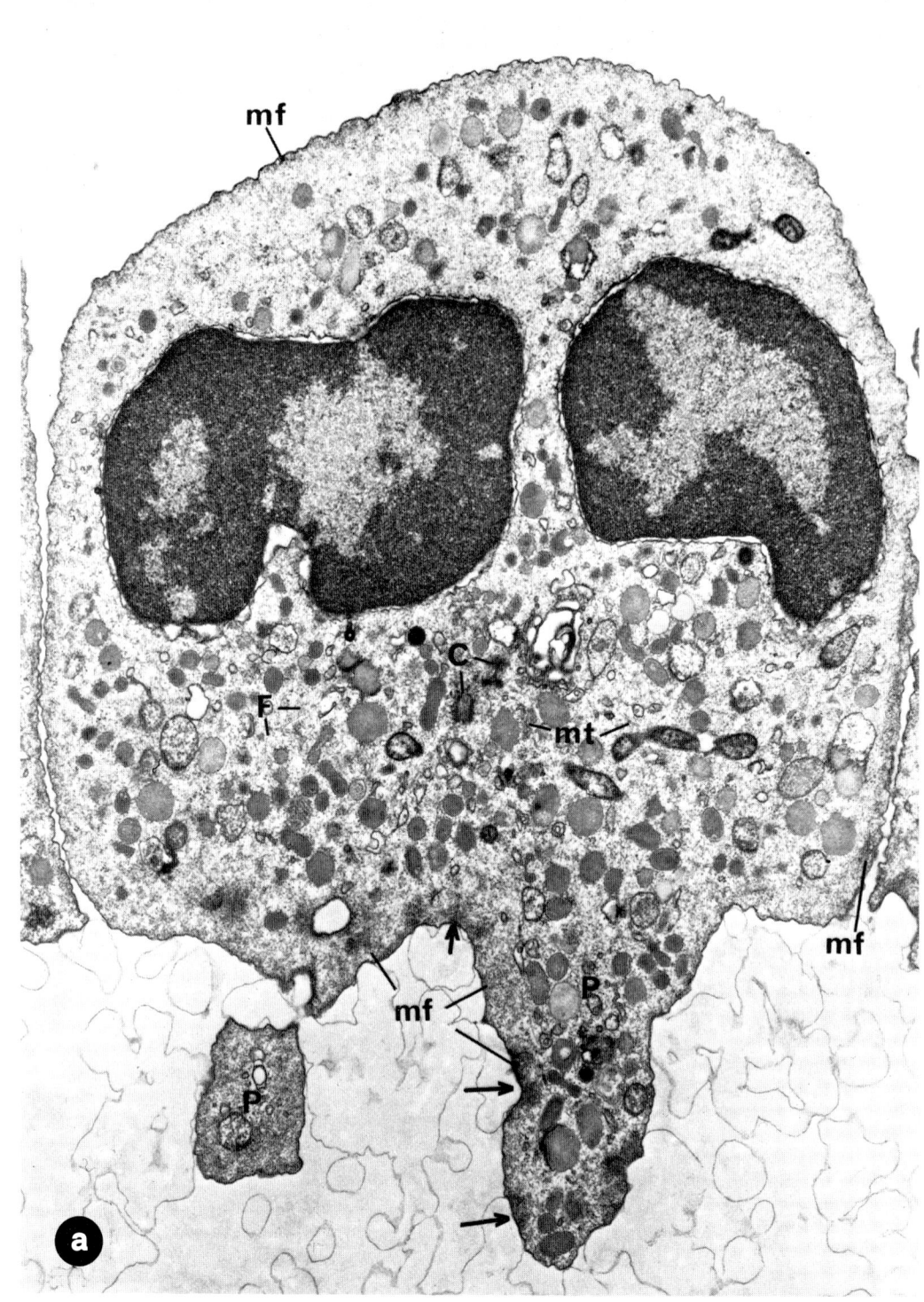

Fig. 32 a) Higher magnification of a neutrophil oriented in a chemotactic gradient consisting of 5% activated serum beneath a micropore filter. The nuclear lobes are in the upper part of the cell while pseudopods extend into the filter. Submembranous microfilaments (**mf**) can be seen at the side and the top of the cell. Aggregates of such filaments are seen in the region of the pseudopod (**P**) (**arrows**). These are illustrated to better advantage in **b**. **C** indicates the centriole, **F** 10 nm filaments, **mt** microtubules ($\times$ 15,340). Courtesy of Dr. John Gallin, National Institute of Allergy & Infectious Diseases, reproduced from ref. 53 with permission of the publisher.

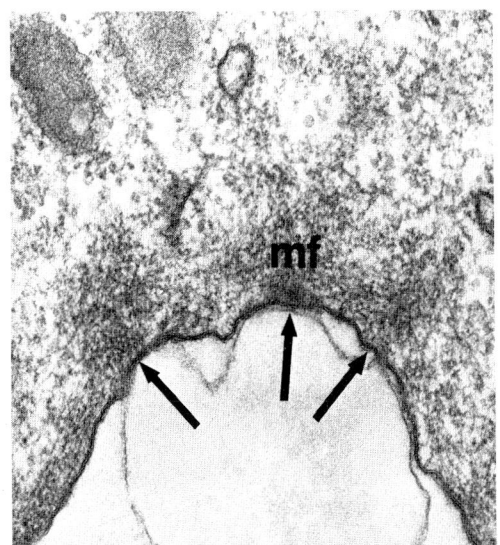
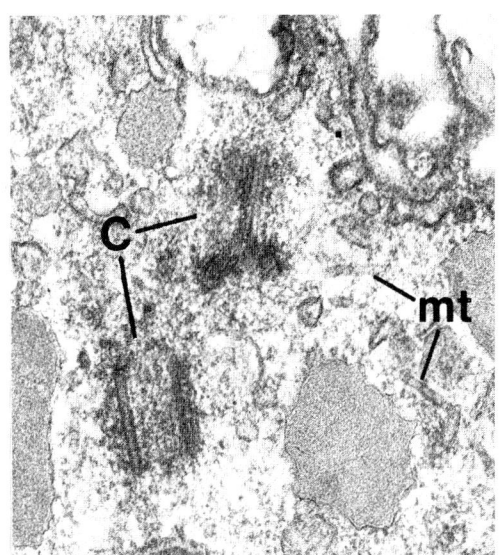

Fig. 32 b) Submembranous microfilaments (**mf**) at the lower end of the neutrophil shown in **a**. Local dense concentrations of microfilaments occur at sites of close contact with the filter matrix (**arrows**) ($\times$ 58,500).
c) Higher magnification of the centriolar region of the cell depicted in **a**. Microtubules (**mt**) radiate from this area. **C**, centriole ($\times$ 58,000).
Courtesy of Dr. John Gallin, National Institute of Allergy & Infectious Diseases, reproduced from ref. 53 with permission of the publisher.

6. PHAGOCYTOSIS AND DEGRANULATION

When the cell has made contact with an object susceptible to being phagocytosed, for example, an opsonized bacterium, a series of morphological events ensue. Pseudopods pass around each side of the particle, meet and fuse (**Fig. 33 a**). The particle is thus enclosed by the cell's invaginated surface membrane, the inner layer of which was originally the external layer of the plasma membrane. Some investigators consider such a phagocytic vacuole or "phagosome" still outside the cell, though continuity with the extracellular medium can no longer be demonstrated. If only a few particles are engulfed, the phagosome appears to move toward the interior of the cell. Cinemicrophotography of the process showed that the cell's granules located near such a phagocytic vacuole disappear almost instantaneously [56]. More recent biochemical studies have confirmed this impression by establishing that the granules discharge within less than 30 seconds [57]. Electron microscopic analysis of cells which were fixed during phagocytosis established that the granules coalesce with the phagocytic vacuole [58]. During this process, the granule membranes fuse with the membrane of the phagosome and the granule content is released into the vacuole (**Figs. 33-36**). Thus the enzymes are discharged directly onto the bacterium without exposing the cell to its own digestive enzymes.

Even massive phagocytosis and almost complete degranulation (**Fig. 35**) do not usually result in cell death. That the same phenomenon takes place *in vivo* has been concluded from studies of cells obtained from various inflammatory tissues and exudates [59] (**Figs. 37 a, b**). However, during massive phagocytosis *in vitro*, small quantities of hydrolytic enzymes appear in the medium. This probably occurs when the phagocytic vacuoles have not completely closed, e.g. when the particles are too large (**Fig. 36 b**). The extreme example of such a situation is seen when neutrophils adhere to and spread over a large opsonized surface. This process has been called "frustrated" phagocytosis [60].

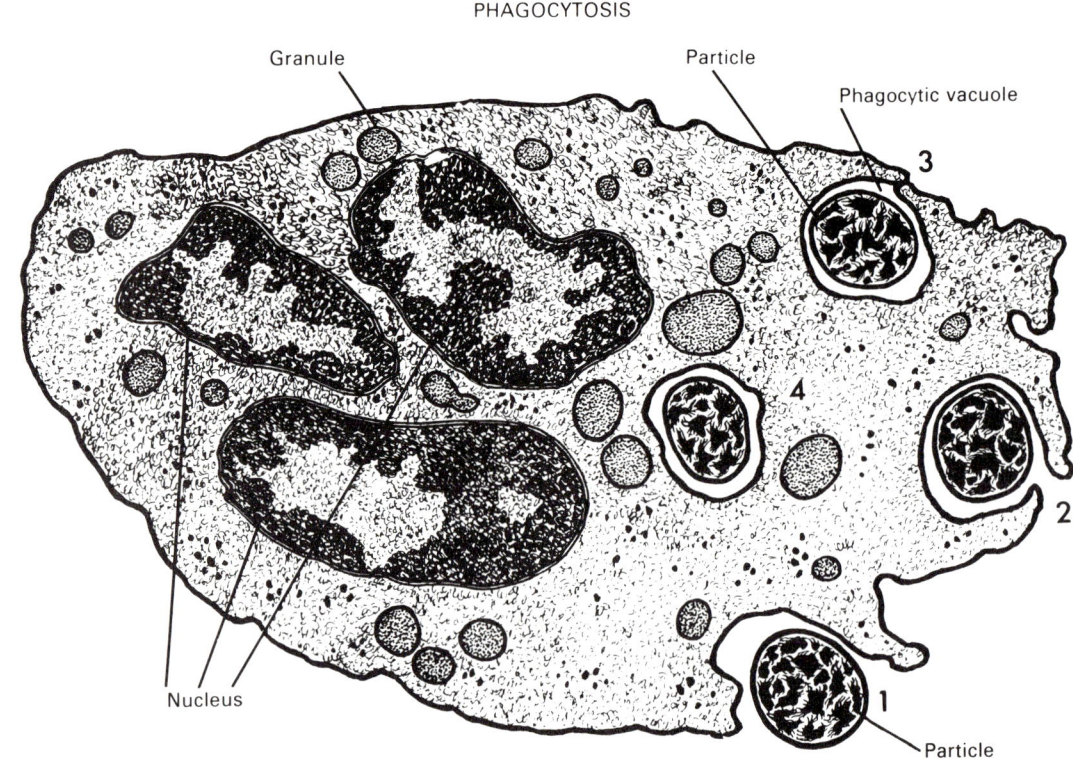

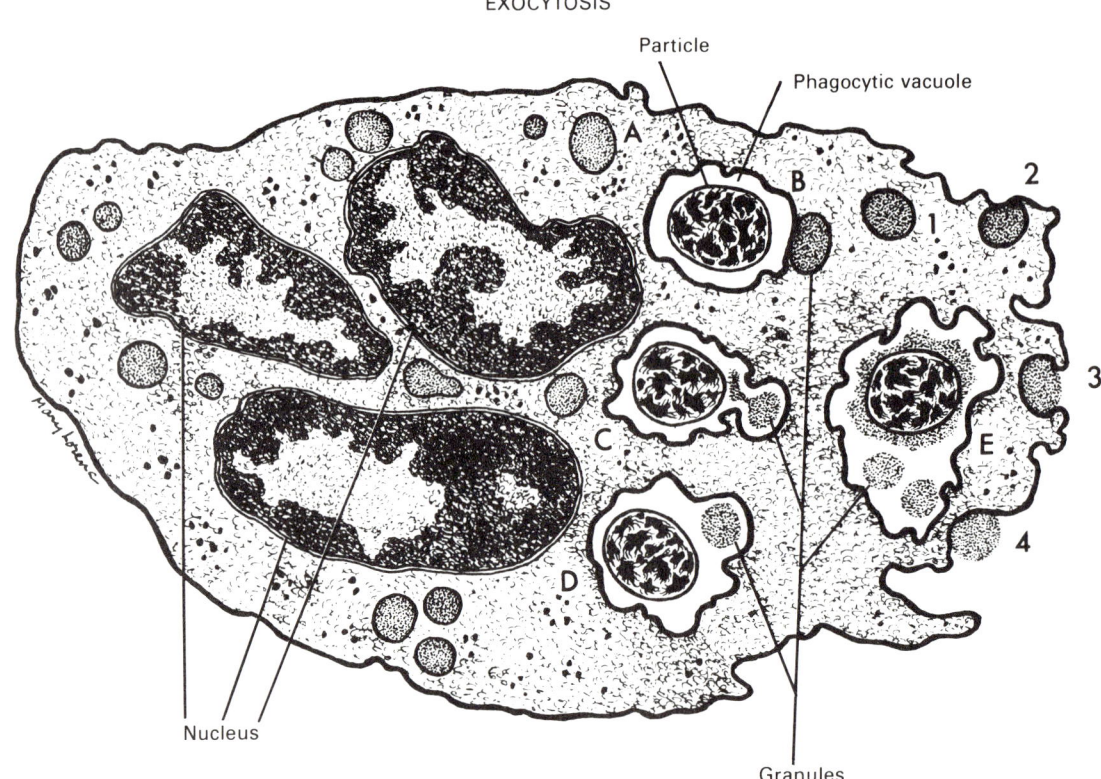

Fig. 33 a) Schematic representation of a neutrophil showing progressive stages of phagocytosis (**1** to **4**).
b) Schematic representation of a neutrophil depicting the mechanism of exocytosis. In sequence **1** to **4**, particulate matter is discharged from the cell with preservation of membrane continuity.
In sequence **A** to **E**, granule content is released into phagocytic vacuole with preservation of membrane continuity. It is believed that this mechanism precludes autodigestion or "suicide" by the cell's own enzymes. Reproduced from ref. 58 with permission of the publisher.

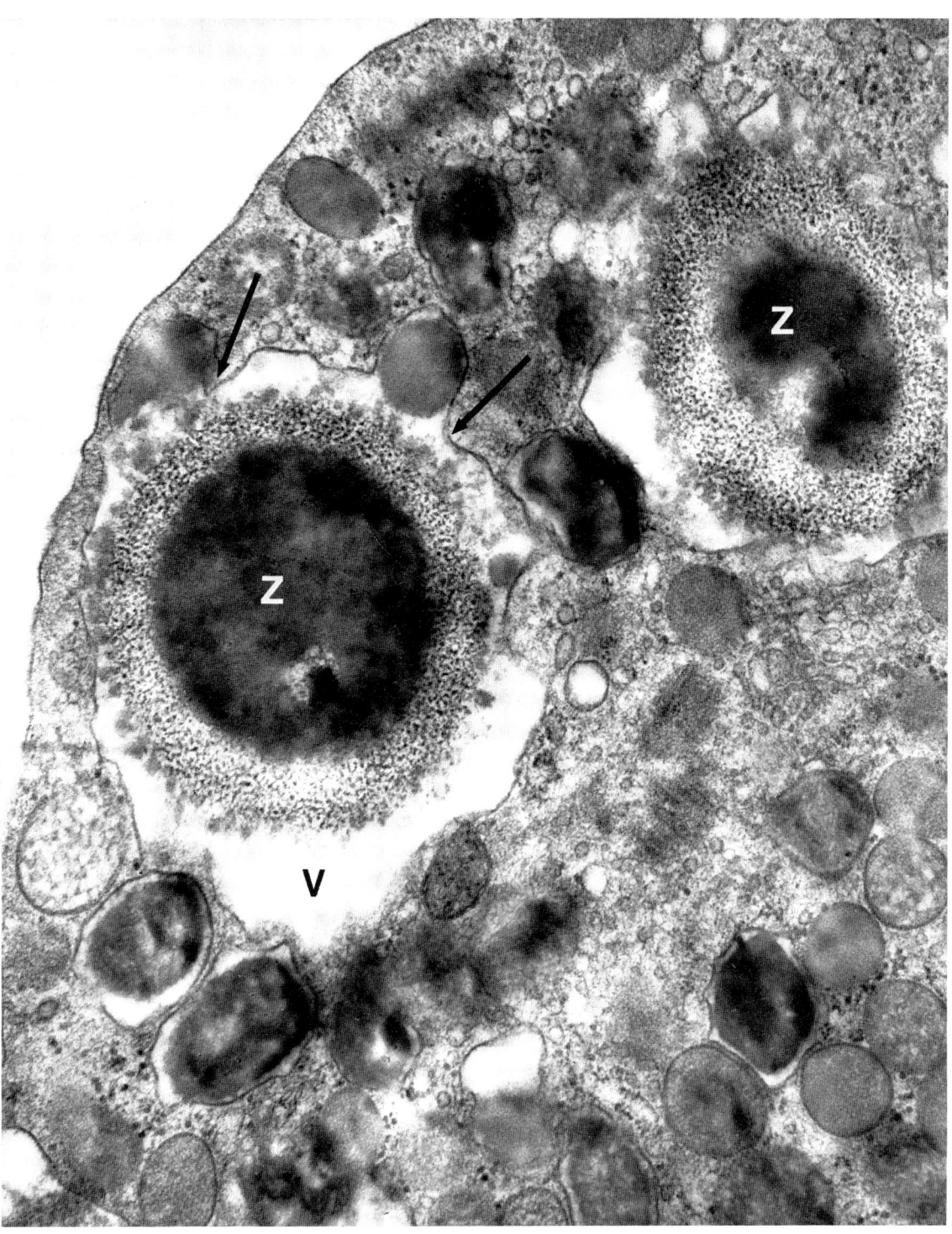

Fig. 34 Reproduction of the original illustration which showed the "degranulation phenomenon" for the first time (from Zucker-Franklin D., Hirsch J.G. - ref. 58 with permission of the publisher). The neutrophils had been incubated with zymosan particles (Z) 1-½ minutes before fixation. Two granules, devoid of membranes, are in the process of entering the phagocytic vacuole (V). Their membranes have fused with the membrane lining the vacuole (**arrows**) ($\times$ 42,000).

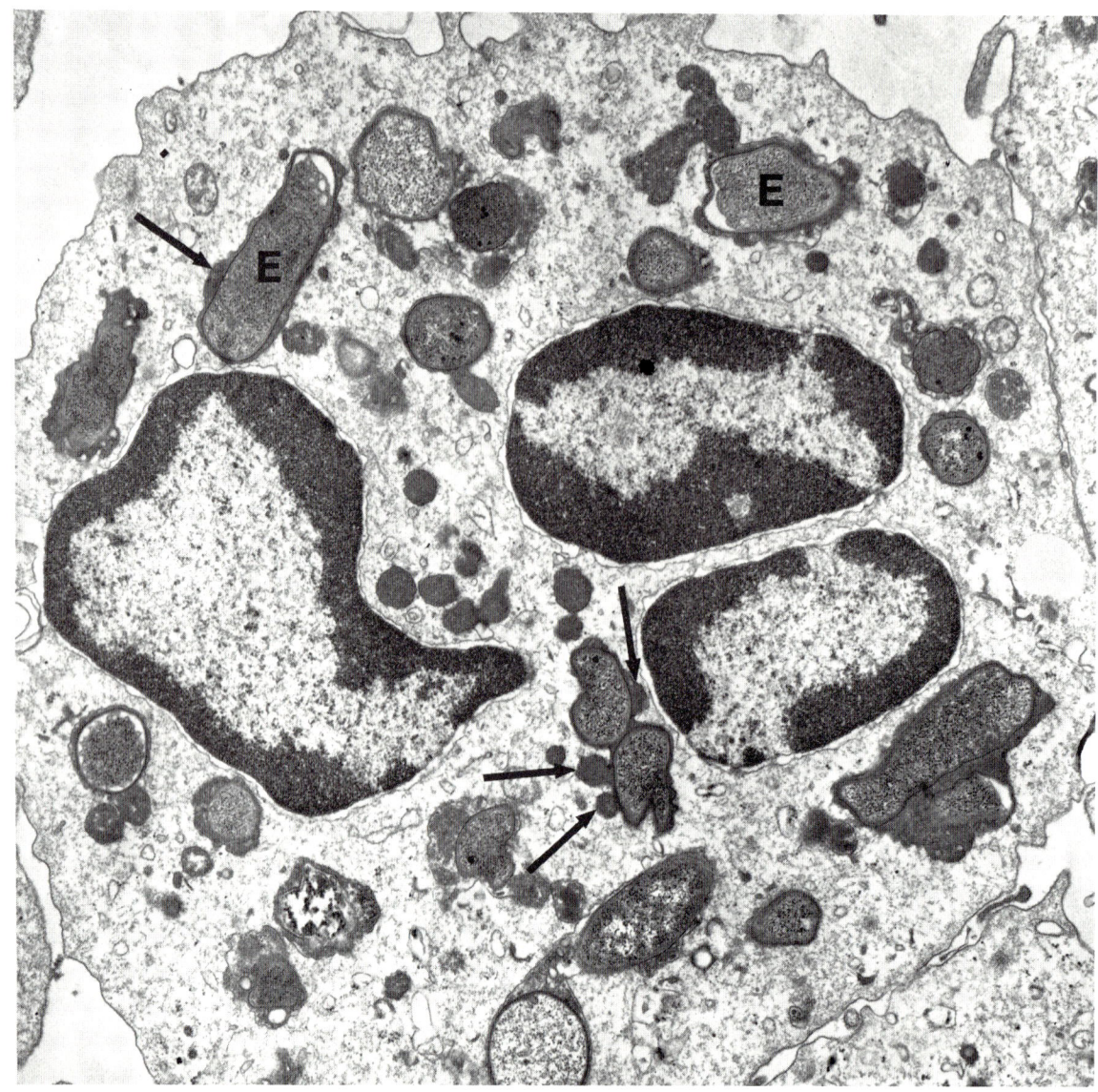

Fig. 35 *Neutrophil from a buffy coat specimen that had been incubated with E. coli (E). Numerous microorganisms are seen within phagocytic vacuoles. The cell is almost completely degranulated, but some lysosomes are still seen in the process of fusion with the phagosomes (arrows) (× 15,000).*

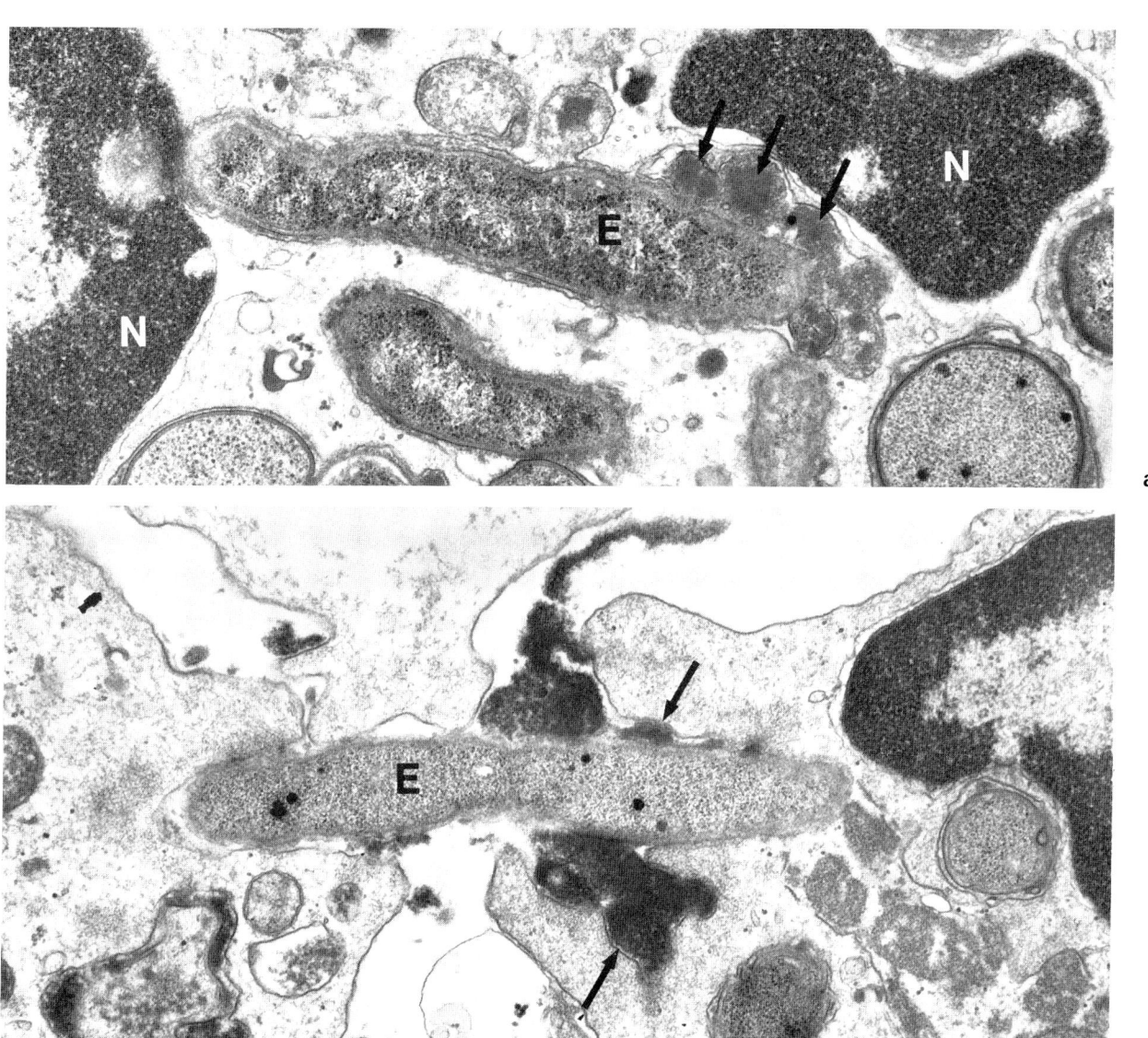

Fig. 36 a) Detail of a neutrophil from the same specimen as **Figure 35** illustrates the degranulation phenomenon to better advantage. **E**, E. coli; **N**, nucleus. **Arrows** indicate content of granules released into the phagocytic vacuole (× 32,000).

b) Example of "frustrated" phagocytosis. Two neutrophils attempting to phagocytose the same microorganism (**E**) without being able to surround and enclose it completely. As a consequence, the neutrophil on the right is discharging the content of its granules into the extracellular medium (**arrows**) (× 30,000).

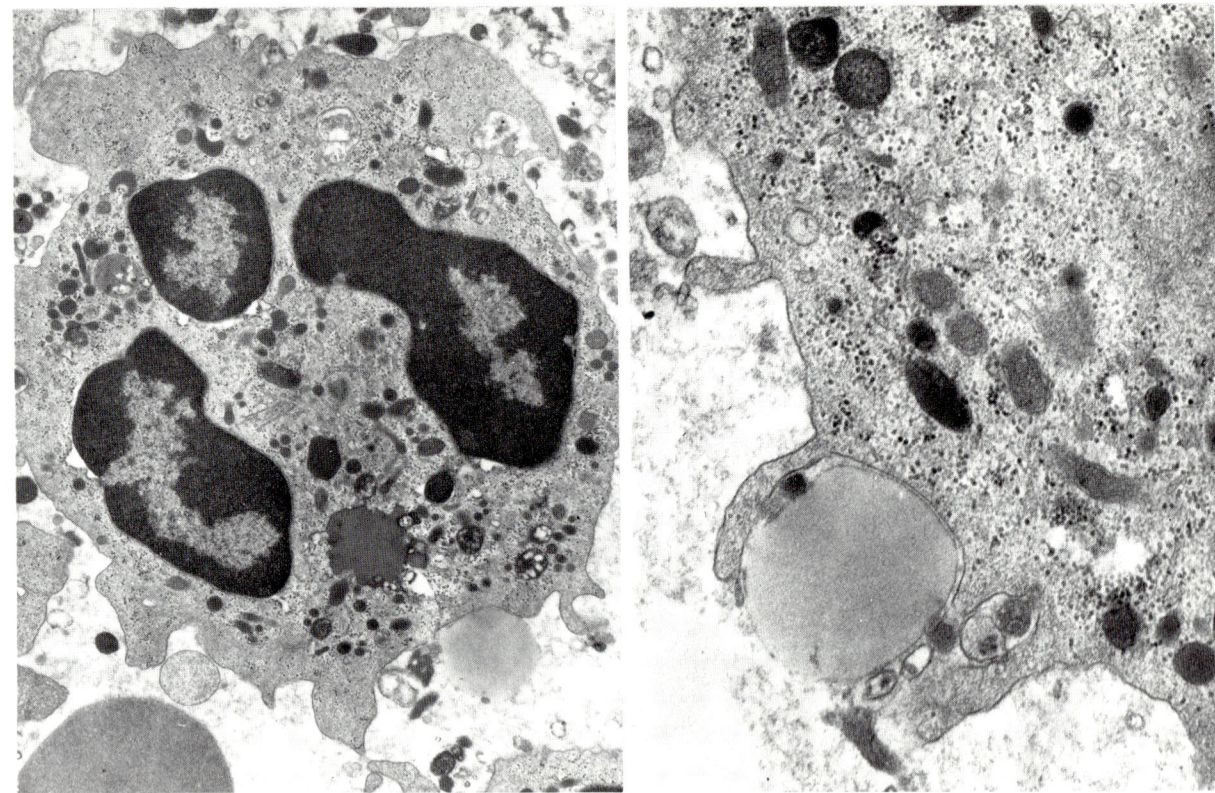

Fig. 37 a) Neutrophil prepared from rheumatoid synovial fluid is surrounded by cellular debris often seen in inflammatory exudates. The cell exhibits several phagolysosomes ($\times$ 12,000).

b) Detail of a neutrophil prepared from the same specimen as **a** shows a cell in the process of phagocytosing cellular debris consisting of a granule and a grey body probably composed of lipid (see lipid inclusions, p. 194) ($\times$ 28,000).
Reproduced from ref. 59 with permission of the publisher.

7. THE L.E. PHENOMENON

The phagocytic property of neutrophils serves, at times, in the diagnosis of non hematologic disorders. The best example of this is the lupus erythematosus (LE) cell phenomenon. LE cells result when leukocytes phagocytose nuclei that have been opsonized with complement fixing antibodies directed against deoxyribonucleoprotein [61-64]. Since antibodies are not capable of penetrating living cells (i.e., antinuclear antibodies [ANA] do not affect the nuclei of intact cells), the LE phenomenon (**Figs. 38 a-g**) is, with rare exceptions, only observed *in vitro* [65-67]. The phagocytic cell could also be an eosinophil or even a monocyte, but, in most instances, it is a neutrophil.

Fig. 38 a) Typical LE cell stained with May Grünwald-Giemsa. The **arrow** indicates the swollen homogenized nuclear mass (probably derived from another granulocyte) which has been phagocytosed by a neutrophil. The nucleus (**N**) of the neutrophil has been characteristically pushed towards the periphery of the cell.

b) Strongly positive LE test from a patient with active SLE. Practically all granulocytes have phagocytosed LE bodies.

c) LE cells stained supravitally with acridine orange observed with blue violet illumination. The phagocytosed nuclei appear in green. The multilobed nuclei of the neutrophils which have engulfed them appear in yellow, while the neutrophil granules are seen in red.

d) An LE cel (**top**) is seen next to a large "plasmocytoid" lymphocyte. Such stimulated lymphocytes are often found in the blood of patients with active SLE but also in other hyperimmune states.

e) Example of a "pseudo" LE cell. LE cells must be distinguished from other types of nucleophagocytosis or from inclusions formed by other substances which the cells have ingested. This particular illustration was obtained from the buffy coat of a patient with mixed cryoglobulinemia. The inclusions were always Feulgen-negative.

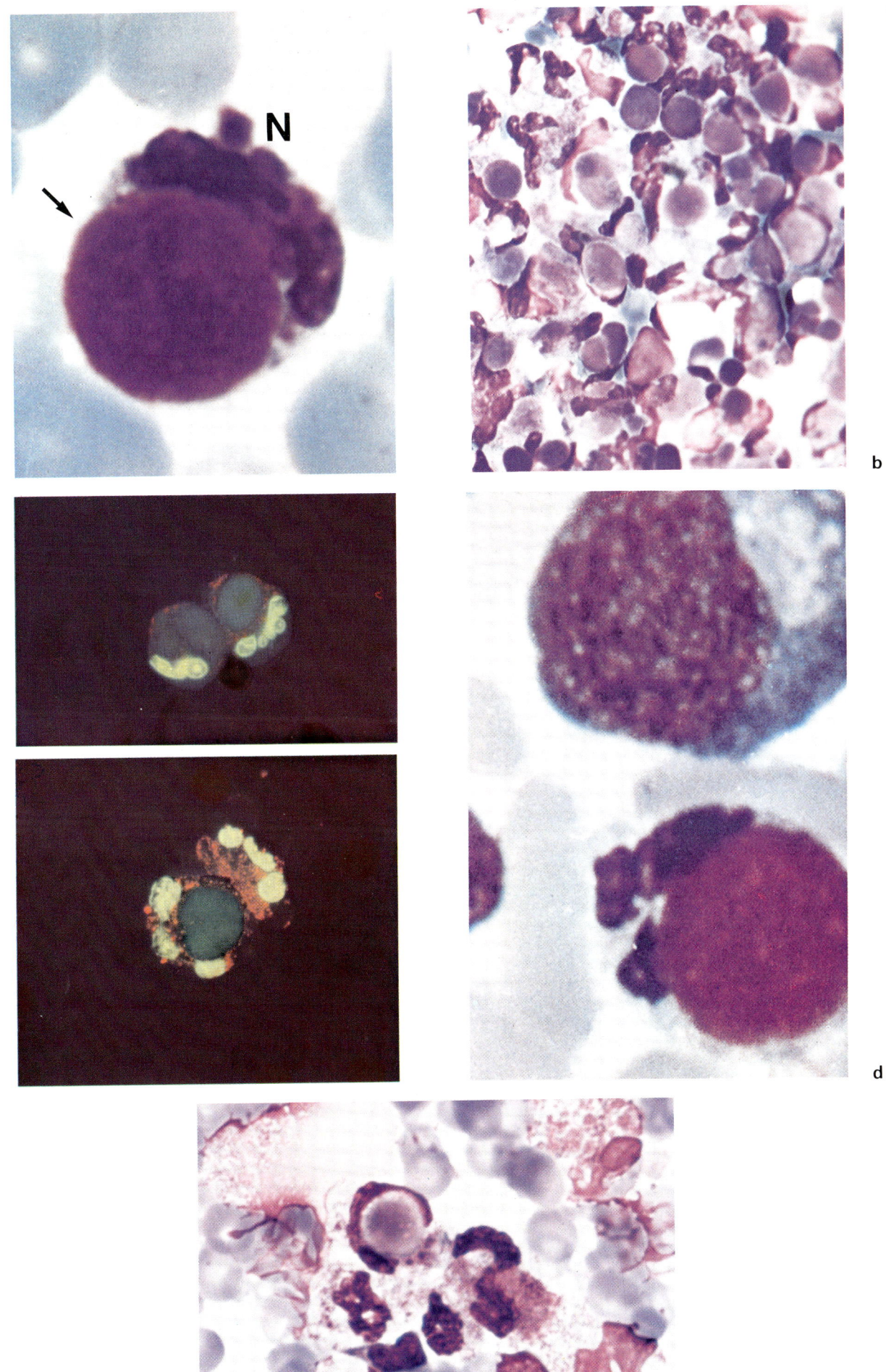

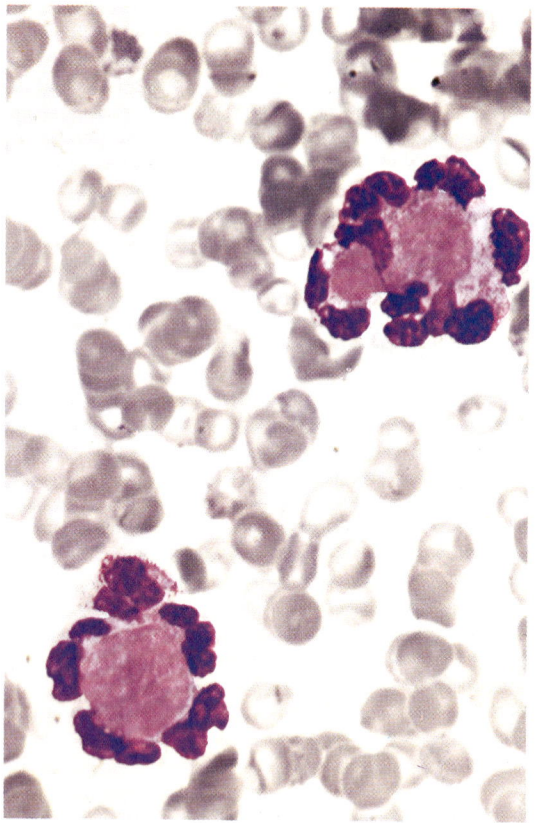 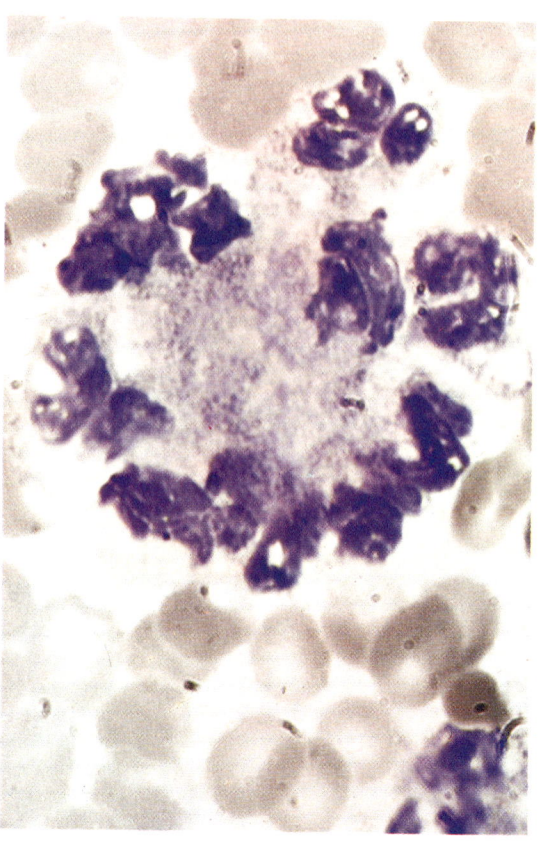

Fig. 38 f) Two typical rosettes from a positive LE preparation. The ground-glass nuclear material is surrounded by phagocytosing granulocytes.

g) Higher magnification of an LE rosette in which the central material has undergone partial degradation.

The phagocytosed nuclei which are usually derived from cells damaged *in vitro*, have a "swollen", "cloudy" or "ground-glass" appearance in contrast to the nuclei ingested by granulocytes in other conditions associated with nucleophagocytosis. In systemic lupus erythematosus (SLE) the antibody is directed specifically against nuclei, which probably undergo some morphologic alterations even before they are taken up by neutrophils. This may also account for the variety in degrees of morphologic changes seen in treated SLE, in LE positive rheumatoid arthritis, and in other conditions associated with somewhat atypical LE cells [68]. Because the LE phenomenon has been of such great clinical usefulness in the diagnosis and management of SLE and related diseases, a vast literature on the subject exists. This has now become largely of historical interest, although many of its aspects continue to stimulate investigators of autoimmune diseases [69-72].

In most modern medical centers, the LE test has been superseded by a battery of immunofluorescent and radioimmunological methods, geared specifically for the detection of anti-DNA antibodies [73-79]. A variety of immunofluorescent nuclear patterns has been recognized (peripheral, homogeneous, speckled, nucleolar, and others). In addition, hemoflagellate kinetoplasts, particularly of *Crithidia luciliae*, have been employed with success for the demonstration of anti-DNA antibodies since they are composed of a concentrated network ("circular") of double stranded DNA unassociated with histone [77-79]. Some of these methods are described in the legends to figures (**Figs. 39-43**).

4 NEUTROPHILS

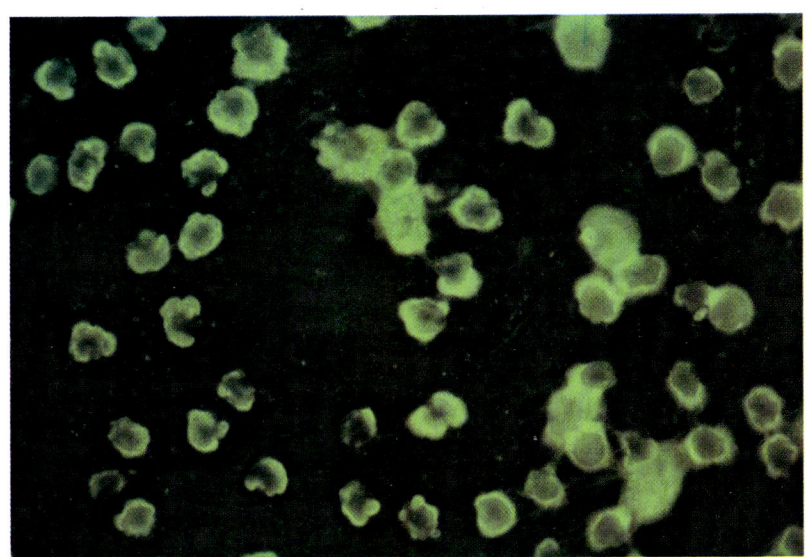

39

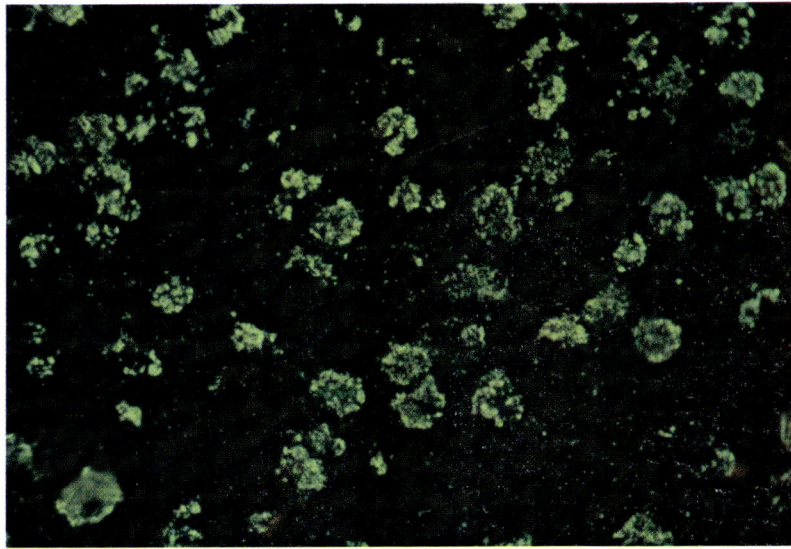

40

Fig. 39 Antinuclear antibody (ANA) test prepared on a frozen section of mouse liver shows a mixed, homogeneous and peripheral pattern indicative of SLE. The antinuclear antibodies in the patient's serum react with DNA of the mouse liver nuclei. This reaction is detected with a fluorescein-conjugated antiserum to human immunoglobulin.

Fig. 40 ANA test illustrating the speckled pattern. This type of reaction is not diagnostic of SLE because it may be elicited by either anti-Sm (SLE) or anti-ENA (MCTD) antigens and requires further analytical procedures. Test carried out on mouse liver section.

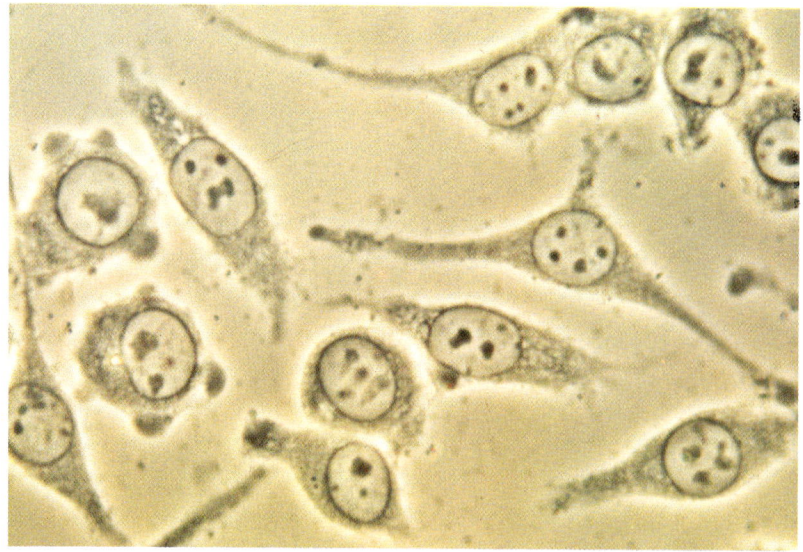

Fig. 41 The fibroblasts used for the reaction in **Figs. 42 a, b** seen by phase microscopy before exposure to the antisera.

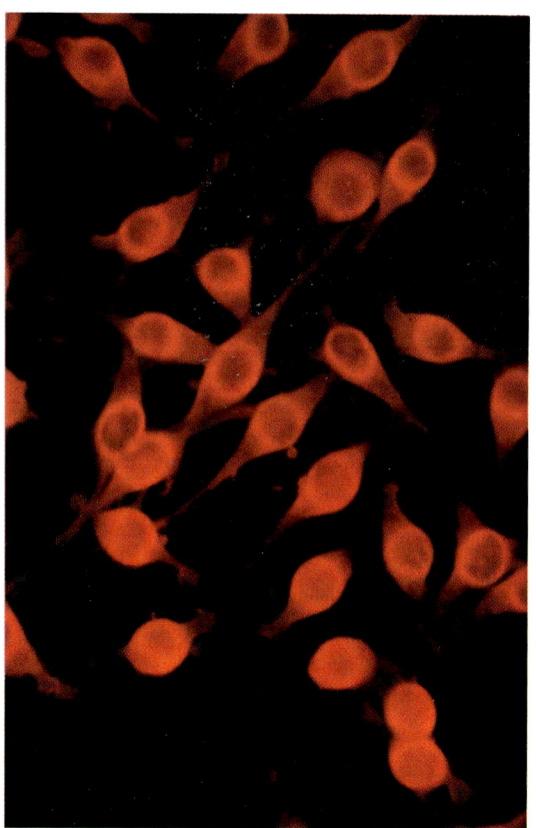
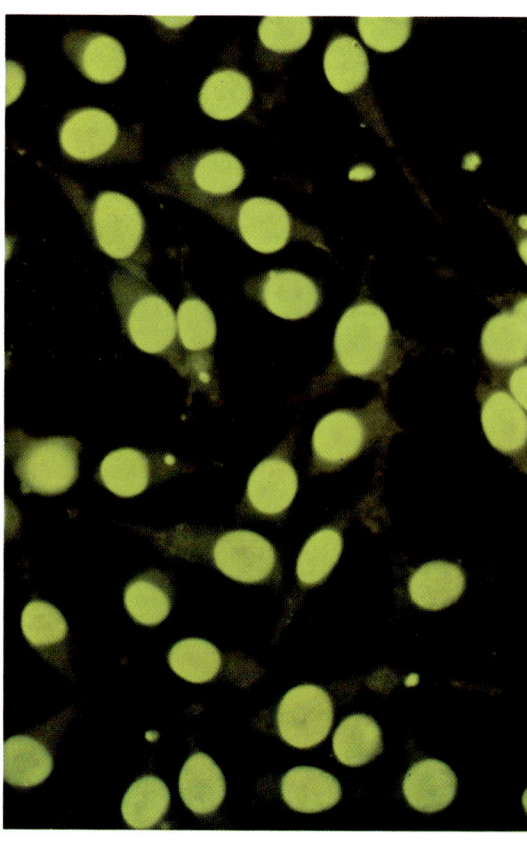

Fig. 42 a) Positive ANA test prepared with rat fibroblasts and reacted with rhodamine-conjugated antiserum; peripheral staining pattern.
b) Positive ANA test prepared as in **a** and reacted with fluorescein-conjugated antiserum; homogeneous staining pattern.

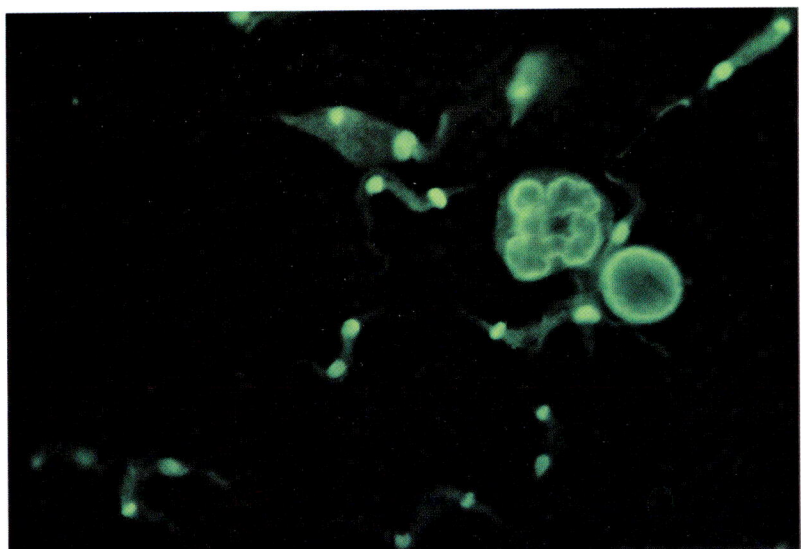

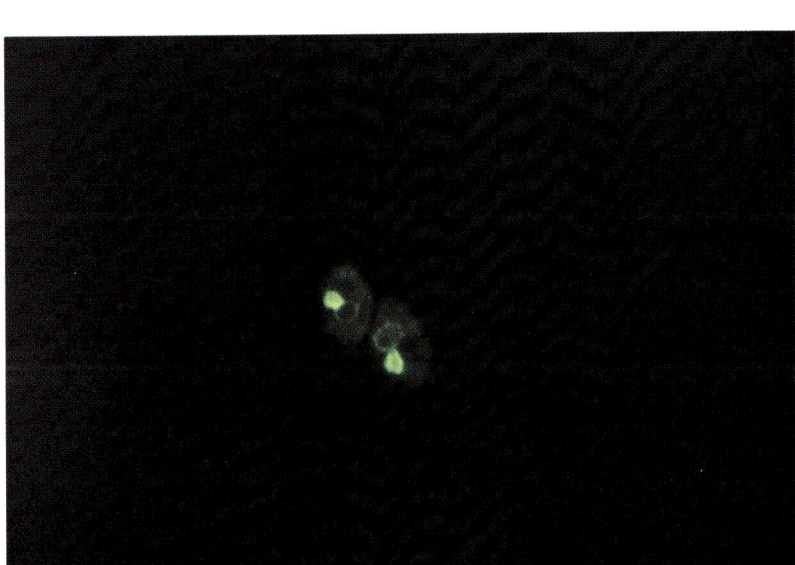

Fig. 43 a) *Anti-DNA antibodies may be conveniently demonstrated by using as a substrate a specific hemoflagellate organelle, the kinetoplast, which consists of circular, native DNA. Three types of immunofluorescence can be seen in this preparation, in which the substrate is peripheral mouse blood heavily parasitized with* Trypanosoma lewisi: *marginal (leukocyte nuclei), homogeneous (Trypanosoma nuclei) and kinetoplastic.*
Preparation kindly supplied by prof. C. Masala, University of Rome.
b) *Anti-DNA antibodies demonstrated by specific immunofluorescence of the kinetoplast of* Crithidia luciliae.

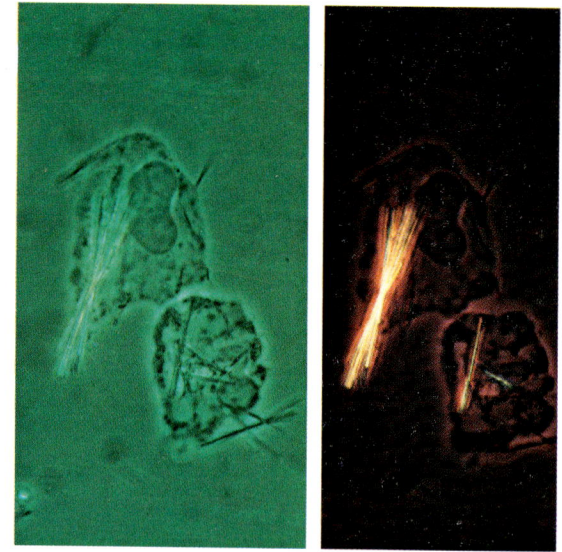

Fig. 44 a) *Phagocytosis of monosodium urate crystals by cells obtained from a gout exudate.*
Left, *phase microscopy;* **right**, *polarization microscopy.*

b) *Phagocytosis of monosodium urate crystals (MSU). Note that the crystal cannot be seen by ordinary light microscopy (first panel); polarization microscopy reveals the crystal but does not resolve the cell (second panel). Compensated phase polarization microscopy resolves both the cell and the crystal while the color change is characteristic for MSU (third and fourth panel).*

c) *Calcium pyrophosphate crystals are easily distinguished from MSU crystals by polarization microscopy.*

8. CRYSTAL PHAGOCYTOSIS

Neutrophil that have phagocytosed crystals, e.g. monosodium urate dihydrate (MSU) or calcium pyrophosphate dihydrate (CPPD) (Figs. 44 a-c), as seen in synovial fluids or other inflammatory exudates obtained from patients with gout and pseudogout respectively, may also provide useful diagnostic clues [80-85] when polarization microscopy with a first order red compensator is used. MSU crystals have a characteristically elongated and thin configuration, and appear colored in yellow or blue, exhibiting so called negative elongation; the more common CPPD crystals have a rhomboid configuration with a weak positive elongation. Hydroxyapatite crystals are primarily identified by means of TEM [87].

Many of the inflammatory manifestations of these diseases hinge on the presence of neutrophils and their ability to phagocytose and degranulate, see below [88, 89]. Indeed, the efficacy of therapeutic agents used in these conditions is often attributed to the inhibitory effects they have on various neutrophil functions [90].

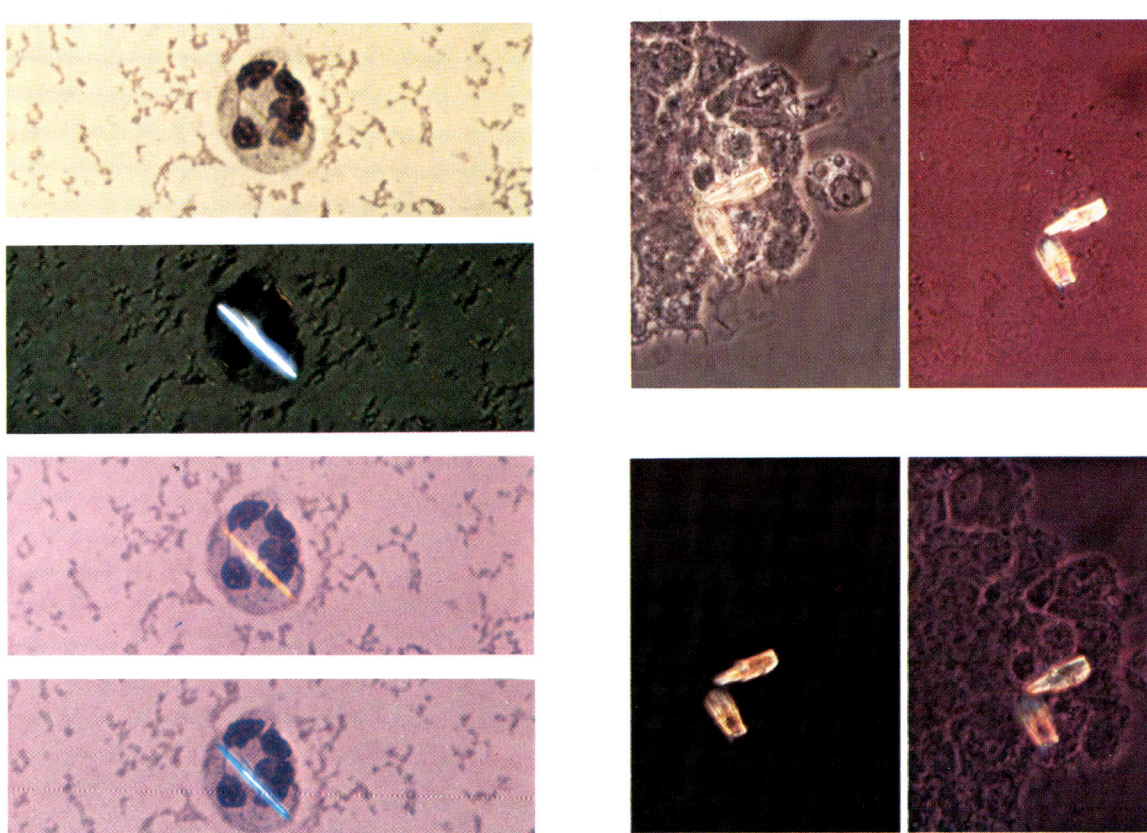

9. NEUTROPHIL METABOLISM

A wealth of new information has been amassed dealing with the biochemical events associated with chemotaxis, adhesion, phagocytosis and degranulation (reviewed in refs. 20, 91-93). In general, the "opsonins" which consist of immunoglobulin and/or complement components react with specific receptors on the PMN's (the cell has receptors for the Fc component of IgG and for C3b) [94-96]. Such contact triggers the membrane and causes the generation of highly reactive oxygen radicals, such as superoxide, singlet oxygen, as well as hydrogen peroxide and hydroxyl ions. These ions may affect microorganisms even before they have been completely engulfed. Concomitantly, there is increased oxygen consumption resulting in increased production of hydrogen peroxide and a 5 to 10 fold increase in direct oxidation of glucose through the hexose monophosphate shunt. Interestingly, inhibition of oxidative phosphorylation does not impair phagocytosis. Indeed, the paucity of mitochondria in mature neutrophils suggests that respiration cannot play an important role. Moreover, the cell contains several cyanide insensitive oxidases (distinct from myeloperoxidase), NADPH oxidase, NADH oxidase and an amino acid oxidase which mediate the consumption of oxygen and cause the generation of the radicals mentioned above.

As illustrated in **Figures 33 a** and **b**, during phagocytosis much of the membrane is invaginated. However, it is not yet generally known that phagocytosis is accompanied by a considerable amount of exocytosis (**Fig. 33 b**).

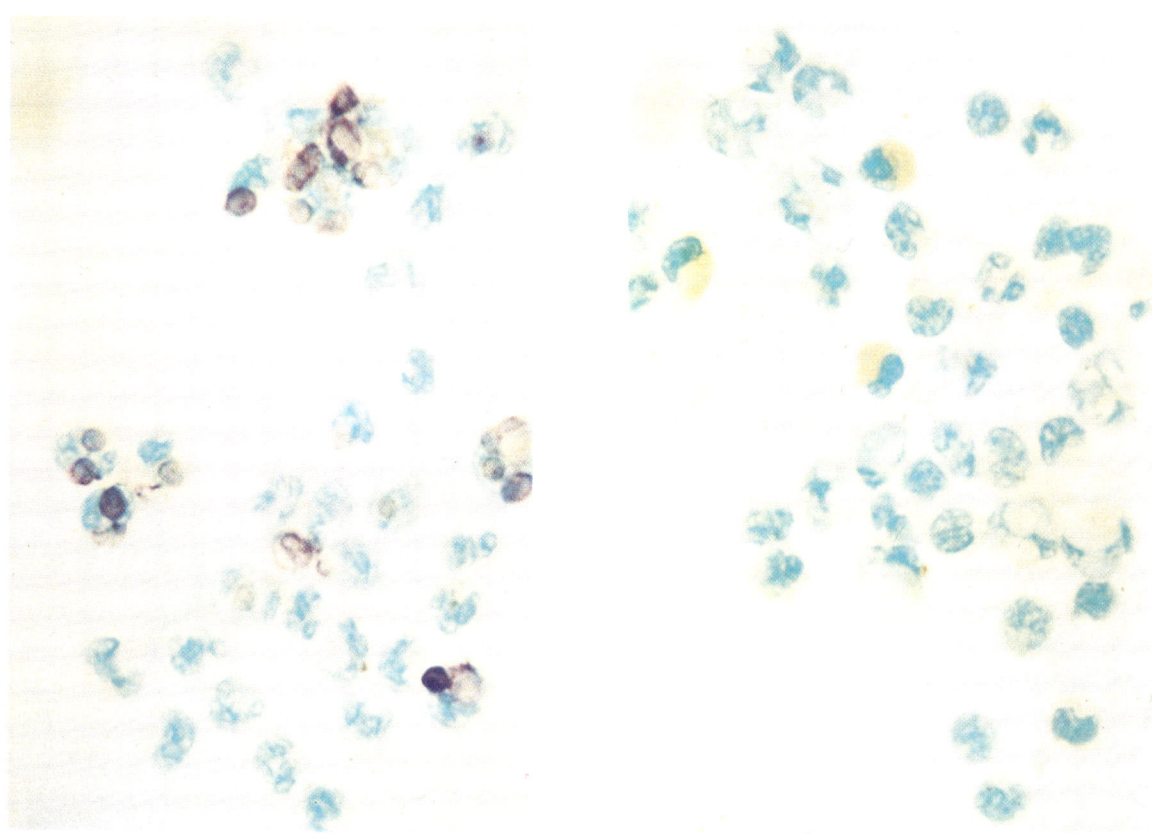

Fig. 45 *NBT test in chronic granulomatous disease (CGD). Activation of NBT reduction by phagocytosis of* Candida albicans *spores. Reduction occurs in 100% of phagocytosing neutrophils in normal controls (a) whereas no reduction is seen in CGD patients (b). Courtesy of Prof. W.H. Hitzig, Kinderspital, Zürich.*

In fact, phagocytosis appears to accelerate non-specific exocytosis [97]. This membrane recycling is associated with an increase in conversion of lysolecithin to lecithin [98]. Moreover, the cell appears to use endogenous triglycerides as a source of fatty acids which are probably reesterified and incorporated into newly formed membranes during periods of rapid membrane turnover [99]. Undoubtedly, cytoskeletal proteins play a role in phagocytosis and the so-called gelation and solation of the cytoplasm which accompanies the process [100-102]. The exact role of microtubules and microfilaments is still controversial, particularly since relevant theories of their function have been based largely on indirect evidence derived from experiments conducted with colchicine and cytochalasin B [103]. These agents affect microtubules and microfilaments respectively but are likely to have also other effects which have remained largely unexplored.

The bactericidal activity of neutrophils has been investigated in many laboratories and is relatively well understood. In essence, the mechanisms whereby PMN's kill bacteria may be either oxygen related and enhanced by the cells' endogenous myeloperoxidase in the presence of an oxidizable cofactor such as a halide [104, 105] or they are associated with lysosomal enzymes.

In addition to the cell's hydrolytic enzymes, lysozyme (muraminidase) may hydrolyze bacterial cell wall mucopolysaccharides, and lactoferrin may deprive microorganisms of iron. To test for the generation of oxygen radicals which should occur during phagocytosis, the dye Nitro-blue tetrazolium (NBT) or chemiluminescence are used [106, 107] (**Fig. 45**). Reduction of Nitro-blue tetrazolium by free oxygen radicals results in a blue-black formazan precipitate [107-109]. The NBT test is useful in the diagnosis of occult infections, or in detecting bactericidal impairment (see p. 196).

Part 2 NEUTROPHIL PATHOLOGY

1. ABNORMALITIES OF THE NUCLEUS

Most nuclear abnormalities are related to nuclear immaturity accompanying reactive hyperplasia or neoplasia of the myeloid system. However, in the secondary (reactive) leukocytoses, cells less differentiated than promyelocytes are usually not found in peripheral blood and the morphology of the immature cells is normal. As a rule, the nuclei of leukemic neutrophils exhibit larger and/or more numerous nucleoli and other bizarre changes such as inclusions, blebs, or filamentous structures. The most common congenital condition involving the neutrophil nucleus is the Pelger-Huët anomaly (**Fig. 46 a**). This was first described as a congenital, non sex-linked, dominant trait associated with round single nuclei in the homozygous state, both in man [110-112] and in rabbits [113], and with characteristic dumbbell-shaped nuclei in the much more frequent heterozygous state. The chromatin texture in these nuclei is characteristically coarse, indicative of the maturity of the cells.

Since such neutrophils are functionally normal, the importance of their recognition lies in the avoidance of unnecessary diagnostic tests often inflicted on individuals who have this anomaly.

The acquired, or pseudo Pelger-Huët anomaly (see **Figs. 46 b, c, d**) may be seen in the preleukemic syndrome, in acute leukemia or other hemopoietic dysplasias when it is often associated with a lack of secondary granules [114-116].

Hypersegmentation of the nucleus also exists in a hereditary form [117]. However, it is much more common as an acquired characteristic which is most frequently associated with megaloblastic anemias caused by folate or vitamin B_{12} deficiency [118]. In fact, the mean nuclear lobe count of neutrophils may be used as a diagnostic screening procedure [119]. Nuclei with 8 or even 10 lobes are sometimes seen (**Fig. 47**). Similar hypersegmentation of the nucleus may also occur during pregnancy or as a result of treatment with antimetabolites, particularly those which impair DNA synthesis. Nuclear hypersegmentation in the blood is usually accompanied by giant metamyelocytes in the marrow (**Fig. 48**). The biochemical steps involved in the transformation of giant metamyelocytes to hypersegmented neutrophils are not known. However, the notion that hypersegmented PMN's reflect cell age is no longer tenable [120].

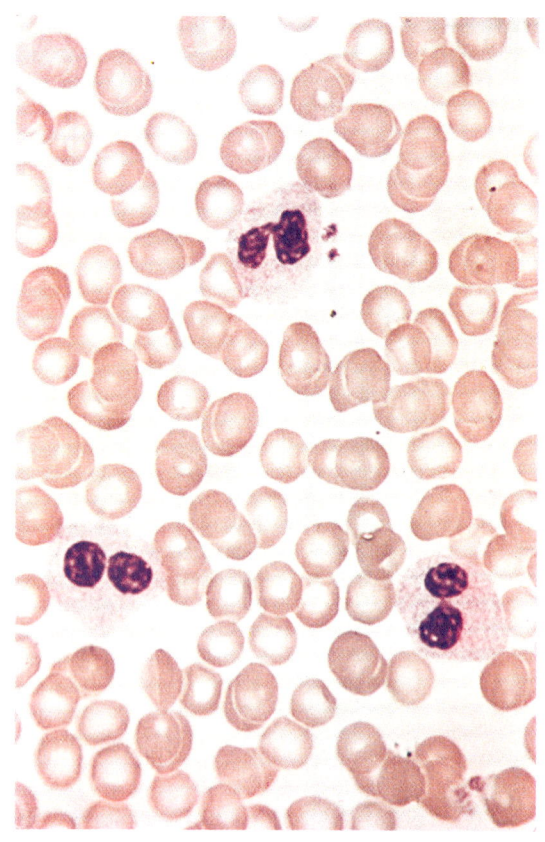
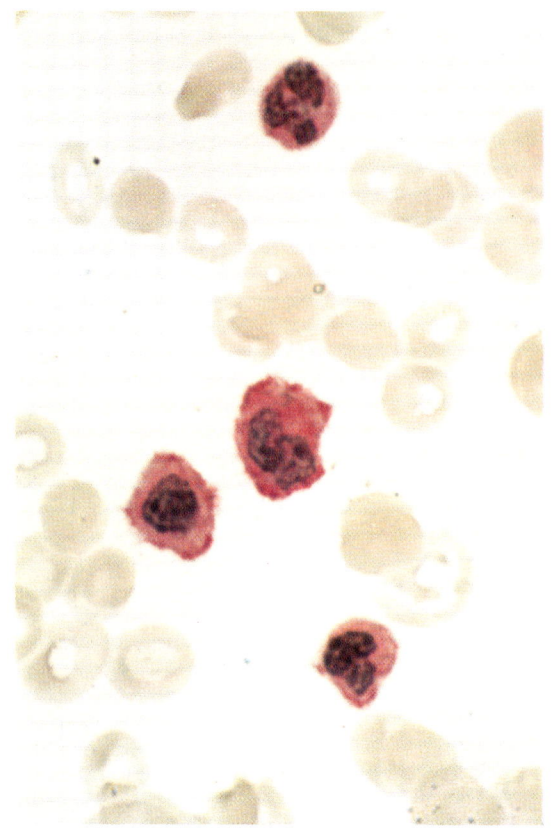
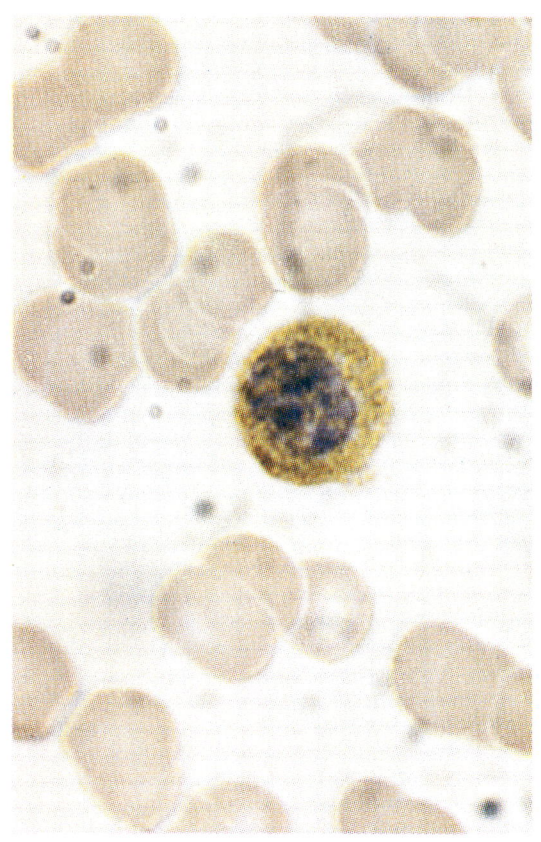
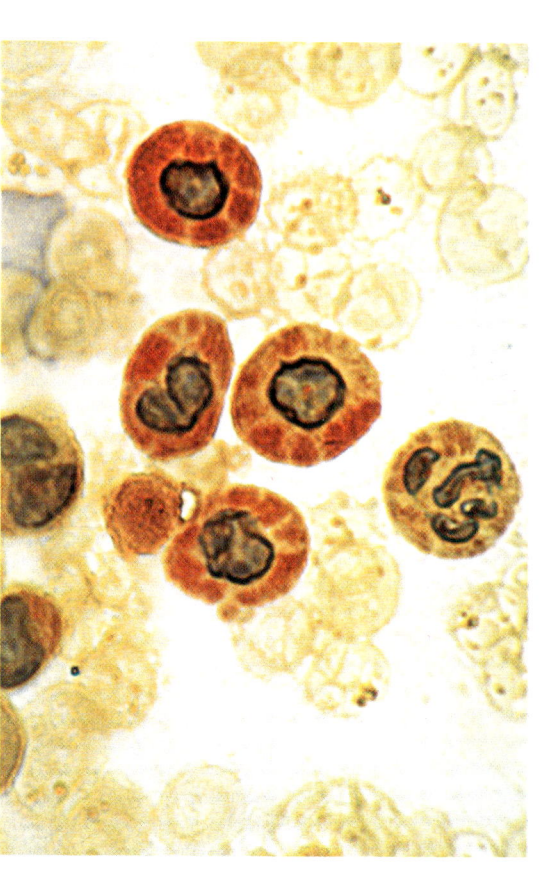

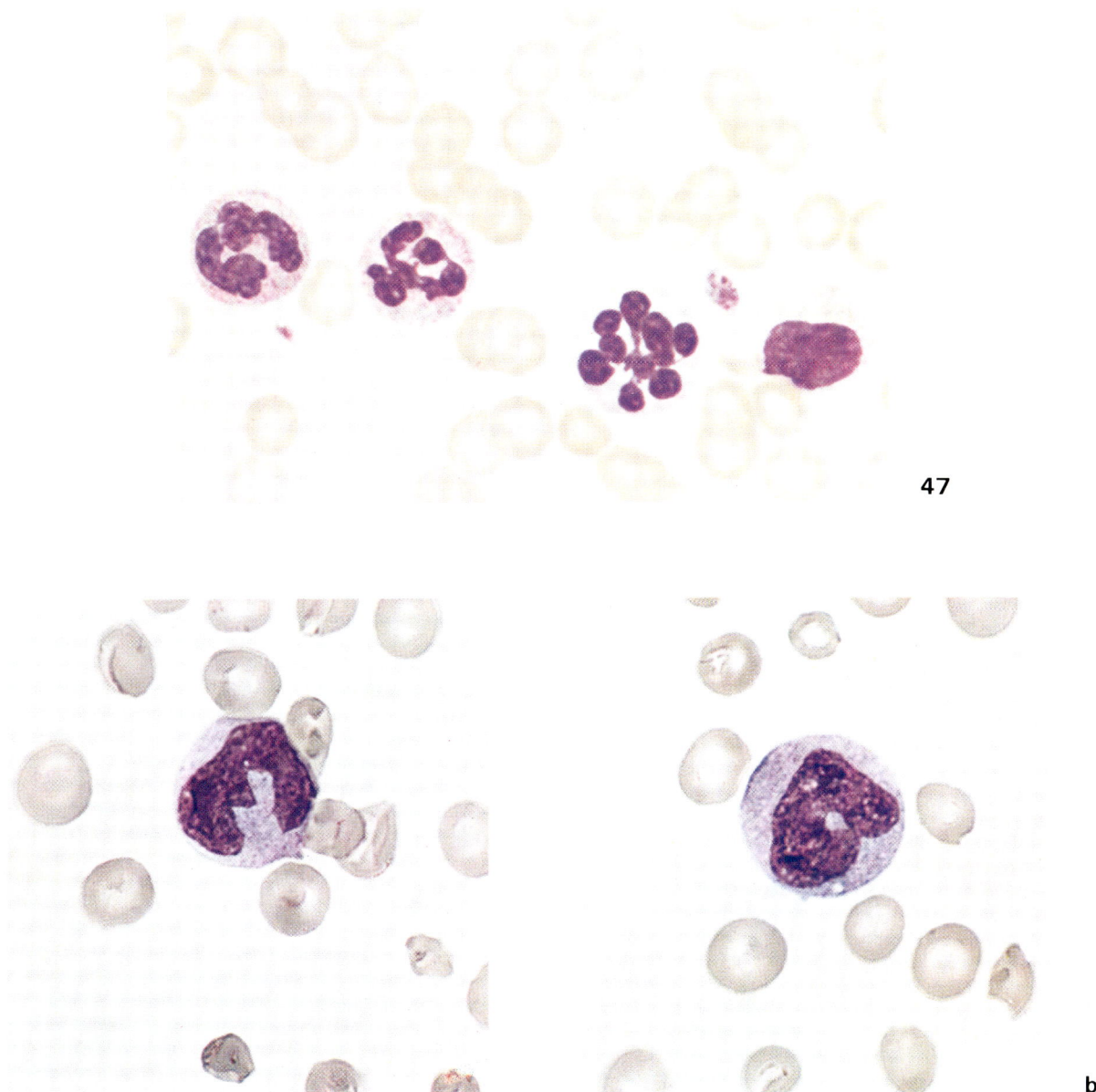

Fig. 47 Hypersegmented nuclei in neutrophils of a patient with folate deficiency.

Fig. 48 a, b) Giant metamyelocytes. This feature of neutrophil maturation is often seen together with the above illustrated nuclear hypersegmentation. Bone marrow of a patient with pernicious anemia (see Chapter 3).

Fig. 46 a) The Pelger-Huët anomaly. The main nuclear characteristics of this anomaly are described in the text.
b, c, d) Cytochemical features of the acquired or pseudo Pelger-Huët anomaly are normal.
b) PAS reaction; **c)** peroxidase reaction; **d)** β-aminopeptidase.
Courtesy of Dr. G.L. Castoldi, University of Ferrara.

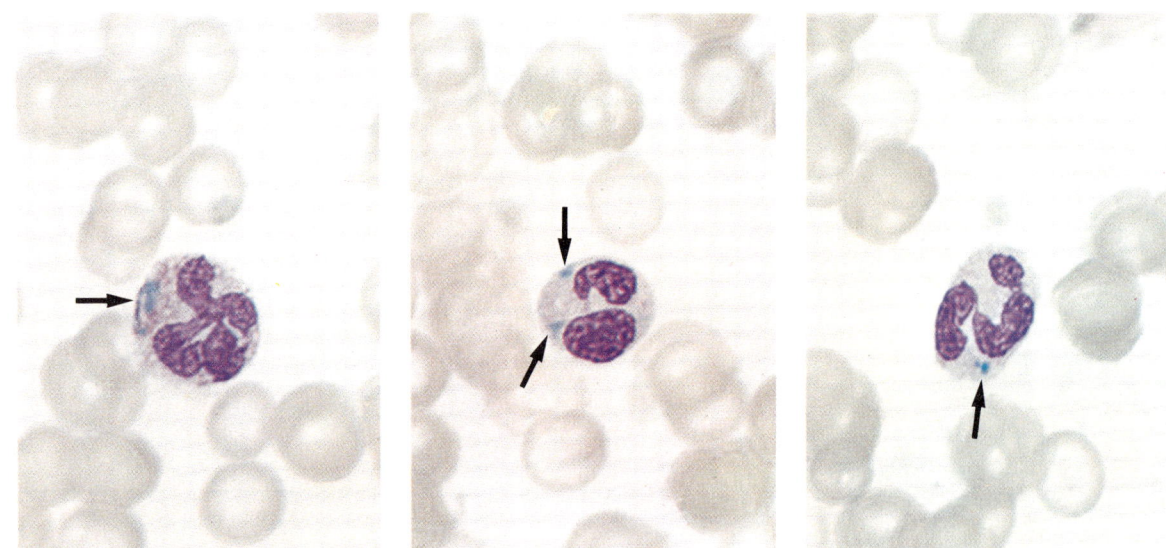

Fig. 49 a, b, c) Döhle bodies. a) A neutrophil showing "toxic" granulations as well as a Döhle body (**arrow**). Note that most of these blue staining inclusions are located peripherally. b) Neutrophil with a bilobed nucleus (pelgeroid) and two Döhle bodies (**arrows**). c) Normal appearing neutrophil with Döhle body (**arrow**). Compare with **Figure 50** which illustrates the ultrastructure of a Döhle body.
Courtesy of Dr. G.L. Castoldi, University of Ferrara.

2. CYTOPLASMIC ABNORMALITIES

Cytoplasmic alterations are much more common than nuclear aberrations. The vast majority are transient and consist of a variety of inclusions associated with "reactive" leukocytosis of infection or other inflammatory responses. The most common of these are toxic granulations and Döhle bodies [18, 121, 122]. Both reflect immaturity of the cytoplasm as a result of diminished number of cell divisions before the neutrophils are released into the circulation. Toxic granules [121] merely reflect the larger number of azurophilic (primary) granules that have not been diluted out by additional mitoses (see normal developmental series) (**Fig. 49 a**). Döhle bodies on the other hand are blue-staining inclusions (**Figs. 49 a-c**) which represent ribosomes or lamellae of rough endoplasmic reticulum [18, 122] (**Fig. 50**).

Very similar inclusions albeit larger and more numerous are seen in the May-Hegglin anomaly (**Fig. 51**), a rare, dominantly inherited disorder which may be associated with a bleeding diathesis because, in some cases, the platelets are also affected [123]. However, although on routine blood smears both Döhle bodies and May-Hegglin inclusions are basophilic and pyroninophilic reflecting their content of RNA, they are ultrastructurally distinguishable. The May-Hegglin inclusions possess particles and rod-like structures not seen in normal cells [124, 125].

2.1. Chediak-Higashi-Steinbrink anomaly

Also referred to as Chediak-Higashi or C-H syndrome, is a rare disorder inherited as an autosomal recessive trait (reviewed in ref. 126). Giant granules are seen in practically all leukocytes and platelets as well as their marrow precursors (**Figs. 52-55**). The affected patients have partial albinism, lymphadenopathy, hepatosplenomegaly, neuropathies, photophobia and susceptibility to infection. Although the disease is extremely rare, in recent years C-H cells have attracted much interest because of their impaired chemotaxis, degranulation and bactericidal activity [127, 128]. Animal models of the syndrome also exist, e.g. in Aleutian mink [129, 130] and in the beige

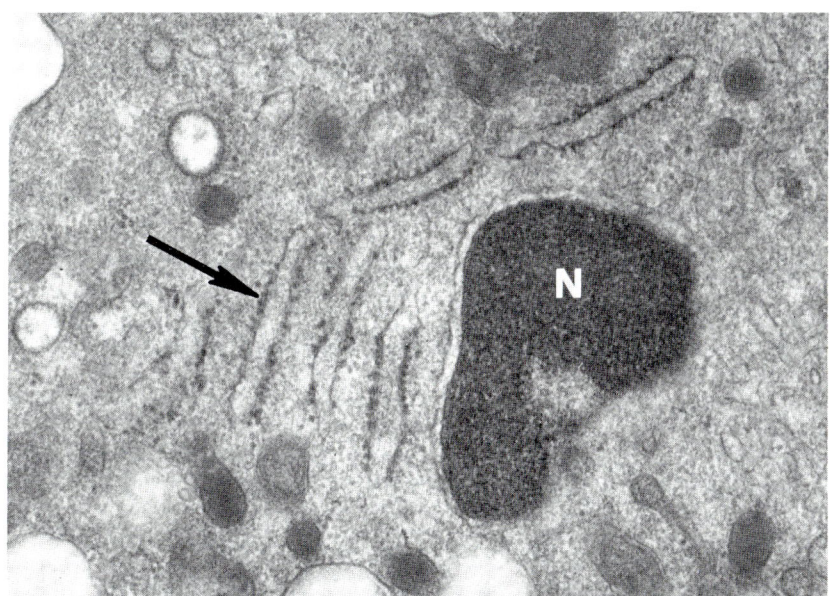

Fig. 50 Döhle body refers to the area occupied by lamellae of rough ER (**arrow**) located in the periphery of an otherwise mature neutrophil. Such areas appear as blue inclusions on light microscopy when stained with Romanovsky dyes (see **Fig. 49**). **N**, nucleus ($\times$ 58,000).

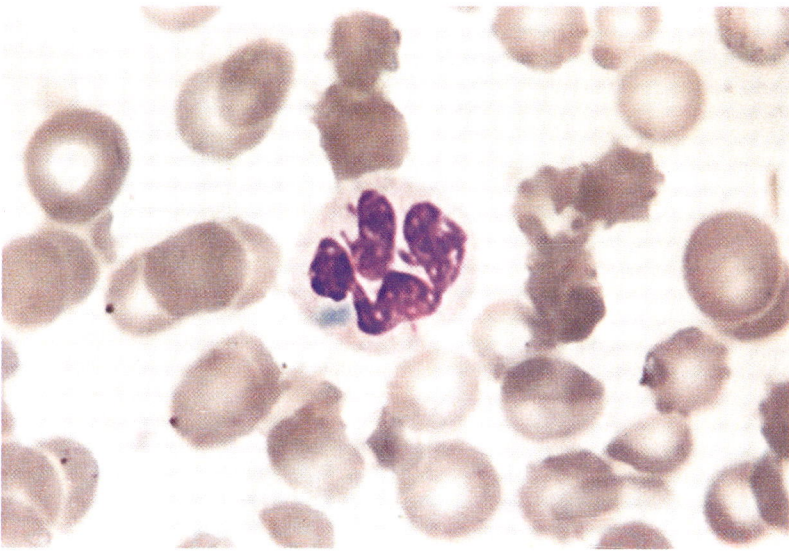

Fig. 51 May-Hegglin anomaly. A large basophilic inclusion is seen in the cytoplasm of this hypersegmented neutrophil.

mouse [131]. The giant inclusions consist of lysosomes that arise by fusion of small azurophilic primary granules in promyelocytes and myelocytes [132]. Similar giant granules are found in all tissues, e.g. the partial albinism is a result of abnormal melanocyte activation.

The neutrophils of the affected patients behave as though they were continuously in a hyperactive state. They ingest particles, release enzymes, and metabolize oxygen at a superactive rate. Yet, when incubated *in vitro*, the cells show delayed killing of microorganisms, probably because of poor fusion of the giant granules with phagocytic vacuoles [133-134]. Although it has been postulated that abnormal membrane activation and premature or "inappropriate" granule fusions are related events which may explain the multiplicity of cellular aberrations, a concept unifying these observations has yet to be delineated.

BLOOD CELLS

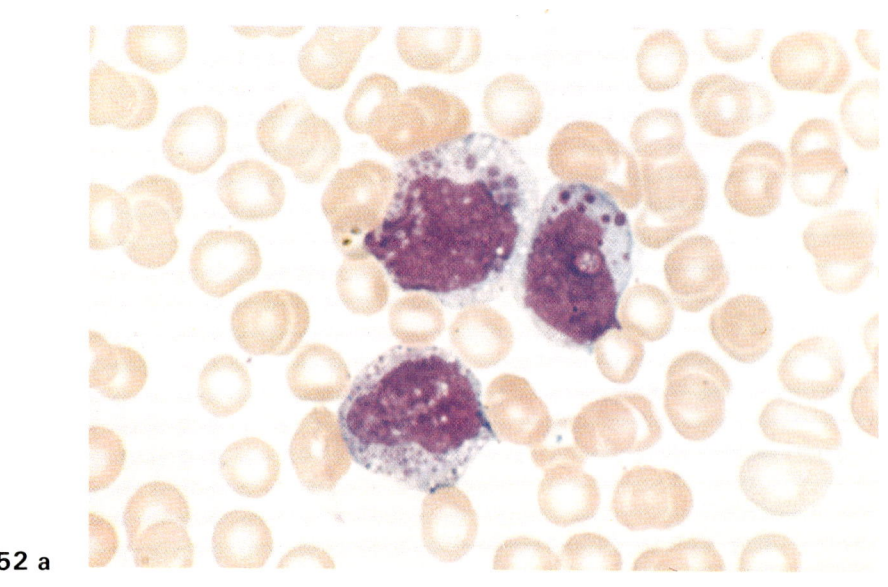

52 a

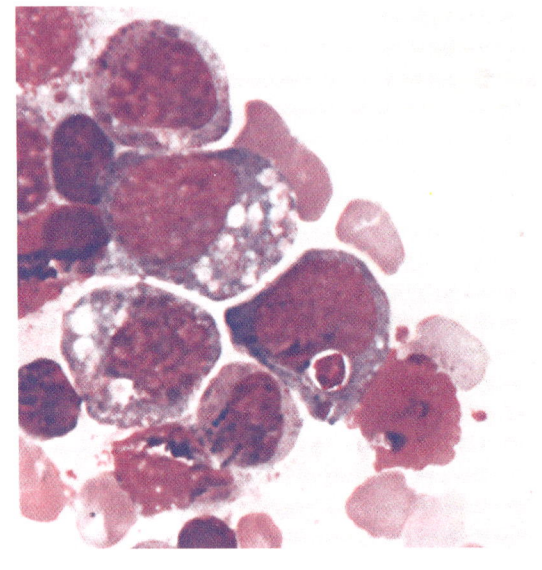
b

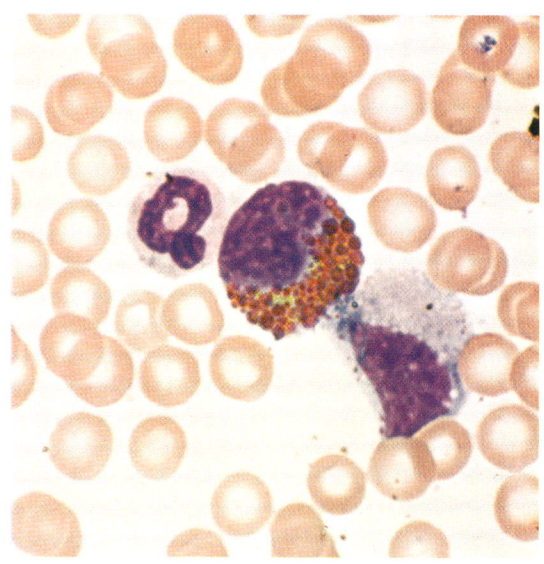
c

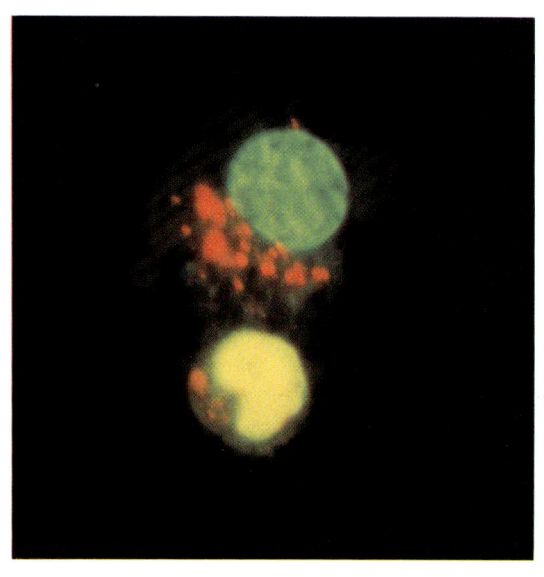
d

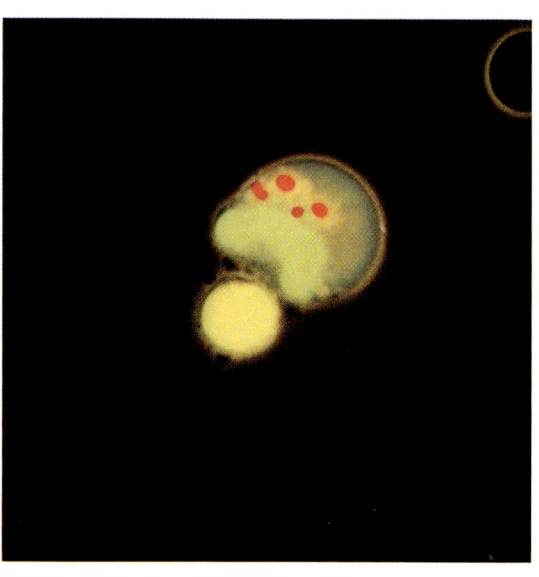
e

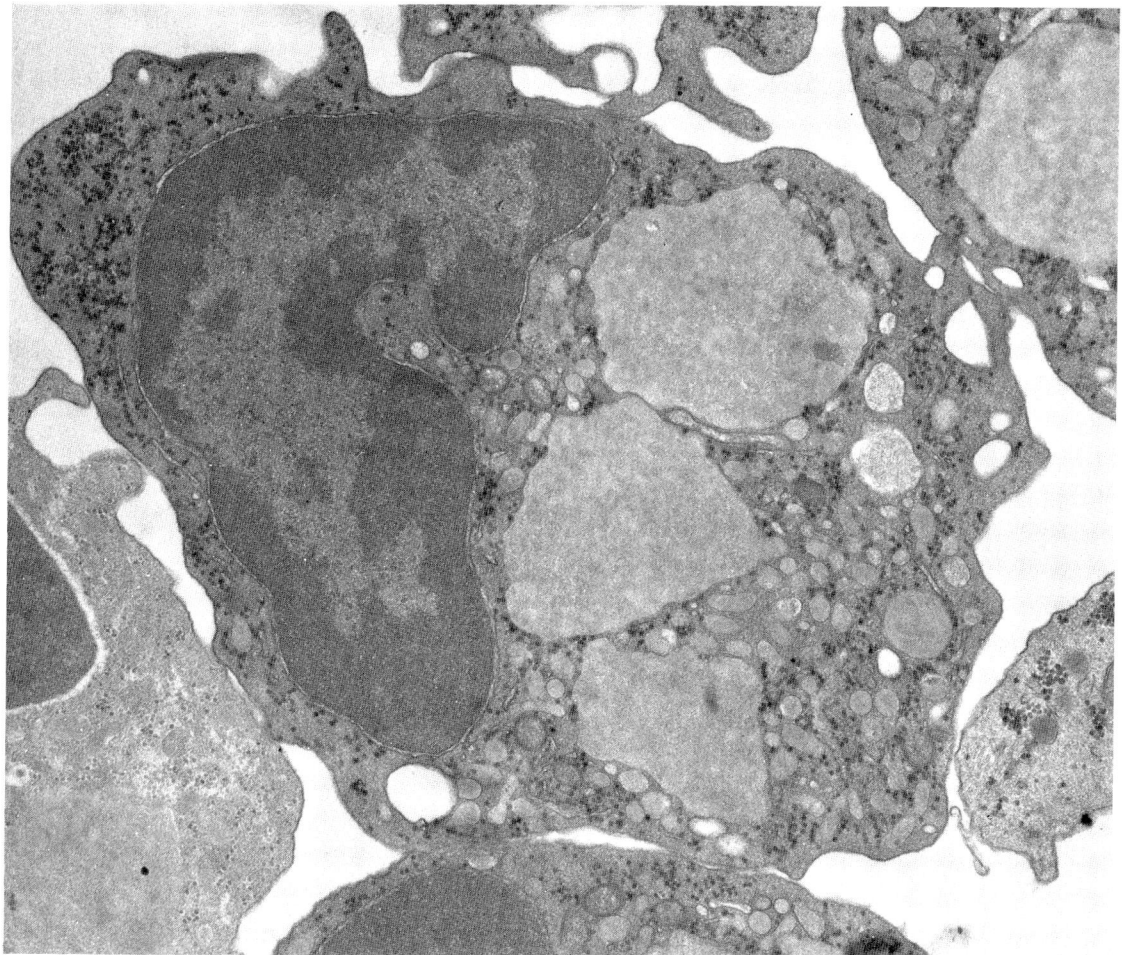

Fig. 53 Neutrophil from the blood of a patient with Chediak-Higashi syndrome shows giant inclusions as well as normal-sized granules. The inclusions contain acid phosphatase and myeloperoxidase (see **Figures 55 a** and **b**).
Courtesy of Dr. J.G. White, Department of Pediatrics, University of Minneapolis.

Fig. 52 Chediak-Higashi-Steinbrink anomaly.
a) Huge granules, probably brought about by fusion of primary lysosomes are seen in all granulated cells. These cells are not fully mature, representative of myelocytes or monocytes.
b) Bone marrow. Vacuolation probably due to loss of the large granules during preparation of specimen.
c) Eosinophil also affected by the same disease process.
d and **e)** Chediak-Higashi-Steinbrink cells stained with acridine orange. The lysosomal nature of the cytoplasmic granules is also suggested by their orange staining with this technique.
Courtesy of Dr. J.G. White, Department of Pediatrics, University of Minneapolis.

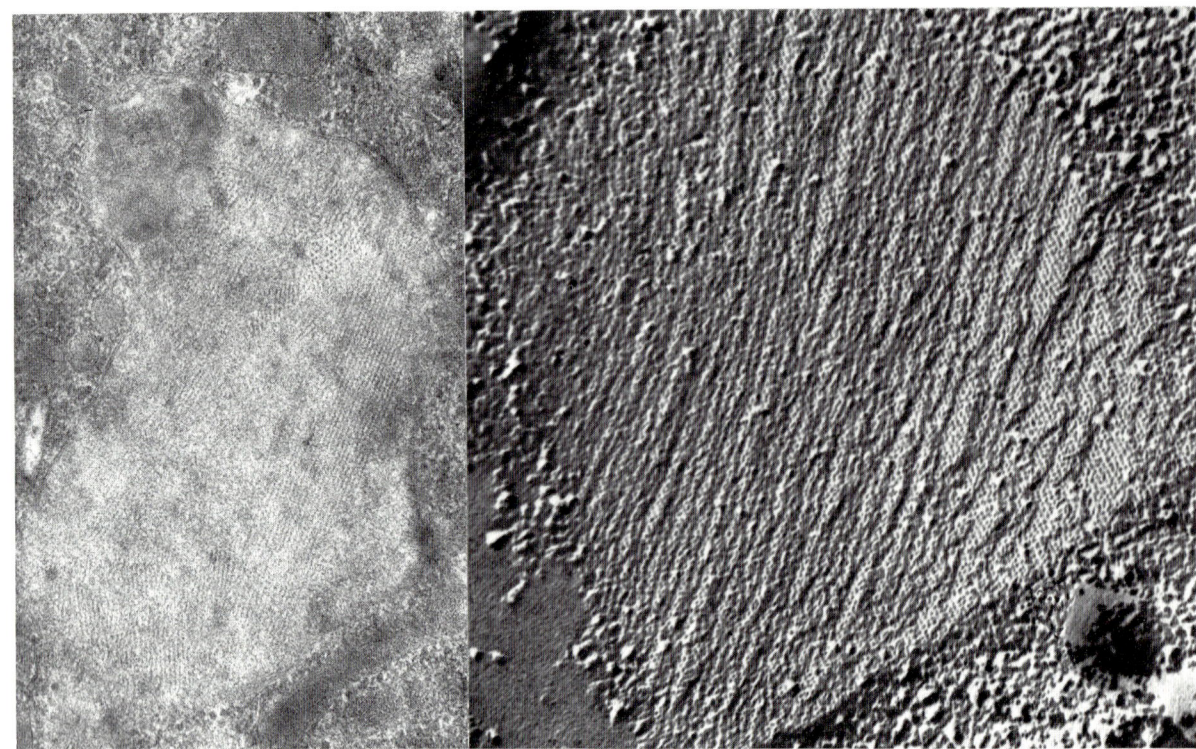

Fig. 54 a) Chediak-Higashi giant inclusion at higher resolution is seen to have a periodic structure (× 140,000).
b) Replica of a freeze-fractured Chediak-Higashi inclusion confirms the lamellated structure (× 140,000). Courtesy of Dr. J.G. White, Department of Pediatrics, University of Minneapolis.

Fig. 55 a) Chediak-Higashi neutrophil illustrating reaction product of myeloperoxidase in giant granules.
b) Chediak-Higashi neutrophil illustrating reaction product of acid phosphatase in a giant granule.
Courtesy of Dr. J.G. White, Department of Pediatrics, University of Minneapolis.

4 NEUTROPHILS

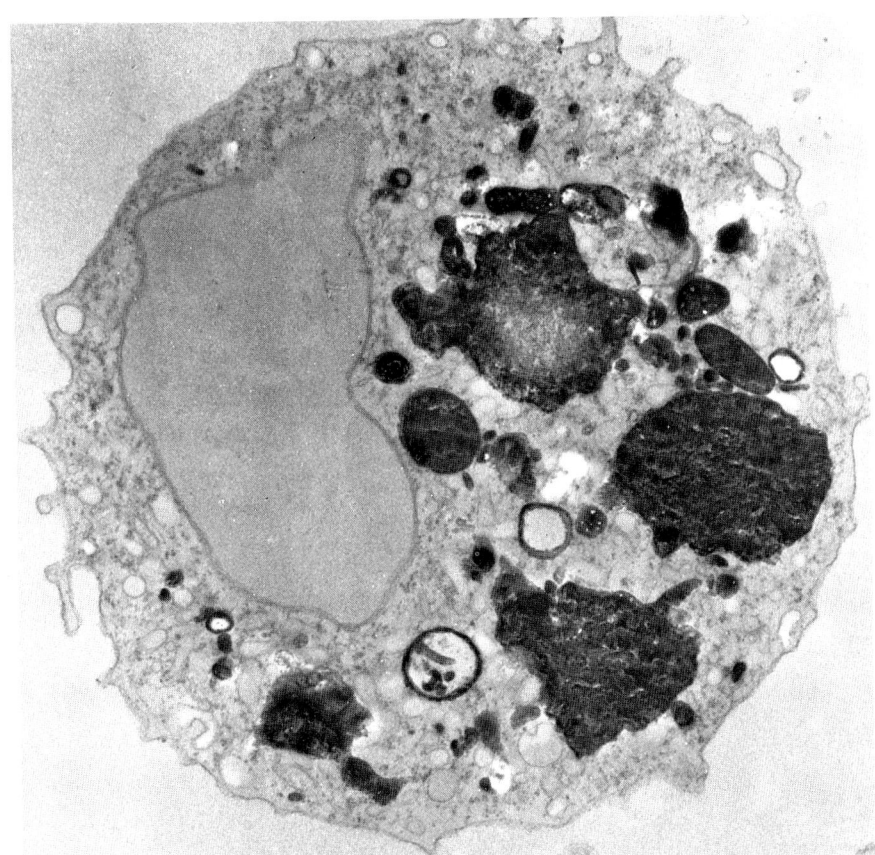

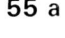

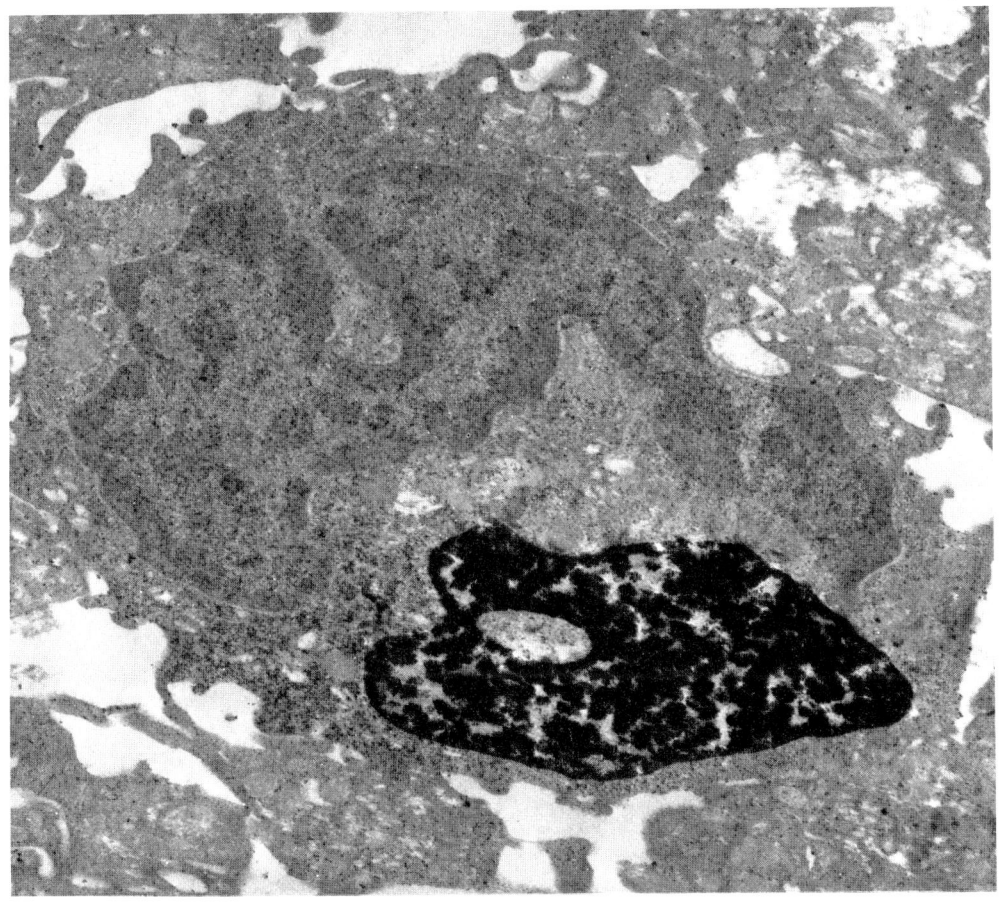

2.2. Alder-Reilly anomaly

Very large granules or inclusions are also seen in the neutrophils of patients with various abnormalities of polysaccharide metabolisms such as the Hürler-Pfaundler syndrome, Morquio's disease, familial amaurotic idiocy, and other genetic syndromes included in the "mucopolysaccharidoses" [135-137]. Inclusions are usually present in all leukocytes and depending on their biochemical makeup, take a variety of stains (**Figs. 56, 57**). Since the diseases are blatantly manifested clinically and the inclusions are seen in almost all tissues, the neutrophils *per se* have not been studied extensively.

2.3. Lipid inclusions

Neutrophils prepared from blood samples that have been stored, or from "stagnant" body fluids such as pleural effusions or synovial exudates [59] may exhibit lipid inclusions (**Figs. 58** and **59**). These have been analyzed and shown to consist predominantly of triglycerides [138]. It has also been observed that the number and size of the inclusions increase with time when blood is kept at room temperature or at 37 °C. Mechanisms that may be responsible for their formation are discussed in ref. 138.

3. DISORDERS AFFECTING NEUTROPHIL NUMBER

The multitude of clinical conditions that are accompanied by neutrophilia or neutropenia cannot be discussed within the frame of an atlas. They are considered in major hematology texts [139, 140]. The histochemical and tissue culture techniques used to distinguish some of the leukocytoses have been illustrated on pp. 28 and 163. Neutropenia is usually not an isolated finding, but associated with anemia and thrombocytopenia (see Chapter 5).

This statement even pertains to situations which may initially be dominated by agranulocytosis. The minimum number of neutrophils in healthy subjects is 1500-1600 per cmm [141]. Adequate defense against infections cannot be maintained with an absolute neutrophil count below 500 per cmm for more than a few days. Peripheral blood neutropenia may be associated with bone marrow hyperplasia as is the case in some patients with hypersplenism or other conditions which damage circulating neutrophils while leaving bone marrow precursors unaffected. However, the vast majority of drug-induced or autoimmune neutropenias involve mature and precursor cells alike. With rare exceptions, morphologic analysis offers no clue in regard to the etiology of the low neutrophil count.

Fig. 58 *Neutrophil prepared from the synovial fluid of a patient with rheumatoid arthritis. The cell contains at least 6 grey globules (arrows). On light microscopy, these may look like "toxic granules" or they may even become vacuolated depending on the fixative and stains used. It is now known that the inclusions consist of lipid (see text) ($\times$ 12,000).*
Reproduced from ref. 59 with permission of the publisher.

Fig. 59 *Neutrophil prepared from normal anticoagulated blood kept at room temperature for 48 hours shows two lipid inclusions (L). The number and size of such inclusions increase with time. The cells remain viable and are able to phagocytose particles (see text) ($\times$ 17,000).*
Reproduced from ref. 138 with permission of the publisher.

4 NEUTROPHILS

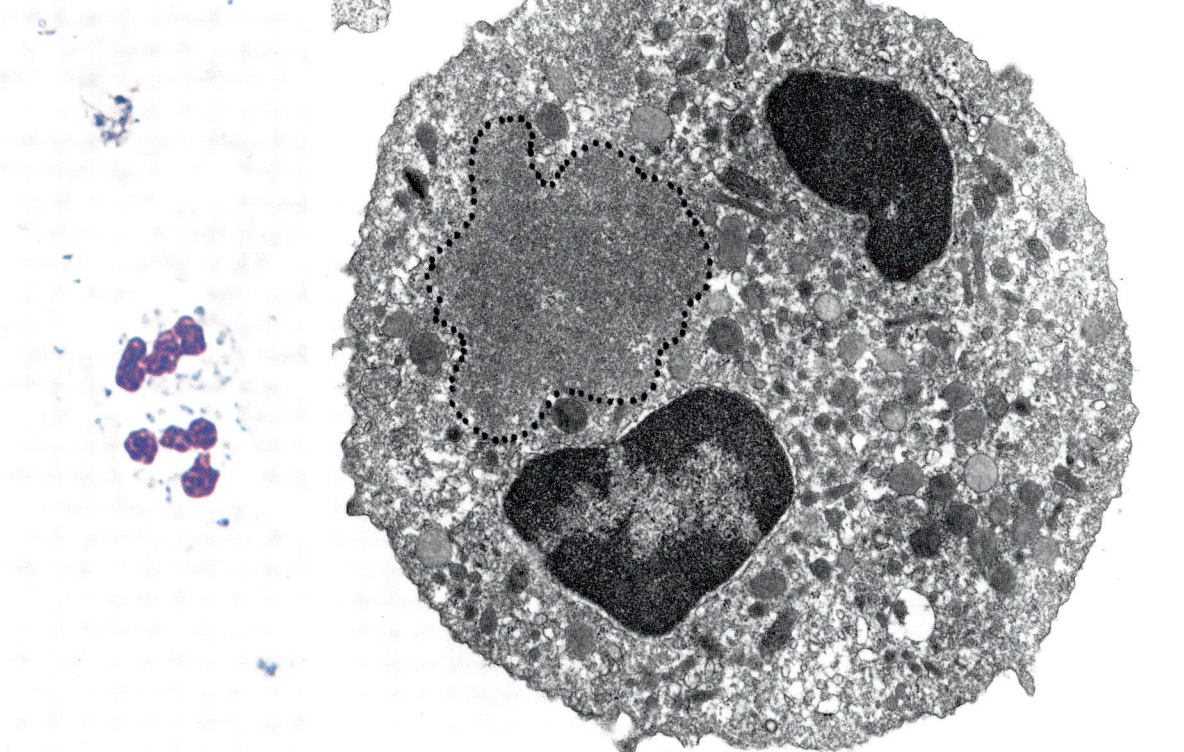

Fig. 56 Alder-Reilly anomaly. Two neutrophils showing large inclusions. These are seen in other cells as well (see text). Courtesy of Dr. G.L. Castoldi, University of Ferrara.

Fig. 57 Ultrastructure of a neutrophil taken from a specimen in which the cells had large basophilic inclusions on routine smears as occurs in the Alder-Reilly anomaly. The area delimited by the stippled line is devoid of granules. The patient was a neonate with hepatosplenomegaly and a poorly defined metabolic abnormality affecting polysaccharides ($\times$ 17,000). Reproduced from ref. 18 with permission of the publisher.

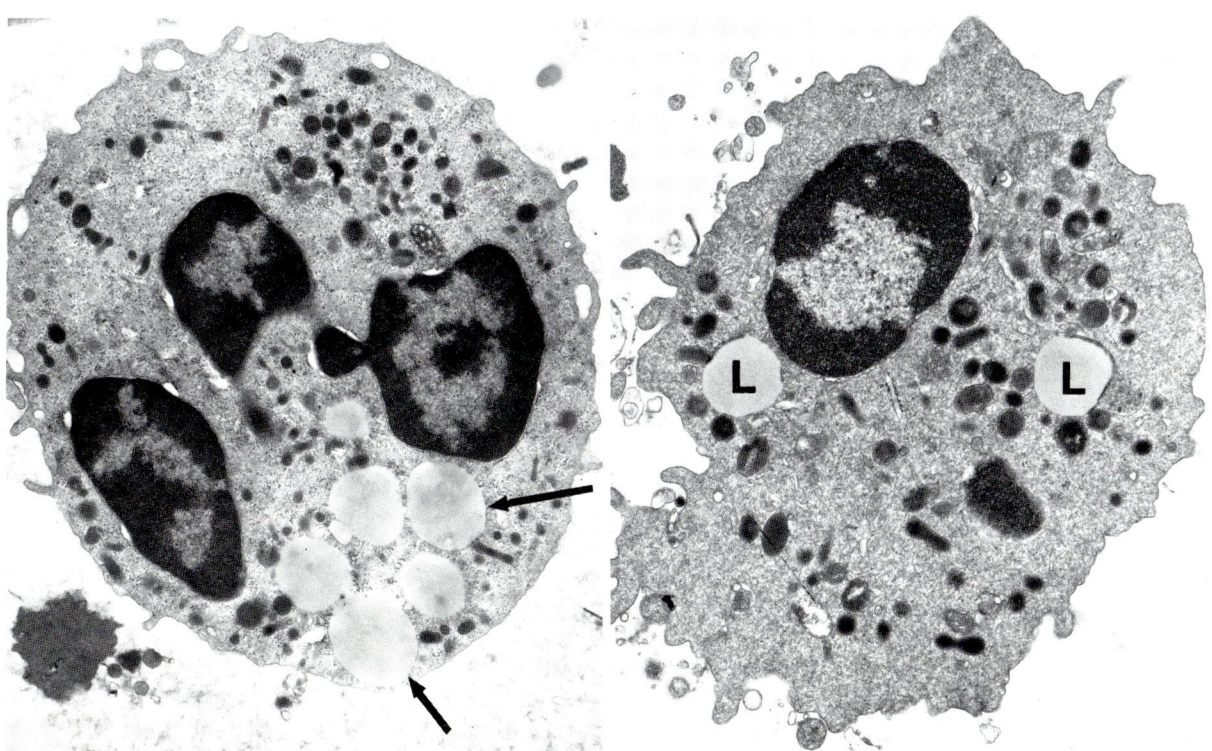

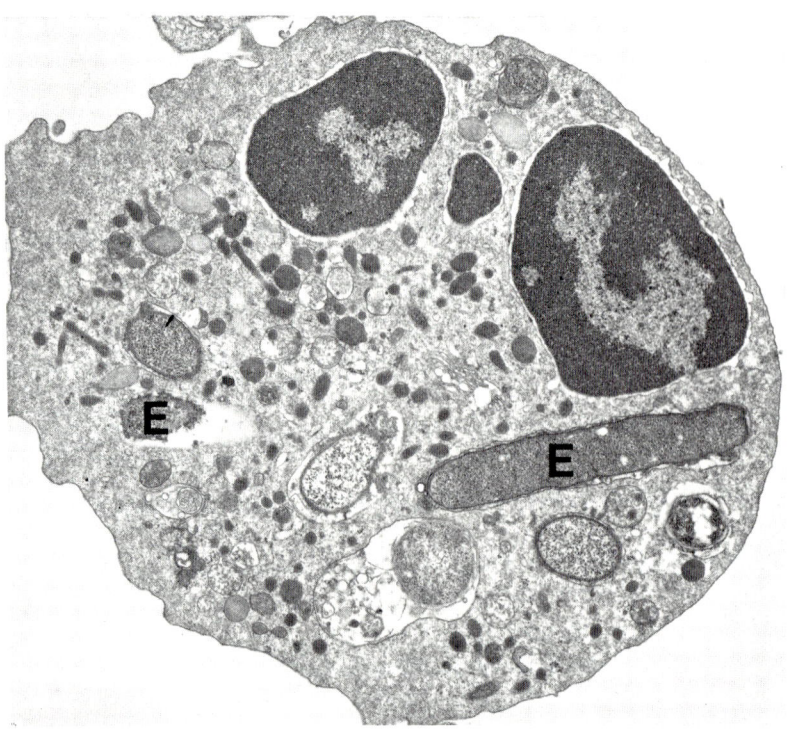

Fig. 60 Neutrophil from a buffy coat specimen that had been treated with the morphine analogue levorphanol before incubation with E. coli for the same length of time as the cell depicted in **Figure 35**. Although this cell was able to phagocytose the microorganisms (**E**), there is very little degranulation and viability studies revealed that the bacteria were not killed (compare with **Figure 35**) ($\times$ 12,000). Reproduced from ref. 146 with permission of the publisher.

4. DISORDERS OF NEUTROPHIL FUNCTION

Even though most disorders of neutrophil function also fail to be detectable by morphologic means, some of them have recently been shown to have structural correlates. This is particularly true when the defect is *intrinsic* to the cell. For instance, chronic granulomatous disease of childhood (CGD) is a genetic disorder in which the leukocytes ingest, but do not kill, catalase-positive microorganisms [142, 143]. Such neutrophils have a deficient oxidase enzyme system which is not activated when the cell membrane is stimulated as is the case in normal cells. The Nitro-blue tetrazolium test is negative (see p. 183). Because of their inability to generate hydrogen peroxide, the cells cannot overcome the catalase activity associated with many aerobic microorganisms, e.g. *Staphylococcus aureus*, most Gram-negative enteric bacteria and some fungi. As a consequence, such organisms multipy within phagocytic vacuoles and may be transported to other sites where new foci of infection are initiated. Microorganisms which do not possess catalase such as pneumococci and streptococci are readily killed by CGD neutrophils [142]. In addition to bacteria-laden neutrophils, the histiocytes at sites of infection as well as those in lymph nodes and the enlarged spleens of these patients may exhibit a gold pigment believed to be derived from phagocytosed material.

The functional impairment of CGD neutrophils, i.e., their failure to generate oxygen radicals or to kill bacteria can be mimicked to some extent *in vitro* by exposing normal neutrophils to drugs that affect membranes (**Fig. 60**) [145, 146]. The postulate that the CGD anomaly involves the membranes of the cells is supported by the observation that some male patients with CGD lack Kx

4 NEUTROPHILS

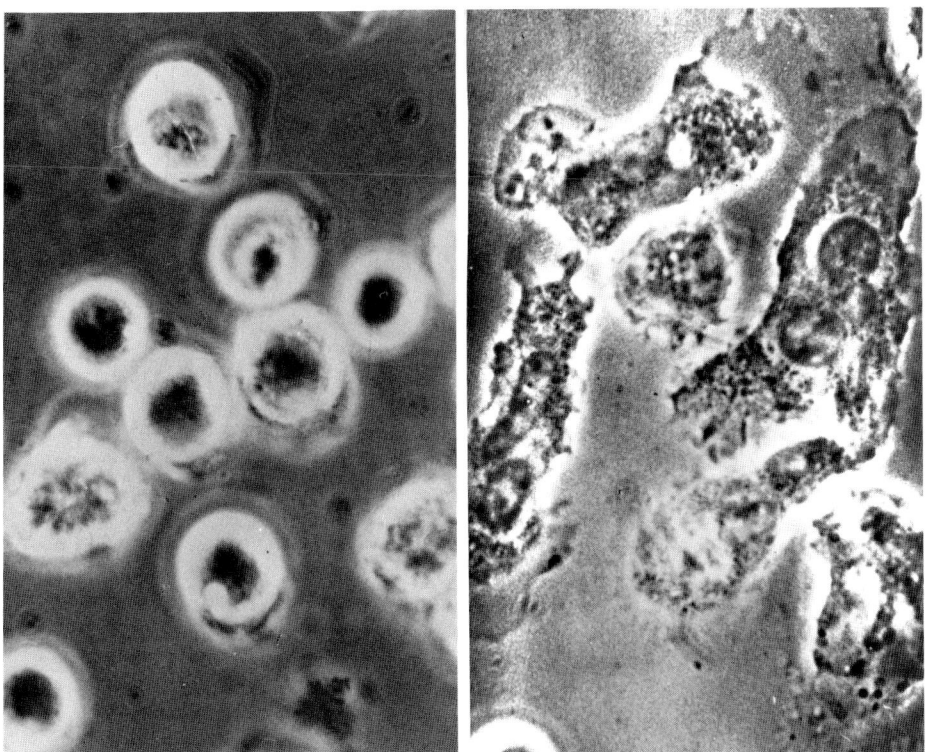

Fig. 61 Abnormal neutrophil adhesion. Failure of neutrophils to anchor to a substratum is seen on the left. The patient's neutrophils remained spherical whereas the normal neutrophils (seen on the right) have spread out and adhered to the substrate.
Courtesy of Dr. Bernard Babior, Tufts-New England Medical Center, Boston, and reproduced with permission of the publisher from ref. 148.

on their erythrocytes and leukocytes, an antigen related to the Kell blood group system. As a consequence, such CGD neutrophils are remarkably susceptible to sensitization with Kell antigens [147].

Defects in cytoskeletal proteins which can also be visualized ultrastructurally will undoubtedly be described in the near future. A patient with recurrent infections whose neutrophils had impaired locomotion, chemotaxis and phagocytosis despite normal oxygen production, granule enzymes, and metabolic parameters proved to have a defect in actin polymerization [101]. As discussed before, the assembly of cytoskeletal proteins into their filamentous form appears to be necessary for normal pseudopod formation and locomotion.

A protein which may be essential for neutrophil adhesion has also been identified. This protein was found lacking in the neutrophils of a patient who had a lifelong history of severe pyogenic infections [148]. Whereas normal PMN's spread on glass, the patient's cells remain spherical and do not attach to any substrate (**Fig. 61**).

In addition to defects intrinsic in neutrophils, abnormal neutrophil responses are seen in many systemic illnesses (e.g. uremia, immunodeficiency diseases, multiple myeloma, rheumatoid arthritis, SLE, hepatic cirrhosis, burns, and diabetes mellitus). A review of these dysfunctions is found in ref. 149.
In most of these instances, the inhibition of one or more neutrophil functions is caused by factors extrinsic to the cell. Occasionally normal function may be restored when the cells are removed from the noxious environment and resuspended in normal plasma.

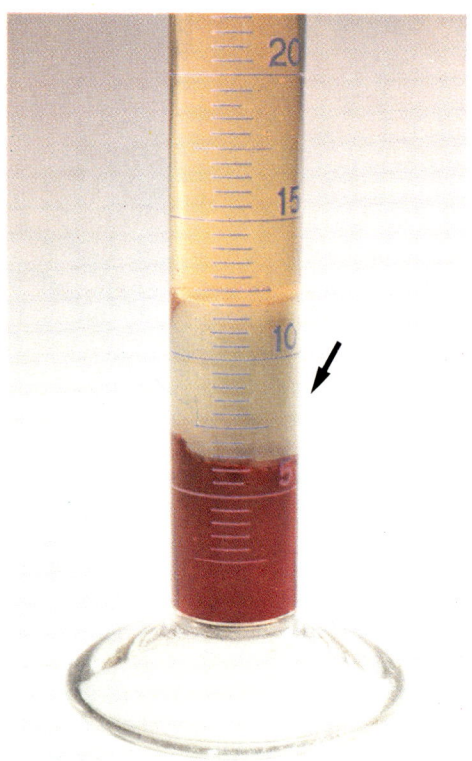
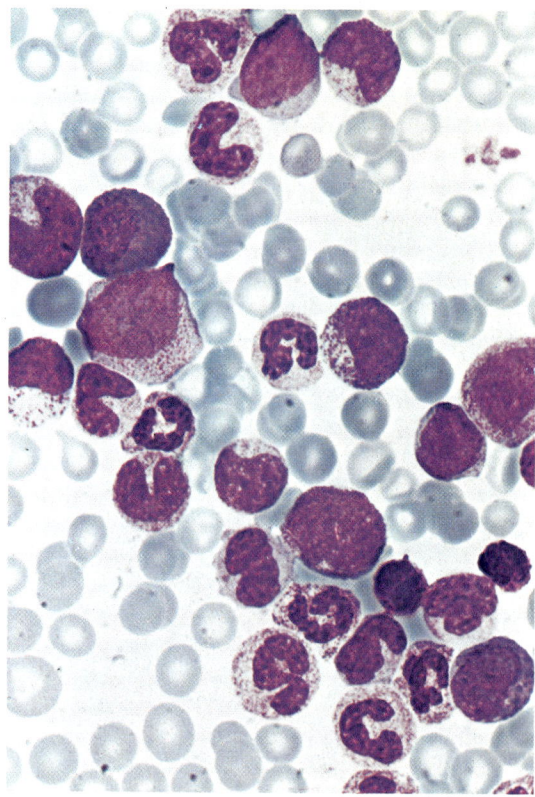

Fig. 62 Illustration of the huge "buffy coat" (**arrow**) which forms when anticoagulated blood of a patient with CML is allowed to stand for a short time.

Fig. 63 Chronic myelogenous leukemia (CML), peripheral blood. All stages of maturation, from the agranular basophilic myeloblast to the mature neutrophil are represented.

5. CHRONIC MYELOGENOUS LEUKEMIA

Chronic myelogenous leukemia (CML) is a hematologic neoplasm characterized by a huge expansion of the total granulocyte mass, including its precursors, while maturation remains more or less orderly (**Figs. 62-64**). In the majority of patients, karyotypic analysis reveals a stable chromosome aberration, the Philadelphia chromosome (Ph^1) [150] in both adult and childhood CML. Ph^1 positive and negative subtypes have been recognized in both age groups [151-154]. That Ph^1 positive CML is the most common variant of the disease became even more obvious when double translocations were uncovered following the introduction of banding techniques (see Chapter 11). Ph^1 positivity is associated with a better prognosis, especially in conjunction with female sex [155]. Karyotypic studies in constitutional mosaics [156, 157], chromosome 22 satellite studies in parents and propositi [158] and G-6-PD isoenzyme studies in female heterozygotes [159, 160] have all proven that CML is a monoclonal disease [161-165]. Cultured marrow fibroblasts have generally been found to be Ph^1 negative [160, 166] and to display a double enzyme phenotype [160]. However, a correlation between leukemia associated antigens and the Philadelphia chromosome in fibroblast-like cells derived from marrow has also been reported [167]. The Philadelphia chromosome positive stem cell clone possesses three noteworthy features: (1) it has a slight proliferative advantage and by the time of diagnosis has usually almost completely replaced normal hematopoiesis [168]; (2) it gives rise to erythroid, monocyte-macrophage, and thrombocyte lineages, even though, as a rule, excessive proliferation is restricted to the granulocytic series; and (3) it appears to be susceptible to cytogenetic instability which becomes evident during the terminal phases of the disease [169]. Thus, CML is best conceived as a monoclonal stem cell neoplasm, initially of low malignancy and maintaining orderly maturation, and in which the clinical onset of disease is preceded by a specific cytogenetic alteration. Although suppression of the Ph^1 positive clone may be achieved temporarily

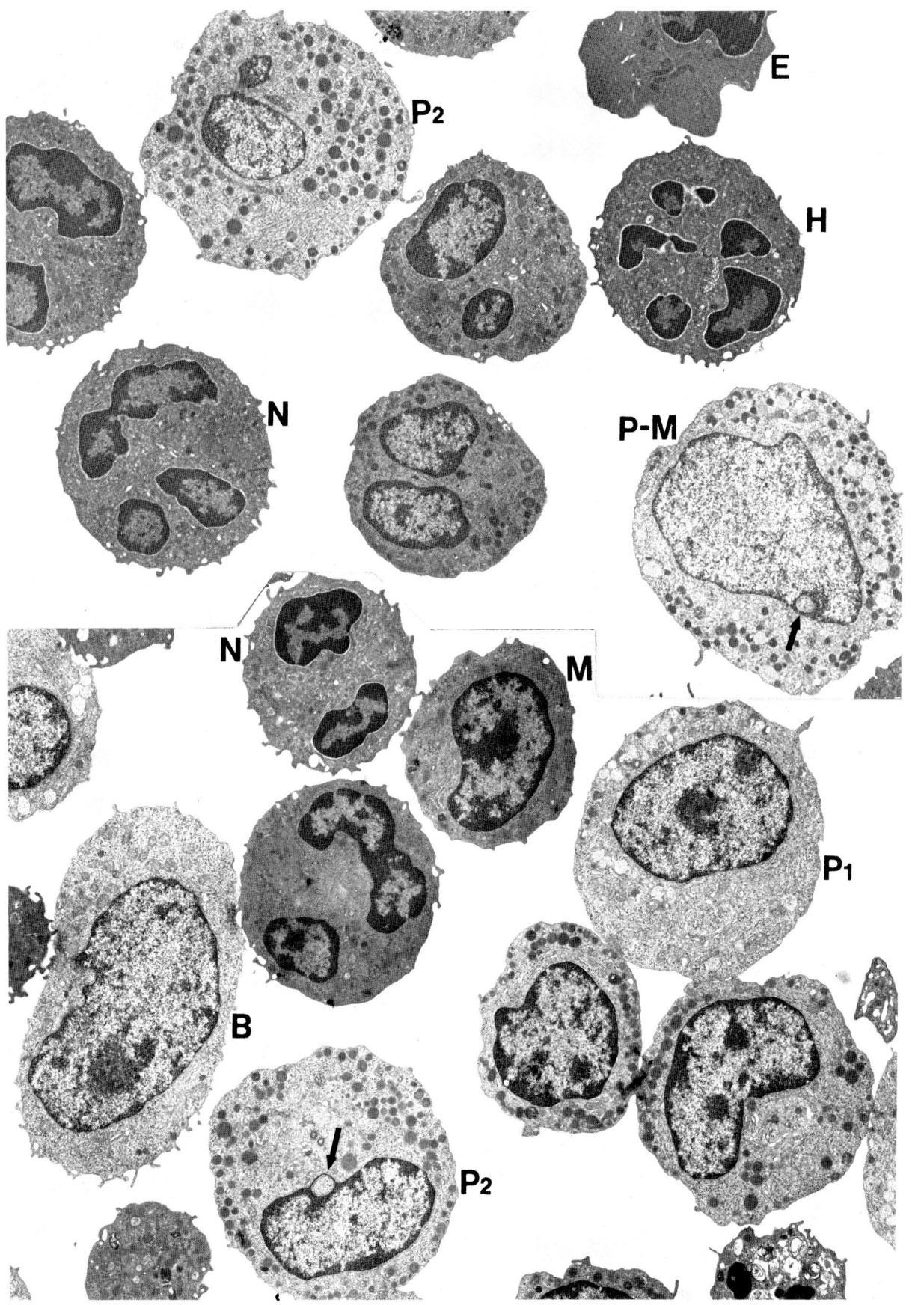

Fig. 64 Survey electron micrograph of the peripheral blood of a patient with Ph¹ positive CML. The entire maturation series is represented. **B**, myeloblast; **P 1**, early promyelocyte; **P 2**, late promyelocyte; **P-M**, a cell with dispersed chromatin and a nuclear bleb **(arrow)**, but a full complement of granules like a myelocyte; **M**, probably a metamyelocyte; **N**, mature PMN; **H**, probably a hypersegmented PMN; **E**, erythroblast. Also note that some of the nuclei exhibit "blebs" **(arrows)** ($\times$ 10,000).

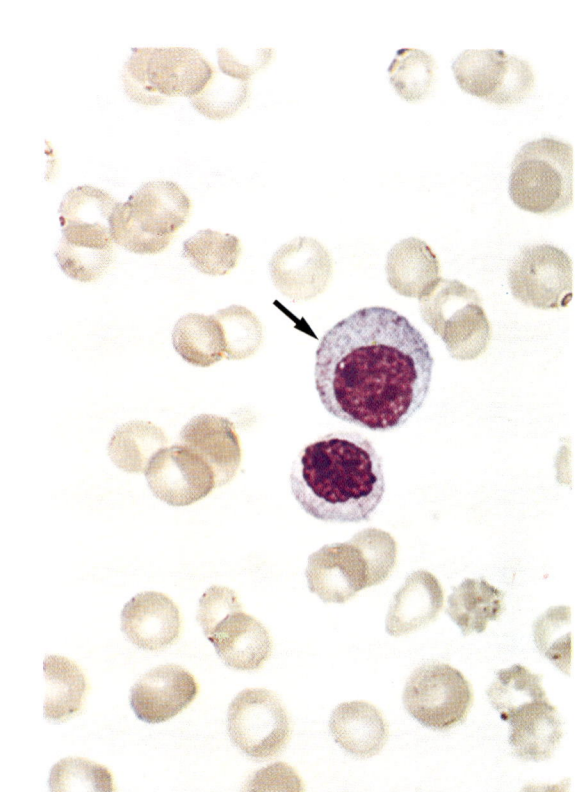

Fig. 65 a, b) *"Pelgeroid" changes seen in granulocytes of a patient with CML. Although the cytoplasm is granulated (**arrows**), the nuclei fail to become segmented.*

[170-175], actual eradication of the disease has only been accomplished after superlethal chemotherapy and/or radiotherapy followed by syngeneic bone marrow transplantation [176]. The failure to detect residual normal committed stem cells *in vitro* as determined by G-6-PD isoenzyme studies has suggested that leukemogenesis is a multistep process [177]. On the other hand, again with the help of G-6-PD markers, it has also been shown that Ph^1 negative cells arose from non-clonal, presumably normal cells, of a patient treated with intensive chemotherapy [178].

5.1. Blood and bone marrow morphology

Typical of the disease is the finding of a continuous spectrum of myeloid precursors as well as mature cells in the circulating blood (**Figs. 63, 64**).

The proportion of myeloblasts and early promyelocytes increases with augmentation of the total granulocyte mass. All myeloid cells are morphologically normal, so that a smear obtained from a patient with CML may show the whole series of granulocytopoiesis (**Figs. 63, 64**).

The frequency of each stage is proportional to its degree of maturity with the exception of metamyelocytes, which are less frequent than myelocytes. A double peaked histogram (myelocytes plus polymorphonuclears) is felt to be diagnostic of CML [179]. The appearance of Pelger-like nuclear changes (**Figs. 65 a, b**) must be regarded with suspicion because they generally herald a more aggressive phase of the disease. Erythroid alterations, such as the presence of erythroblasts, anisopoikilocytosis, basophilic stippling and dacriocytes strongly indicate myelofibrosis (see p. 252). A certain degree of eosinophilia and basophilia is usually seen (see Chapter 6, p. 282 and Chapter 7, p. 307).

The most typical cytochemical alteration in CML is the absence, or near absence, of neutrophil alkaline phosphatase (LAP) activity [180-182], which has become

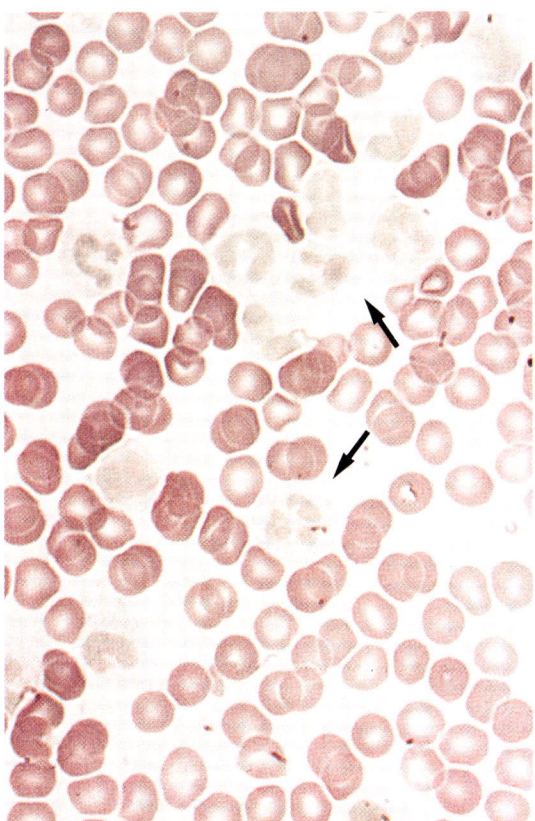
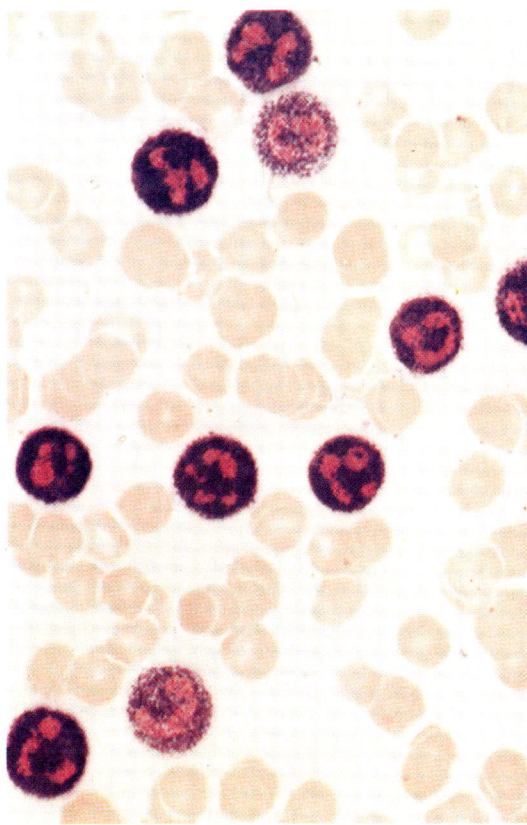

Fig. 66 *Negative reaction for alkaline phosphatase in patient with CML (**a**). **Arrows** indicate neutrophils which did not stain cytochemically, as contrasted with the neutrophils seen in **b** which were obtained from a patient with polycythemia vera (see text).*

an important diagnostic criterion especially in the early stages of the disease (**Figg. 66 a, b**). LAP is contained in the secondary specific granules. Its disappearance in CML is not related to the absence of specific granules which have been often observed to be present in LAP negative cases [183-185]. It is possible that the enzyme is present in a latent form [186]. Activation of such a latent enzyme is probably the explanation for the observation that a transfusion of LAP negative CML cells into an infected neutropenic recipient caused the cells to become LAP positive [187].

Initially, CML bone marrow is markedly hyperplastic (**Figs. 67 a-c**) but in the course of the disease the marrow may show secondary myelofibrosis. The most prevalent cell in untreated marrow is the myelocyte (**Figs. 67 a-e**), which also shows the greatest number of mitoses. Positive histochemical reactions obtained in CML are illustrated in **Figures 68 a-e**. As a rule, some unusual cells are encountered in the marrow of patients with CML. Among these is a storage cell with a bluish, ground-glass, wrinkled cytoplasm, practically indistinguishable from Gaucher cells by conventional staining techniques and light microscopy (**Fig. 69 a**) [188]. By polarization microscopy the anisotropic, birefringent properties of ingested cerebrosides are striking (**Fig. 69 c**). While in Gaucher's disease there is a primary deficiency of β-glucocerebrosidase, making the cells unable to break down membrane lipid derived from ingested effete erythrocytes (see p. 336), in CML the accumulation of the cerebrosides may reflect inadequate enzyme reserves in the face of a vastly increased intramedullary cell turnover [189]. This interpretation is supported by a similar finding in thalassemia and some dyserythropoietic anemias [190, 191]. Another unusual cell is the so-called blue macrophage which is a macrophage that has phagocytosed the nuclei of effete granulocytes (**Fig. 70**). This cell is not to be confused with the sea-blue histiocyte (see Chapter 8, p. 339) [192, 193].

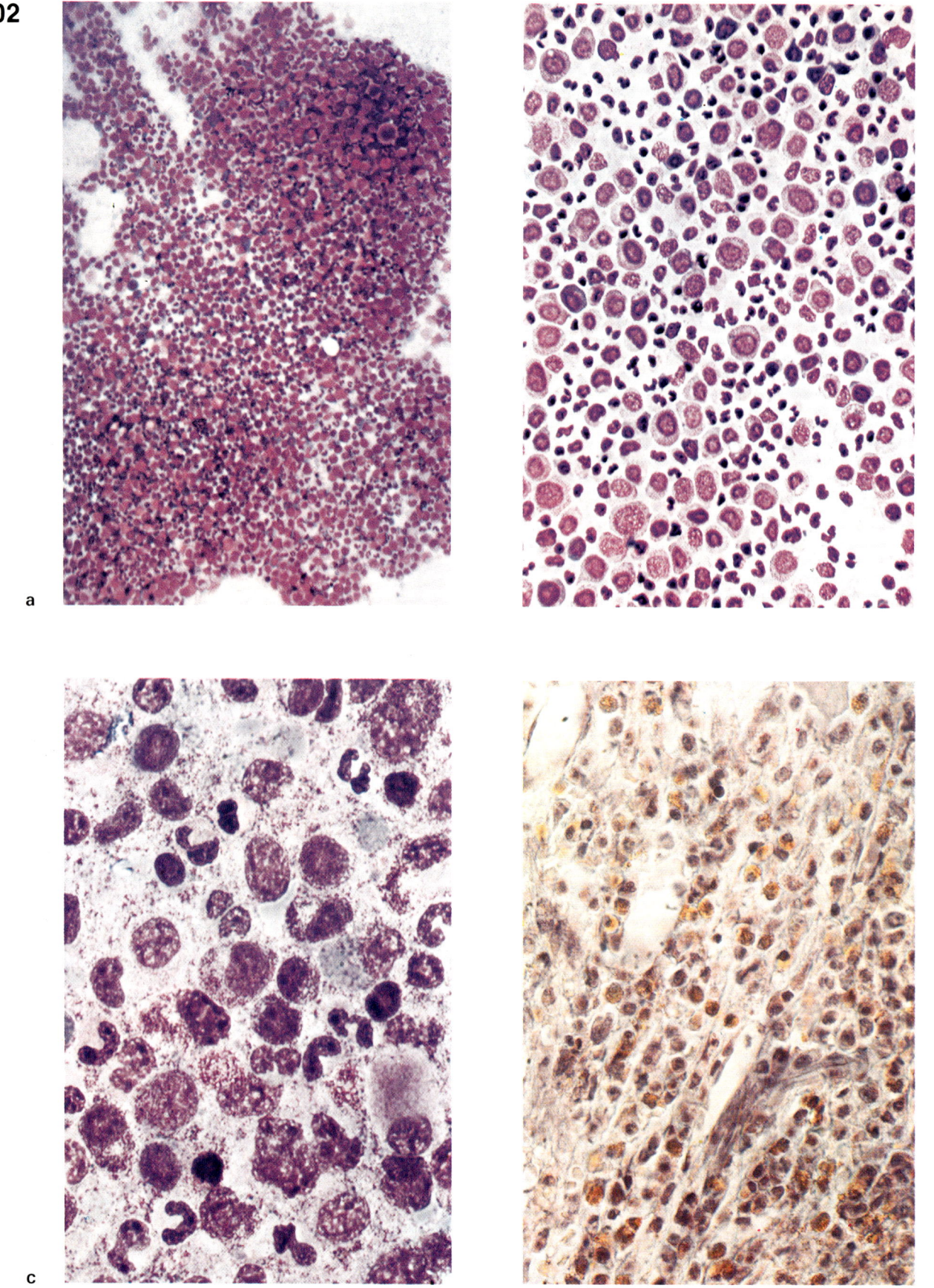

Fig. 67 a, b) CML. Bone marrow aspirates usually show a very "full" hypercellular marrow with a markedly increased myeloid : erythroid ratio. This may not be diagnostic.
c) CML. Myelocytes and mature neutrophils predominate in the marrow.
d) CML. Bone marrow biopsy showing marked eosinophilia.

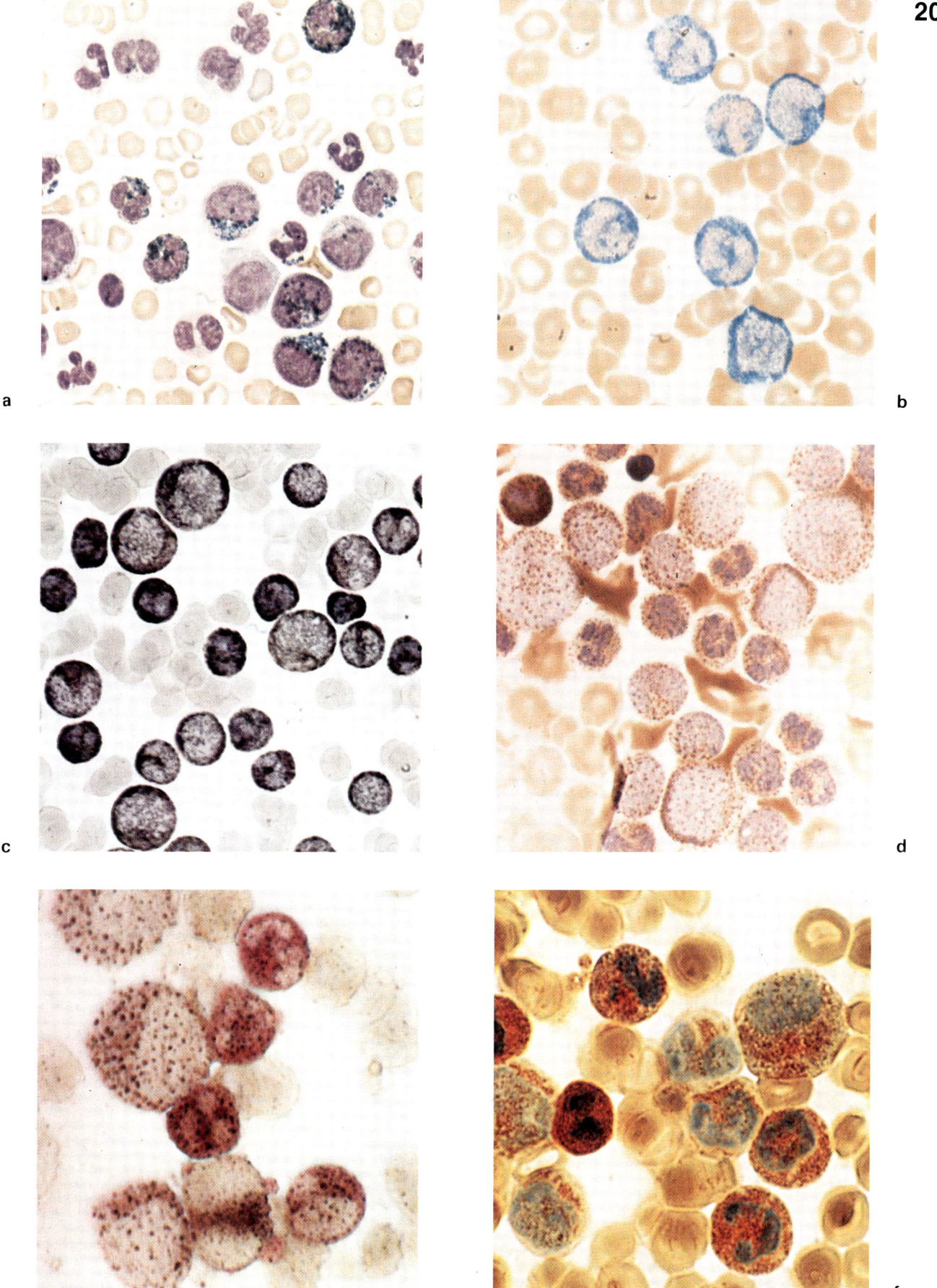

Fig. 68 CML, peripheral blood cytochemistry. While the alkaline phosphatase reaction is usually negative or weak, the following cytochemical reactions remain positive. **a**) peroxidase; **b**) naphthol-AS-D-chloroacetate esterase; **c**) Sudan black; **d, e**) low and high power of acid phospatase; **f**) β-aminopeptidase.

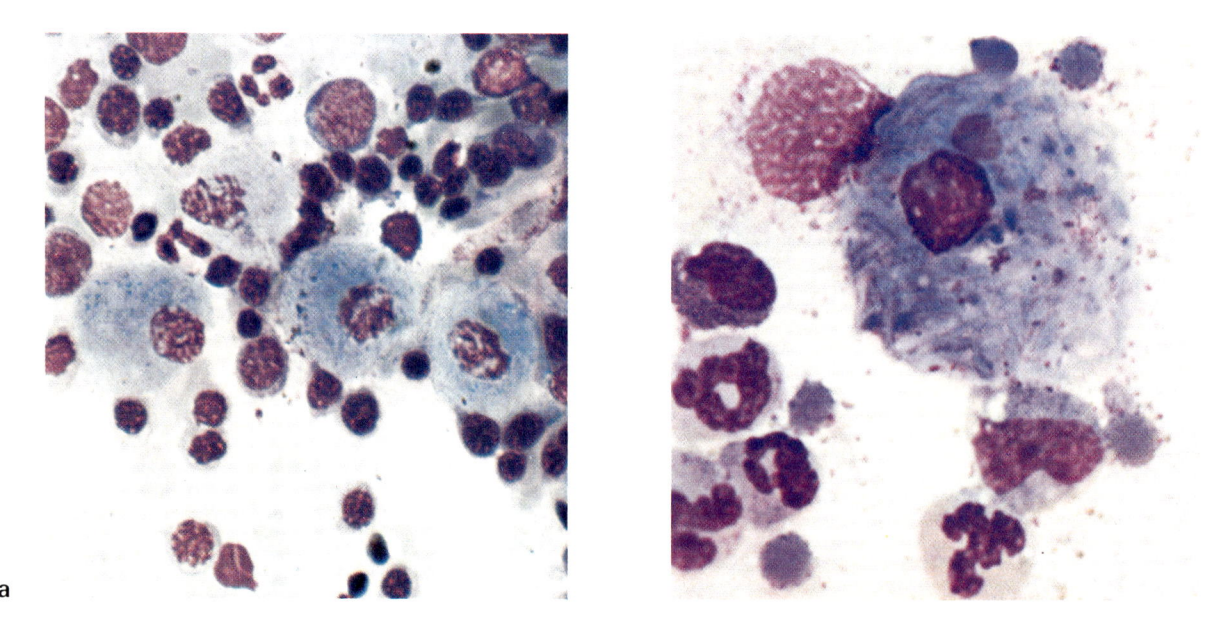

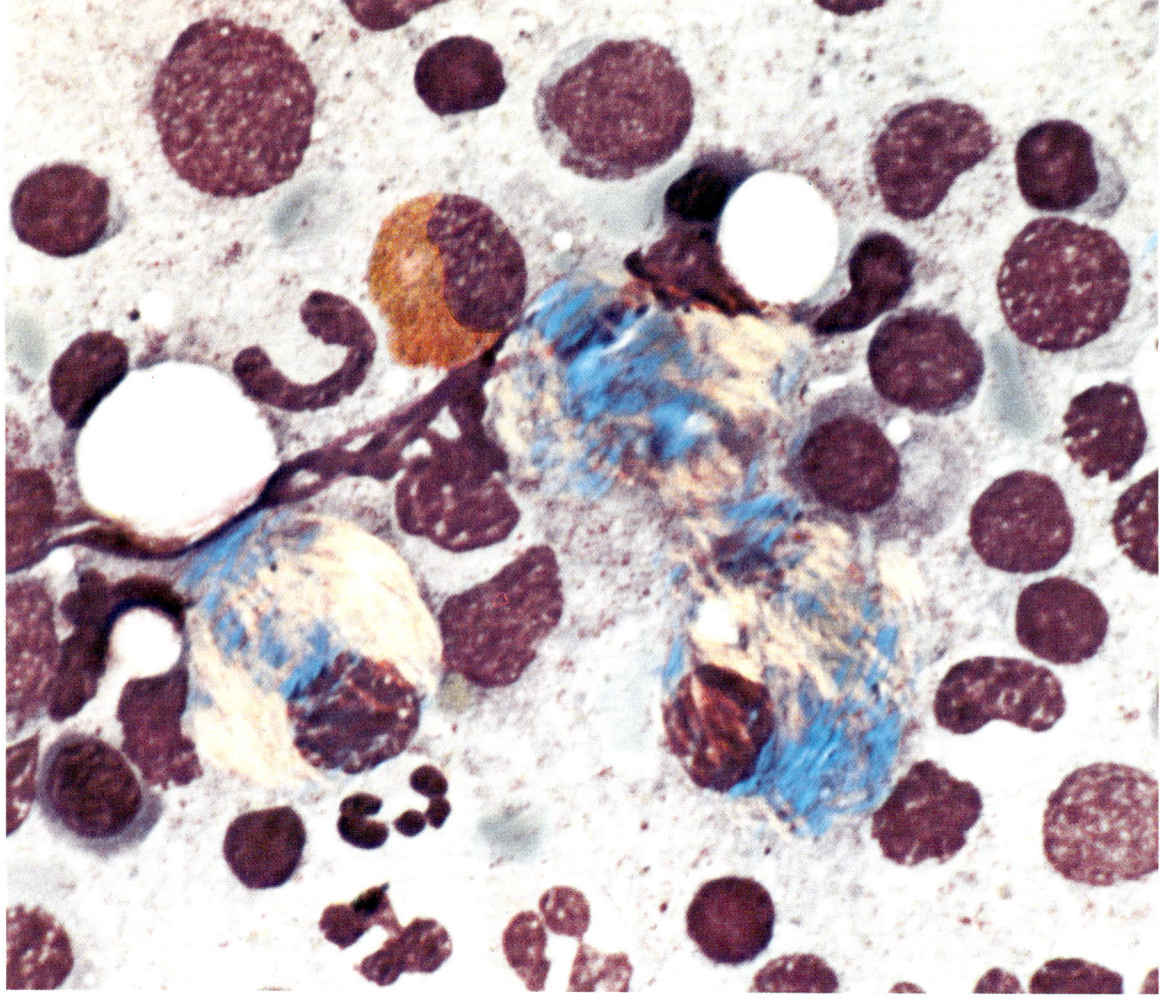

Fig. 69 a, b) Gaucher-like cells in CML bone marrow may be seen in about 15% of patients.
c) Gaucher-like cells in CML bone marrow seen by polarization microscopy which resolves the glucocerebroside inclusions to better advantage because of their birefringent properties.

4 NEUTROPHILS

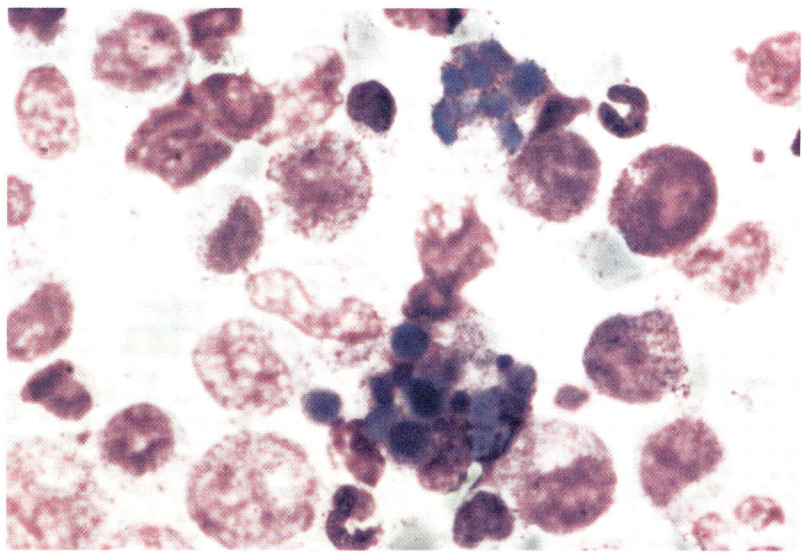

Fig. 70 Example of the so-called blue macrophages seen in CML marrow. They represent histiocytes that have phagocytosed the nuclei of effete granulocytes ("ineffective granulocytopoiesis"). They should not be confused with the "sea-blue" histiocytes (see Chapter 8).

Gaucher-like cells and blue macrophages should be looked upon as morphologic indicators of ineffective granulocytopoiesis. It is not unusual to find CML associated with marked increase in megakaryocytes, eosinophils or basophils (**Fig. 71 a**).
In fact, it is often difficult to distinguish severe eosinophilia in CML from the hypereosinophilic syndrome or eosinophilic leukemia or the severe basophilia sometimes associated with CML from true basophilic leukemia.
This problem has been discussed in detail in Chapter 6, pp. 276, 282 and in Chapter 7, pp. 307-308 respectively.

5.2. Blast transformation in Chronic Myelogenous Leukemia (CML)

The terminal phase of CML may be characterized by a poorly defined clinical and hematologic stage when the disease becomes refractory to previously effective therapy, and the total granulocyte mass expands to the point where it impairs vital processes, or the disease may end in a "blast cell crisis". The term metamorphosis is sometimes used to include the whole spectrum of termination including the so-called accelerated phase of the disease [194]. The accelerated phase is characterized by lymphadenopathy, massive splenomegaly, an increase in bone marrow blasts over 10%, new cytogenetic abnormalities and unresponsiveness to chemotherapy. About 50% of CML's terminate this way; the remainder develops the "blast" crisis. The "blast" cells are not morphologically distinguishable on routine smears, but have been shown to represent one of two major subtypes by other means: lymphoid (L) or myeloid (M). Their relative incidence is about 1 : 4 [195]. Their respective phenotypes are summarized in **Figure 72**.

It should be noted that most L forms have essentially the same overall phenotype as common ALL which includes also a proportion of cells with cytoplasmic μ or IgM heavy chains (i.e. "pre-B-ALL", see Chapter 9). No cases with the phenotype of T-ALL or B-ALL have so far been described. Some cases (10%) of blast crisis present as quite complex mixtures of lymphoblasts and myeloid cells or many shift from predominant "lymphoid" to predominant "myeloid" during the course of disease evolution. In such "mixed" cases staining with antibodies followed by separation on the Fluorescence Activated Cell Sorter can clearly reveal the presence of the lymphoid component (**Fig. 73**). The blasts may also represent progenitors of the megakaryocytic or erythroid series. Recent studies have

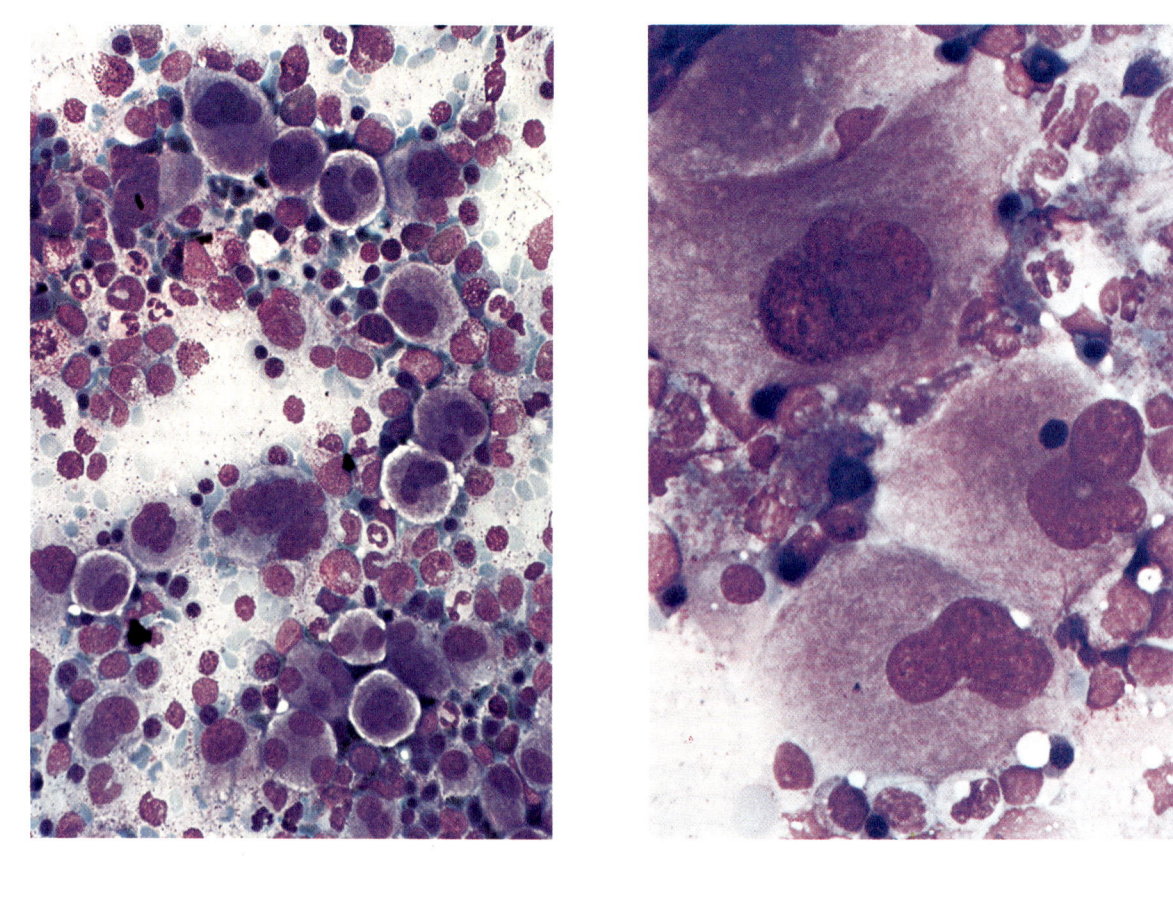
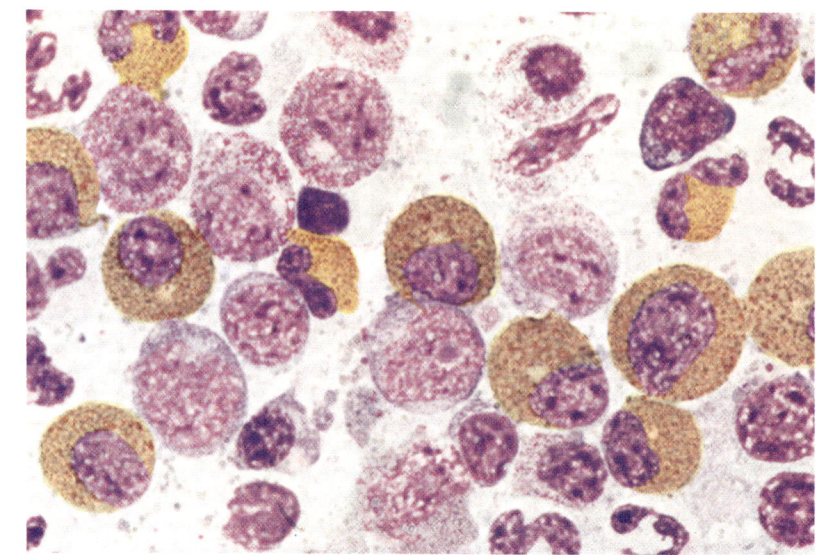

Fig. 71 a, b) CML showing megakaryocytosis.
c) Marked eosinophilia seen in the bone marrow of a patient with Ph¹-positive CML. This is sometimes difficult to distinguish from eosinophilic leukemia or the "hypereosinophilic" syndromes (see Chapter 6).

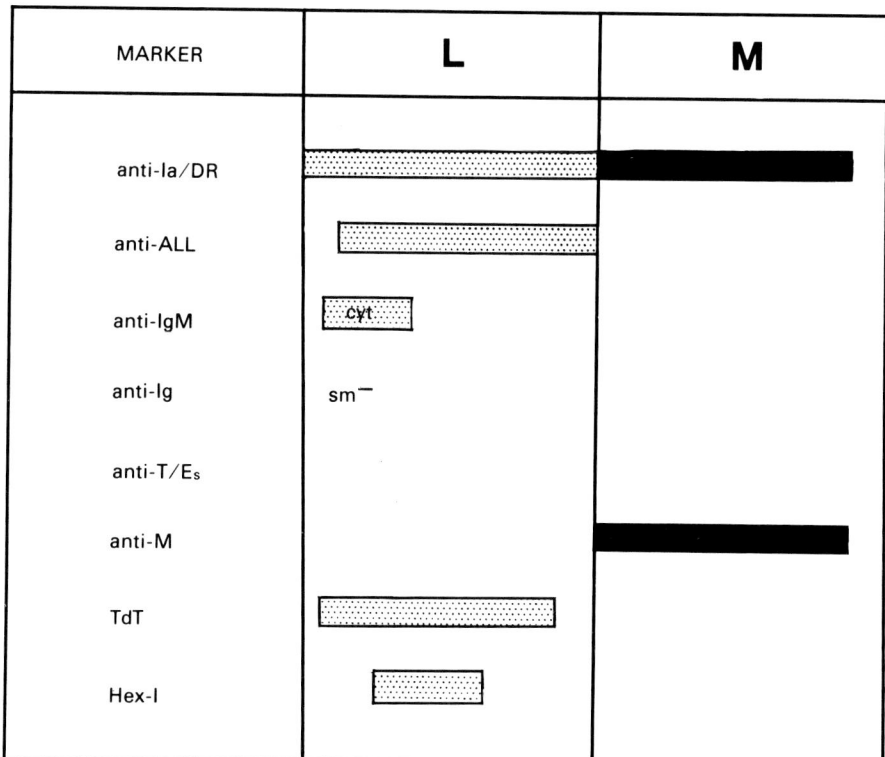

Fig. 72 Composite antigenic and enzymatic phenotypes in blast crisis of Ph¹-positive CML. For discussion and references see similar phenotypic maps in Chapter 9, Parts 1 and 2.
Abbreviations: **L**, lymphoid; **M**, myeloid; **Cyt**, cytoplasmic μ chains; **sm⁻**, surface membrane (immunoglobulin) negative; **anti-T**, anti-thymus derived lymphocytes; **E$_s$**, sheep erythrocyte rosettes; **anti-M**, anti-myeloid serum; **TdT**, terminal deoxynucleotidyl transferase; **Hex-I**, elevated isoenzyme I of hexosaminidase.
Taken from a survey of 223 patients in blast crisis. Courtesy of Dr. M.F. Greaves, Imperial Cancer Research Fund, London.

shown that cryptic erythroid cells may be detected by staining the blast cells with anti-glycophorin (Greaves and Robinson, unpublished observations). Classification of blasts into "L" and "M" subtypes has prognostic relevance, e.g. studies utilizing terminal deoxynucleotidyl transferase (TdT) [196] and membrane antigens [197] indicate a substantially higher remission induction rate and overall survival of the "L" variety treated with chemotherapy that includes vincristine and prednisolone.

The unequivocal demonstration of "early" or "immature" lymphoid phenotypes during the "blast" crisis of CGL (including Ph¹ negative cases, ref. 195) suggests that the initial leukemic transformation occurred in a common progenitor of lymphocytes and myeloid cells (i.e. a pluripotential stem cell) [198, 199, 202]. This view, first proposed by Boggs [200], is supported by glucose 6-phosphodiesterase studies [201] which indicate monoclonality of at least some lymphoid cells in CGL. Cytogenetic studies confirm that different myeloid lineage cells (monocytic, erythroid, platelet, as well as granulocytic) are included in the dominant Ph¹ positive stem cells progeny (see Chapter 11) [203]. Most T and B lymphocytes do not, however, have the Ph¹ chromosome which may reflect the fact that most of these cells are long lived and derived from cells which may have been able to give rise to progeny before the Ph¹ chromosome abnormality developed. The appearance of the bone marrow during CML metamorphosis and blast cell crises is illustrated in **Figure 74**.

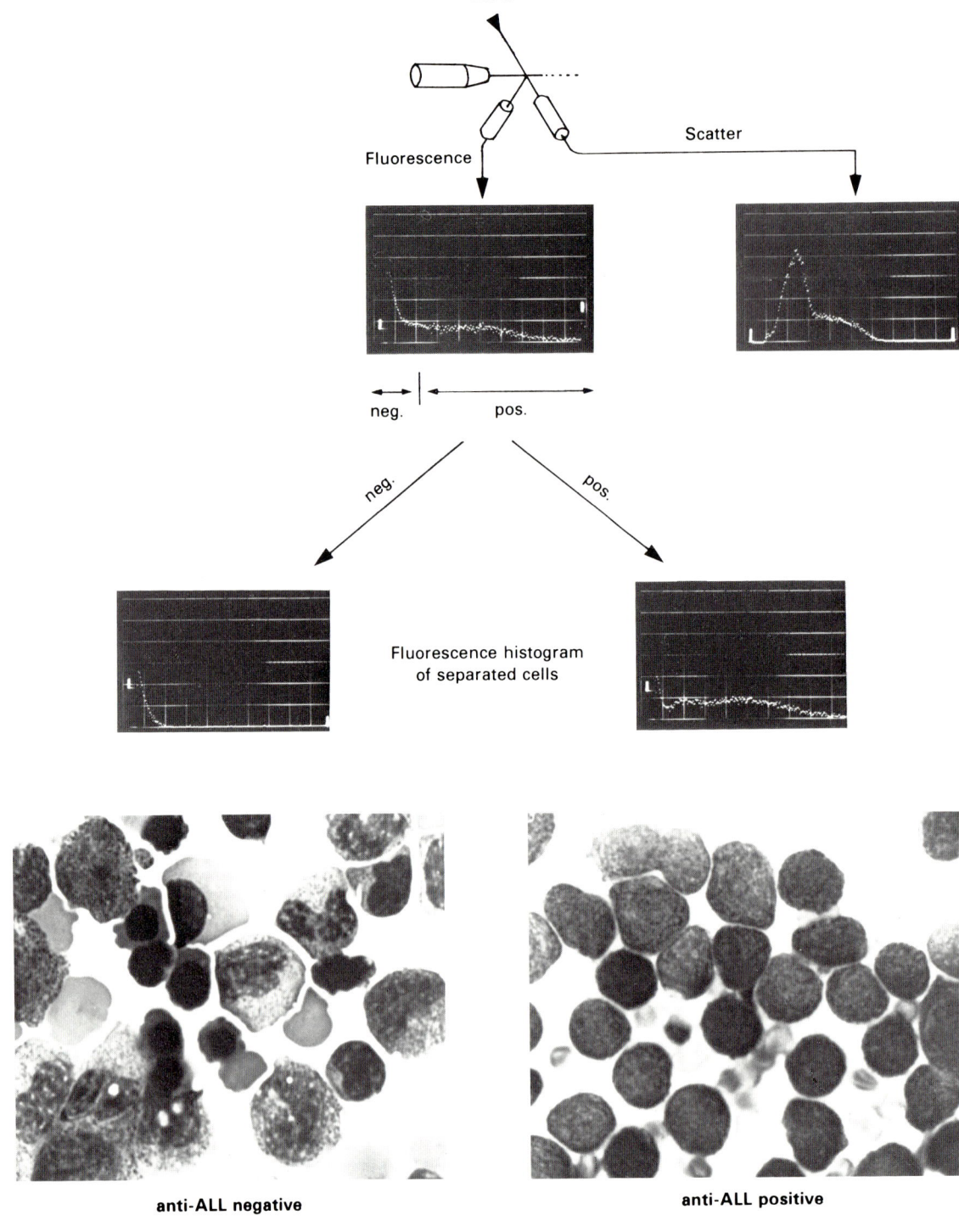

Fig. 73 Separation of lymphoblasts in blast crisis of Ph^1-positive CML. Leukemic cells from a patient in blast crisis were stained with anti-cALL (see Chapter 9, Part 2) and the population separated on the Fluorescence Activated Cell Sorter into positive and negative fractions as shown. Cytocentrifuge preparations were stained with May Grünwald-Giemsa. Note that the lymphoblast population is localized in the anti-cALL-positive fraction, whereas the negative fraction contains myeloid and erythroid cells.
Courtesy of Dr. M.F. Greaves, Imperial Cancer Research Fund, London.
Taken from ref. 202.

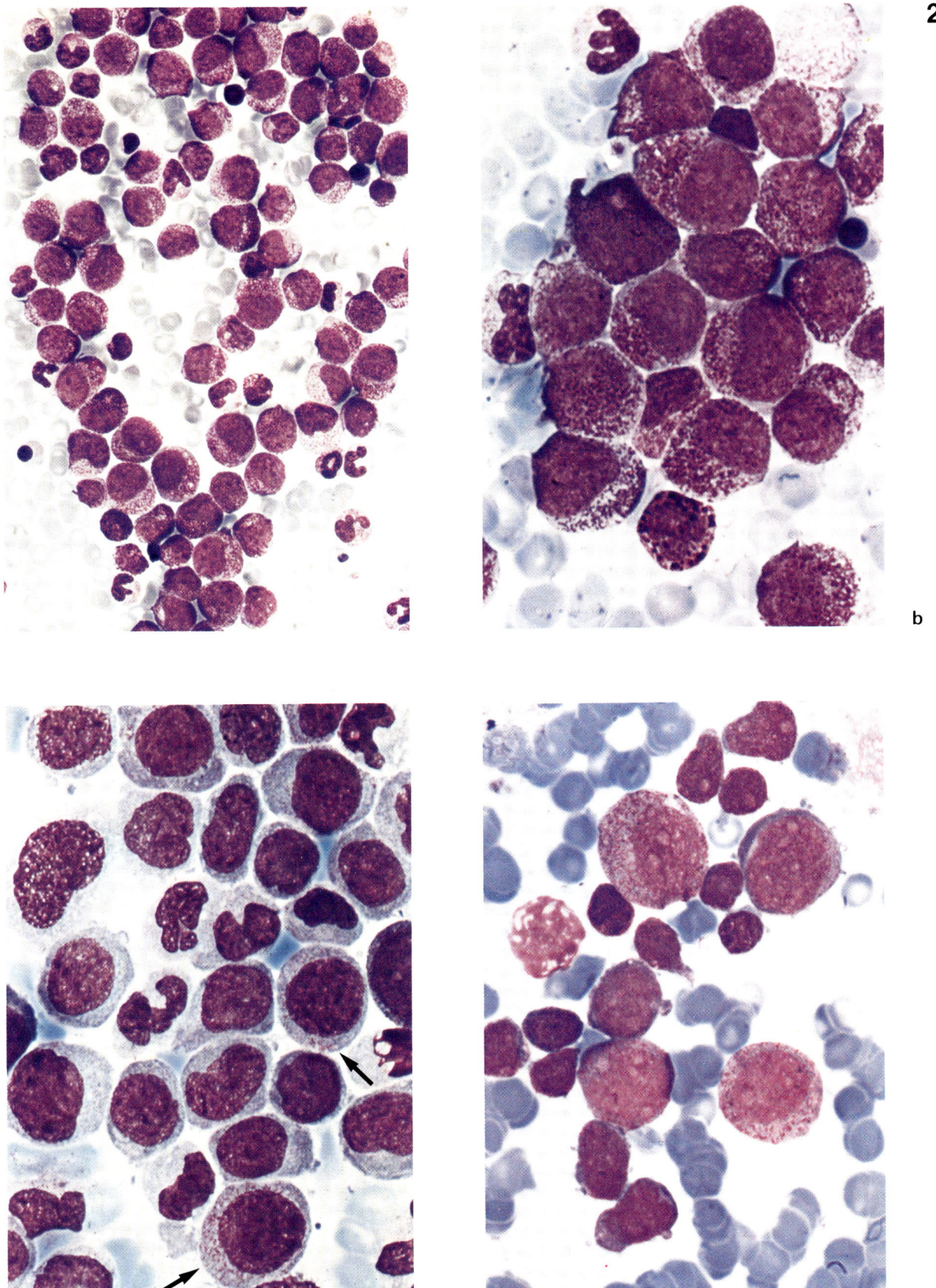

Fig. 74 A series of illustrations depicting the morphologic changes seen in the blood and marrow of patients with CML who enter the "aggressive phase", "metamorphosis" or "blast cell crisis".

a) Excess of promyelocytes, large nucleoli and an increase in the percentage of blasts suggests that CML has entered a "more aggressive" phase.

b) A typical granular metamorphosis of CML.

c) Blast cell crisis, myeloid type. Presence of some azurophilic granules (**arrows**) in early promyelocytes are indicative of myeloid commitment.

d) Blast cell crisis, "mixed" type; some cells appear lymphoid, others are clearly myeloid (see **Fig. 73**).

BLOOD CELLS

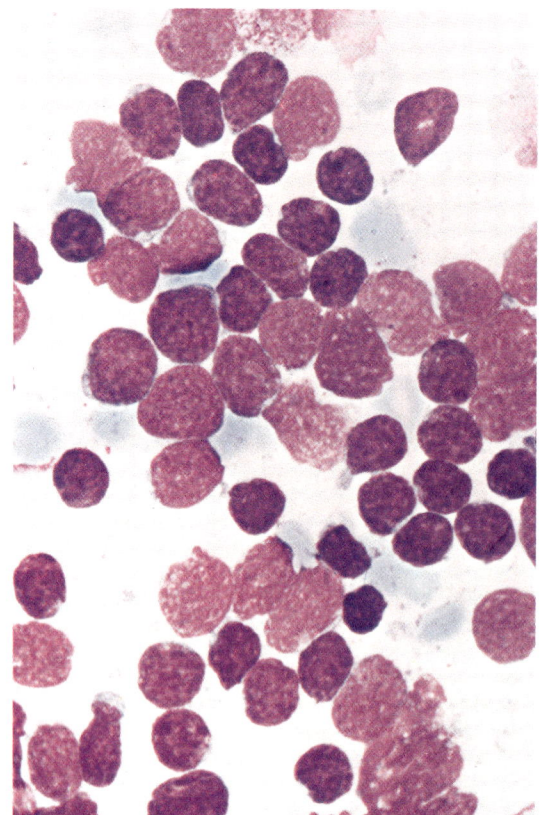
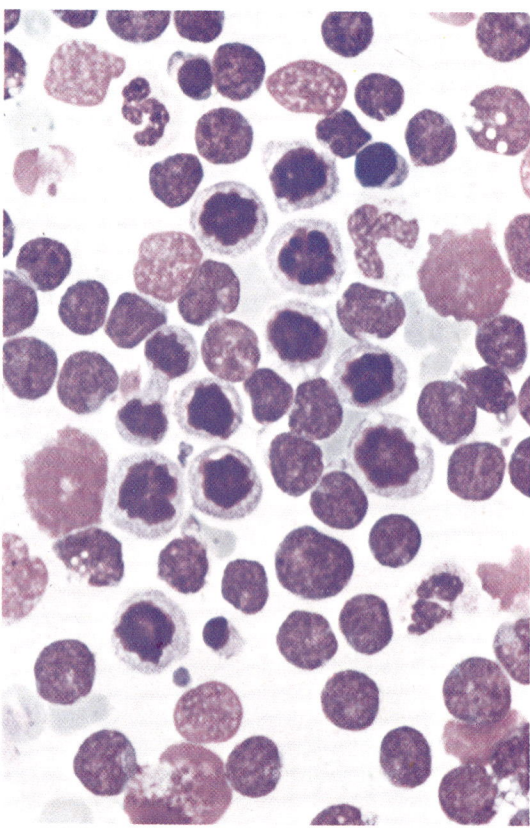
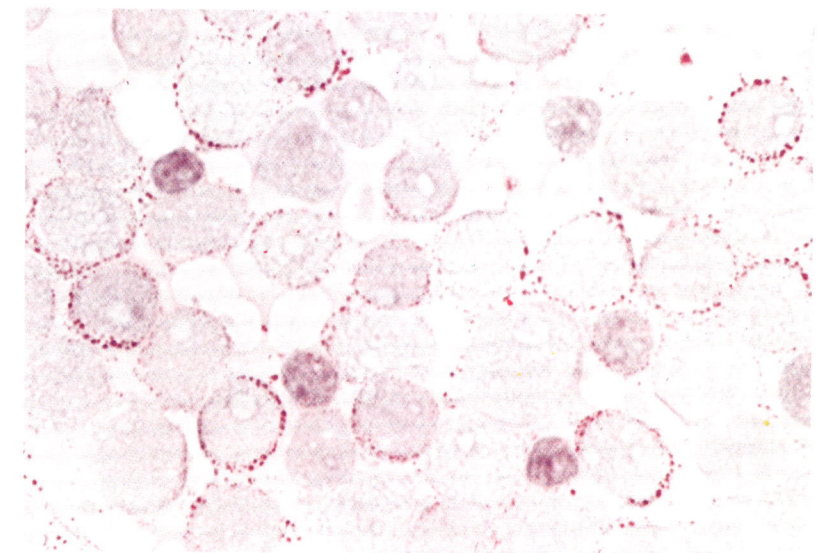

Fig. 74 e) *Blast cell crisis, lymphoid type.*

f) *Bone marrow of lymphoid blast crisis 24 hours after administration of vinicristine. An imposing metaphasic arrest is visible (see also p. 235).*

g) *Lymphoid crisis, PAS reaction. The majority of the cells are positive, with a microgranular pattern.*

h) *Blast cell crisis, myelomonocytic type, packed marrow.*

i) *Blast crisis of the megakaryoblastic type.*

j) *The appearance of vacuolated erythroblasts which are characteristically PAS-positive, herald the onset of blast crisis.*

k) *Typical granular PAS-positivity of an erythroblast from the marrow of the case shown in* **j**.

4 NEUTROPHILS

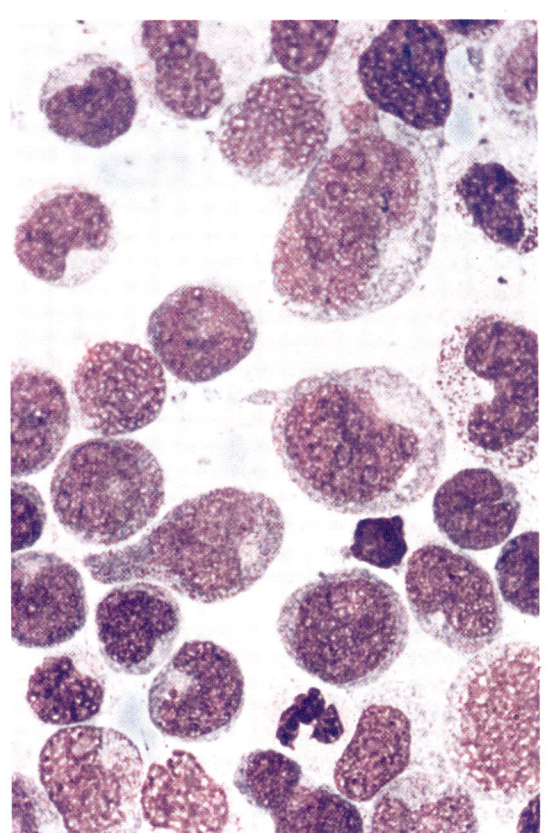
h

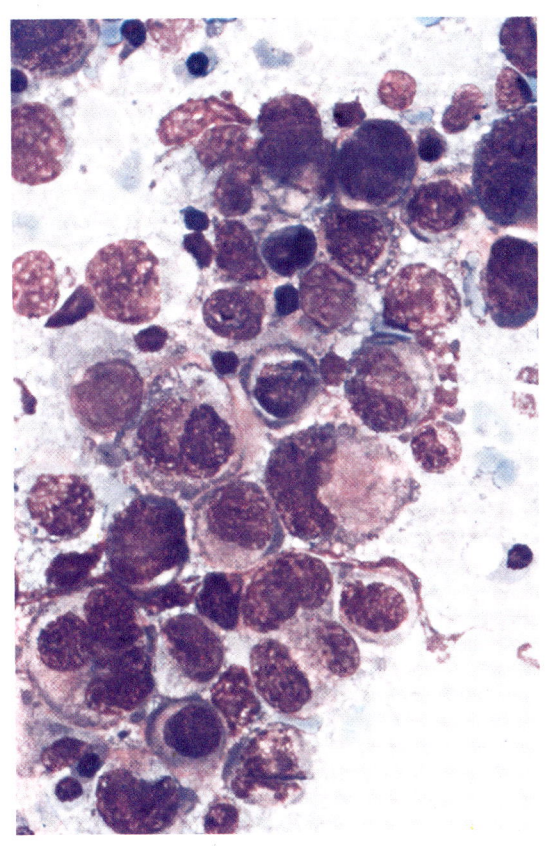
i

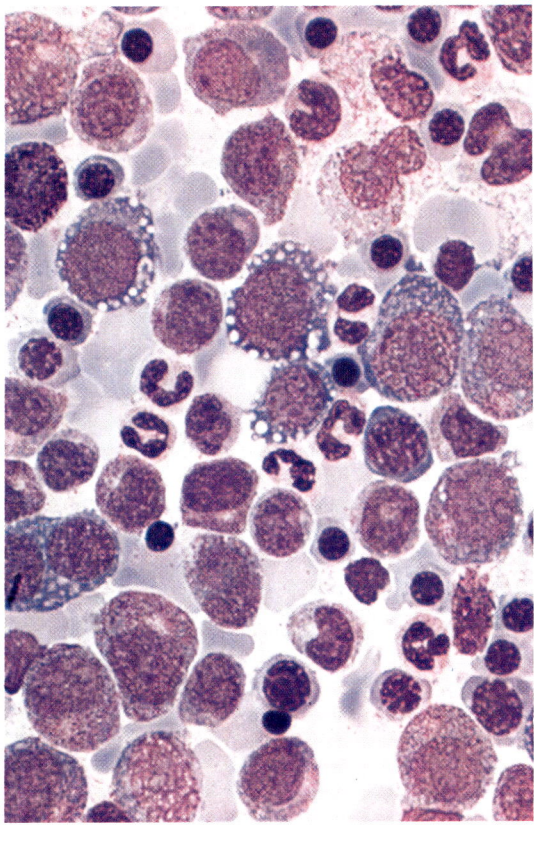
j

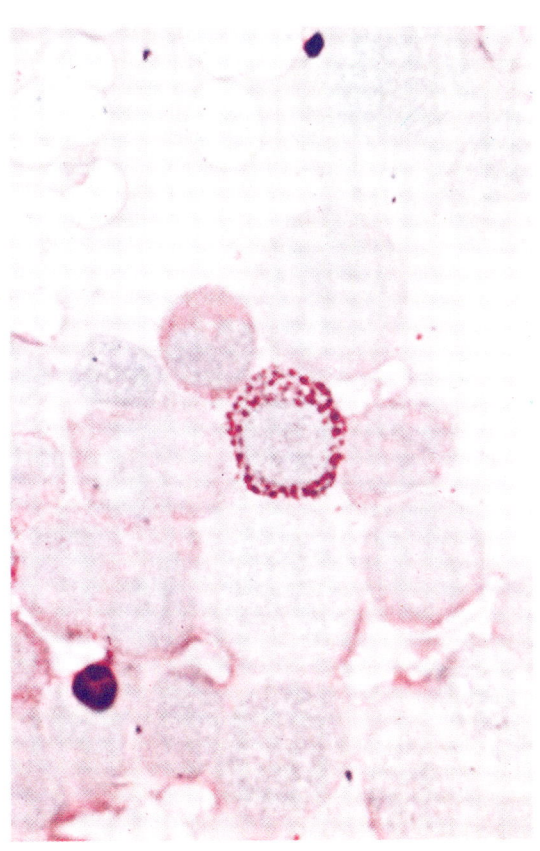
k

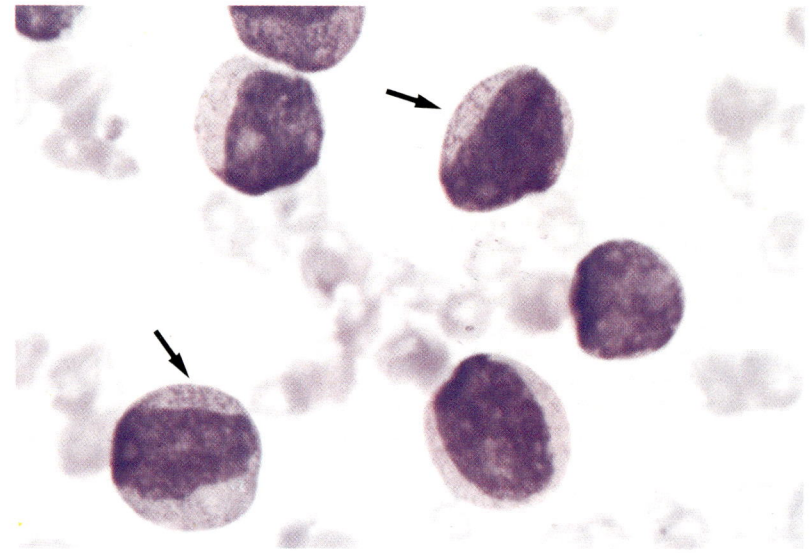

Fig. 75 AML, M1 type.
a) Blood, undifferentiated blasts large nucleoli. A few non specific granules (**arrows**) suggest myeloid type, however cytochemical analysis is necessary for confirmation (see also **Figs. 75 b-g**).

6. THE ACUTE MYELOGENOUS LEUKEMIAS

6.1. General considerations

In general, the connotation "acute" signifies poorly differentiating, non-maturing cells with short doubling time, neoplastic progression, suppression of normal hematopoiesis and a short clinical course. However, there are numerous cases in which the presence of undifferentiated blasts, in the marrow, even when the percentage is high, is associated with pancytopenia in the periphery, and a rather chronic clinical course. Such cases have been variously defined as oligoblastic [204, 205], smoldering [206, 207], indolent [208, 209], subacute [210, 211] and even chronic [212-214]. Various subgroups both of oligoleukemia and preleukemia have been identified on the basis of *in vitro* soft agar cultures [215, 216].

Although the cells appear "frozen" at various stages of early development, there is an increasing tendency to believe that leukemogenesis occurs at the level of the pluripotent stem cell [217].

Cytogenetic [218, 219] and enzymatic [220] evidence is in favor of a monoclonal disorder although some controversy exists. Studies using G-6-PD isoenzymes have suggested heterogeneity in contrast to the relative homogeneity usually seen in CML [221]. In some patients the disease appears to be expressed only in precursors restricted to myelocytic differentiation, whereas in others it involves stem cells which may differentiate into erythroid as well as myeloid elements [165].

Cytogenetic studies of cells obtained from patients in remission show that the bulk of residual hemopoiesis is non-leukemic [222-225], suggesting clonal competition between residual normal stem cells and newly arising AML cells [226]. The degree of maturation blockage may be incomplete [227, 228], especially in some of the myelodysplastic syndromes [226, 229, 230], but, in typical, overt AML, it usually affects all cells. The suppression of normal hemopoiesis in AML is still largely unexplained, but is not believed to be due to simple "crowding out" [231, 232]. A number of *in vitro* studies seem to suggest that AML cells are capable of maturation and differentiation. For instance, the cells of a patient with promyelocytic leukemia (APL) showed differentiation in diffusion chambers [233]. In other experiments, APL blasts were converted into adherent, macrophage-like cells [234]. Granulocyte maturation was also achieved with cells of murine myelogenous leukemia in the presence of several inducers [235].

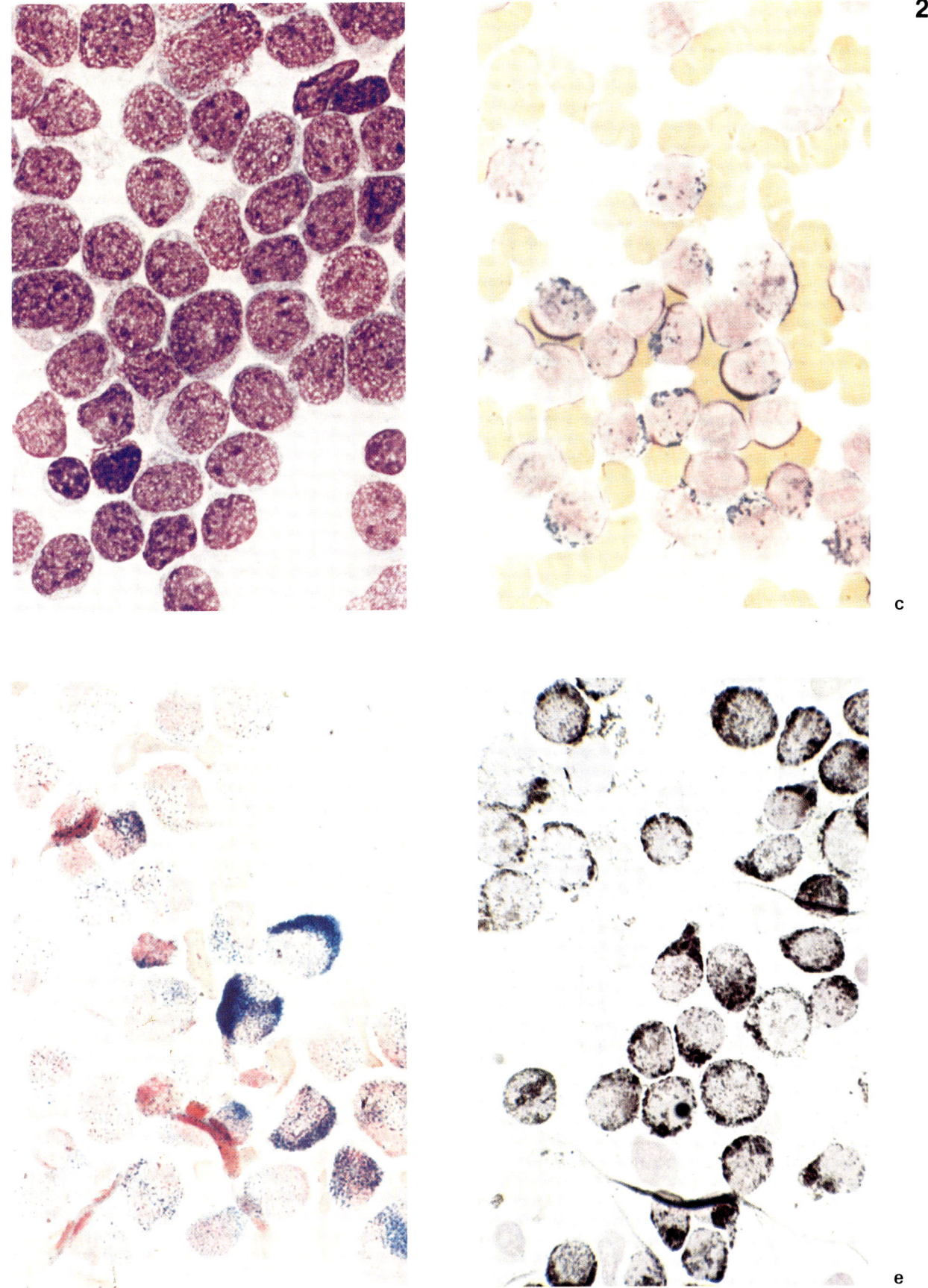

Fig. 75 b) Bone marrow of patient with AML (M1 type), Giemsa stain.
c) Same specimen as **b** stained for peroxidase. Positive stain indicates myeloid type.
d) Same specimen as **b** stained for naphthol-AS-D-chloroacetate esterase.
e) Same specimen as **b**. Sudan black reaction is positive.

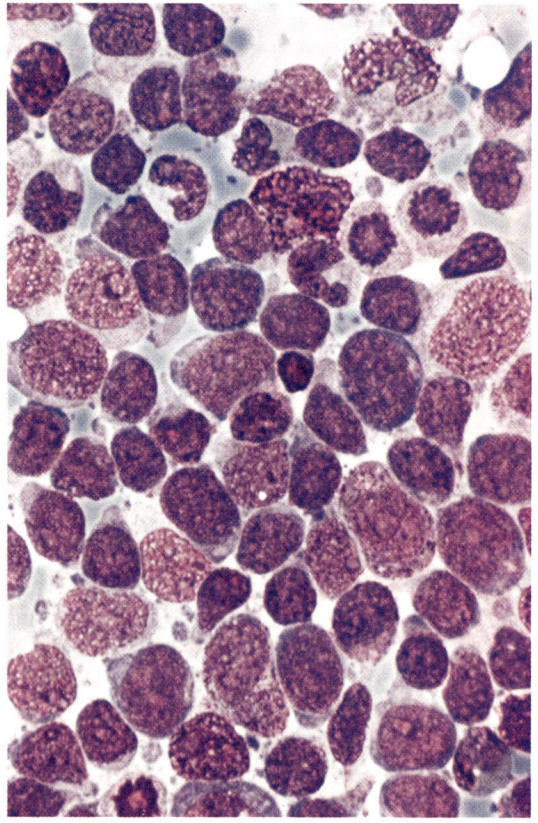 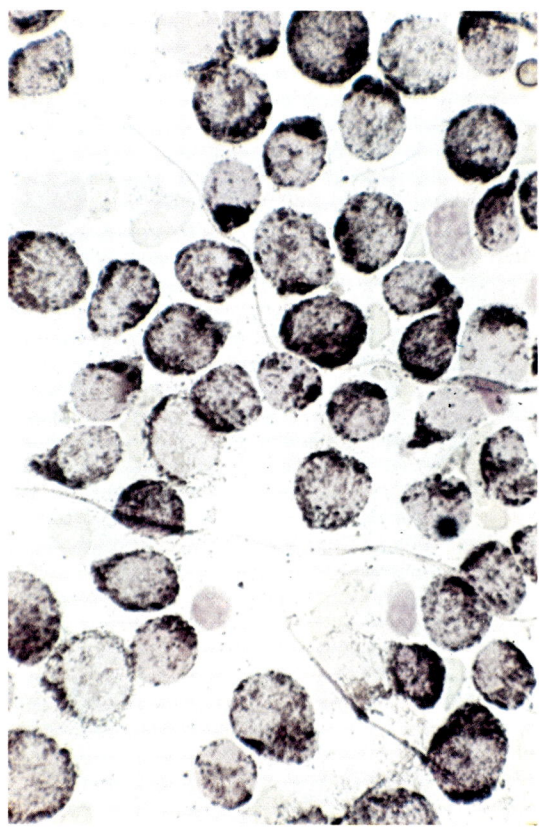

Fig. 75 f) Another example of M1 AML which is difficult to distinguish from acute lymphoblastic leukemia (ALL, L1), were it not for strongly positive cytochemical reactions for myeloid enzymes.
g) Same specimen as **f** stained with Sudan black.

A continuous myeloid cell line has been established from a patient with APL (HL-60). These cells were able to differentiate to maturity in culture without change in their intrinsic cytogenetic abnormalities [236]. Such observations have raised the hope of many investigators that "regulatory" therapy may eventually replace blastolysis [237].

6.2. Classifications of Acute Leukemia (AL)

The two classifications of AL which include the lymphocytic leukemias (see Chapter 9) most widely accepted are the WHO classification and the FAB classification (see p. 415). Each has its merits and drawbacks. The FAB classification will be used here.

Six main types (M 1 - M 6) are defined according to (a) the direction of differentiation, i.e. into which cell series, and (b) the degree of maturation of the cells (see **Figs. 75-85**).

M 1 is defined as *myeloblastic leukemia without maturation*. The blast cells are either non-granular, or contain a few azurophilic granules and/or Auer rods. Auer rods are elongate inclusions which are peroxidase-positive, naphthol-ASD-chloracetate esterase (NASDCA)-positive which is not inhibited by NaF, and Sudan black positive (**Figs. 75 a-g, 76** and **77**).

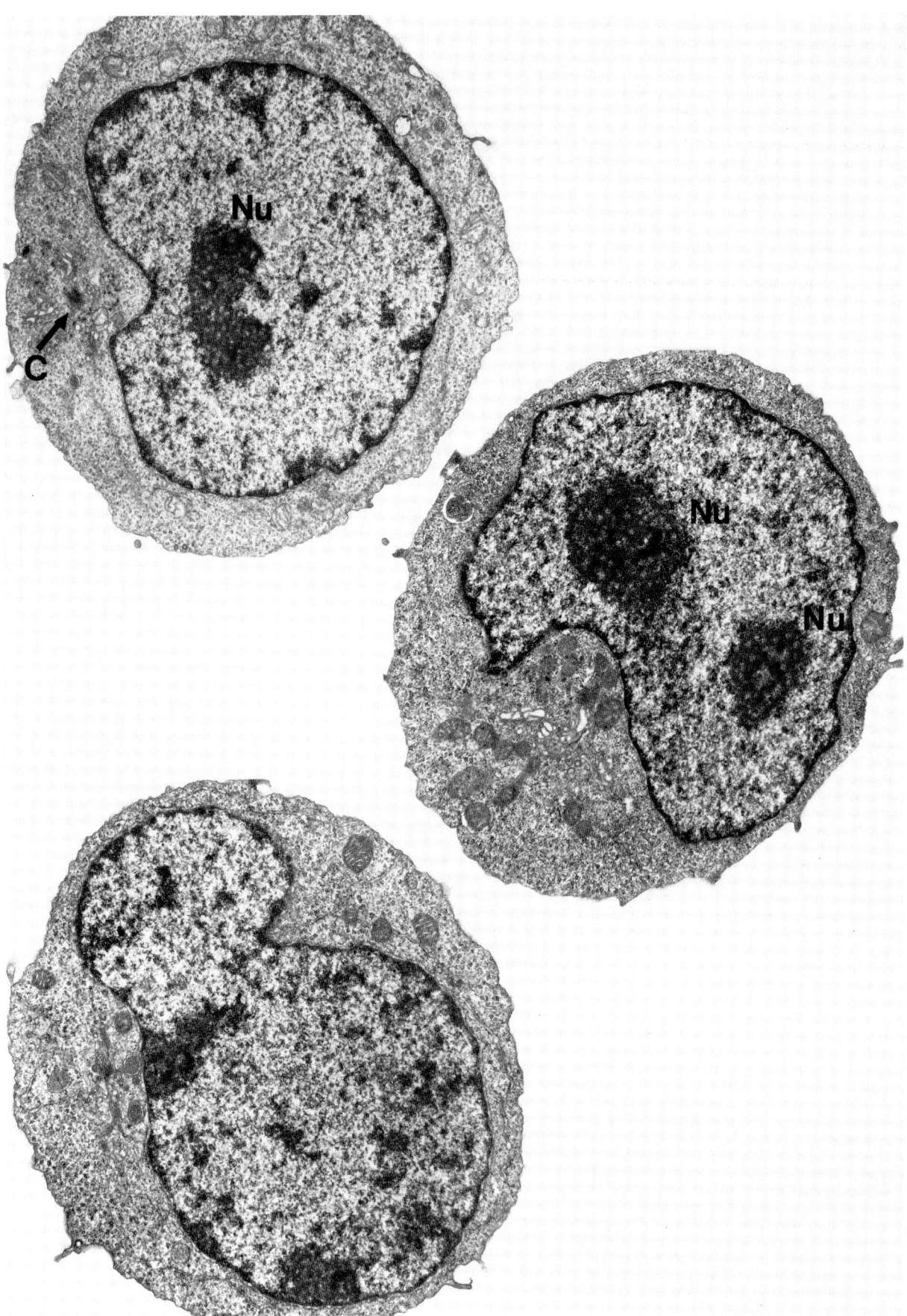

Fig. 76 Three myeloblasts from the bone marrow of a patient with AML. The cells were selected to illustrate their relative monotony, even on the ultrastructural level. **C**, centriole; **Nu**. nucleolus (× 12,000).

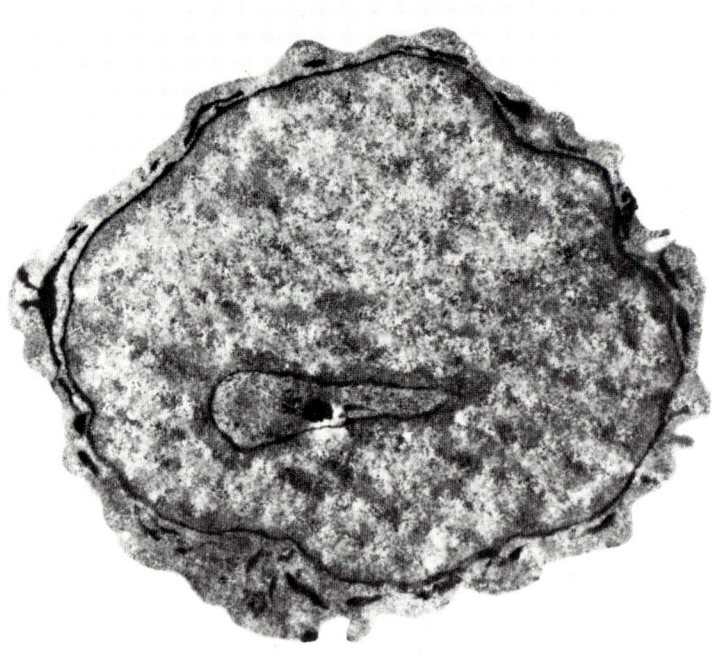

Fig. 77 *Primitive cell of a patient with acute leukemia shows reaction product for peroxidase in the perinuclear space and some profiles of ER distinguishing this cell as a myeloblast rather than a lymphoblast. Courtesy of Dr. Marcel Bessis, Institut de Pathologie Céllulaire, Hôpital du Bicetre, Paris, France.*

M 2, or *myeloblastic leukemia with maturation*, is characterized by maturation at or beyond the promyelocyte stage, with myelocytes, metamyelocytes and mature granulocytes (often demonstrating abnormal features) to be found in varying proportions. All the cytochemical reactions mentioned above are even more strongly positive (**Figs. 78 a-e**).

M 3, or *hypergranular promyelocytic leukemia (APL)*, is composed of atypical promyelocytes with a cytoplasm densely packed with azurophilic granules of various dimensions (**Figs. 79 a-f, 80** and **81**). A pseudonucleus may be simulated by these dense, coalescent granule collections. Bundles ("faggots") of slender Auer rods (see p. 232) are often present. Granules and rods are, by definition, "myeloid enzyme" positive. Recently a variant for of APL has been recognized in which the cells are characterized by bilobed, multilobed or reniform nuclei, but the cytoplasm has minimal or no atypically recognizable granulations; these may be identified by transmission electron microscopy [238]. Both variants are characterized by a translocation involving the long arms of chromosomes 15 and 17 [t (15;17) (q25;q22)] (see Chapter 11). An example of such a case is shown in **Figures 79 g, h**.

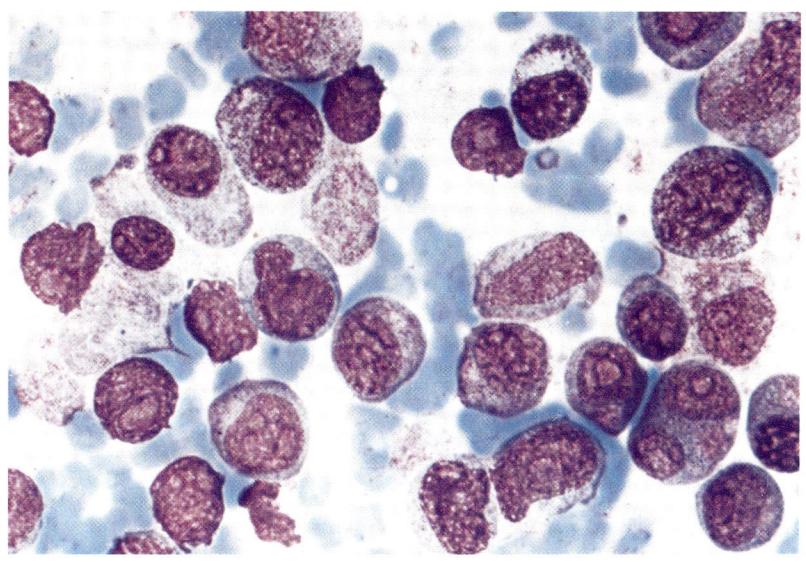

Fig. 78 AML, M2 type.
a) Blasts with large nucleoli and a few cytoplasmic granules. These cells are less differentiated than M3 promyelocytes.

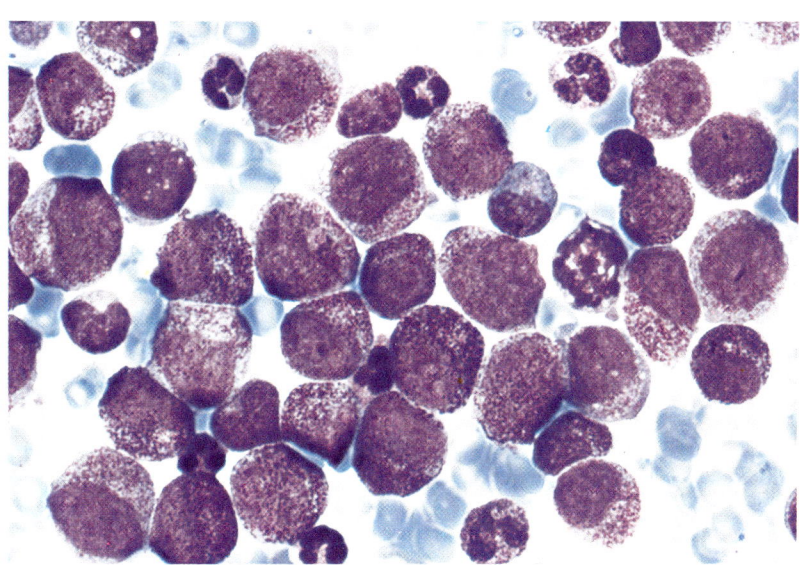

Fig. 78 b) Another example of M2 with somewhat greater differentiation.

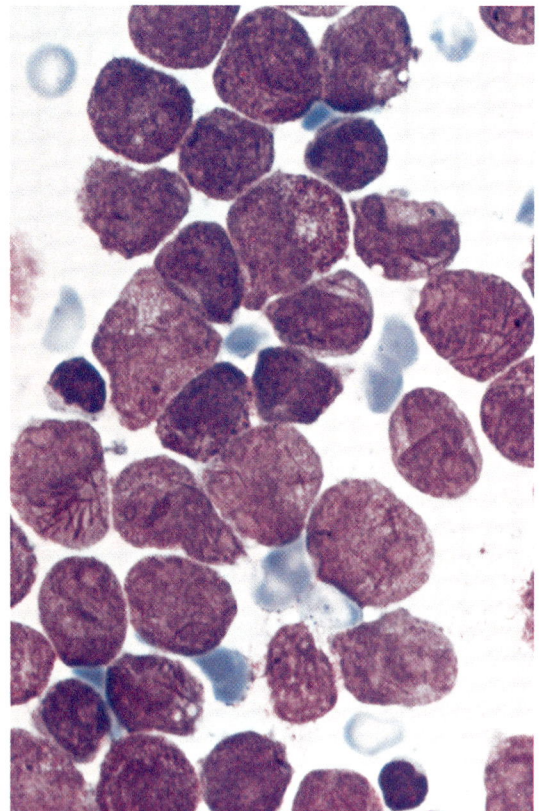
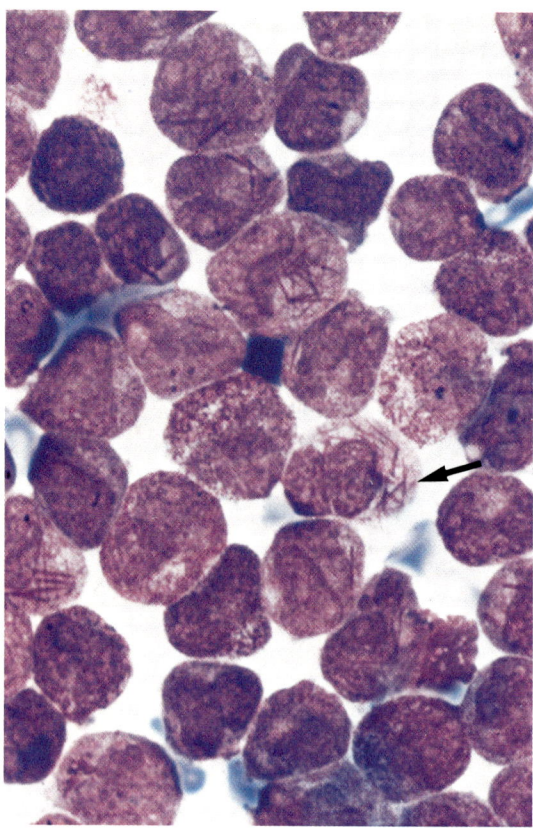

Fig. 79 AML, M 3 type.
a, b, c) Acute promyelocytic leukemia (APL). The marrow is replete with granulocyte precursors arrested at the promyelocyte stage. There are numerous slender Auer rods which are often seen in bundles (**arrows**). This variant is clearly distinguishable from the M 2 variant of AML on morphological and clinical grounds (see text).

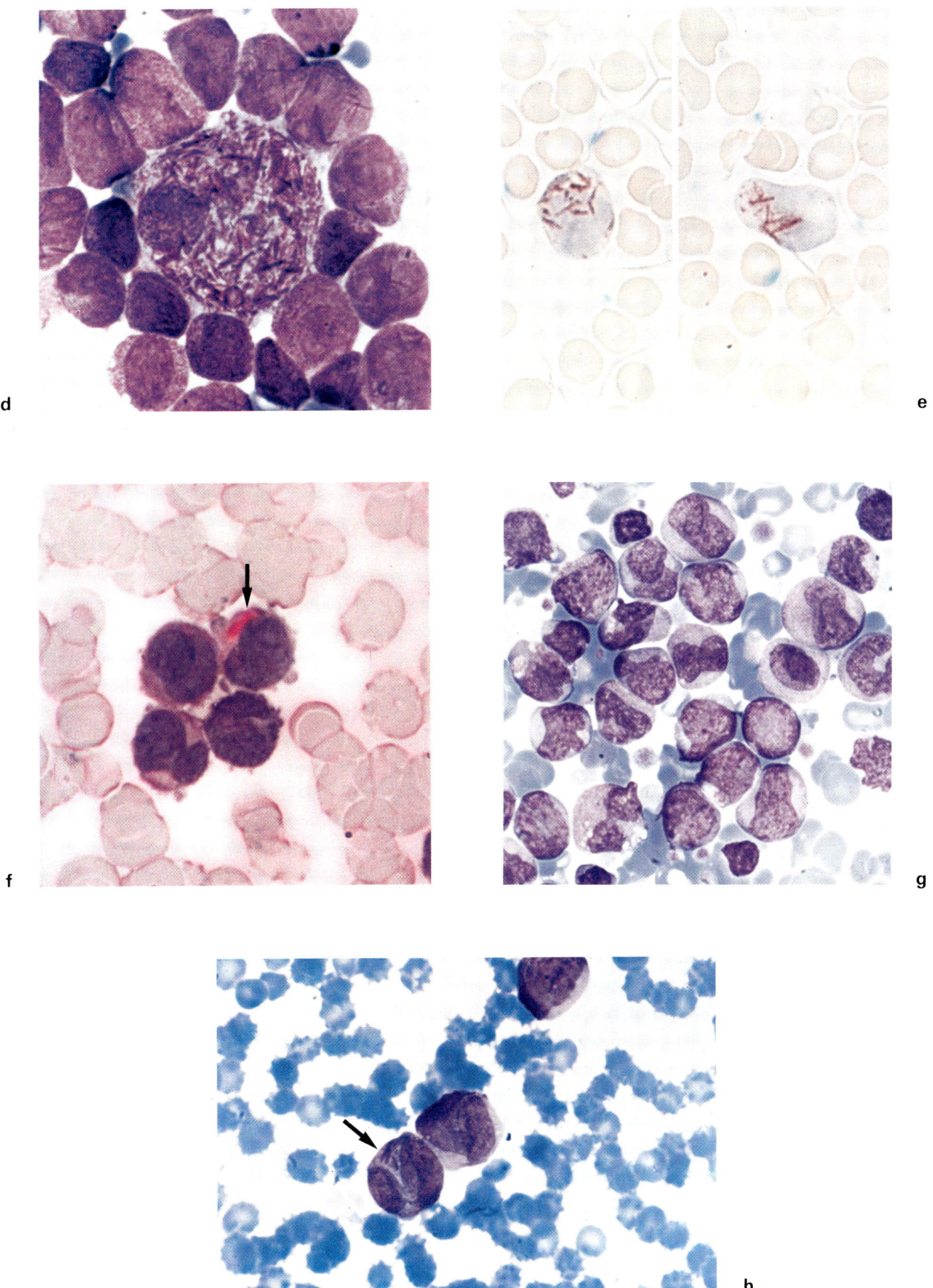

Fig. 79 d) Auer rods released by disintegrating promyelocytes may be phagocytosed by marrow macrophages. This is an example of such an "APL macrophage".

e) Auer rods are strongly positive for naphthol-AS-D-chloroacetate esterase. This supports the concept that they are derived from coalescing azurophilic primary granules.

f) Auer rods are also stained by the PAS-reaction (**arrow**).

g, h) "Microgranular" APL (M 3). In this example, all cells display a monocyte-like morphology. **Arrow** indicates an Auer rod.

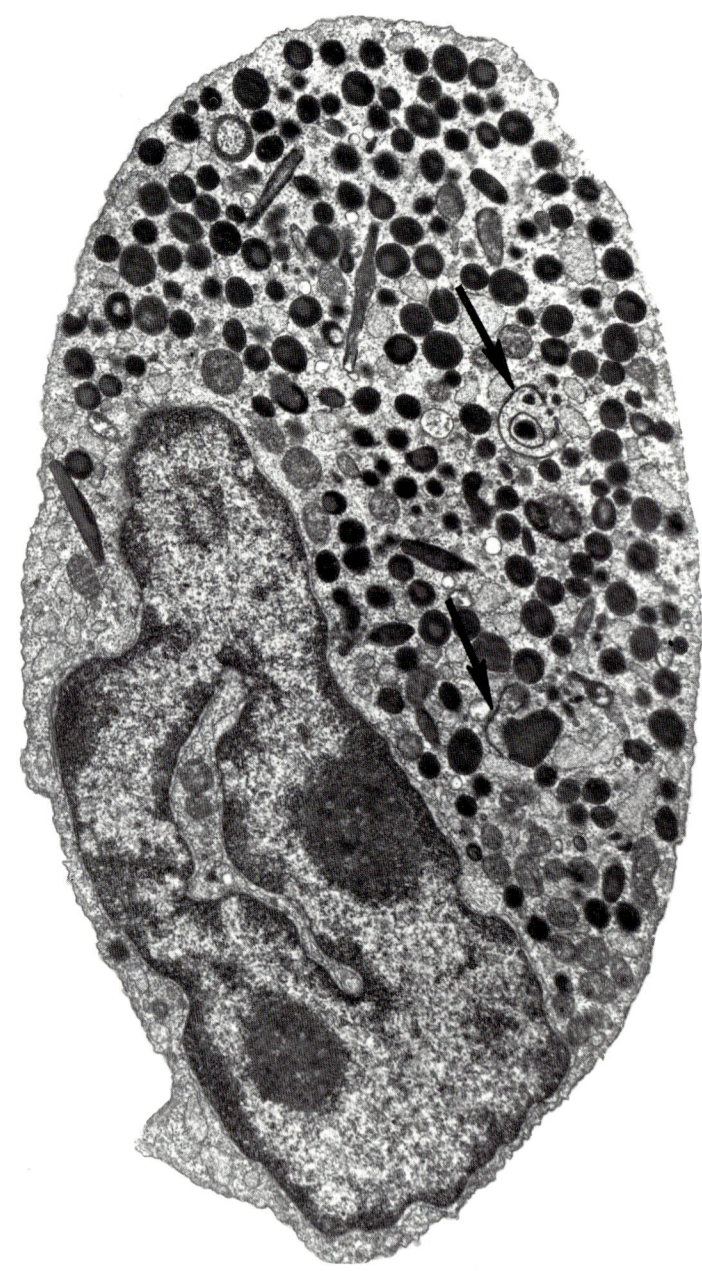

Fig. 80 "Hypergranulated" promyelocyte from a case of APL. Note that there are at least 4 needle-like structures probably representing sections of slender Auer bodies. The nucleus is peculiarly convoluted for this stage of differentiation and there are two large nucleoli. Ring-like and serpentine inclusions are also noteworthy (**arrows**) (× 12,500).

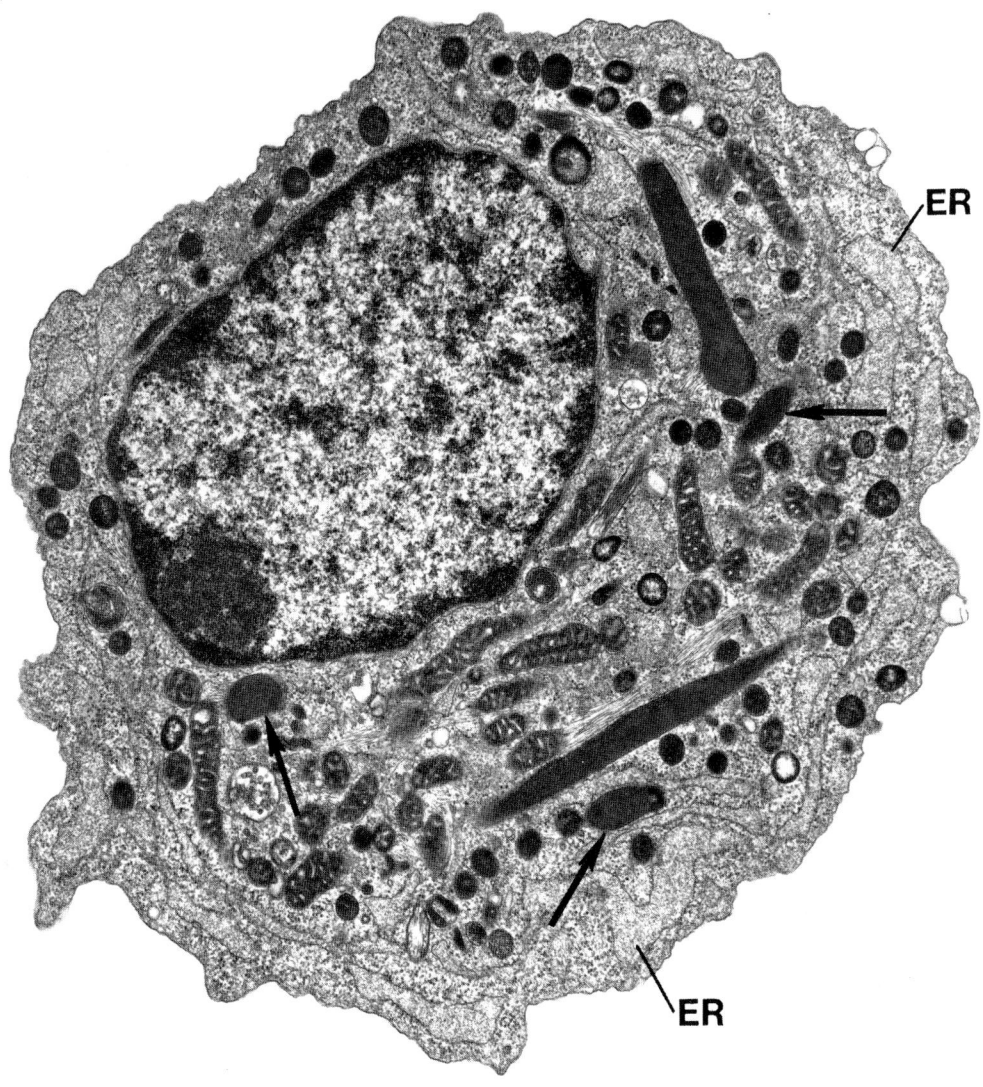

Fig. 81 Early promyelocyte from the blood of a patient with APL. The Auer rods that have been sectioned longitudinally are obvious. **Arrows** indicate additional Auer rods which have been cross-sectioned. Note that the cisternae of rough **ER** are distended with material, presumably the substance which will be packaged into granules. There are numerous mitochondria ($\times$ 16,000).

BLOOD CELLS

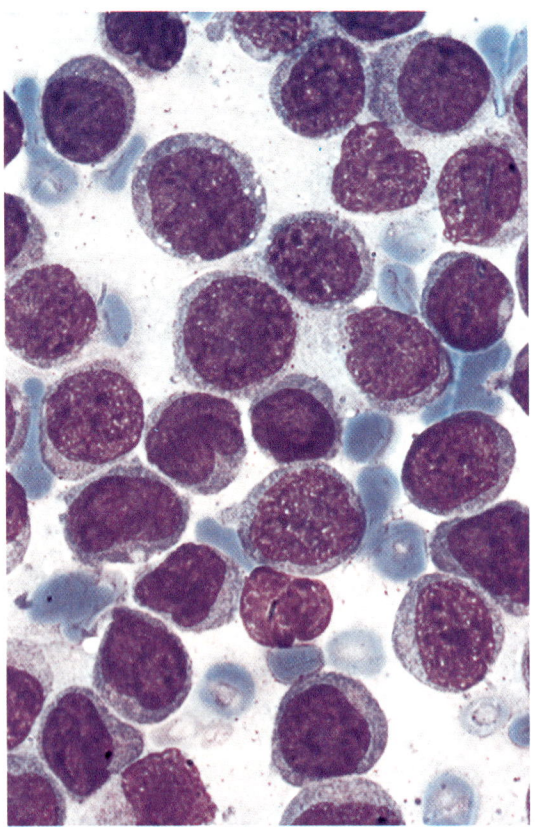 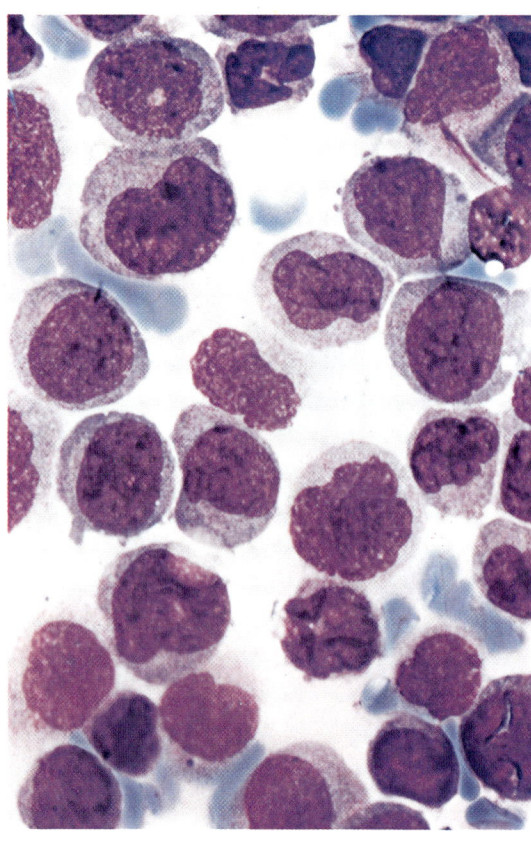

Fig. 82 AML, M 4 type.
a, b) Acute myelomonocytic leukemia exhibits variable percentages of myelo- and monocytic precursor cells. Two examples are illustrated. A common feature is a prevalence of monocytoid morphology in the blood with more "myeloid" appearing cells in the marrow. Cytochemical analysis may be helpful.

M 4, or *myelomonocytic leukemia (AMML)*, is characterized by simultaneous granulocytic and monocytic differentiation; the proportion of promonocytes and monocytes exceeds 20% of the nucleated cells in marrow and/or blood (**Figs. 82 a-e**). Cytochemical analysis is imperative for diagnosis, and the most clear-cut results are obtained by double esterase incubation methods using α-naphthyl-acetate esterase and naphthol-ASD-chloracetate esterase. When stained with Fast Red Violet, myeloid cells will appear red and when stained with Fast-Garnet-GBC monocytoid cells will stain brown.

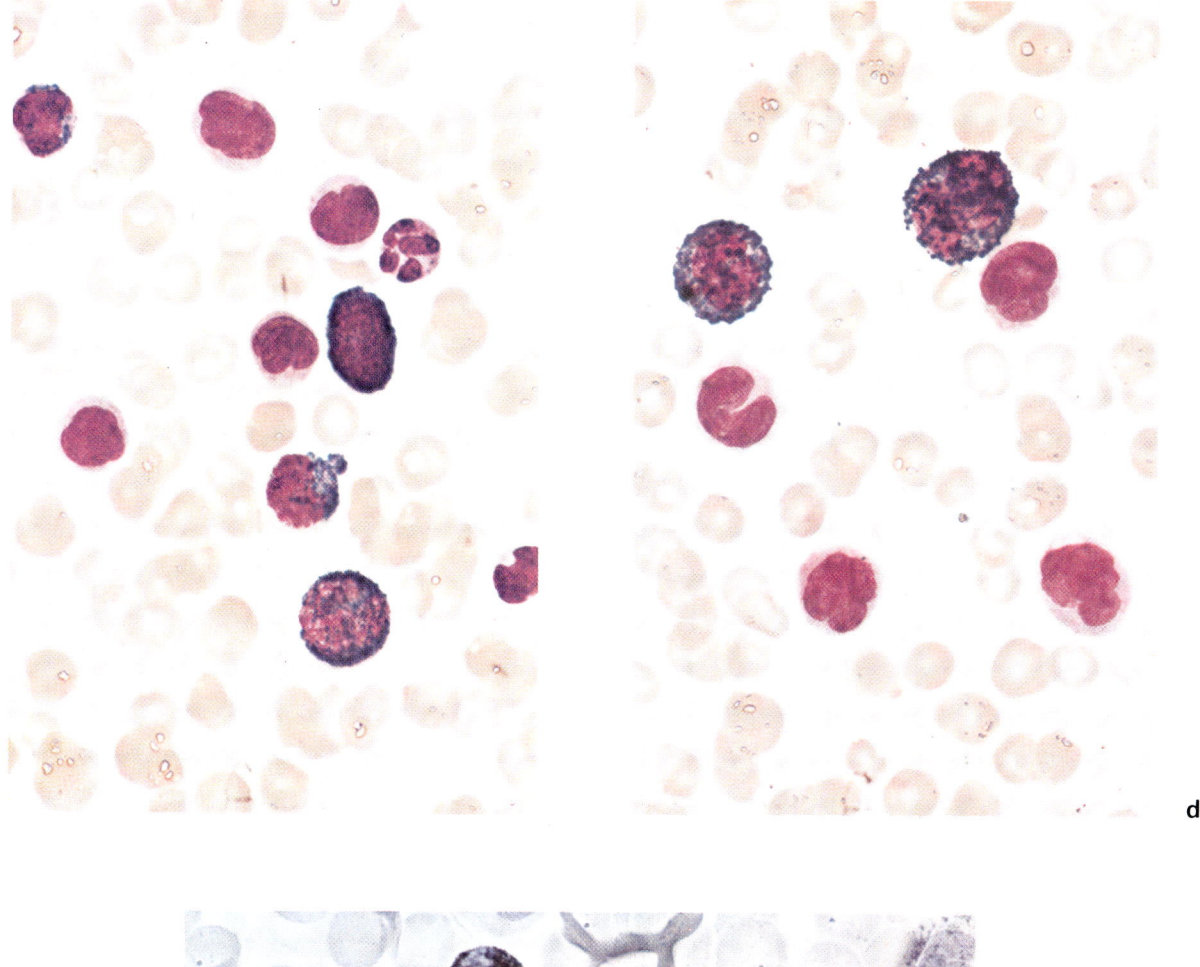
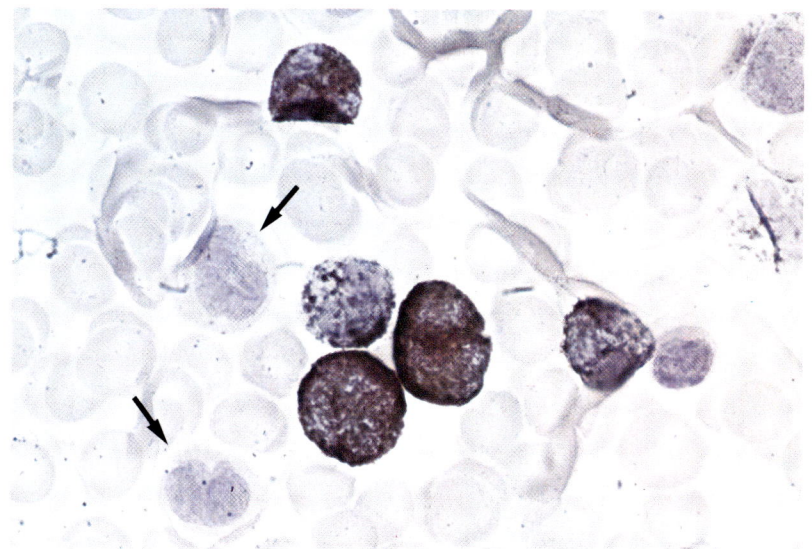

Fig. 82 c, d) Peroxidase-positive myeloid cells are distinguished from peroxidase-negative monocytoid cells.
e) Sudan black reaction also distinguishes positive granulocyte series from negative monocytoid cells. However, there is a great deal of overlap in these reactions, in some cases suggesting the common origin of these two cell lines. **Arrows** indicate monocytoid cells.

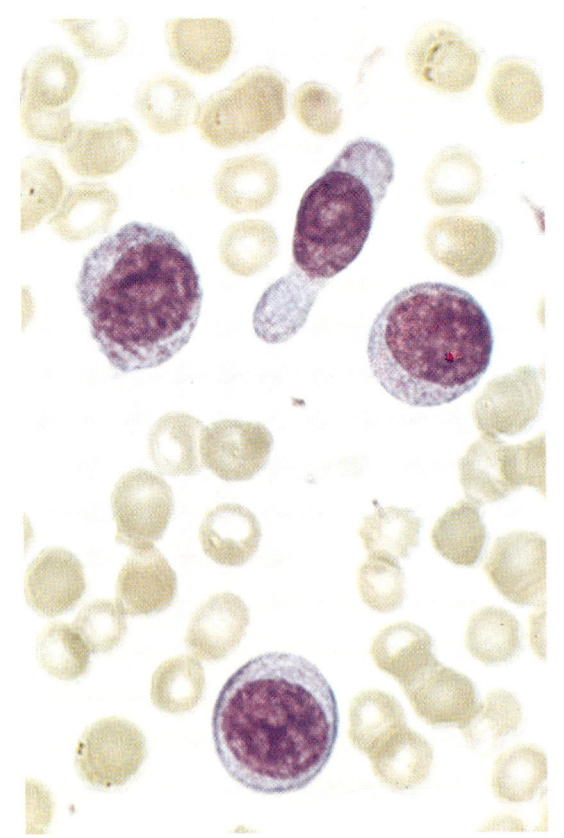
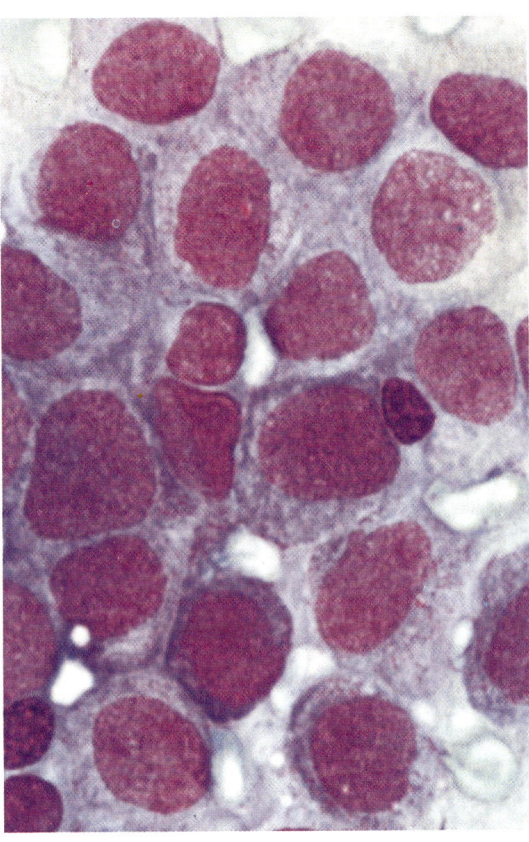
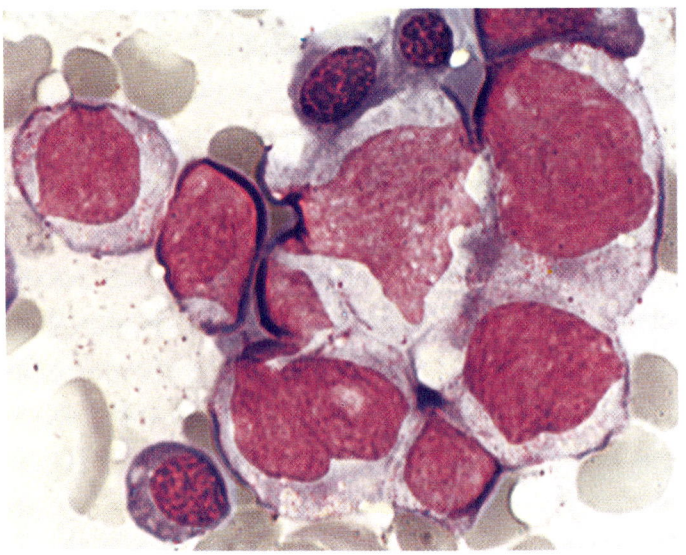

Fig. 83 AML, M 5 type. **a)** Monoblastic leukemia, peripheral blood. **b)** Monoblastic leukemia, bone marrow. **c)** Monocytic leukemia, bone marrow.

M 5, or (pure) monocytic leukemia (AMoL), is divided into two subtypes, the poorly differentiated (monoblastic) and the more differentiated, with promonocytes and monocytes. These cells must be shown to have fluoride inhibitable esterase activity (**Figs. 83 a, b,i, j**).

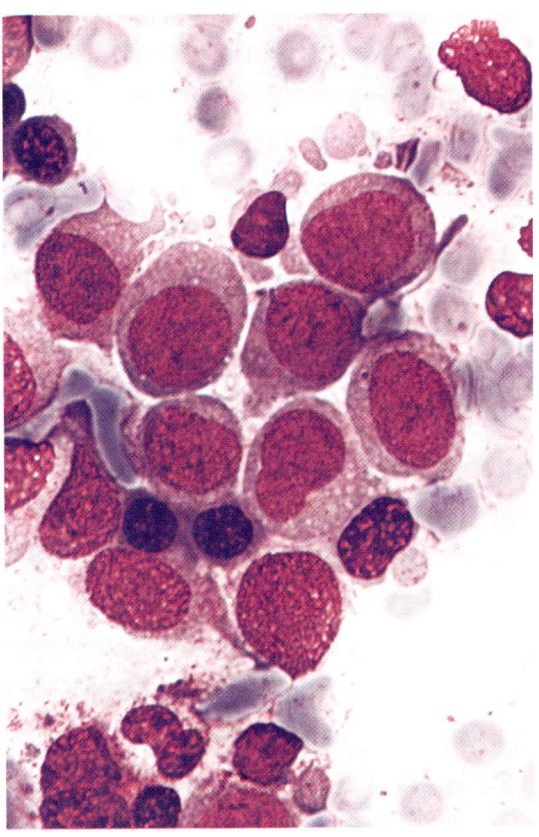
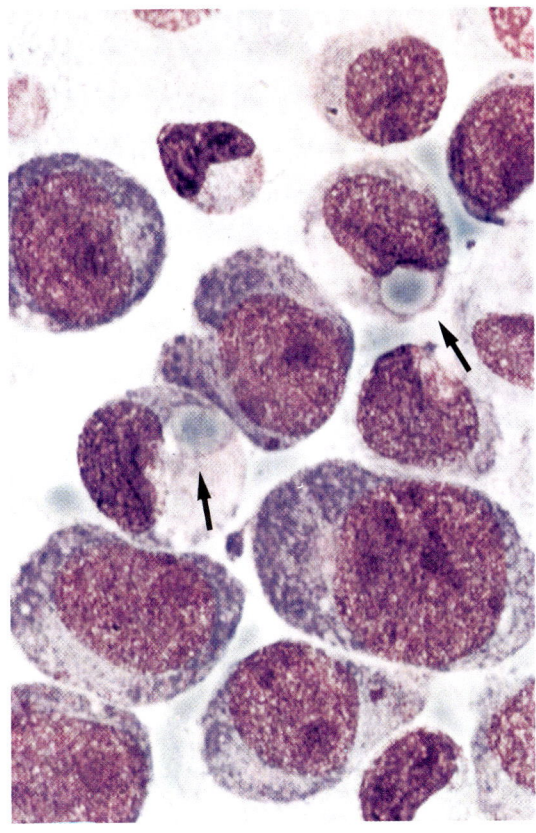
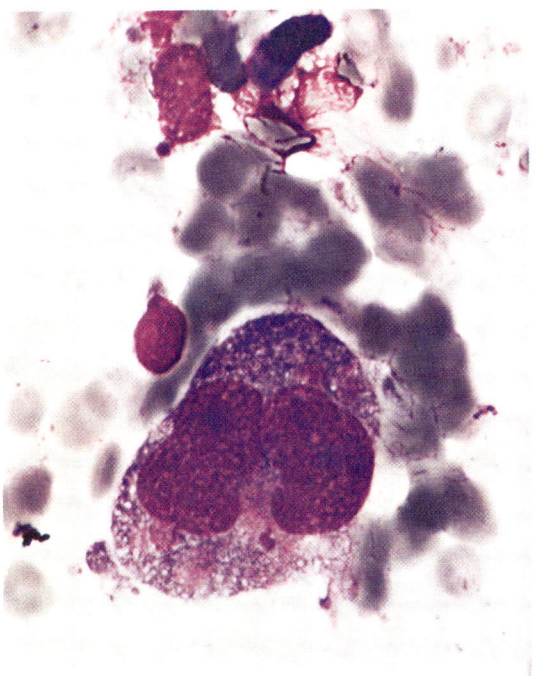
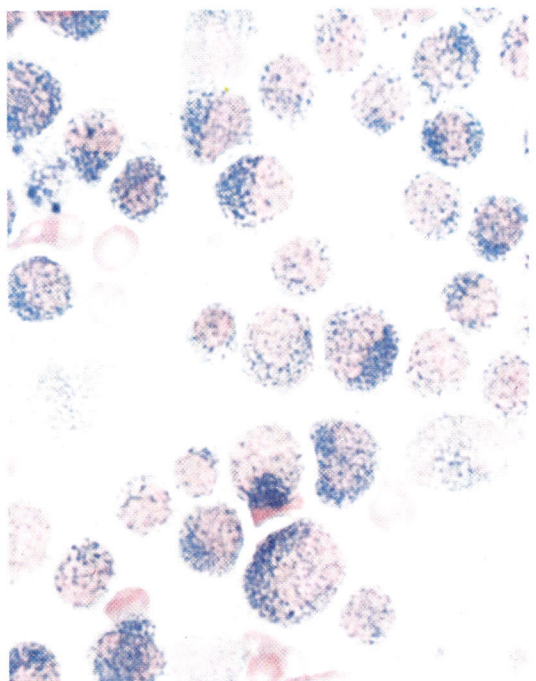

Fig. 83 d) *Monocytic leukemia, marrow.*
e) *Monoblastic leukemia without differentiation (type M 5 a). The cells have agranular, basophilic cytoplasm and not uncommonly display active erythrophagocytosis (**arrows**).*
f) *Aberrant monoblast reminiscent of a Reed-Stenberg cell in the marrow of a patient with AMoL. The diagnosis of AML, M 5 may hinge on cytochemical analyses: 1) positive naphthol-AS-D-acetate esterase reaction inhibited by NaF; 2) strong alpha-naphthyl esterase positivity; 3) lysozyme secretion as detected by the* Lysodeikticus *lysis.*
g) *Blast cells show strong naphthol-AS-D-acetate esterase positivity.*

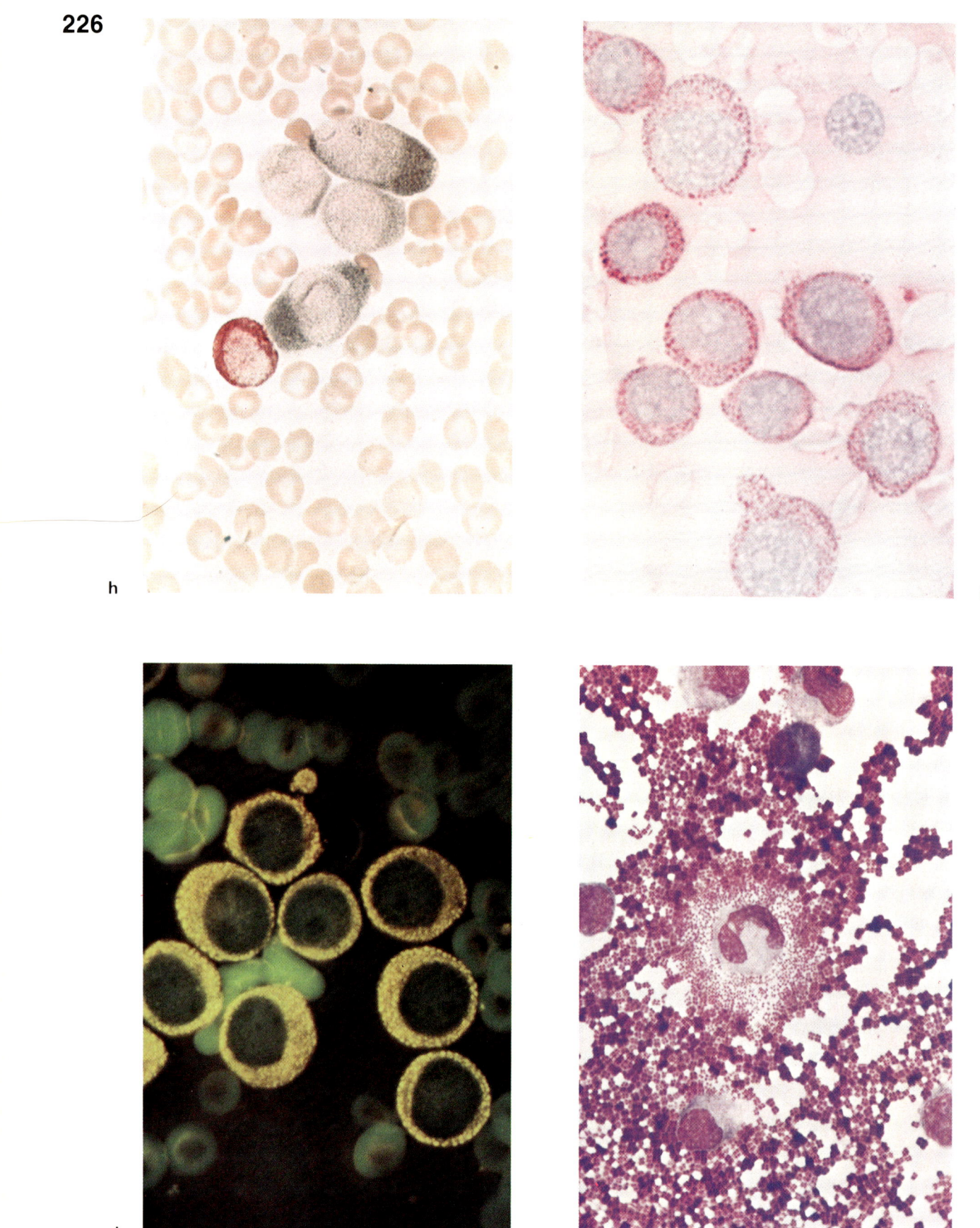

Fig. 83 h) A solitary myeloid cell is positive for naphthol-AS-D-chloroacetate esterase while the monocytoid cells are positive for alpha-naphthyl acetate esterase.
i, j) PAS reaction is positive in all cells, with both conventional (i) and fluorescent Schiff reagents (j).
k) Lysodeikticus lysis produced by a monocytoid cell. Courtesy of Dr. Liso, University of Bari.

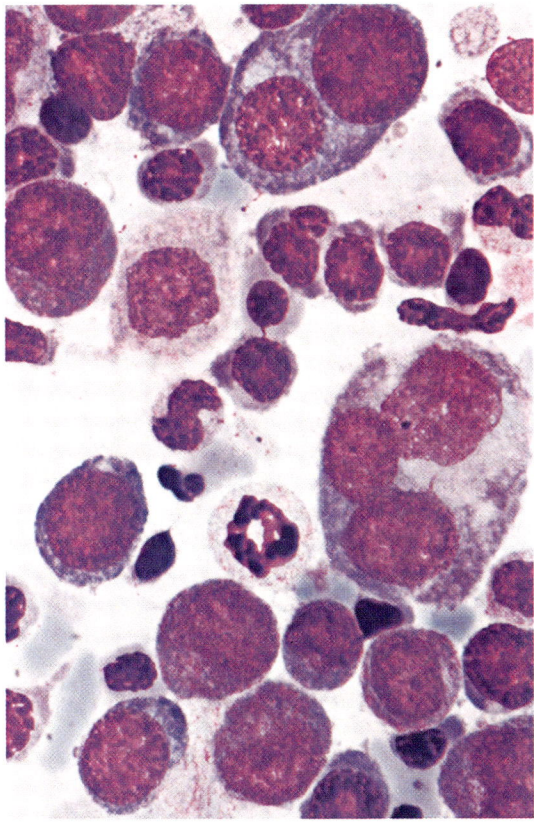
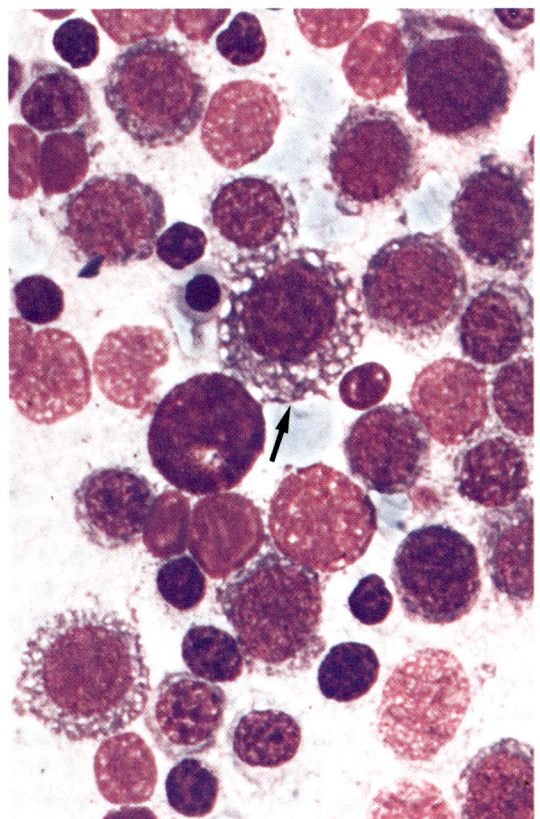
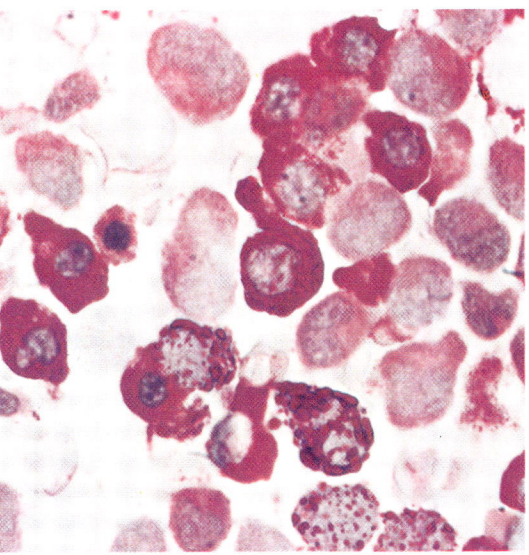
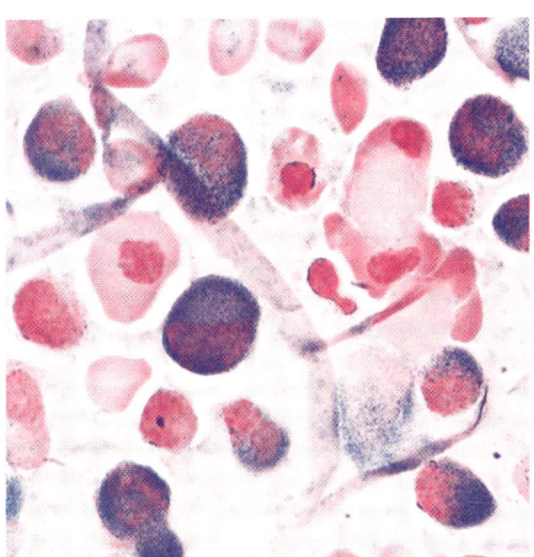

Fig. 84 *AML, M 6 type.*
a) *Marrow, erythroleukemia (often referred to as Di Guglielmo's syndrome); bizarre erythroid precursors with giant multinucleated cells are recognizable.*
b) *Marrow, erythroleukemia illustrating vacuolated erythroid precursors (**arrow**).*
c) *Erythroid cells in erythroleukemia are strongly positive with the PAS reaction.*
d) *Erythroleukemia, marrow. While the erytroid precursors are all strongly PAS-positive, only the myeloid progenitors are naphthol-AS-D-chloroacetate esterase positive.*

M 6 is characterized by a high (50%) bone marrow erythroblastosis; the erythroblasts are often atypical, with nuclear irregularity, giant polynuclear cells and megaloblastosis (**Figs. 84 a-c**). A strong PAS reaction of the erythroblastic cytoplasm (and of some erythrocytes) is the rule (**Fig. 84 c**). Abnormal megakaryocytes may be present. The percentage of myeloblasts and early promyelocytes is variable but, when less than 30%, erythroleukemia must be considered. M 6 generally progresses to M 1, M 2 or M 4.

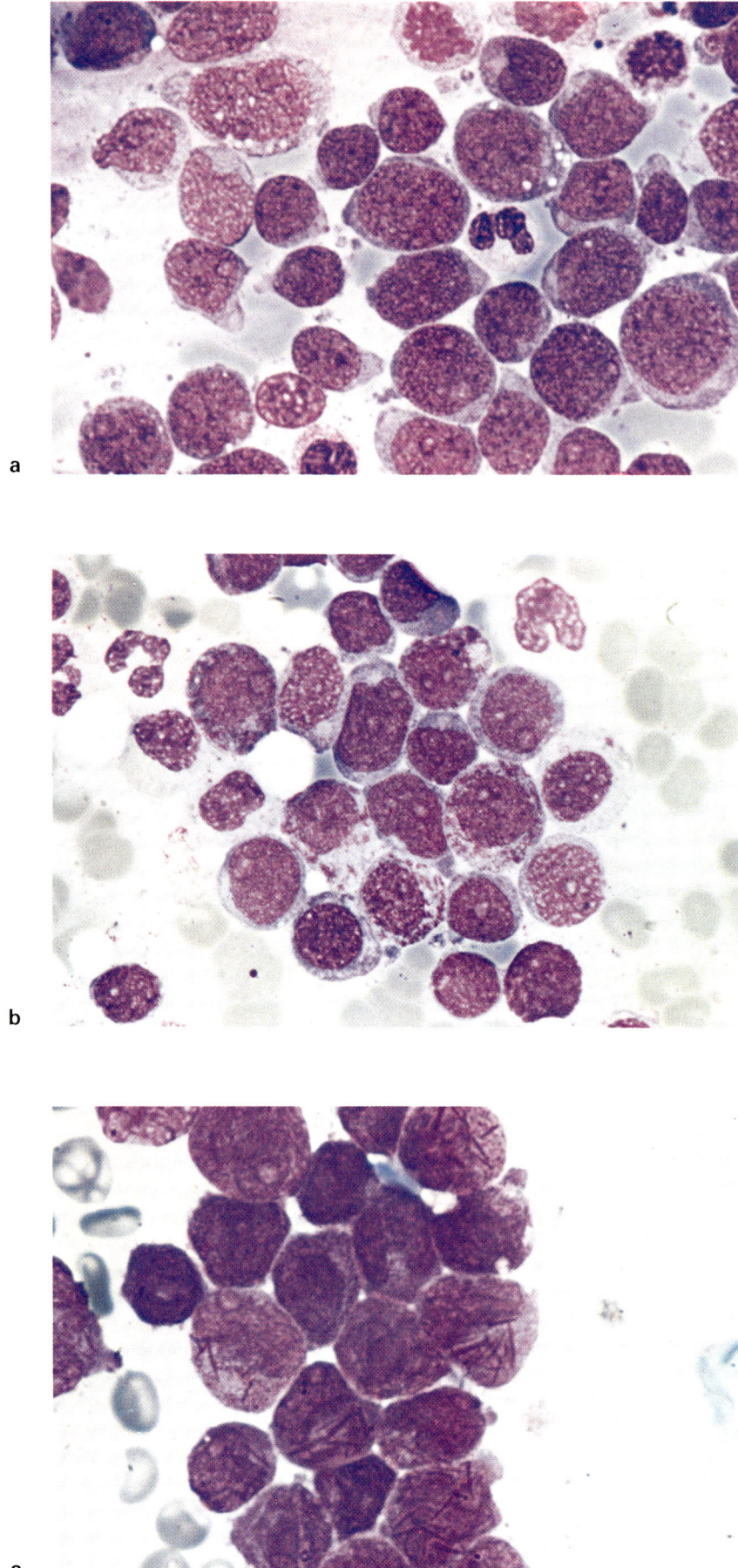

Fig. 85 *Representative illustrations of the six types of AML according to the FAB scheme.*
a, b, c) *M 1, M 2, M 3 types.*

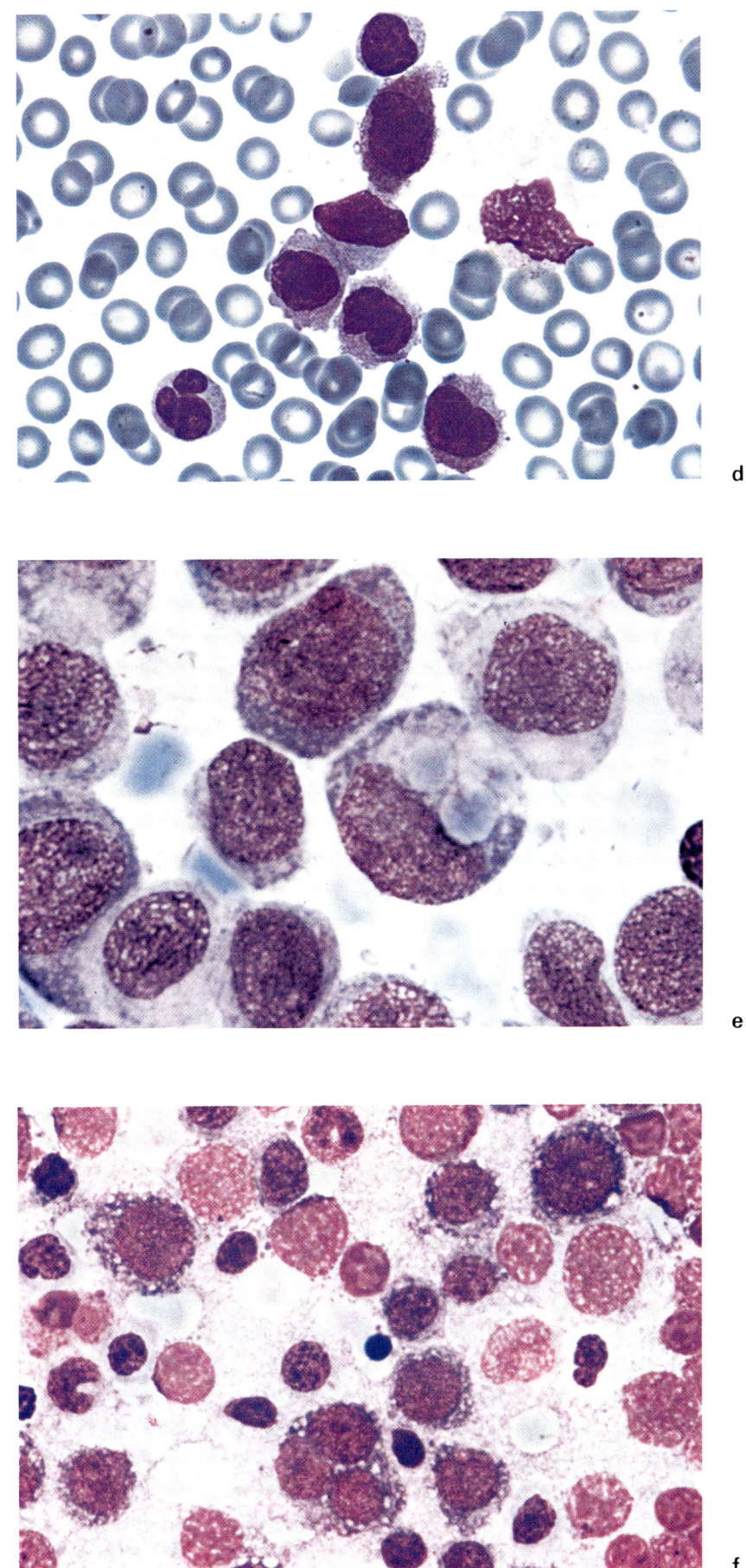

Fig. 85 *Representative illustrations of the six types of AML according to the FAB scheme.*
d, **e**, **f**) *M 4, M 5, M 6 types.*

6.3. Dysmyelopoietic syndromes (DMPS)

The term of dysmyelopoietic syndromes (DMPS) includes a group of "refractory" anemias most generally associated with quantitative and qualitative defects in the production of granulocytes and platelets [239]. DMPS are considered stem cell disorders, which often precede the development of AML [226]. Morphological, tissue culture and cytogenetic studies are helpful in the diagnostic workup.

Four groups of DMPS have been recognized. Among these are acquired idiopathic sideroblastic anemia (AISA; see Chapter 3) which is considered preleukemic; refractory anemia with excess of blasts (RAEB); chronic myelomonocytic syndromes (CMMS), as well as other, less well defined disease entities. The main feature of RAEB is an increased number (10-30%) of leukemic cells, mainly myeloblasts and promyelocytes. Recently micromegakaryocytes have been recognized as an additional diagnostic feature [240]. CMMS are seen in patients over 50 years of age. The most constant finding in these patients is a significant monocytosis associated with high levels of serum and urinary lysozyme.

Finally, there is a group of patients who do not fit either category, but who share with RAEB and CMMS patients the ill-defined symptoms, protracted course and unresponsiveness to conventional therapy. Some of the characteristic features of the dysmyelopoietic syndromes are listed in Table 1 and representative illustrations are shown in **Figure 86**.

Table 1 DYSMYELOPOIETIC SYNDROMES

	Acquired idiopathic sideroblastic anemia (AISA)	Erythroleukemia (EL)	Refractory anemia with excess of blasts (RAEB)	Chronic myelomonocytic leukemia (CMML)
Neutrophilic alterations (hypogranularity, etc.)	—	—	++	+
Monocytosis	—	—	—	+
Ringed sideroblasts	++	+	—	—
PAS-positive erythroblasts	—	++	±	—
Megaloblasts	—	++	+	—
Dyserythropoiesis	+	++	+++	—
Serum lysozyme increased	—	—	—	+
Emergence of PNH clone	±	±	±	±
Acute leukemic transformation	+	+++	++	+++

Fig. 86 a, b) Refractory anemia with excess of blasts (RAEB). Dyserythropoiesis is prominent.
c) Peripheral blood in chronic myelomonocytic leukemia.
d) A cluster of immature megakaryocytes in a case of RAEB. Ultrastructural demonstration of platelet peroxidase may be helpful for identification (see Chapter 10).
e, f, g, h) Examples of abnormal megakaryocytes seen in the marrow of patients with RAEB.

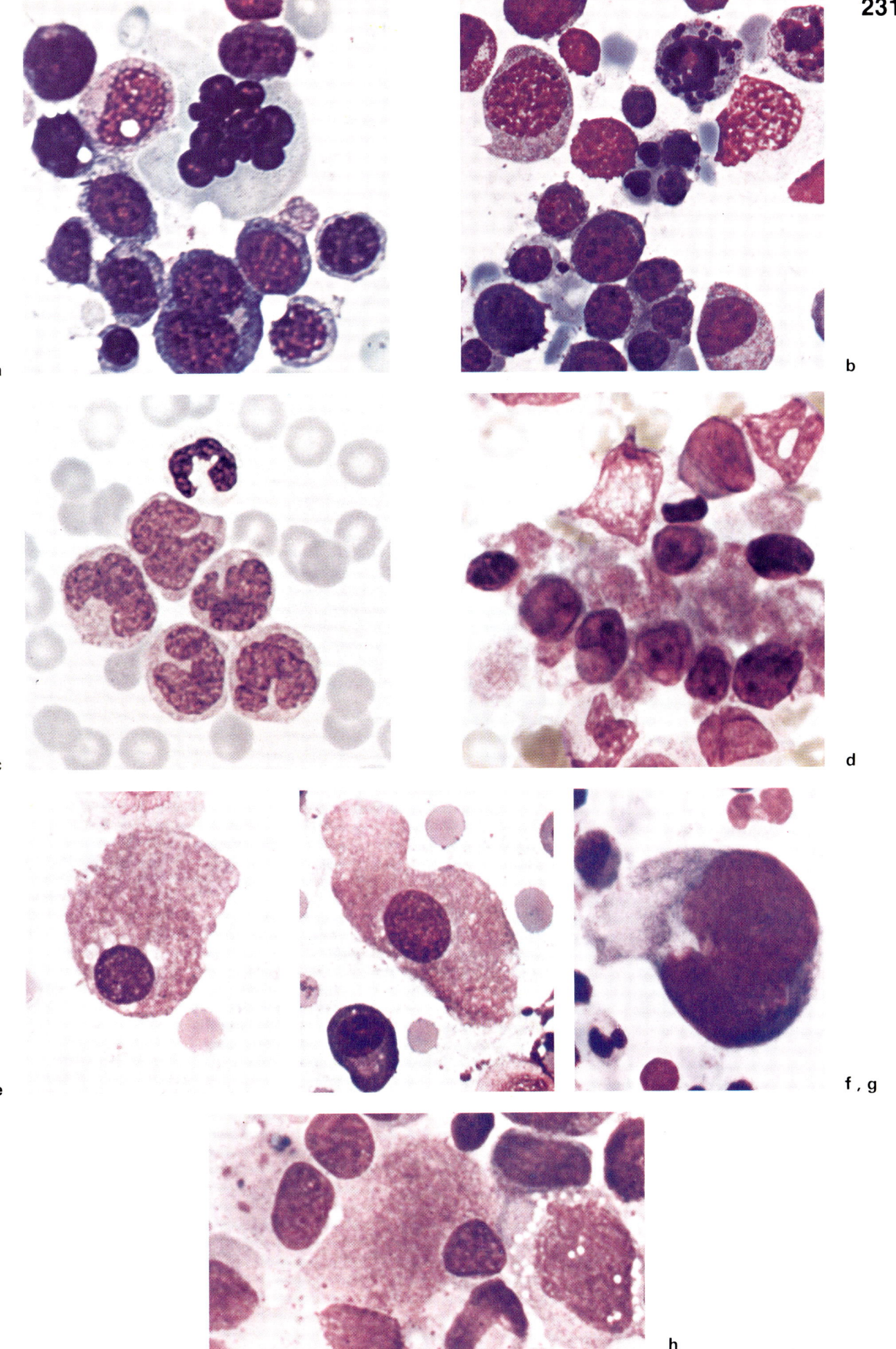

7. ADDITIONAL PHENOTYPIC CHARACTERISTICS AND MORPHOLOGIC ABNORMALITIES ASSOCIATED WITH MYELOGENOUS LEUKEMIAS

Membrane antigens have been studied in acute myeloid leukemias although not as extensively as in ALL. Antigens shared by monocytes and granulocytic cells may be expressed in AML, AMML and AMonL but not in ALL [241]. The majority of the former acute myeloid leukemias also express HLA-DR (Ia-like) antigens [242-244] which parallels the presence of these antigens on CFU-GM (see p. 149).

Although Terminal deoxynucleotidyl Transferase (TdT) is generally considered an enzyme marker for immature lymphocytes and their precursors (see p. 422, Chapter 9), occasional cases of AML, AMML or AMonL may be TdT positive [245, 246]. In some but not all cases the enzyme is restricted to a small "lymphoid" component as revealed by immunofluorescence tests [247].

Well prepared, Wright and Giemsa stained blood smears and bone marrow aspirates are still the mainstay in the diagnosis of the acute leukemias; however, precise classification which is of theoretical as well as clinical importance requires a combination of morphologic, cytochemical, immunologic and cytogenetic analyses [248-258].
Many of the morphologic criteria, e.g. the shape of the nucleus, the size of the nucleoli or the greater or lesser delicacy of the chromatin network have been shown to be features of immature cells, not necessarily leukemic. The most important morphologic marker for AML "blasts" is the presence of azurophilic granules. These granules may not be equatable with normal myeloperoxidase-containing lysosomes, but if they can be delineated with Sudan black, ASD chloroacetate esterase or peroxidase stains, myeloid derivation of the cell may be assumed. Moreover, even in the absence of granules, the enzymes may be detected ultrastructurally in the perinuclear space [11] or cisternae of rough ER (**Fig. 77**).

7.1. The Auer body

The Auer body is an eosinophilic rod-like structure which, when present, affords some aid in the diagnosis of AML (**Figs. 87 a-c**). Histochemical studies on the light and electron microscopic level have shown it to contain acid phosphatase [259, 260] as well as a number of other enzymes [261, 262]. Although the structures may be the result of abnormal granule production, they may also form as a consequence of fusion between granules and other organelles, i.e. as in the formation of autophagic vacuoles (**Figs. 87 b and c**). In the very undifferentiated AML (M 1), there is usually only one rod per cell whereas in APL a multitude of slender, needle-like rods may at times be seen to form faggots [263-265]. The procoagulant activity which results in thrombosis as well as catastrophic disseminated intravascular coagulation leading to hemorrhage, and which is characteristically associated with APL, may be attributable to the granule enzymes released by disintegrating cells.

Other morphologic aberrations, such as disorderly development of granules [228], unexplained nuclear and cytoplasmic inclusions and heterogeneity in size and staining characteristics are numerous. Some of these are illustrated in **Figures 83 f** and **88**. Some aspects of the acute monocytic leukemias (M 5) and of erythroleukemias (M 6) are also considered in Chapters 8 and 3 respectively.

Fig. 87 a) *Auer rod (arrow) in AML blast stained with May-Grünwald-Giemsa.*
b) *Leukemic promyelocyte showing a large Auer rod, a detail of which is illustrated at higher resolution in c. Also note peculiarly shaped nucleus with nucleolus and large area of filaments (F) between nuclear segments (× 12,000).*
c) *Detail of Auer rod delimited by the rectangle in b. Note that the structure is membrane-bound and filled with longitudinally arranged filamentous material. However, crystalloid and membrane-like components can also often be resolved. This suggests that some of the inclusions are formed by autophagy, i.e. fusion of lysosomes with other cellular organelles (× 85,000).*

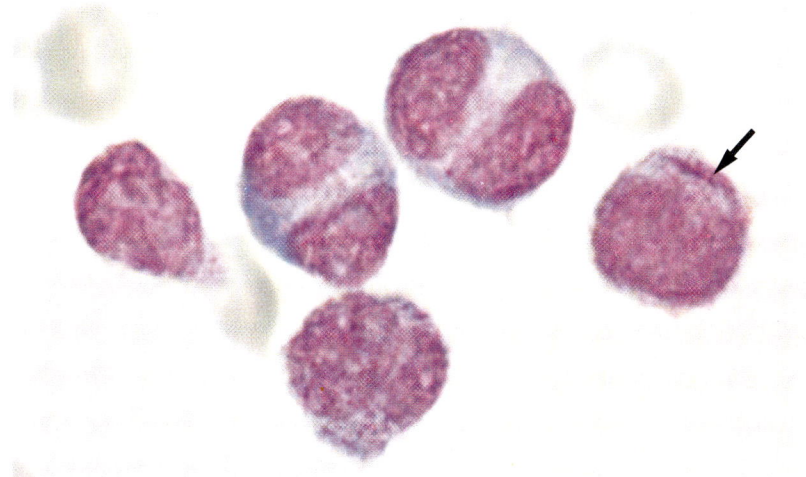

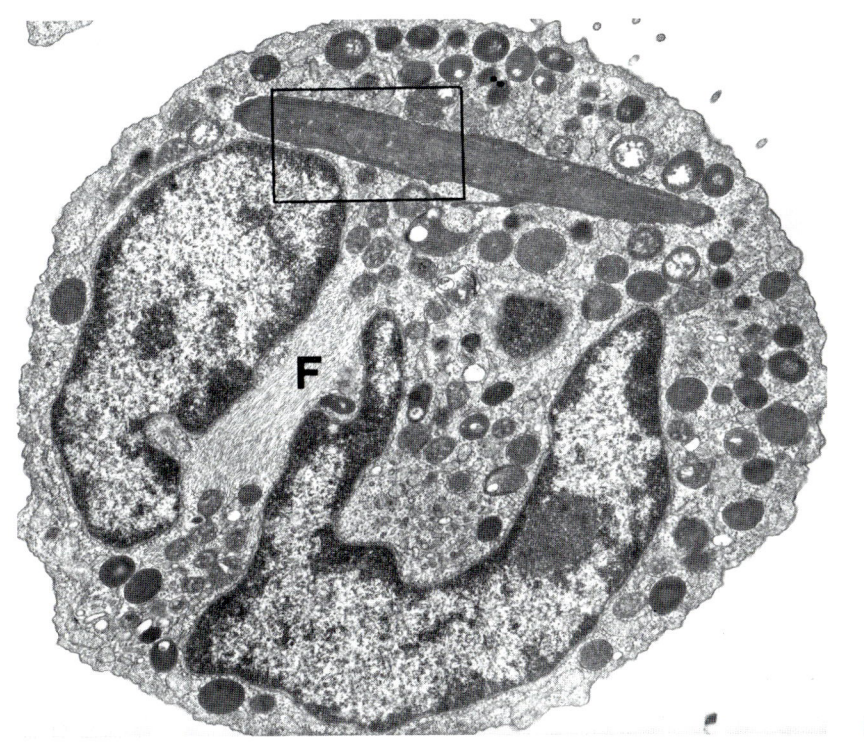

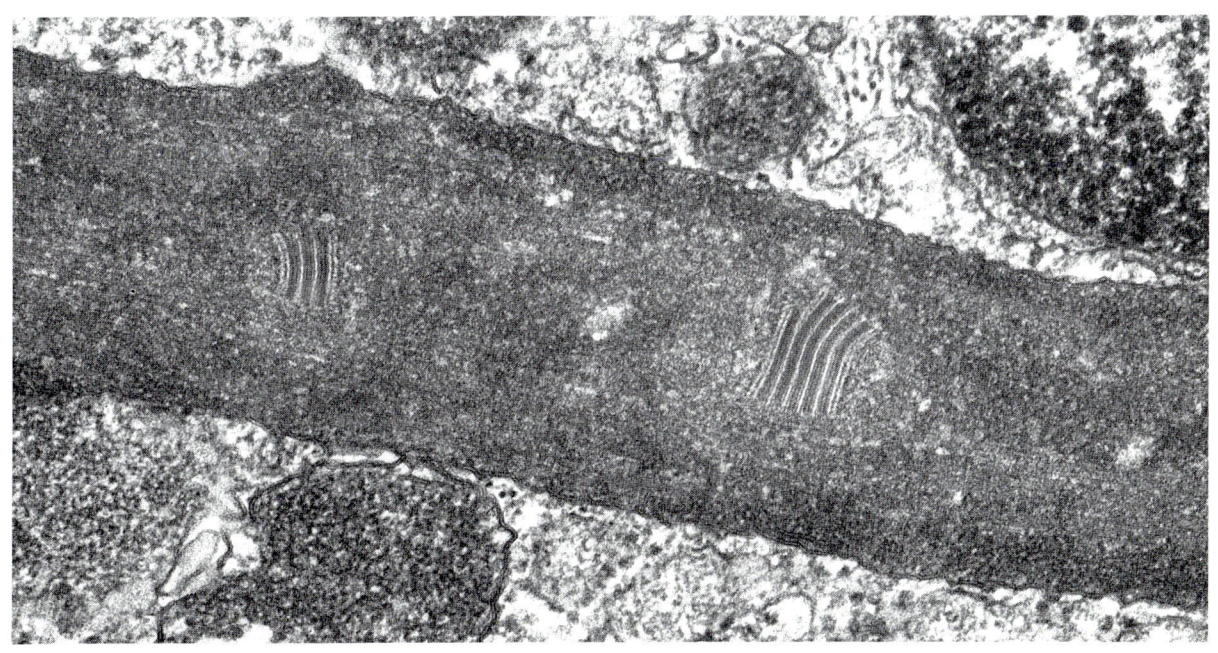

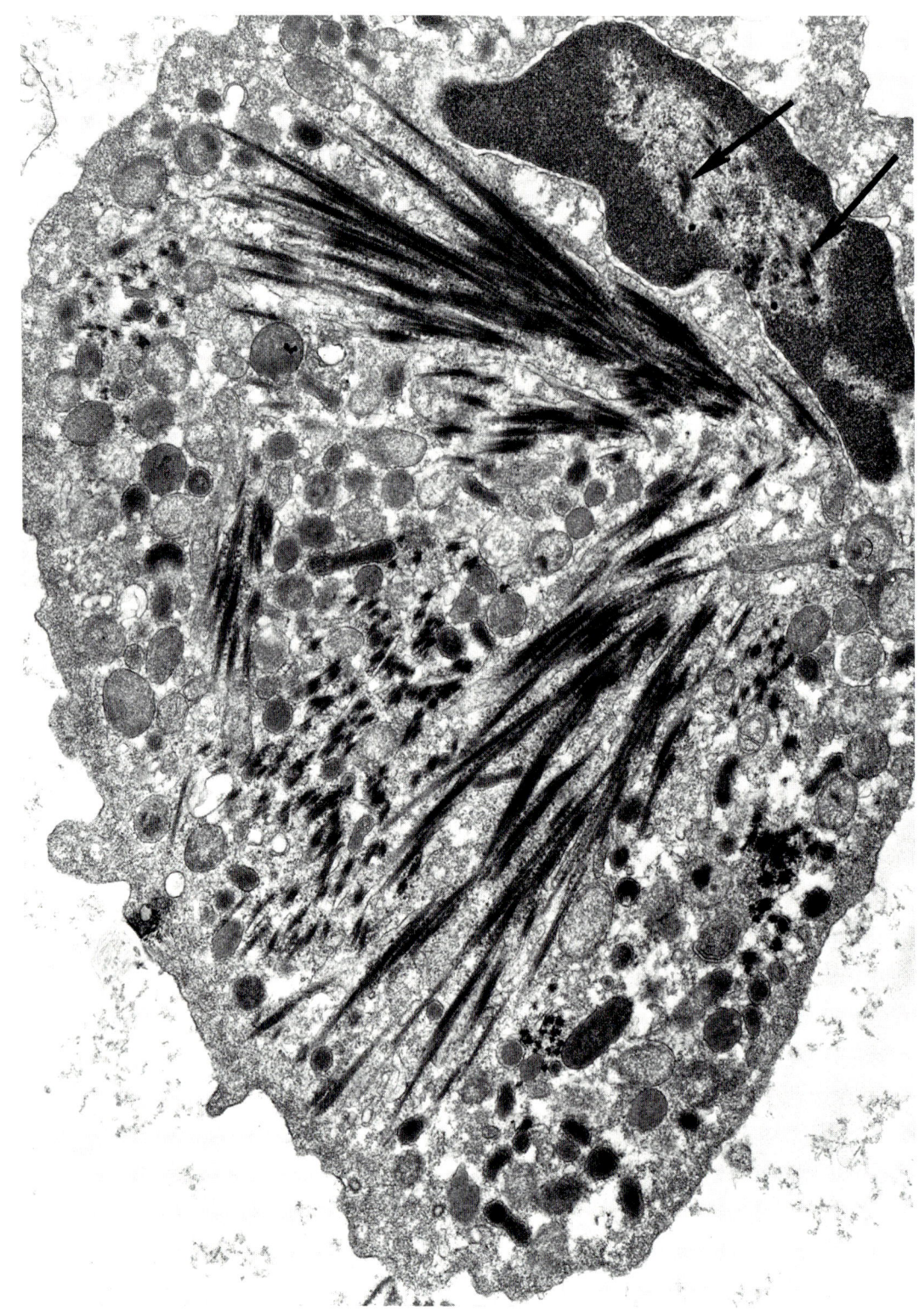

Fig. 88 Neutrophil from the bone marrow of a patient with unclassified hemopoietic dysplasia. Bundles of filaments resembling actin paracrystals are present throughout the cytoplasm as well as in the nucleus - where in this illustration they are seen in cross section (arrows). The nucleus has the chromatin distribution of a mature PMN and the granules appear normal ($\times$ 25,000).

4 NEUTROPHILS

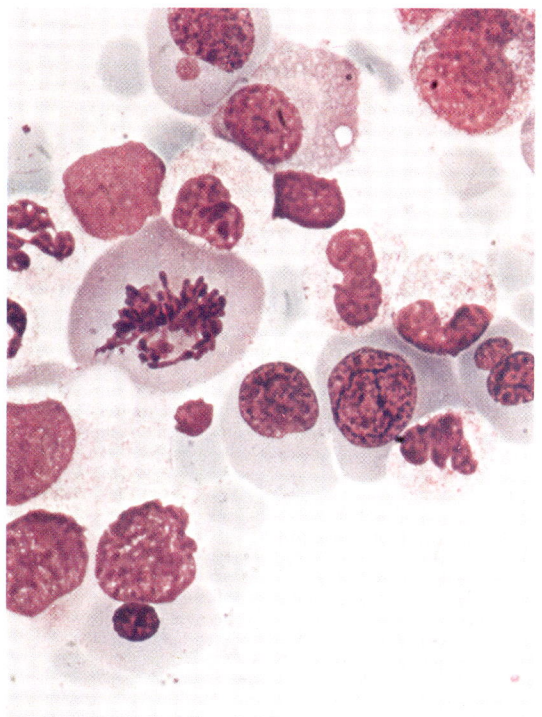
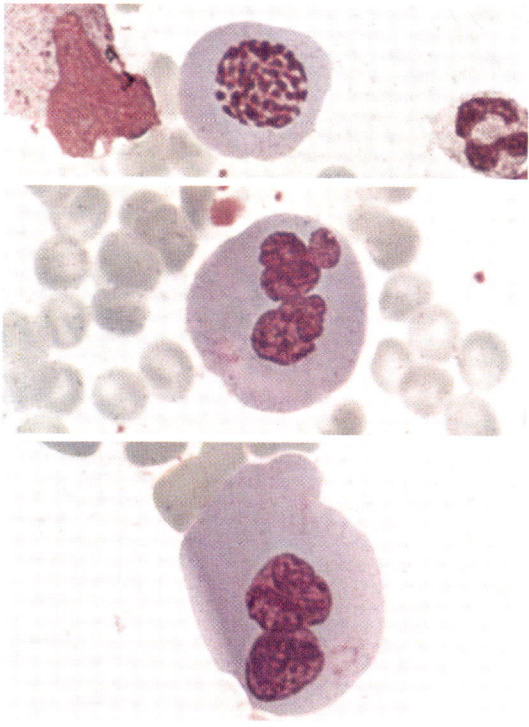
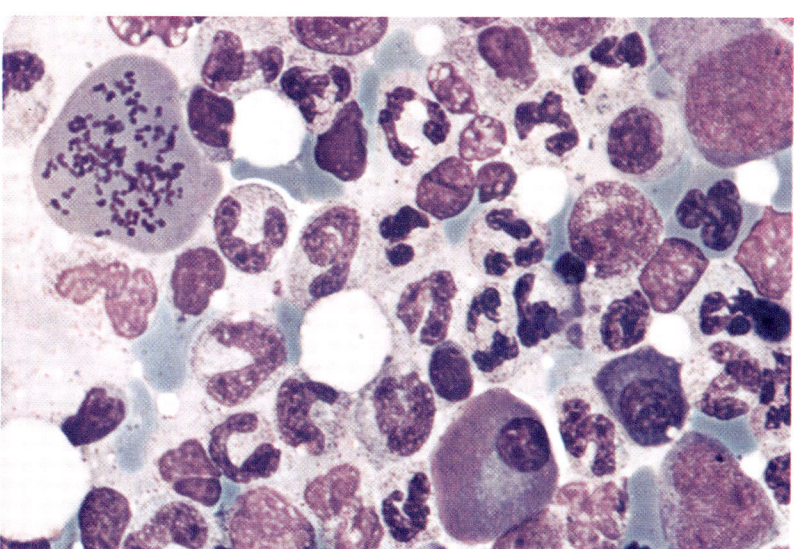

Fig. 89 a, b) *Extreme megaloblastic transformation induced by cytarabine.*
c) *Marrow aspirate illustrating effect of chemotherapy. Giant cell is seen in metaphase arrest. Excess of large metamyelocytes and vacuolated cells.*

8. BONE MARROW MORPHOLOGY AFTER THERAPY

Antileukemic therapy causes a wide variety of morphologic alterations in the bone marrow. These concern both leukemic and normal cells since all modalities of treatment are aimed at basic metabolic or biochemical aspects underlying cellular physiology. The greater susceptibility of the neoplastic cells is dependent on their rapid proliferation. The most striking effects are caused by antimetabolites and *Vinca* alkaloids. Both agents cause almost grotesque morphologic changes. In the case of the antifols, these consist mostly of severe megaloblastosis (**Figs. 89 a**, **b**). Vincristine, on the other hand, depolymerizes microtubules and therefore causes mitotic arrest in metaphase (**Fig. 89 c**). This is particularly striking when the lymphoid type of blast crisis in AML is treated with this drug (see **Fig. 74 f**). The aim of antileukemic therapy is complete remission as defined by normalization of the marrow, peripheral hemogram and clinical signs and symptoms. The bone marrow status is assessed through the analysis of two criteria, cellularity (C) and composition, with special regard to absence or percentage of leukemic cells (M). Five categories are recognized for each criterium, ranging from 0 to 4. Thus a totally infiltrated and intensely hypercellular marrow is rated as C_3M_4, while a complete remission with no recognizable leukemic cells may be rated as C_3M_1. A tabulation of these criteria as currently employed by CALGB (Cancer and Acute Leukemia, Group B; June 1975 modification of 1969 criteria) is given under (see also ref. 266).

Table 2 EVALUATION OF THE BONE MARROW STATUS IN ACUTE LEUKEMIA BEFORE AND AFTER TREATMENT

Rating	Blast cells (%)	Lymphocytes + blast cells (%)	Blast cells (%)	Blast cells + promyelocytes (%)
M_0				
M_1	0 - 5.0	0 - 40.0	0 - 5.0	0 - 10.0
M_2	5.1 - 25.0	40.1 - 70.0	5.1 - 25.0	10.1 - 30.0
M_{2x}	0 - 25.0	70.0	0 - 25.0	0 - 30.0
M_3	25.1 - 50.0	70.0	25.1 - 50.0	30.1 - 55.0
M_4	50.0	—	50.0	55.0

REFERENCES

1. Metcalf D.: *Hemopoietic colonies: in vitro cloning of normal and leukemic cells*. Springer-Verlag, Berlin-Heidelberg-New York, 1977.
2. Metcalf D.: *Detection and analysis of human granulocyte-monocyte precursors using semi-solid cultures*. Clin. Haemat., 8, 263, 1979.
3. Verheugt F.U.A. Von der Borne A.E.G. Kr., Decary F., Engelbriet C.P.: *The detection of granulocyte alloantibodies with an indirect immunofluorescence test*. Brit. J. Haemat., 36, 533, 1977.
4. Andersson L.C., Gahmberg C.G.: *Surface glycoproteins of human white blood cells. Analysis by surface labeling*. Blood, 52, 57, 1978.
5. Janossy G., Francis G.E., Capellaro D., Goldstone A.H., Greaves M.F.: *Cell sorter analysis of leukemia associated antigens on human myeloid precursors*. Nature, 276, 176, 1978.
6. Murphy P.: *The neutrophil*. Plenum, New York-London, 1976.
7. Ferrata A.: *Morfologia normale e patologica del sangue*. Soc. Ed. Libraria, 1912.
8. Ferrata A., Storti E.: *Le malattie del sangue*. Vallardi Ed., Milano, 1958.
9. Bessis M.: *Les cellules du sang*. Masson, Paris, 1972.
10. Bessis M.: *Blood smears reinterpreted*. Springer International, New York, 1977.
11. Bessis M., Maigne J.: *Le diagnostic de variétés de leucémies aiguës par la reaction des peroxydases au microscope électronique. Son interêt et ses limites*. Rév. Franç. d'Etudes Cliniques et Biologiques, 15, 691-698, 1970.
12. Undritz E.: *Hämatologische Tafeln Sandoz*. Sandoz AG, Basel, 1972.
13. Rohr K.: *Das menschliche Knochenmark*. Georg Thieme Verlag, Stuttgart, 1960.
14. Bainton D.F., Ullyot J.L., Farquhar M.G.: *The development of neutrophilic polymorphonuclear leukocytes in human bone marrow*. J. Exp. Med., 134, 907, 1971.
15. Bainton D.F.: *Neutrophil granules*. Brit. J. Haemat., 29, 17, 1972.
16. Scott R.E., Horn R.G.: *Ultrastructural aspects of neutrophil granulocyte development in humans*. Lab. Invest., 23, 202-215, 1970.
17. Baehner R.L.: *Microbe ingestion and killing by neutrophils normal mechanisms and abnormalities*. Clin. Haemat., 4, 609, 1975.
18. Zucker-Franklin D.: *Physiological and pathological variations in the ultrastructure of neutrophils and monocytes*. Clin. Haemat., 4, 485, 1975.
19. Cline M.J., Golde D.W.: *Granulocytes and monocytes: functional disorders*. In: Hoffbrand A.V., Brain M.C., Hirsch J. (eds.): *Recent Advances in Haematology*. Churchill Livingstone, Edinburgh-London-New York, p. 69, 1977.
20. Stossel T.P., Cohen H.J.: *Neutrophil function normal and abnormal*. In: Gordon A.S., Silber R., Lo Bue J. (eds.): *The Year in Hematology*. Plenum Press, New York-London, p. 192, 1977.

21. Bainton D.F., Farquhar M.G.: *Origin of granules in polymorphonuclear leukocytes: two types derived from opposite faces of the Golgi complex of developing granulocytes.* J. Cell. Biol., *28*, 277, 1966.
22. Baggiolini M.: *The enzymes of the granules of polymorphonuclear leukocytes and their functions.* Enzyme, *13*, 132, 1972.
23. Ohlsson G., Olsson I., Spitznagel J.K.: *Localization of chymotrypsin-like cationic protein, collagenase and elastase in azurophilic granules of human neutrophilic polymorphonuclear leukocytes.* Hoppe-Seyler Z. Physiol. Chem., *358*, 361, 1977.
24. Pryzwansky B., Rausch P.G., Spitznagel J.K., Herion J.C.: *Immunocytochemical distinction between primary and secondary granule formation in developing human neutrophils: correlations with Romanowsky stains.* Blood, *53*, 179, 1979.
25. Zucker-Franklin D.: *Electron microscopic studies of human granulocytes: structural variations related to function.* Seminars in Hematology, *5*, 109-133, 1968.
26. Zucker-Franklin D.: *Electron microscope study of the degranulation of polymorphonuclear leukocytes following treatment with streptolysin.* Am. J. Path., *47*, 419, 1965.
27. Tolksdorf M.: *Diagnosis of X chromatin by leukocyte test.* In: Schwarzacher H.G., Wolf U. (eds.): *Methods in Human Cytogenetics.* Springer Verlag, Berlin-Heidelberg-New York, p. 238, 1978.
28. Mittwoch U.: *The incidence of drumsticks in patients with three X chromosomes.* Cytogenetics, *2*, 241, 1963.
29. Mittwoch U.: *Sex chromosomes.* Academic Press, New York-London, 1967.
30. Zech L.: *Investigation of metaphase chromosomes with DNA-binding fluorochromes.* Exper. Cell. Res., *58*, 463, 1969.
31. Pearson P.L.: *The uniqueness of the human karyotype.* In: Caspersson T., Zech L. (eds.): *Chromosome Identification: Technique and Applications in Biology and Medicine.* Nobel Symposium, Vol. 23, Academic Press, New York, p. 145, 1973.
32. Schwarzacher H.G.: *Analysis of interphase nucleus.* In: Schwarzacher H.G., Wolf U. (eds.): *Methods in Human Cytogenetics.* Springer-Verlag, Berlin-Heidelberg-New York, p. 209, 1978.
33. Kosenow W.: *Nuclear appendages in leukocytes and the sex pattern of chromosomes.* In: Braunsteiner H., Zucker-Franklin D. (eds.): *The Physiology and Pathology of Leukocytes.* Grune & Stratton, New York, p. 196, 1962.
34. Cohn Z.A., Morse S.I.: *Functional and metabolic properties of polymorphonuclear leukocytes. Observation on the requirements and consequence of particle ingestion.* J. Exp. Med., *111*, 667, 1960.
35. Trubowitz S., Feldman D., Morgenstern S.W., Hunty M.: *The isolation, purification and properties of the alkaline phosphatase of human leukocytes.* Biochem. J., *80*, 369, 1961.
36. Kaplow L.S.: *Cytochemistry of leukocyte alkaline phosphatase: use of complex naphthol AS phosphates in azo dye-coupling techniques.* Am. J. Clin. Path., *39*, 439-449, 1963.
37. Hayhoe F.G.J., Quaglino D., Dell R.: *The cytology and cytochemistry of acute leukemia.* H.M. Stationary Office, London, pp. 17-68-86, 1964.
38. Dewald B., Rindler-Ludwig R., Bretz U., Baggiolini M.: *Subcellular localization and heterogeneity of neutral protease in neutrophilic polymorphonuclear leukocytes.* J. Exp. Med., *141*, 709, 1975.
39. Boggs D.R.: *Physiology of neutrophil proliferation, maturation and circulation.* Clin. Haemat., *4*, 535, 1975.
40. Rytomaa T.: *Chalones and blood cells.* In: Silber R., Lo Bue J., Gordon A. (eds.): *The Year in Hematology.* Plenum Medical Book Co., p. 321, 1978.
41. Kurland J., Moore M.A.S.: *The regulatory role of the macrophage in normal and neoplastic hemopoiesis.* In: Baum S.J., Ledney G.D. (eds.): *Experimental Hematology Today.* Springer-Verlag, Berlin-Heidelberg-New York, p. 51, 1977.
42. Kurland J.I., Broxmeyer H.E., Pelus L.M., Bockman R.S., Moore M.A.S.: *Role for monocyte-macrophage derived colony stimulating factor and prostaglandin E in the positive and negative feedback control of myeloid stem cell proliferation.* Blood, *52*, 388, 1978.
43. Chamberlain J.K., Lichtman M.A.: *Marrow cell egress: specificity of the site of penetration into the sinus.* Blood, *52*, 919, 1978.
44. Lichtman M.A., Chamberlain J.K., Santillo A.: *Factors thought to contribute to the regulation of egress of cells from marrow.* In: Silber R., Lo Bue J., Gordon A.S. (eds.): *The Year in Hematology.* Plenum, p. 243, 1978.
45. Marchesi V.T., Florey H.W.: *Electron microscopic observations on the emigration of leukocytes.* Q. J. Physiol., *45*, 343, 1968.
46. Majno G., Palade G.E.: *Studies on inflammation. I. The effect of histamine and serotonin on vascular permeability. An electron microscopic study. II. The site of action of histamine and serotonin along the vascular tree: a topographic study.* J. Biophys. Biochem. Cytol., *11*, 571 and 607, 1961.
47. Boyden S.: *The chemotactic effect of mixtures of antibody and antigen on polymorphonuclear leukocytes.* J. Exp. Med., *115*, 453, 1962.
48. Zigmond S.H., Hirsch J.G.: *Leukocyte locomotion and chemotaxis: new methods for evaluation and demonstration of cell-derived chemotactic factor.* J. Exp. Med., *137*, 387, 1973.
49. Gallin J.I., Gallin E.K., Schiffmann E.: *Mechanism of leukocyte chemotaxis.* In: Advances in inflammation research. Keissmann G., Samuelsson B., Paoletti R. (eds.). Raven Press, New York, *1*, 123, 1979.
50. Ramsey W.S., Grant L.: *Chemotaxis.* In: Zweifach B.W., Grant L., Mc Cluskey R.T. (eds.): *The Inflammatory Process.* Vol. 1, 2nd Edition, Chapter 5, Academic Press, New York, p. 287, 1974.
51. Gallin J.I., Wolff S.M.: *Leukocyte chemotaxis physiological considerations and abnormalities.* Clin. Haemat., *4*, 567, 1975.
52. Showell H.J., Freer R.J., Zigmond S.H., Schiffman E., Aswanikumar S., Corcoran B., Becker E.L.: *The structure-activity relations of synthetic peptides as chemotactic factors and inducers of lysosomal enzyme secretion for neutrophils.* J. Exp. Med., *143*, 1154, 1976.
53. Malech H.L., Root R.K., Gallin J.I.: *Structural analysis of human neutrophil migration.* J. Cell Biol., *75*, 666, 1977.
54. Ward P.A.: *The regulation of leukotactic mediators.* In: Sorkin E. (ed.): *Chemotaxis, Its Biology and Biochemistry.* Antibiotics and Chemotherapy, 19, 333. Karger, Basel, 1974.
55. Ward P.A.: *Leukotaxis and leukotactic disorders.* Am. J. Path., *77*, 520, 1974.
56. Hirsch J.G.: *Cinemicrophotographic observations on granule lysis in polymorphonuclear leukocytes during phagocytosis.* J. Exp. Med., *116*, 827, 1962.
57. Segal A.W., Dorling J., Coade S.: *Kinetics of fusion of the cytoplasmic granules with phagocytic vacuoles in human polymorphonuclear leukocytes.* J. Cell Biol., *85*, 42, 1980.
58. Zucker-Franklin D., Hirsch J.G.: *Electron microscopic studies on the degranulation of rabbit peritoneal leukocytes during phagocytosis.* J. Exp. Med., *120*, 569, 1964.
59. Zucker-Franklin D.: *The phagosomes in rheumatoid synovial fluid leukocytes – a light, fluorescence and electron microscope study.* Arth. & Rheum., *9*, 24, 1966.
60. Henson P.M.: *The immunologic release of constituents from neutrophil leukocytes. I. The rate of antibody and complement on non-phagocytoseable surfaces or phagocytoseable particles.* J. Immunol., *107*, 1535, 1971.
61. Hargraves M.M., Richmond H., Morton R.: *Presentation of two bone marrow elements: the "Tart" cell and "LE" cell.* Proc. Staff Meet. Mayo Clin., *23*, 25, 1948.
62. Hargraves M.M.: *The LE phenomenon.* Adv. Intern. Med. Year Book Publ., Chicago, 1954.
63. Marmont A.: *Beobachtungen über das sogenannte LE Phänomen.* Schw. Med. Wschr., *82*, 1111, 1952.
64. Heller P., Zimmerman H.J.: *Nucleophagocytosis. Studies on 336 patlents.* Arch. Intern. Med., *97*, 403, 1956.

65. Marmont A.: *The transfusion of active LE plasma into non-lupus recipients with a note on the LE-like cell.* Ann. N.Y. Acad. Sci., *24*, 838, 1965.
66. Bencze G., Cserhati S., Kovacs J., Tiboldi T.: *Production of LE cells in vivo by transfusions of systemic lupus erythematosus plasma.* Ann. Rheum. Dis., *17*, 426, 1958.
67. Chomet B., Kirshen M.M., Schlefer G., Mudrick P.: *The finding of LE (Lupus Erythematosus) cells in smears of untreated freshly drawn peripheral blood.* Blood, *8*, 1107, 1953.
68. Godman G.C., Deitch A.D., Klemperer P.: *The composition of the LE bodies of systemic lupus erythematosus II proteins.* J. Exp. Med., *106*, 593, 1957.
69. Barnes G.W., Sullivan M.A., Beutner E.H., Witebsky E.: *In vitro and in vivo interaction of nuclear antibodies with corresponding antigens.* Experientia, *21*, 485, 1965.
70. Marmont A.M., Pluma A.M., Capponi G.: *Eine einfache, empfindliche und sichere Methode zur Auslösung des LE Phänomens durch mechanische Schädigung der Leukocyten des substrates mit besonderer Berücksichtigung der Befunde bei Lupus erythematodes und Polyarthritis chronica.* Schw. Med. Wschr., *39*, 1, 1957.
71. Zinkham W.H., Conley C.L.: *Some factors influencing the formation of LE cells. Method for enhancing LE cell production.* Bull. Johns Hopkins Hosp., *88*, 102, 1956.
72. Damasio E., Marcolongo R., Marmont A.M.: *Recenti acquisizioni sugli anticorpi antinucleari e sul fattore reumatoide. Definizioni, ricerca, significato clinico ed immunopatologico.* La Med. Int., *22*, 1975.
73. Feltkamp T.E. (ed.): *The significance of the determination of anti-DNA, and DNA/anti-DNA complexes.* Scand. J. Rheum. (Suppl.), *11*, 1, 1975.
74. Gonzalez E.N., Rothfield N.: *Immunoglobulin class and pattern of nuclear fluorescence in systemic lupus erythematosus.* New Engl. J. Med., *274*, 1333, 1966.
75. Barnett S.V., Bakemeier R.P., Leddy J.P., Vaugham J.H.: *Gamma 2, Gamma 1 A, and Gamma 1 M antinuclear factors in human sera.* J. Clin. Invest., *43*, 1104, 1964.
76. Notman D.D., Kurata N., Tan E.M.: *Profiles of antinuclear antibodies in systemic rheumatic diseases.* Ann. Int. Med., *83*, 464, 1975.
77. Aarden L.A., De Groot E.R., Feltkamp T.E.W.: *Immunology of DNA. III. Crithidia luciliae, a simple substrate for the determination of anti-ds DNA with the immunofluorescence technique.* Ann. N.Y. Acad. Sci., *254*, 505, 1975.
78. Chubick A., Sontheimer R.D., Gillian S.N., Ziff M.: *An appraisal of tests for native DNA antibodies in connective tissue diseases. Clinical usefulness of Crithidia luciliae assay.* Ann. Int. Med., *89*, 186, 1978.
79. Marmont A., Damasio E., Giordano D., Cerri R., Banchi L.: *Some modern aspects of systemic lupus erythematosus with special reference to the treatment with cyclophosphamide of lupus nephritis.* In: Weissman G., Samuelsson B., Paoletti R. (eds.). Adv. Inflamm. Res., *1*, 591, 1979.
80. Mc Carty D.J.: *Mechanisms of the crystal deposition diseases gout and pseudogout.* Ann. Int. Med., *78*, 767, 1973.
81. Schumacher H.R., Phelps P.: *Intravascular changes in human polymorphonuclear leukocytes after urate crystal phagocytosis. An electron microscopic study.* Arthr. Rheum., *14*, 513, 1971.
82. Mc Carty J., Kozin F.: *An overview of cellular and molecular mechanisms in crystal induced inflammation.* Arthr. Rheum., *18*, 757, 1975.
83. Schumacher H.R., Fishbein P., Phelps P., Tse R., Krauser R.: *Comparison of sodium urate and calcium phosphate crystal phagocytosis by polymorphonuclear phagocytes.* Arthr. Rheum., *18*, 783, 1975.
84. Wallingford W.R., Mc Carty D.J.: *Differential membranolytic effects of microcrystalline sodium urate and calcium pyrophosphate dihydrate.* J. Exp. Med., *133*, 100, 1971.
85. Mc Carty D.J.: *Calcium pyrophosphate dihydrate crystal deposition disease: nomenclature and diagnostic criteria.* Ann. Int. Med., *87*, 240, 1977.
86. Coatter R.A.: *The use of the compensated polarizing microscope.* Clin. Rheum. Dis., *3*, 91, 1977.
87. Dieppe P.A., Huskisson E.G., Crocker P., Willoughby D.A.: *Apatite deposition disease. A new arthropathy.* Lancet, *i*, 266, 1976.
88. Phelps P.: *Polymorphonuclear leukocyte motility in vitro. IV. Colchicine inhibition of chemotactic activity formation after phagocytosis of urate crystals.* Arthr. Rheum., *13*, 1, 1970.
89. Naff G.B., Byers P.H.: *Complement as a mediator of inflammation in acute gouty arthritis. I. Studies on the reaction between human serum complement and urate crystals.* J. Lab. Clin. Med., *81*, 747, 1973.
90. Malawista S.E.: *The action of colchicine in acute gouty arthritis.* Arthr. Rheum., *18*, 835, 1975.
91. Weissmann G. (ed.): *Mediators of inflammation.* Plenum Press, New York, 1974.
92. Rossi F., Dri P., Bellavite P., Zabucchi G., Berton G.: *Oxidative metabolism of inflammatory cells.* In: Weissman G. et al. (eds.): *Advances in Inflammation Research.* Vol. 1. Raven Press, New York, 1979.
93. Spitznagel J.K.: *Bactericidal mechanisms of the granulocyte.* In: Greenwalt T.J., Jamieson G.A. (eds.): *The Granulocyte.* Vol. 13 of Progs. in Clin. & Biol. Research. Alan R. Liss, Inc., New York, p. 103, 1977.
94. Lay W.H., Nussenzweig V.: *Receptors for complement on leukocytes.* J. Exp. Med., *129*, 991, 1968.
95. Atkinson J.P., Frank M.M.: *Role of complement in the pathophysiology of hematologic diseases.* In: Brown E.B. (ed.): *Progress in Hematology.* Grune & Stratton, New York-San Francisco-London, p. 211, 1977.
96. Ehelenberger A.G., Nussenzweig V.: *Phagocytosis: role of C3 receptors and contact-inducing agents.* In: Gordon A.S., Silber R., Lo Bue J. (eds.): *The Year in Hematology.* Plenum Press, New York-London, p. 221, 1977.
97. Berlin R.D., Fera J.P., Pfeiffer J.R.: *Reversible phagocytosis in rabbit polymorphonuclear leukocytes.* J. Clin. Invest., *63*, 1137-1144, 1979.
98. Elsbach P., Zucker-Franklin D., Sansaricq C.: *Increased lecithin synthesis during phagocytosis by normal leukocytes and by leukocytes of a patient with chronic granulomatous disease.* New Engl. J. Med., *280*, 1319, 1969.
99. Elsbach P., Farrow S.: *Cellular triglyceride as a source of fatty acid for lecithin synthesis during phagocytosis.* Biochim. Biophys. Acta, *176*, 438, 1969.
100. Stossel T.P., Pollard T.D.: *Myosin in polymorphonuclear leukocytes.* J. Biol. Chem., *248*, 8288, 1973.
101. Boxer L.A., Hedley-Whyte E.T., Stossel T.P.: *Neutrophil actin dysfunction and abnormal neutrophil motility.* New Engl. J. Med., *293*, 1093, 1974.
102. Boxer L.A., Stossel T.P.: *Interaction of actin, myosin and an actin-binding protein of chronic myelogenous leukemic leukocytes.* J. Clin. Invest., *57*, 964, 1976.
103. Zurier R.B., Weissmann G., Hoffstein S.: *Mechanisms of lysosome release from human leukocytes. Effects of cyclic AMP and cyclic GMP autonomic antagonists and agents which affect microtubule function.* J. Clin. Invest., *53*, 297, 1974.
104. Klebanoff S.J.: *Iodination of bacteria: a bactericidal mechanism.* J. Exp. Med., *126*, 1063-1078, 1967.
105. Klebanoff S.J.: *Antimicrobial systems of polymorphonuclear leukocytes.* In: Balanta J.A., Dayton D.H. (eds.): *The Phagocytic Cell and Host Resistance.* Raven Press, New York, p. 45, 1975.
106. Nakamura R.M.: *Immunopathology. Clinical laboratory concepts and methods.* Little Brown, Boston, 1974.
107. Quie P.G., Mills E.L., Holmes B.: *Molecular events during phagocytosis by human neutrophils.* In: Brown E.B. (ed.): *Progress in Hematology.* Grune & Stratton, New York-San Francisco-London, p. 193, 1977.
108. Allen R.C., Yevich S.J., Orth R.W.: *The superoxide anion and singlet molecular oxygen. Their role in the microbicidal activity of the polymorphonuclear leukocyte.* Biochem. Biophys. Res. Commun., *60*, 909, 1974.
109. Matula G., Paterson P.Y.: *Spontaneous in vitro reduction of nitroblue tetrazolium by neutrophils*

of adult patients with bacterial infection. New Engl. J. Med., 285, 211-317, 1971.
110. Pelger K.: *Demonstratie van een paar zeldzaam voorkomende typhen van bloedlichaampjes en bespreking der patienten.* Discuss. Med. Tijdschr. Geneesk., 11, 1264, 1932.
111. Huët G.J.: *Familial anomaly of leukocytes.* Discuss. Med. Tijdschr. Geneesk.
112. Begemann W.H., Campagne A.: *Homozygous form of Pelger-Huët's nuclear anomaly in man.* Acta Haemat., 7, 295, 1952.
113. Harm H.: *Beitrage zur morphologie und Genetik der Pelger Anomalie bei Menschen und Kaninchen.* Z. Menschl. Vererb., 30, 501, 1952.
114. Pierre R.S.: *Preleukemic states.* Semin. Hemat., 11, 73, 1974.
115. Linman J.W., Bagby C.C.: *The preleukemic syndrome: clinical and laboratory features, natural course and management.* Blood Cells, 2, 11, 1976.
116. Heimpel H.: *Conventional morphological examination of blood and bone marrow cells in the diagnosis of preleukemic syndromes.* In: Schmalzl F., Hellriegel K.P. (eds.): *Preleukemia.* Springer-Verlag, Berlin-Heidelberg-New York, p. 4, 1979.
117. Undritz E., Schali H.: *Eine neue Sippe mit erblich konstitutioneller Hochsegmentierung der Neutrophilen Kerne und des Knochenmarkbildes beim homozygoten Träger dieser Anomalie.* Schweiz. Med. Wschr., 94, 1365, 1964.
118. Herbert V.: *Megaloblastic anemias – mechanism and management.* Disease-a-Month, Yearbook Publishers, Chicago, August 1965.
119. Orfanakis N.G., Ostlund R.E., Bishop G.R., Athens J.W.: *Normal blood leukocyte concentration values.* Am. J. Clin. Path., 53, 647, 1970.
120. Fliedner T.H., Cronkite E.P., Killmann S.A., Bond V.P.: *Granulocytopoiesis. II. Emergence and pattern of labelling of neutrophilic granulocytes in humans.* Blood, 24, 683-700, 1964.
121. Gordin R.: *Toxic granulation in leukocytes.* Acta Med. Scand. (Suppl.), 270, 1, 1952.
122. Mc Call C.E.: *Lysosomal and ultrastructural changes in human toxic neutrophils during bacterial infection.* J. Exp. Med., 129, 267, 1969.
123. Buchanan J.G., Pearce L., Wetherly-Mein G.: *The May-Hegglin anomaly.* Brit. J. Haemat., 10, 508, 1964.
124. Cawley J.C., Hayhoe F.G.: *The inclusions of the May-Hegglin anomaly and Döhle bodies of infection: an ultrastructural comparison.* Brit. J. Haemat., 22, 491, 1972.
125. Jordan S.W., Larsen W.E.: *Ultrastructural studies of the May-Hegglin anomaly.* Blood, 25, 921, 1965.
126. Blume R.S., Wolff S.M.: *The Chediak-Higashi syndrome: studies in four patients and a review of the literature.* Medicine, 51, 247, 1972.
127. Wolff S.M., Dale D.C., Clark R.A., Root R.K., Kimball H.R.: *The Chediak-Higashi syndrome: studies of host defenses.* Ann. Int. Med., 76, 293, 1972.
128. Clark R.A., Kimball H.R., Padgett G.A.: *Granulocyte chemotaxis in the Chediak-Higashi syndrome of mink.* Blood, 39, 644, 1972.
129. Davis W.C., Spicer S.S., Greene W.B., Padgett G.A.: *Ultrastructure of bone marrow granulocytes in normal mink and mink with the homologue of the Chediak-Higashi trait of humans: I. Origin of the abnormal granules present in the neutrophils of mink with C-H trait.* Lab. Invest., 24, 303, 1971.
130. Davis W.C., Spicer S.S., Greene W.B., Padgett G.A.: *Ultrastructure of cells in bone marrow and peripheral blood of normal mink and mink with the homologue of the Chediak-Higashi trait of humans: II. Cytoplasmic granules in eosinophils, basophils, mononuclear cells and platelets.* Am. J. Path., 63, 411, 1971.
131. Oliver C., Essner E.: *Distribution of anomalous lysosomes in the beige mouse: a homologue of Chediak-Higashi syndrome.* J. Histochem. Cytochem., 21, 218, 1973.
132. White J.G.: *The Chediak-Higashi syndrome: a possible lysosomal disease.* Blood, 10, 143-156, 1966.
133. Clawson C.C., Repine J.E., White J.G.: *Chediak-Higashi syndrome: quantitative defect in bactericidal capacity.* Blood, 38, 814, 1971.
134. Stossel T.P., Root R.K., Vaughan M.: *Phagocytosis in chronic granulomatous disease and the Chediak-Higashi syndrome.* New Engl. J. Med., 286, 120, 1972.
135. Alder A.: *Uber konstitutionell bedingte Granulations-veränderungen der Leukocyten.* Dtsch. Arch. Klin. Med., 183, 372, 1939.
136. Reilly W.A., Lindsay S.: *Gargoylism (lipochondrodystrophy): a review of clinical observations in eighteen cases.* Am. J. Dis. Child., 75, 595, 1948.
137. Groover R.V.: *The genetic mucopolysaccharidoses.* Semin. Hemat., 9, 371, 1972.
138. Lutas E.M., Zucker-Franklin D.: *Formation of lipid inclusions in normal human leukocytes.* Blood, 49, 309, 1977.
139. Finch S.C.: *Granulocyte disorders: benign quantitation abnormalities of granulocytes.* In: Williams W.J. et al. (eds.): Hematology. 2nd Edition, Chapts. 83 and 84. Mc Graw Hill, 1977.
140. Wintrobe M. et al.: *Clinical Hematology.* 7th Edition. Lea & Febiger, Philadelphia, p. 1270, 1974.
141. Zacharski L.R., Elveback L.R., Linman J.W.: *Leukocyte counts in healthy adults.* Am. J. Clin. Path., 56, 148, 1971.
142. Quie P.G., White J.G., Holmes B., Good R.A.: *In vitro bactericidal capacity of human polymorphonuclear leukocytes: diminished activity in chronic granulomatous disease of childhood.* J. Clin. Invest., 46, 668, 1967.
143. Douglas S.D., Davis W.C., Fudenberg H.H.: *Granulocytopathies: pleomorphism of neutrophil dysfunction.* Am. J. Med., 46, 901, 1969.
144. Athens J.W., Haab O.P., Raab S.O., Mauer A.M., Ashenbrucker H., Cartwright G.E., Wintrobe M.M.: *Leukokinetic studies. IV. The total blood circulating and marginal granulocyte pools and the granulocyte turnover rate in normal subjects.* J. Clin. Invest., 40, 989, 1961.
145. Wurster N., Elsbach P., Simon E.J., Pettis P., Lebow S.: *The effects of the morphine analogue levorphanol on leukocytes. Metabolic effects at rest and during phagocytosis.* J. Clin. Invest., 50, 1091, 1971.
146. Zucker-Franklin D., Elsbach P., Simon E.J.: *The effect of the morphine analogue levorphanol on phagocytozing leukocytes.* Lab. Invest., 25, 415, 1971.
147. Marsh W.L., Oyen R., Nichols M.E., Allen F.H.: *Chronic granulomatous disease and the cell blood groups.* Brit. J. Haemat., 29, 247, 1975.
148. Crowley C.A., Curnutte J.T., Rosin R.E., André-Schwartz J., Gallen J.J., Klempner M., Snyderman R., Southwick F.S., Stossel T.P., Babior B.M.: *An inherited abnormality of neutrophil adhesion.* New Engl. J. Med., 302, 1163, 1980.
149. Miller M.E.: *Pathology of chemotaxis and random motility.* Seminars in Hemat., 12, 59, 1975.
150. Nowell P.C., Hungerford D.A.: *Chromosome studies on normal and leukemic human leukocytes.* J. Natl. Cancer Inst., 25, 85, 1960.
151. Kardinal G.G., Bateman J.R., Weiner J.: *Chronic granulocytic leukemia. Review of 536 cases.* Arch. Int. Med., 136, 305, 1976.
152. Catovsky D.: *Ph¹ positive acute leukemia and chronic granulocytic leukaemia: one or two diseases.* Brit. J. Haemat., 42, 493, 1979.
153. Brodeur G.M., Dow L.W., Williams D.L.: *Cytogenetic features of juvenile chronic myelogenous leukemia.* Blood, 53, 812, 1979.
154. Gunz F., Baikie A.G.: *Leukemia.* Grune & Stratton, 1974.
155. Lawler S.D., Lobb D.S., Wiltshaw E.: *Philadelphia chromosome positive bone marrow cell showing loss of the Y in males with chronic myeloid leukaemia.* Brit. J. Haemat., 27, 247, 1974.
156. Fitzgerald P.H., Pickering A.F., Eiby J.R.: *Clonal origin of the Philadelphia chromosome and chronic myeloid leukaemia. Evidence from a sex chromosome mosaic.* Brit. J. Haemat., 21, 473, 1971.
157. Moore M.A.S., Ekert H., Fitzgerald M.G., Carmichael A.: *Evidence for the clonal origin of chronic myeloid leukemia from a sex chromosome mosaic.* Blood, 43, 15, 1974.
158. Gaharton G., Lindstein J., Zech H.: *Clonal origin*

of the Philadelphia chromosome from either the paternal or the maternal chromosome number 22. Blood, 43, 837, 1974.
159. Bark R.D., Fialkow P.J.: *Clonal origin of chronic myelocyte leukemia.* New Engl. J. Med., *289,* 307, 1976.
160. Fialkow P.J., Jacobson R.J., Papayannopoulou T.: *Chronic myelocytic leukemia: clonal origin in a stem cell common to the granulocyte, erythrocyte, platelet and monocyte-macrophage.* Am. J. Med., *63,* 125, 1977.
161. Lawler S.D.: *The cytogenetics of chronic granulocytic leukaemia.* Clin. Haemat., *6,* 55, 1977.
162. Galton D.H.: *The chronic leukaemias.* In: Hoffbrand A.V., Brain M.C., Hirsch J. (eds.): *Recent advances in haematology.* Churchill Livingstone, Edinburgh-London-New York, p. 219, 1977.
163. Whang-Peng J., Young R.C.: *Cytogenetic studies in leukemia.* In: Silber R., Lo Bue J., Gordon A.S. (eds.): *Year Book in Hematology.* Plenum, New York-London, p. 375, 1978.
164. Rowley J.B.: *Chromosomes in leukemia and lymphoma.* Semin. Hemat., *15,* 301, 1978.
165. Fialkow P.J.: *Clonal and stem cell origin of blood cell neoplasm.* In: Lo Bue J., Gordon A.S., Silber R., Muggia F.M. (eds.): *Contemporary Hematology/Oncology.* Plenum, New York-London, p. 1, 1980.
166. Greenberg B.F., Wilson F.D., Woo L., Jenks H.M.: *Cytogenetics of fibroblastic colonies in Ph¹ positive chronic myelogenous leukemia.* Blood, *51,* 1039, 1978.
167. Lozzio G.B., Lozzio B.B., Wust C.J., Kim J.: *Correlation of leukemia associated antigens and Ph¹ chromosome in fibroblastic cells derived from bone marrow.* Blood, *52,* 673, 1978.
168. Golde D.W., Bargaleta G., Sparkes R.S., Cline M.J.: *The Philadelphia chromosome in human macrophages.* Blood, *49,* 367, 1977.
169. Killman S.A., Muller-Berat C.N.: *Chronic myeloid leukemia: preleukemia or leukemia?* In: Stacher A., Höcker P. (eds.): *Erkrankungen der Myelopoese.* Urban Schwarzenberg, Munich-Berlin-Vienna, p. 307, 1976.
170. Djaldetii M., Padeh B., Pinkhas J., Devries A.: *Prolonged remission in chronic myeloid leukemia after one course of Busulfan.* Blood, *27,* 103, 1966.
171. Maurice P.A., Ferrier A.P., Freund M.: *Leucémie myelocytaire chronique. "Guerison" apparente depuis plus de 9 ans consecutive à une hypoplasie médullaire thérapeutique.* Schweiz. Med. Wschr., *101,* 1781, 1971.
172. Perreau P., Garais J.: *Survival in chronic myeloid leukaemia following aplasia caused by busulphan.* Sem. Hôp., *45,* 964, 1969.
173. Cunningham I., Gee T., Dowling M., Chaganti R., Bailey R., Jopfan S., Bowden L., Turnbull A., Knapper W., Clarkson B.: *Results of treatment of Ph¹ positive chronic myelogenous leukemia with an intensive treatment regimen (L 5 protocol).* Blood, *53,* 375, 1979.
174. Sharp J.G., Joguer M.W.: *Karyotypic conversion in Ph¹ positive chronic myeloid leukemia with combination chemotherapy.* Lancet, *i,* 1370, 1979.
175. Smalley R.V., Vogel J., Huguley C.M. Jr., Miller D.: *Chronic granulocytic leukemia: cytogenetic conversion of the bone marrow with cycle specific chemotherapy.* Blood, *50,* 107, 1977.
176. Fefer A., Cheever M.A., Thomas E.D., Boyd C., Ramberg R., Glucksberg H., Buckner C.D., Storb R.: *Disappearance of Ph¹ positive cell in four patients with chronic granulocytic leukemia after chemotherapy, irradiation and bone marrow transplantation from an identical twin.* New Engl. J. Med., *300,* 333, 1979.
177. Fialkow P.J., Steinmann L., Najfeld V., Robinson W.A.: *Chronic myelocytic leukemia (CML). Failure to detect residual normal committed cells in vitro.* Blood, *53,* 264, 1979.
178. Singer J.W., Arlin Z., Adamson J.W., Majfeld V., Kempin F., Clarkson B., Fialkow P.J.: *Restoration of non clonal presumably normal hematopoiesis accompanying a chemotherapeutic conversion of Ph¹ positive chronic myelogenous leukemia (CML) to Ph¹ negative.* Blood (abstr.), in press.
179. Spiers A.S.D.: *Clinical aspects of chronic myeloid leukemia.* Clin. Haemat., *6,* 9, 1977.
180. Kober R.D., Seaman A., Osgood E.E., van Bellinghen P.: *Myeloproliferative diseases: diagnostic value of the leukocyte alkaline phosphatase test.* Am. J. Clin. Path., *30,* 295, 1958.
181. Mitus W.S., Bergna L.J., Mednicoff I.B., Dameshek W.: *Alkaline phosphatase of mature neutrophils in chronic forms of the myeloproliferative syndrome.* Am. J. Clin. Path., *30,* 285, 1958.
182. Marmont A., Correale L., Negrini A.C.: *La fosfatasi alcalina leucocitaria in ematologia.* Arch. Maragliano (Genova), *19,* 231, 1963.
183. Chikappa G., Boecker A.R., Carsten A.L., Conkling K., Cook L., Kronkite E.P., Bundwoody S.: *Return of alkaline phosphatase in chronic myelocytic leukemia cells in diffusion chambers cultures.* Proc. Soc. Exp. Biol. Med., *143,* 212, 1973.
184. Dallegri F., Sessarego M., Ghio R., Patrone F.: *Alkaline phosphatase activity in neutrophils of chronic myelocytic leukemia grown in liquid culture.* Acta Haemat., *62,* 12, 1979.
185. Greenberg J.S., Hassam L.R., Karpas A.: *Leukocyte alkaline phosphatase elevation in human acute leukaemia derived cell lines cultured in diffusion chambers.* Scand. J. Haemat., *19,* 242, 1977.
186. Bottomley R.H., Lovig C.A., Holt R., Griffin M.J.: *Comparison of alkaline phosphatase from human normal and leukemic leukocytes.* Cancer Res., *29,* 1866, 1969.
187. Shiffer C.A., Aisner J., Dacy P.A., Wiernik P.H.: *Increased leukocyte alkaline phosphatase activity following transfusion of leukocytes from a patient with a chronic myelogenous leukemia.* Am. J. Med., *66,* 519, 1979.
188. Albrecht M.: *"Gaucher Zellen" bei chronisch myeloischer Leukämie.* Blut, *13,* 169, 1966.
189. Kattlove H.E., Williams H.E., Williams C., Gaynor E., Spivack M., Bradley R.M., Brady K.U.: *Gaucher cells in chronic myelocytic leukemia, an acquired abnormality.* Blood, *33,* 379, 1969.
190. van Dorpe L., Broeckaert-Vanorshoven A., Desmet V., Verwilghen R.L.: *Gaucher-like cells and congenital dyserythropoietic anemia type II (HEMPAS).* Brit. J. Haemat., *25,* 165, 1973.
191. Lewis S.M., Verwilghen R.L.: *Dyserythropoiesis: definition, diagnosis and assessment.* In: Lewis S.M., Verwilghen R.L. (eds.): *Dyserythropoiesis.* Academic Press, London-New York-San Francisco, p. 3, 1977.
192. Sawitsky A.: *The sea blue histiocyte syndrome: a review of genetic and biochemical studies.* Semin. Hemat., *9,* 285, 1972.
193. Quattrin N., De Rose L., Quattrin S., Cecio A.: *Sea blue histiocytosis. A clinical cytologic and nosographic study on 23 cases.* Klin. Wschr., *56,* 17, 1978.
194. Karanas A., Silver R.T.: *Characteristics of the terminal phase of chronic granulocytic leukemia.* Blood, *32,* 445, 1968.
195. Greaves M.F.: *Analysis of lymphoid phenotypes in acute leukemia: their clinical and biological significance.* In: *Cell markers in acute leukemia.* Cancer Treatment Reports, 1980.
196. Marks S.M., Baltimore D., Mc Cathrey R.: *Terminal transferase as a predictor of initial responsiveness to Vincristine-Prednisone in blastic chronic myelogenous leukemia.* New Engl. J. Med., *298,* 812, 1978.
197. Janossy G., Woodruff R.K., Pippard M.J., Prentice G., Hoffbrand A.V., Paxton A., Livrer T.A., Bunch C., Greaves M.F.: *Relation of "lymphoid" phenotypes and response to chemotherapy incorporating Vincristine-Prednisone in the acute phase of Ph¹ leukemia.* Cancer, *43,* 426, 1979.
198. Janossy G., Roberts M., Greaves M.F.: *Target cell in chronic myeloid leukemia and its relationship to acute lymphoid leukemia.* Lancet, *ii,* 1058, 1976.
199. Greaves M.F., Verbi W., Reeves B.R., Hoffbrand A.V., Drysdale H.C., Jones L., Sacker L.S., Samaratunga I.: *"Pre-B" phenotypes in blast crisis of Ph¹ positive leukemia. Evidence for a pluripotential stem cell target?* Leuk. Res., *3,* 181, 1979.
200. Boggs D.R.: *Editorial: Hematopoietic stem cell theory in relation to possible lymphoblastic conversion of chronic myeloid leukemia.* Blood, *44,* 449, 1974.
201. Fialkow P.J., Denman A.M., Singer J., Jacobson R.J.,

Lowenthal M.N.: *Human myeloproliferative disorders: clonal origin in pluripotential stem cells*. In: Clarkson B., Marks P.A., Till J.E. (eds.): *Differentiation of Normal and Neoplastic Hemopoietic Cells*. Cold Spring Harbor Publ., p. 131, 1978.

202. Janossy G., Woodruff R.K., Paxton A., Greaves M.F., Capellaro D., Kirk B., Innes E.M., Eden O.B., Lewis C., Catovsky D., Hoffbrand A.V.: *Membrane marker and cell separation studies in Ph[1] positive leukemia*. Blood, *51*, 861, 1978.

203. Rosenthal J., Canellos G.P., De Vita V.T., Gralnick H.R.: *Characteristics of blast cells in chronic granulocyte leukemia*. Blood, *49*, 705, 1977.

204. Bernard J.: *Natural defense mechanisms in human acute leukaemia (a preliminary study)*. In: Libansky L., Donner L. (eds.): *Present Problems in Haematology*. Excerpta Medica, Amsterdam, p. 20, 1974.

205. Flandrin G., Daniel M.T.: *La leucémie oligoblastique*. In: Bernard J. (ed.): *Actualités hématologiques*. Masson, Paris-New York-Barcelona-Milan, p. 83, 1979.

206. Rheingold J.J., Kaufman R., Adelson E., Lear A.: *Smoldering acute leukemia*. New Engl. J. Med., *268*, 812, 1963.

207. Knospe W.H., Gregory S.A.: *Smoldering acute leukemia*. Arch. Int. Med., *127*, 910, 1971.

208. Branda R.F., Jacob H.S., Douglas S.D., Moldow F., Pnumala R.R.: *Destruction and abnormal lysosome disruption in cultured bone marrow: association with indolent acute leukemia*. Blood, *48*, 23, 1976.

209. Marmont A., Fusco F.A.: *Leucemie acute oligoblastiche e bradievolutive. Profilo terapeutico*. Rec. Progr. Med., *59*, 345, 1975.

210. Sexauer J., Kass L., Schnitzer B.: *Subacute monocytic leukemia*. Am. J. Med., *57*, 853, 1974.

211. Cohen J.R., Creger W.P., Greenberg P.L., Schrire S.L.: *Subacute myeloid leukemia. A clinical review*. Am. J. Med., *66*, 959, 1979.

212. Geary C.G., Catovsky D., Wiltshaw J., Milnes G.R., Scholes M.C., Van Noorden S., Wadsworth S., Muldal S., Mac Iver J.E., Galton D.A.: *Chronic myelomonocytic leukaemia*. Brit. J. Haemat., *30*, 289, 1975.

213. Broun G.O.: *Chronic myelomonocytic leukemia*. Am. J. Med., *47*, 785, 1969.

214. Hartmann D., Obrecht J.P.: *Cytotoxic drugs in the treatment of preleukemic syndromes*. In: Schmalzl F., Hellriegel K.P. (eds.): *Preleukemia*. Springer-Verlag, Berlin-Heidelberg-New York, 1975.

215. Spitzer F., Dhmavir S.V., Diche A., Smith T., Mc Credie K.B.: *Subgroups of oligoleukemia as identified by in vitro agar culture*. Leuk. Res., *9*, 29, 1979.

216. Verma D.S., Spitzer G., Dicke K.A., Mc Credie K.B.: *In vitro agar culture patterns in preleukemia and their clinical significance*. Leuk. Res., *3*, 41, 1979.

217. Golde D.W.: *Pathogenesis of acute myeloid leukemia*. In: Cline M.J. (moderator): *Acute leukemia biology and treatment*. Ann. Int. Med., *91*, 758, 1979.

218. Jensen M.K., Killmann S.A.: *Chromosome studies in acute leukaemia: evidence for chromosomal abnormalities common to erythroblasts and leukaemic white cells*. Acta Med. Scand., *181*, 47, 1967.

219. Blackstock A.M., Garson O.M.: *Direct evidence for involvement of erythroid cells in acute myeloblastic leukemia*. Lancet, *ii*, 1178, 1974.

220. Wiggans R.G., Jacobson R.J., Fialkow P.J., Woolley P.V. III, Mc Donald J.S., Schein P.S.: *Probable clonal origin of acute myeloblastic leukemia following radiation and chemotherapy of colon cancer*. Blood, *52*, 659, 1978.

221. Fialkow P.J., Singer J.W.: *Acute non lymphocytic leukemia: expression in cells restricted to granulocytic and monocytic differentiation*. New Engl. J. Med., *301*, 1, 1979.

222. Reisman L.E., Zuelzer W.W., Thompson R.I.: *Further observation on the role of aneuploidy in acute leukemia*. Cancer Res., *24*, 1448, 1964.

223. Clarkson B.D.: *Acute myelocytic leukemia in adult*. Cancer, *30*, 1572, 1972.

224. Whang-Peng J., Young R.C.: *Cytogenetic studies in leukemia*. In: Silber R., Lo Bue J., Gordon A.S. (eds.): *The Year in Hematology*. Plenum, New York-London p. 375, 1978.

225. Rowley J.D.: *The cytogenetics of acute leukaemia*. Clin. Hemat., *7*, 385, 1978.

226. Mertelsman R., Moore M.A.S., Clarkson B.D.: *Sequential marrow culture studies and terminal deoxynucleotidyl transferase activities in myelodysplastic syndromes*. In: Schmalz F., Hellriegel K.P. (eds.): *Preleukemia*. Springer-Verlag, New York, p. 106, 1979.

227. Moore M.A.S., Williams N., Metcalf D.: *In vitro colony formation by normal and leukemic human hematopoietic cells: characterization of the colony forming cells*. J. Natl. Cancer Inst., *50*, 603, 1973.

228. Bainton D., Friedlander L.M., Shohet S.B.: *Abnormalities in granule formation in acute myelogenous leukemia*. Blood, *49*, 693, 1977.

229. Golde D.W., Cline M.G.: *Human preleukemia: identification of a maturation deficit* in vitro. New Engl. J. Med., *288*, 1083, 1973.

230. Greenberg P.L., Mara B.: *The preleukemic syndrome. Correlation of in vitro parameters of granulopoiesis with clinical features*. Am. J. Med., *66*, 951, 1979.

231. Miller A.M., Page P.L., Harwell B.W., Robinson S.H.: *Inhibition of growth of normal murine granulocytes by co-cultured acute leukemic cells*. Blood, *50*, 799, 1977.

232. Quesenberry P.J., Rappaport J.M., Fountebuoni A., Sullivan A., Zuckerman K., Ryan M.: *Inhibition of normal murine hematopoiesis of leukemic cells*. New Engl. J. Med., *299*, 71, 1978.

233. Boecker W.R., Ohl S., Hossfeld D.K., Schmidt C.G.: *Differentiation of Auer-rod positive leukemic cells in diffusion chamber culture*. Lancet, *1*, 267, 1978.

234. Rovera G., Santoli D., Damsky C.: *Human promyelocytic leukemia cells in culture differentiate into macrophage like cells when heated with a phospho-diesterase*. Proc. Natl. Acad. Sci., *76*, 2779, 1979.

235. Sachs L.: *Control of normal cell differentiation and the phenotypic reversion of malignancy in myeloid leukaemia*. Nature, *274*, 535, 1978.

236. Gallagher R., Collins S., Trujillo K., Mc Credie K., Ahearn M., Tsai S., Metzgar R., Aulakh G , Ting R. Ruscetti F., Gallo R.: *Characterization of the continuous differentiating myeloid cell line (HL 60) from a patient with acute promyelocytic leukemia*. Blood, *54*, 713, 1979.

237. Sachs L.: *Diagnostic and therapeutic implications of cell cultures for human leukemias*. In: Gross R., Hellriegel K.P. (eds.): *Strategies in clinical hematology*. Springer-Verlag, Berlin-Heidelberg-New York, p. 15, 1979.

238. Golomb H.M., Rowley J.D., Vardiman J.W., Testa J.R., Butler A.: *"Microgranular" acute promyelocytic leukemia: a distinct clinical, ultrastructural and cytogenetic entity*. Blood, *55*, 253, 1980.

239. Sultan C.: *Dysmyelopoietic syndromes*. In: Gralnick H.R. (moderator): *Classifications of acute leukemia*. Ann. Int. Med., *87*, 740, 1977.

239. Sultan C., Pierre R.V., Hast R., Imbert M.: *Refractory anemias and dysmyelopoietic syndromes (DMPS)*. Hematology-Transfusion, Education Program Amer. Soc. Hemat., 1980.

239. *Preleukemic states*. Blood Cells, *1*, 2, 1976.

239. Schmalzl F., Hellriegel K.P. (eds.): *Preleukemia*. Springer Verlag, Berlin-Heidelberg-New York, 1979.

240. Dreyfus B.: *Preleukemic states. II. Refractory anemia with an excess of myeloblasts in bone marrow*. Blood Cells, *2*, 36, 1976.

241. Roberts M., Greaves M.F.: *Maturation-linked expression of a myeloid cell surface antigen*. Brit. J. Haemat., *38*, 439, 1978.

242. Schlossman S.M., Chess L., Humphreys R.E., Strominger J.L.: *Distribution of Ia-like molecules on the surface of normal and leukemic human cells*. Proc. Natl. Acad. Sci. U.S.A., *73*, 1288, 1976.

243. Billing R., Ting A., Tarasaki P.I.: *Human B-lymphocyte antigens expressed by lymphocytic and myelocytic leukemia cells*. J. Natl. Cancer Inst., *58*, 199, 1977.

244. Greaves M.F., Janossy G.: *Patterns of gene expression and the cellular origins of human leukaemias*. Biochem. Biophys. Acta., *516*, 193, 1978.

245. Hutton J.J., Coleman M.S., Keneklis T.P., Bollum F.J.: *TdT as a tumor cell marker in leukaemia and lymphoma: results from 1,000 patients*. In: Fox M. (ed): *Advances*

in *Medical Oncology*. Pergamon Press, Oxford, p. 165, 1979.
246. Hoffbrand A.V., Ganeshaguru K., Llewellin P., Janossy G.: *Biochemical markers in leukaemia and lymphoma*. In: Gross R., Hellriegel K.P.: *Recent Results in Cancer Research*, 69, 25. Springer-Verlag, Berlin, 1979.
247. Bradstock K., Hoffbrand A.V., Ganeshaguru K., Llewellin P., Patterson K., Wonke B., Pizzolo G., Prentice G., Bennett M., Bollum F.J., Janossy G.: *Terminal deoxynucleotidyl transferase expression in acute non-lymphoid leukaemia – an analysis by immunofluorescence*. Brit. J. Haemat., 1980.
248. Bennet J.M., Catovsky D., Daniel M.G., Flandrin G., Galton D.A.G., Gralnik H.R., Sultan C.: *Proposals for the classification of the acute leukemias*. Brit. J. Haemat., 33, 451, 1976.
249. Gralnick H.R., Galton D.A.G., Catovsky D., Sultan C., Bennet J.M.: *Classification of acute leukemia*. Ann. Int. Med., 87, 740, 1977.
250. Mathé G., Rappaport H.: *Histological and cytological typing of neoplastic disease of haemopoietic and lymphoid tissues*. WHO, Geneva, 1976.
251. Hayhoe F.G.J., Quaglino D., Dell R.: *The cytology and cytochemistry of acute leukaemias. A study of 140 cases*. M.R.C. Special Report Series N. 304, London HMSO, 1964.
252. Bennet J.M., Reed C.E.: *Acute leukemia cytochemical profile: diagnostic and clinical implications*. Blood Cells, 1, 101, 1975.
253. Shaw M.T.: *The cytochemistry of acute leukaemia: a diagnostic and prognostic evaluation*. Semin. Oncol., 3, 219, 1976.
254. Thierfelder S., Rodt H., Thiel E.: *Immunological diagnosis of leukemias and lymphomas*. Springer-Verlag, Berlin-Heidelberg-New York, 1977.
255. Catovsky V.: *Cell markers in acute lymphoblastic leukaemia and lymphoproliferative disorders*. In: Hoffbrand A.V., Brain M.C., Hirsch J. (eds.): *Recent Advances in Haematology*. Churchill-Livingstone, Edinburgh-London-New York, p. 201, 1977.
256. Necheles T.: *The acute leukemia*. Thieme, Stuttgart, 1979.
257. Gordon D.S., Hutton J.J., Smalley R.V., Meyer L.M., Vogler W.R.: *Terminal deoxynucleotidyl transferase and membrane receptors in adult acute leukemia*. Blood, 52, 1079, 1978.
258. Gordon D.S., Hubbard M.: *Surface membrane characteristics and cytochemistry of the normal cells in adult acute leukemia*. Blood, 52, 681, 1978.
259. Goldberg A.: *Acid phosphatase activity in Auer bodies*. Blood, 24, 305, 1964.
260. White J.G.: *Fine structural demonstration of acid phosphatase in Auer bodies*. Blood, 29, 667, 1967.
261. Harada N.: *Histochemical studies on the Auer body*. Science, 14, 129, 1951.
262. Fischer R., Hennekeuser H.H., Kaufer C.: *Der Cytochemische Nachweis von Naphthol-AS-D-Chloroacetat-Esterase in Auer Stäbchen*. Klinische Wochschr., 44, 1401, 1966.
263. Stavem P.: *Hypergranular acute promyelocytic leukaemia with intravascular coagulation*. Scand. J. Haemat., 2, 249, 1973.
264. Bernard J., Lasneret J., Chome J., Levy J.P., Boiron M.: *A cytological and histological study of acute promyelocytic leukaemia*. J. Clin. Path., 13, 628, 1963.
265. Breton-Gorius J., Houssay D.: *Auer bodies in acute promyelocytic leukemia: demonstration of their fine structure and peroxide localization*. Lab. Invest., 28, 135, 1973.
266. Cavalli F.: *Prognostische Faktoren und Therapie der akuten Läukemien beim Erwachsenen*. Huber Verlag, Bern-Stuttgart-Wien, 1980.

5
Aplastic, hypoplastic and metaplastic myelopathies

A.M. MARMONT and E. DAMASIO

Division of Hematology, S. Martino's Hospital, Genova, Italy

This brief Chapter encompasses a wide variety of syndromes with divergent etiologies and clinical manifestations which extend beyond the boundaries of the Chapters devoted to individual hematopoietic cell lines. In most instances, all three cell lineages, erythroid, myeloid and megakaryocytic, are involved, although single line deficiencies occur (see below). What these conditions have in common is an "empty" bone marrow (**Figs. 1-4**) which is particularly deficient in precursors of the cells that are missing in the blood. Instead, the marrow biopsy specimens (aspirates may yield "dry taps") show variable numbers of fibroblasts, mononuclear leukocytes, plasma cells, osteoblasts, and fat. The remaining hematopoietic cells may display a variety of morphologic abnormalities, some of which have been illustrated (Chapter 3, pp. 75 and 134; Chapter 4, p. 194; Chapter 10, p. 600). The causes for bone marrow failure [1-3] are usually classified into three categories:

1. defects *intrinsic* to the stem cells,
2. defects attributable to the "micro-environment" prevailing in the medullary cavity,
3. missing or damaging factors *extrinsic* to the hematopoietic cells or their connective tissue matrix.

The last category includes myelosuppressive chemicals, X-irradiation, immune reactions and many drugs which may either affect the cells directly or act via a number of disparate immune mechanisms.

1. ACQUIRED APLASTIC ANEMIA

The most severe form of aplastic anemia is manifested by a pancytopenic state in which the neutrophil count is less than $5 \times 10^9/l$, the platelet count less than $20 \times 10^9/l$ and the reticulocytes make up less than 1.0% of the white blood cell count. The marrow is hypocellular and contains mostly non-hematopoietic cells [5]. A low reticulocyte count is considered the most serious prognostic sign [6]. Although, as outlined above, a multitude of causes has been identified [7-14], the vast majority of aplastic anemias are still considered "idiopathic".

Three different pathogenetic mechanisms have been postulated [14]:
– type I is associated with a basic stem cell defect comparable to the anemia of W/W^v mice (see ref. 15),
– type II is associated with a defective micro-environment like the anemia of Sl/Sl^d mice (ref. 15), and
– type III is associated with an autoimmune response involving cytotoxic lymphocytes [16], autoantibodies [17, 18] and other, more indirect, immunoregulatory mechanisms affecting hematopoiesis [1, 4, 12]. In some instances, immunosuppressive therapy proves to be beneficial and is always indicated before bone marrow transplantation is undertaken [19-22]. The bone marrow in aplastic anemia has two prominent features: parenchymal hypoplasia and an inflammatory cell infiltrate (**Figs. 5-7**). Sometimes, the severity of the disease correlates with the number of infiltrating lymphocytes or the number of CFU-C's obtainable in culture [23-25]. The inflammatory infiltrate consists mostly of mononuclear leukocytes. Macrophages predominate in the acute aplastic anemias when they function as scavengers for damaged hemopoietic cells [25].

Lymphocytes and plasma cells are characteristically seen in the more chronic variant of aplastic anemia (see **Fig. 6**). Megaloblastic and dyserythropoietic alterations affecting the erythroid series are the rule (see Chapter 3, p. 75) (see **Fig. 12**). The congenital type of aplastic anemias known by the eponym Fanconi's anemia is associated with karyotypic and multiple somatic abnormalities [26].

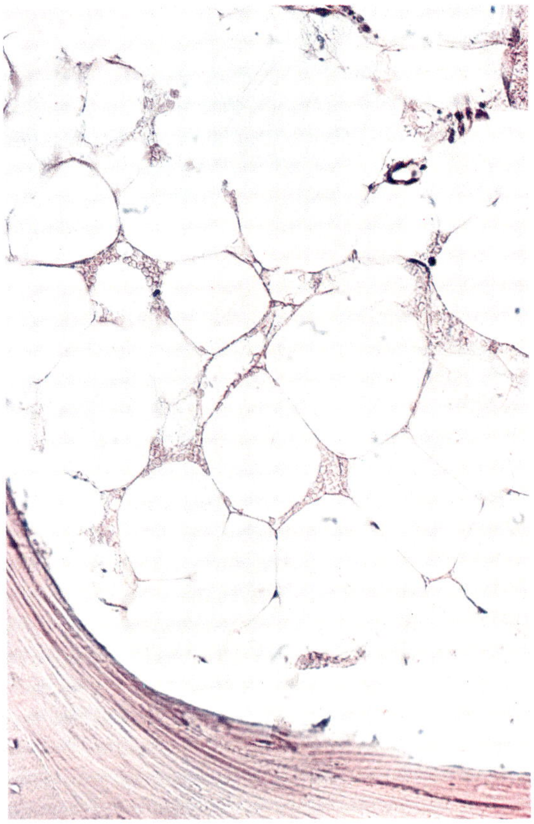

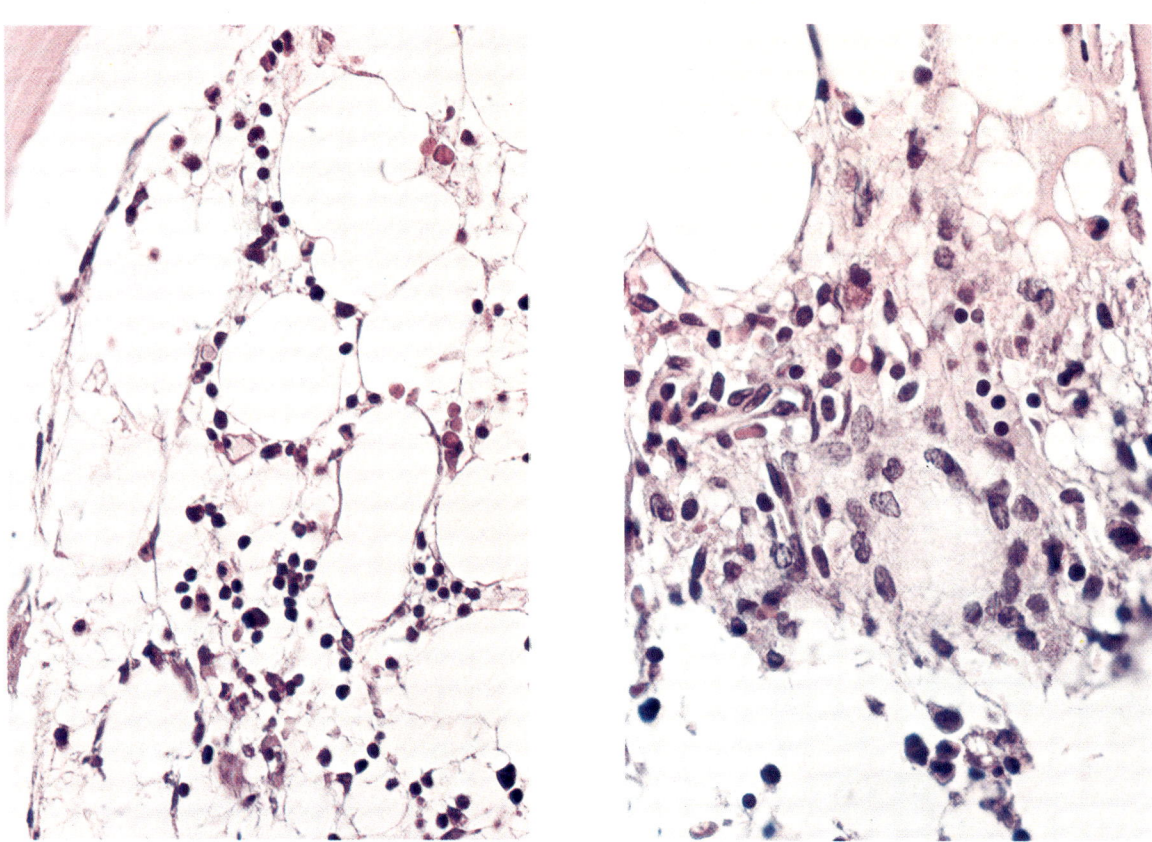

Fig. 1 Depleted "empty" marrow from a patient with severe aplastic anemia (pancytopenia) shows only fibrous tissue and fat (H & E).

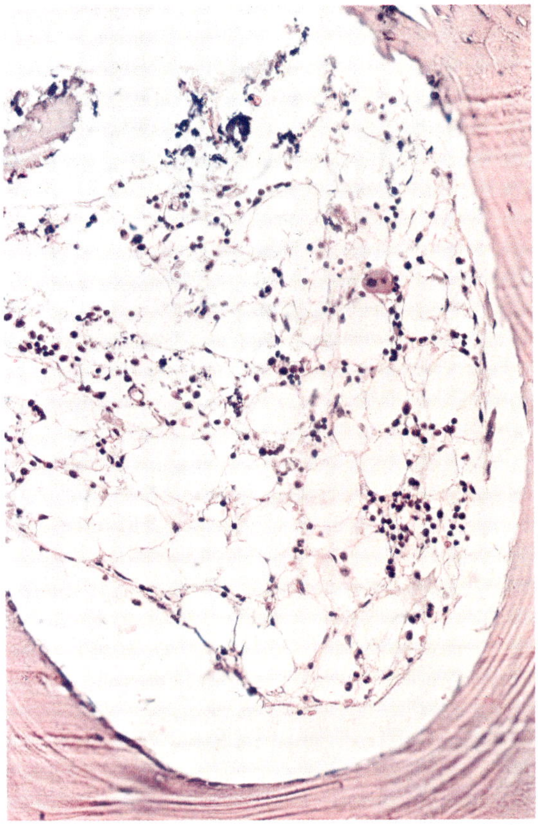

Fig. 2 Needle biopsy of aplastic marrow depicts a few scattered lymphocytes (H & E).

Fig. 3 Hypoplastic marrow, somewhat less depleted than specimen shown in **Figs. 1** and **2** (H & E)

Fig. 4 Biopsy of marrow from a patient with pancytopenia shows no hematopoiesis. The cells represent mostly infiltrating lymphocytes (H & E).

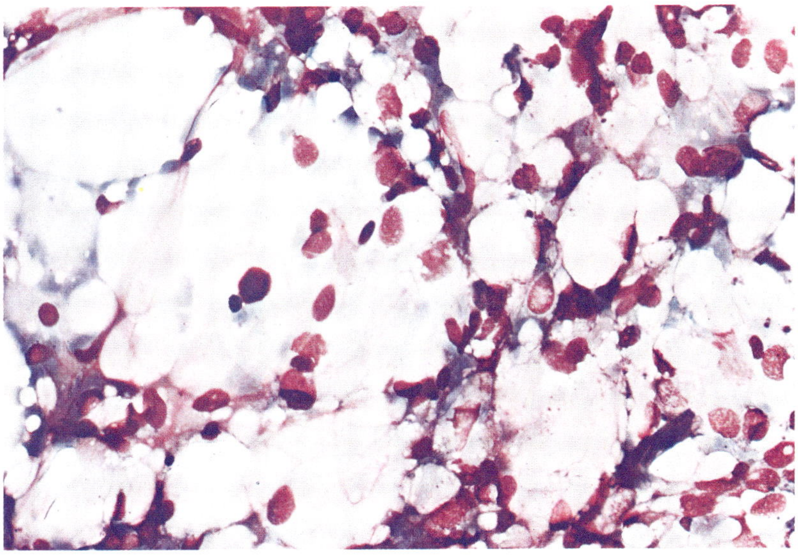

Fig. 5 *Inflammatory reaction in the bone marrow of a patient with severe aplastic anemia. Poorly preserved hematopoietic cells are seen among macrophages, fibroblasts, fat cells and lymphocytes.*

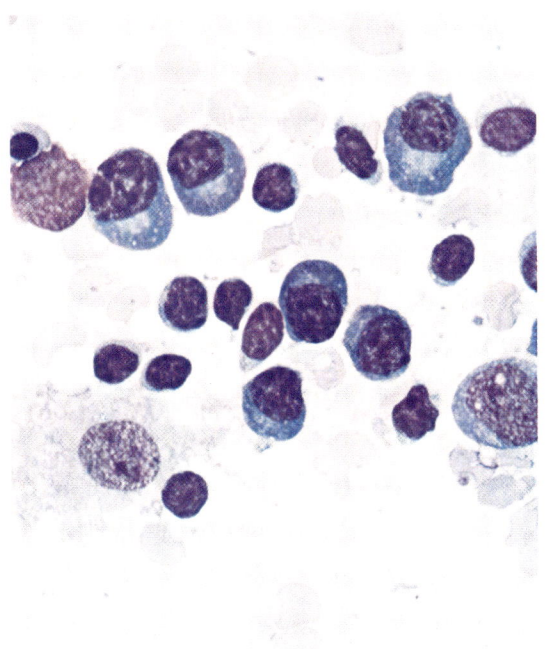
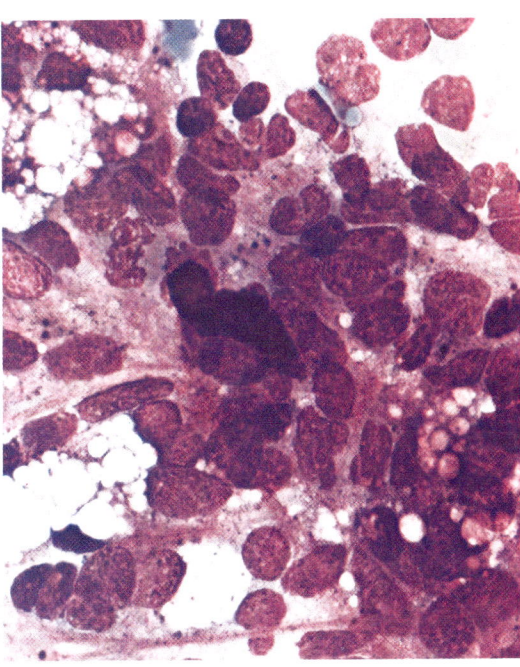

Fig. 6 *Example of a marrow aspirate obtained from a patient with severe aplastic anemia shows primarily lymphocytes and plasma cells.*

Fig. 7 *Mononuclear cell infiltrate in the marrow of a patient with severe aplastic anemia has assumed the morphology of a granuloma*

2. PURE RED CELL ANEMIA (PRCA)

Selective damage to the erythron with partial or complete disappearance of erythroblasts in the marrow in the presence of intact granulocytic and megakaryocytic cell series (**Figs. 8, 9, 10**) also has various disparate etiologies [27]. The congenital disease, known as the Diamond-Blackfan syndrome, appears to have a familial incidence (reviewed in ref. 28) which is occasionally associated with skeletal and other congenital abnormalities. At the time of this writing, there is still controversy as to whether serum factors [29, 30] and/or lymphocytes [31] are involved in the suppression of erythropoiesis in these patients. Most likely, the defect is at the level of the stem cell, possibly of the BFU-E [1], but the responsiveness of the disease to corticosteroids and/or

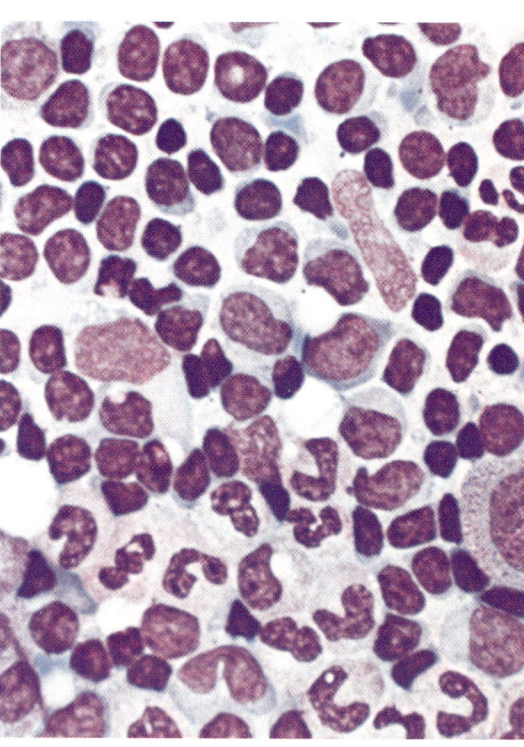

Fig. 8 Bone marrow aspirate from a patient with pure red cell anemia reveals hyperplasia consisting completely of the myeloid cell series with complete absence of erythroid precursors.

Fig. 9 A lymphoid infiltrate in the bone marrow of a patient with pure red cell anemia.

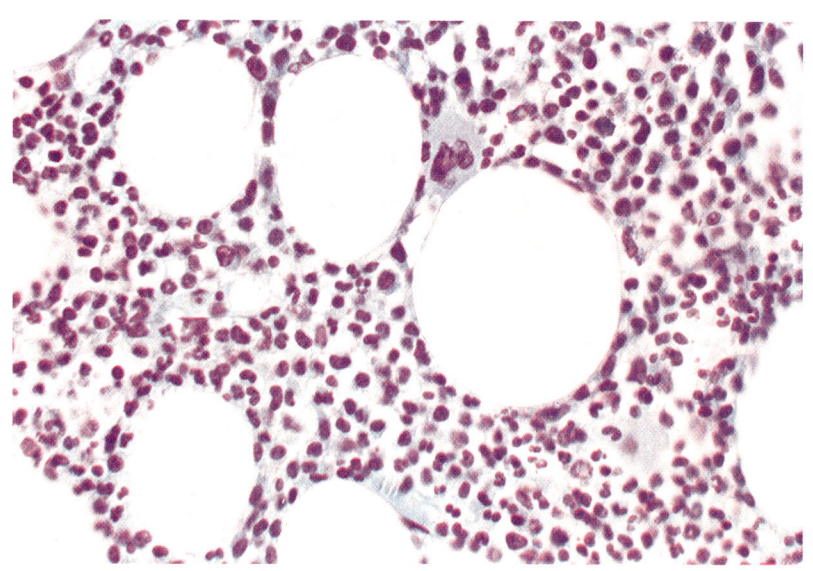

Fig. 10 Biopsy section of marrow from a patient with pure red cell anemia. The "full" marrow is devoid of erythroblasts.

immunosuppressants is suggestive of a superimposed autoimmune response [31] (see **Figs. 11 a, b**). Acquired pure red cell anemia may be seen in the preleukemic state [32] but may be also associated with some tumors, particularly those involving the thymus [33]. Frequently, remission of this type of anemia follows thymectomy. However, there are also some case reports of patients who have developed PRCA following thymectomy [34, 35].

Both in idiopathic and thymoma-associated PRCA, it is sometimes possible to detect antibodies directed against erythroid precursors (Type I) [36, 37]. In rare instances, antibodies may even be directed against erythropoietin (Type II) [38]. As already stated, the bone marrow of patients with PRCA is usually quite cellular with marked hyperplasia of the myeloid series and an abundance of megakaryocytes. Marrow lymphocytosis is common, but there are few plasma cells.

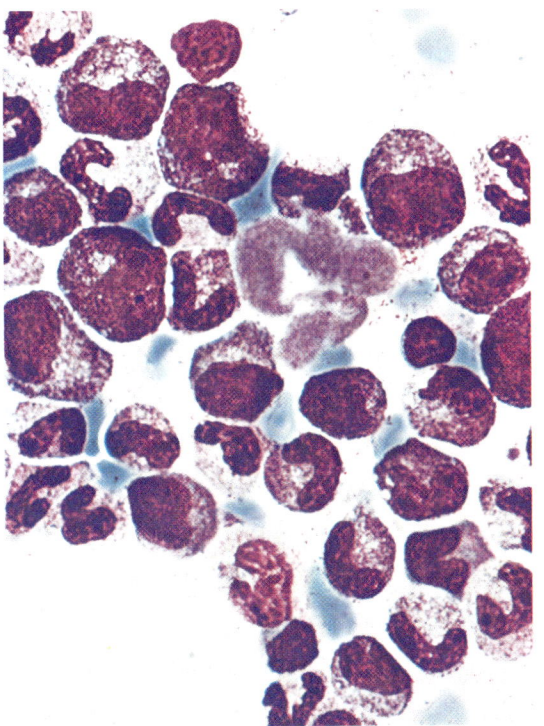
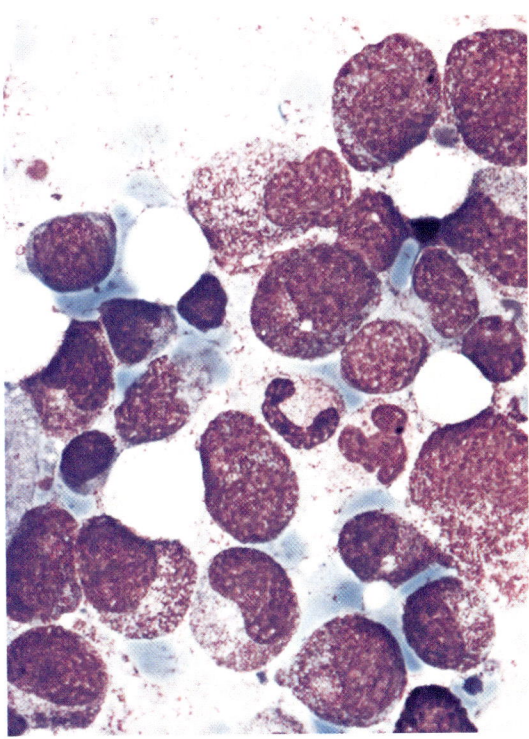

Fig. 11 a) *Marrow aspirate from a patient with Diamond-Blackfan syndrome. Marked predominance of myeloid series which shows normal maturation and almost complete absence of erythroid precursors.*
b) *Diamond-Blackfan syndrome. Myeloid hyperplasia may simulate CML. Note lack of erythroid series.*

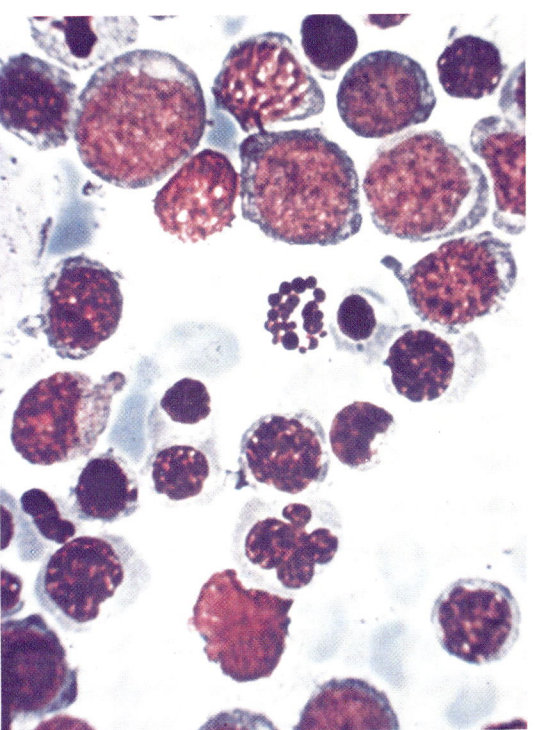
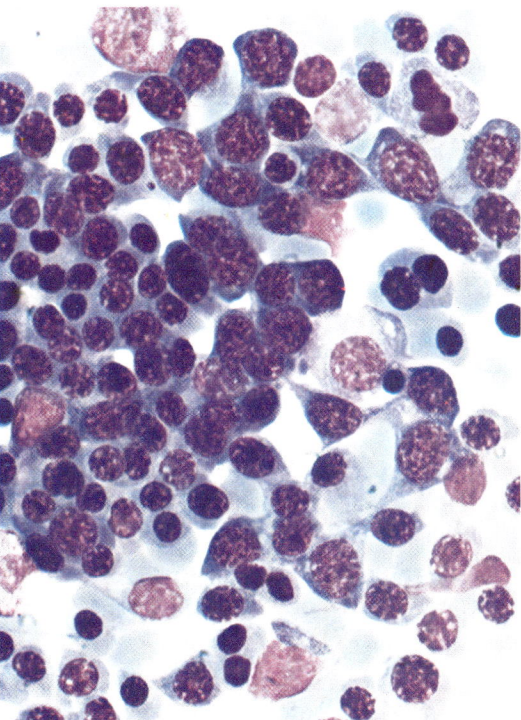

Fig. 12 *Erythroid dysplasia in aplastic anemia.*

Fig. 13 *Recovery phase seen in the marrow of a patient with pure red cell anemia following treatment with immunosuppressive agents. The marrow aspirate exhibits marked erythroid hyperplasia.*

The acute form of PRCA is usually associated with giant erythroid precursors (**Fig. 12**) [39].

Treatment with corticosteroids or immunosuppressive agents may be remarkably effective (**Fig. 13**) [18, 27, 36].

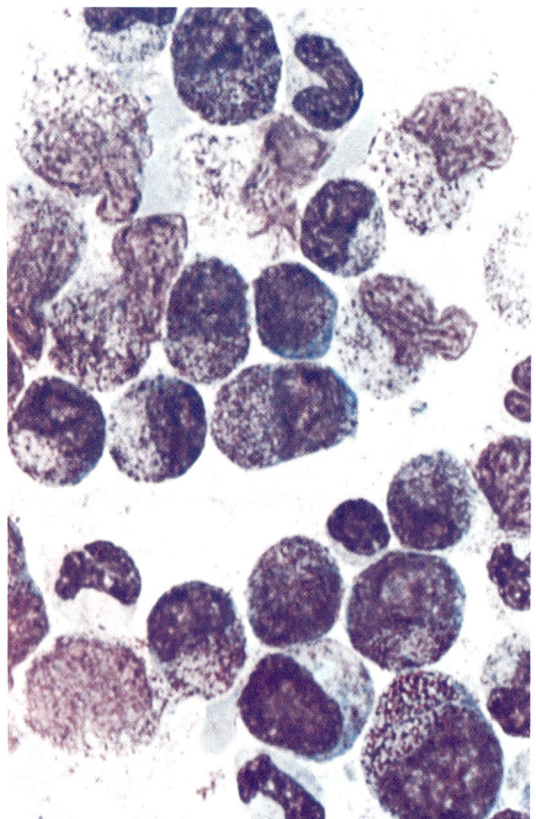 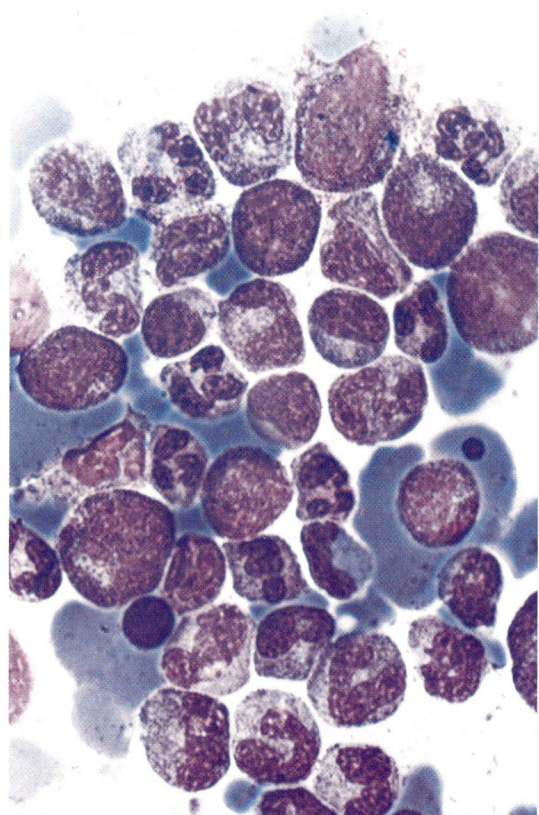

Fig. 14 a) Marrow showing promyelocyte arrest which accompanied severe peripheral blood neutropenia.
b) Marrow of the same patient during recovery phase. Mature neutrophils have reappeared.

3. AGRANULOCYTOSIS

The causes for agranulocytosis are also manifold and may cause both "peripheral" and "central" granulocytopenia.

Immunologic, drug-induced and "idiopathic" mechanisms may damage mature cells or their precursors at any stage of differentiation or maturation. Most of the chemotherapeutic agents currently used lead to bizarre morphologic changes (**Figs. 14** and **15**). Some medications have a predictable myelosuppressive effect and the degree of marrow depression is in proportion to the amount of the drug used. Others elicit idiosyncratic reactions which depend on host factors.

In addition, there are congenital and cyclic neutropenias. Serum inhibitors of CFU-C have been demonstrated both in autoimmune [40] and drug-associated [41] conditions.

Fig. 15 Examples of bone marrow specimens obtained from patients with peripheral blood agranulocytosis.
a) Cause unknown, marrow shows abundance of highly immature promyelocytes.
b) Agranulocytosis caused by pyramidone. Promyelocyte arrest. Note that the erythroid precursor (**arrow**) is normal.
c) Agranulocytosis in the rigenerative, promyelocytic stage. Synchronous amplification causes a leukemoid pattern, however APL can be excluded by the absence of extreme hypergranularity and Auer rods.
d) Another "leukemoid" pattern from the same marrow aspirate. A wave of peripheral neutrophilia could be observed two days later.

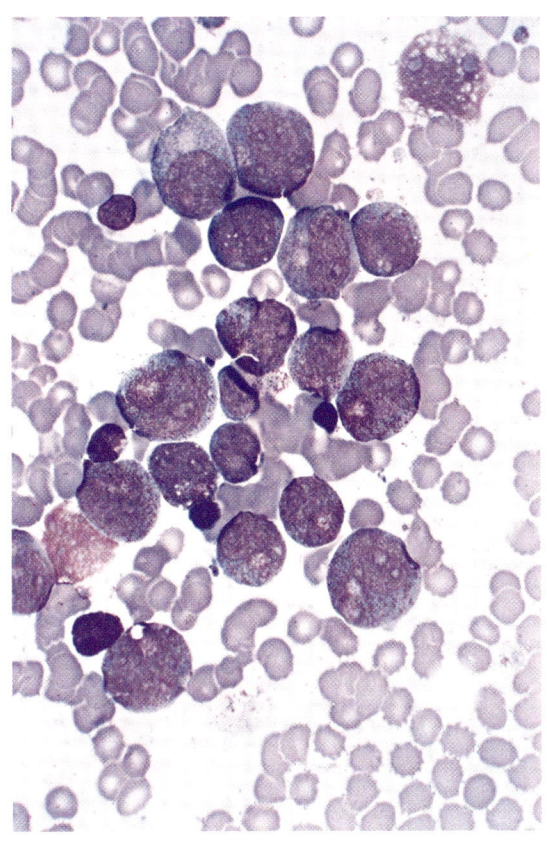
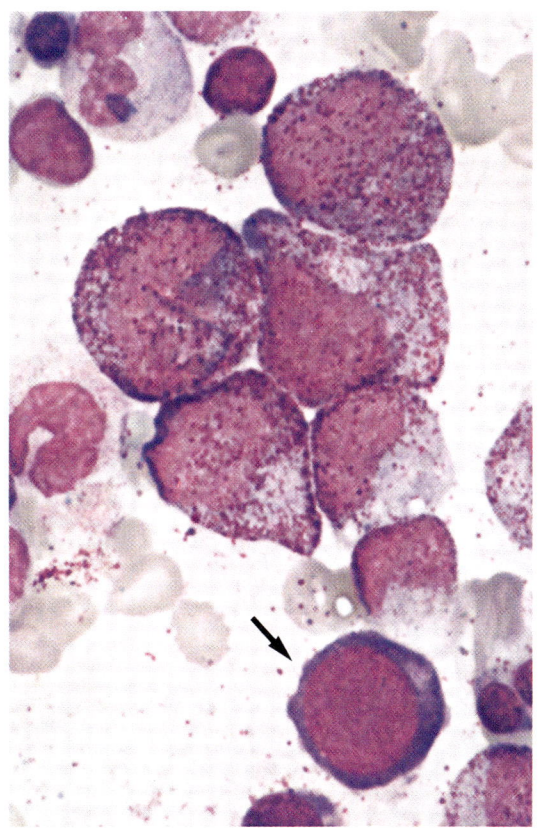
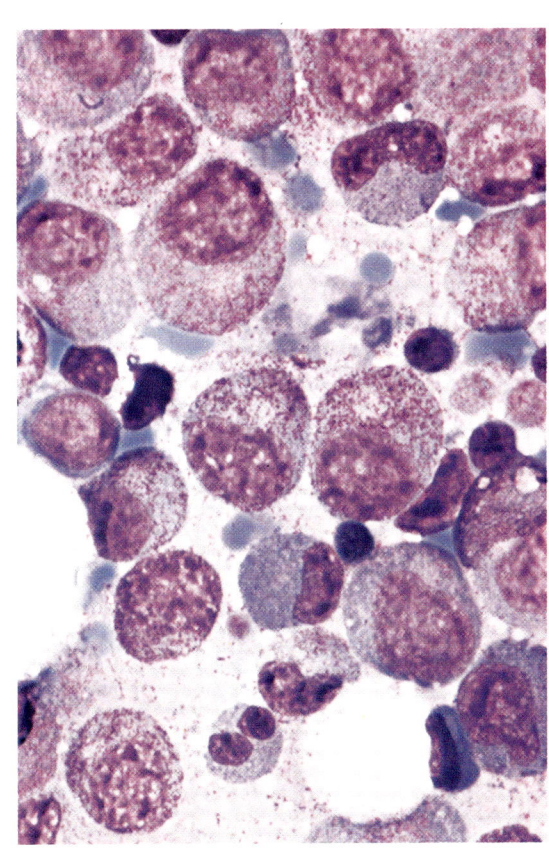
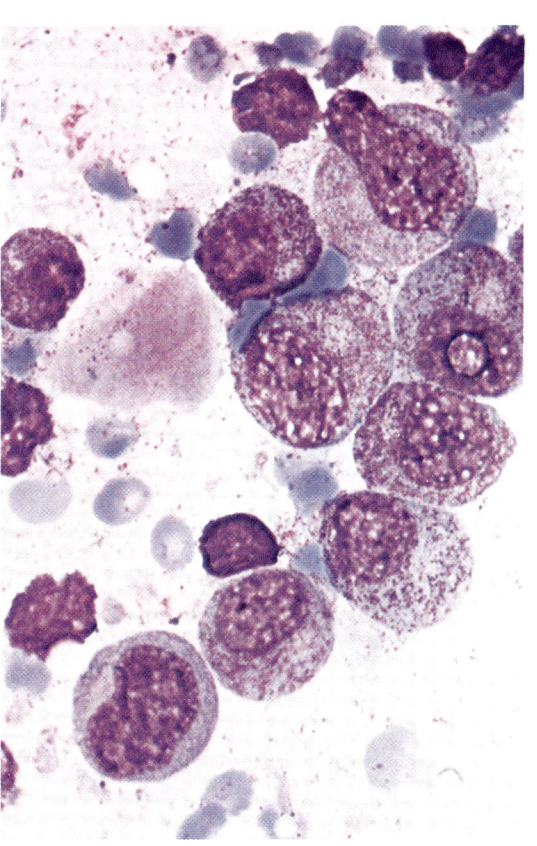

4. THE MYELOFIBROSIS-OSTEOSCLEROSIS SYNDROME (MOS)

This syndrome is considered to be a myeloproliferative disorder which may involve all three cell series and eventuates in myelofibrosis, osteomyelosclerosis or megakaryocytic leukemia [42]. The clinical and laboratory manifestations of this syndrome are so diverse that the disease has been described under 49 different names [43, 44]. The one adapted here was proposed by the Dahlem Workshop held in 1974 [43] which lists more than 1,200 publications.

Myelofibrosis differs from osteomyelosclerosis in that the former presents with more myeloproliferative and inflammatory activity, whereas the latter is characterized by more bone formation and impaired osteoclast function. Osteomyelosclerosis is a consequence rather than an alternative to myelofibrosis. Moreover, it is currently believed that hematologic neoplasia is primary and that fibrosis and sclerosis are secondary events. Perhaps the most helpful study in this area has been the one demonstrating in a female with MOS and G-6-PD isoenzyme heterogeneity that the erythrocytes, granulocytes and megakaryocytes were monoclonal whereas skin and marrow derived fibroblasts were not [45]. In addition, karyotypic anomalies have been found in granulocytic and erythrocytic precursors but not in marrow fibroblasts [46]. The morphologic and functional abnormalities of the hemopoietic cells have been postulated to be the source of factors which may stimulate fibroblast proliferation and lead to fibrosis.

Myelofibrosis may be the final common pathway resulting from all kinds of marrow injury. Although it is, at times, difficult to tell MOS from CML, careful assessment of clinical and laboratory manifestation usually permits a correct diagnosis. In MOS reticulocytosis and circulating normoblasts are generally present; dacryocytes are more frequent than in any other blood disorder (**Fig. 17**); platelet levels are often high and the platelets and megakaryocytes show various pathologic changes described in Chapter 10, p. 600, **Figures 45-49**. Bone marrow aspiration is usually unrewarding and biopsy is necessary for diagnosis. The biopsies show the gamut of fibrosis and sclerosis (**Figs. 16 a, b**). The terminal phase of the disease is dominated by myeloid metaplasia in the spleen, liver, lymph nodes and often other organs as well.

5. MYELOPHTHISIS

This is a term applied to a process in which the bone marrow is suppressed and/or replaced by cells which are not ordinarily present in the medullary cavity. The most common cause is metastatic carcinoma (**Fig. 18**). However, other conditions, such as Hodgkin's disease, primary xanthomatosis and other lesions which invade bone may result in myelofibrosis. In addition, protozoan infestations, viral and bacterial infections may sometimes depress hematopoiesis and have a similar outcome (see also Chapter 3, p. 134).

Fig. 17 Dacriocytes associated with macrocytosis in a case of MOS.

Fig. 18 Biopsy of bone illustrating myelophthisis due to metastatic carcinoma of the breast.

5 APLASTIC MYELOPATHIES

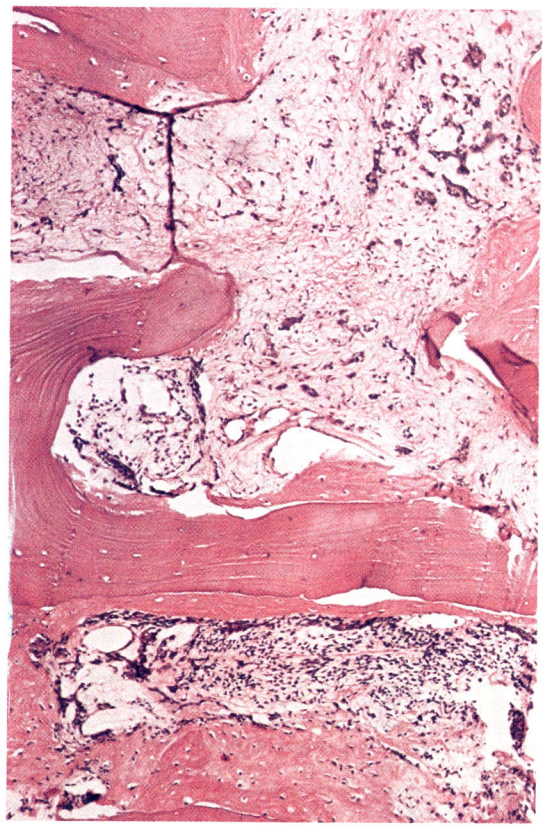
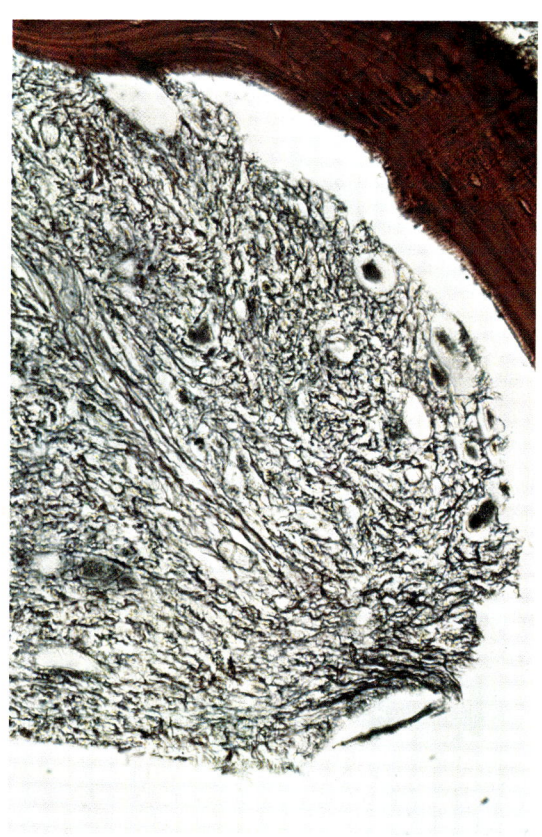

Fig. 16 a) Bone marrow biopsy illustrating myelofibrosis (H & E).
b) Reticulin stain of bone marrow biopsy depicting fibrosis.

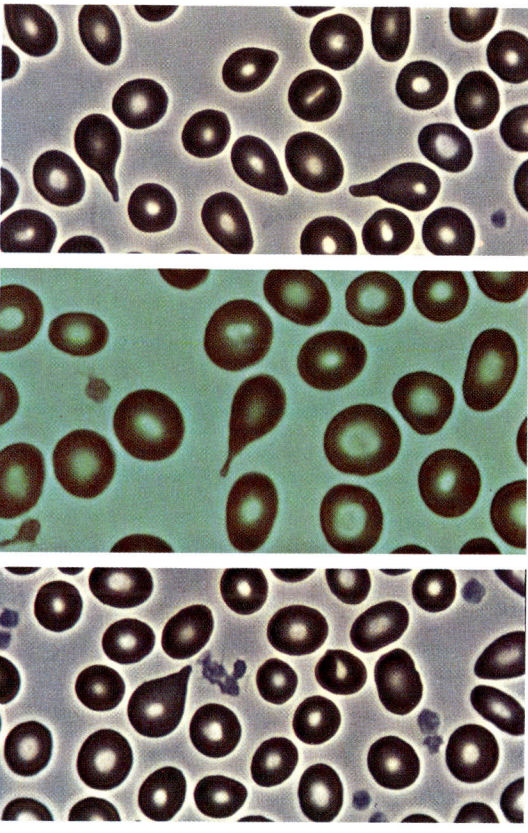
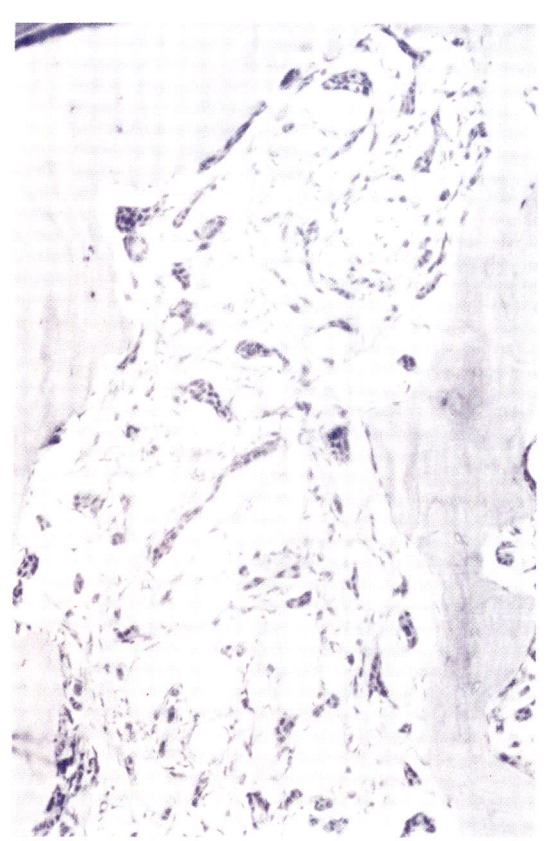

REFERENCES

1. Alter B.P., Upp Potter N.P., Li F.P.: *Classification and etiology of the aplastic anemias*. Clin. Haemat., 7, 431, 1978.
2. Boggs D.R., Boggs S.S.: *The pathogenesis of aplastic anemia: a defective pluripotent hematopoietic stem cell with inappropriate balance of differentiation and self replication*. Blood, 48, 71, 1976.
3. Boggs D.R., Boggs S.S.: *Possible pathogenic mechanisms in aplastic anemia and related disorders*. Transplantation Proc., 10, 125, 1978.
4. Heimpel H., Gordon-Smith E.C., Heit W., Kubanek B.: *Aplastic anemia*. Springer, Berlin-Heidelberg-New York, 1979.
5. Camitta B.M., Thomas E.D.: *Severe aplastic anemia: a prospective study on the effect of androgens or transplantation on haematological recovery and survival*. Clin. Haemat., 4, 587, 1978.
6. Lohman H.P., Niethammer D., Kern P., Heimpel H.: *Identification of high risk patients with aplastic anaemia in selection for allogeneic bone marrow transplantation*. Lancet, ii, 647, 1976.
7. Wade D.L., Beeley L.: *Adverse reactions to drugs*. Heinemann, London, 1976.
8. De Gruchy G.C.: *Drug induced blood disorders*. Blackwell, London, 1976.
9. Williams D.M., Lynch R.E., Cartwright G.E.: *Drug-induced aplastic anemia*. Semin. Haemat., 10, 195, 1973.
10. Marmont A.M.: *Emopatie farmacologiche a patogenesi immunologica*. Acta med. romana (Rome), 16, 163, 1978.
11. Yunis A.A.: *Chloramphenicol-induced bone marrow suppression*. Semin. Haemat., 10, 225, 1973.
12. Parkman R.: *The immunopathology of marrow failure*. Clin. Haemat., 7, 475, 1978.
13. Camitta B.M., Nathan D.G., Forman E.N., Parkman R., Rappaport J.M., Orellana T.D.: *Posthepatitic severe aplastic anemia: an indication for early bone marrow transplantation*. Blood, 43, 473, 1974.
14. Kagan W.W., Ascensao J.L., Fialk M.A., Coleman M., Vallera J., Good R.A.: *Studies on the pathogenesis of aplastic anemia*. Am. J. Med., 66, 444, 1979.
15. Harrison D.E.: *Use of genetic anaemias in mice as tools for haematological research*. Clin. Haemat., 8, 238, 1979.
16. Hoffman R., Zanjani E.D., Lutton J., Zalusky R., Wasserman L.R.: *Suppression of erythroid colony formation by lymphocytes from patients with aplastic anemia*. New Engl. J. Med., 296, 10, 1977.
17. Cline M.J., Golde D.W.: *Immune suppression of hematopoiesis*. Am. J. Med., 64, 301, 1978.
18. Marmont A.M.: *Immune suppression of hematopoiesis, with special reference to aplastic anemia and its treatment*. 11th Europ. Congr. Acad. Allerg. Clin. Immunol., Vienna, 1980 (in press).
19. Baran D.T., Griner P.F., Klemperer M.R.: *Recovery from aplastic anemia after treatment with cyclophosphamide*. New Engl. J. Med., 295, 1522, 1976.
20. Gluckman E., Devergie A., Faille A., Barrett A.J., Bonneau M., Boiron M., Bernard J.: *Action du sérum antilymphocytaire dans les aplasies médullaires graves*. Nouv. Presse Méd., 7, 493, 1978.
21. Speck B., Gluckman E., Haak H.L., Van Rood J.J.: *Treatment of aplastic anaemia by antilymphocyte globulin with or without marrow infusion*. Clin. Haemat., 7, 611, 1978.
22. Bagby G.C., Goodnight S.H., Mooney W.M., Richert-Boe K.: *Prednisone-responsive aplastic anemia: a mechanism of glucocorticoid action*. Blood, 54, 322, 1979.
23. Frisch B., Lewis S.M.: *The bone marrow in aplastic anemia: diagnostic and prognostic feaures*. J. Clin. Path., 27, 39, 1974.
24. Te Velde J., Haak H.L.: *Aplastic anaemia. Histological investigation of methacrylate embedded bone marrow biopsy specimens; correlation with survival after conventional treatment in 15 adult patients*. Brit. J. Haemat., 35, 61, 1977.
25. Duhamel G., Muratore R., Bryon P.A., Horchowsky N.: *Les lesions histologiques de la moelle dans l'aplasie médullaire. Resultats d'un protocol commun portant sur 216 biopsies*. Nouv. Rév. Franç. Hémat., 20, 17, 1978.
26. Latt S.A., Stetten G., Juergens L.A., Buchanan G.R., Gerald P.S.: *Induction by alkylating agents of sister chromatid exchanges and chromatic breaks in Fanconi's anemia*. Proc. Natl. Acad. Sci., 72, 4066, 1975.
27. Krantz S.B., Zaentz S.D.: *Pure red cell aplasia*. In: Gordon A.S., Silber R., Lo Bue J. (eds.): *The Year in Hematology*, Plenum Press, New York-London, p. 153, 1977.
28. Diamond L.K., Allen D.M., Magill F.B.: *Congenital (erythroid) hypoplastic anemia*. Am. J. Dis. of Child., 102, 503, 1961.
29. Ortega J.A., Shore M.A., Dukes P.P., Hammond D.: *Congenital hypoplastic anemia. Inhibition of erythropoiesis by sera from patients with congenital hypoplastic anemia*. Blood, 45, 83, 1975.
30. Geller G., Krivit W., Zalusky R., Zanjani E.D.: *Lack of erythropoietic inhibitory effect of serum from patients with congenital pure red cell aplasia*. J. Pediatr., 2, 189, 1975.
31. Hoffman R., Zanjani E.D., Zalusky R., Lutton J.D., Wasserman L.R.: *Diamond-Blackfan syndrome. Lymphocyte-mediated suppression of erythropoiesis*. Science, 193, 899, 1976.
32. Dumont J.: *Erythroblastopénie chronique de l'adulte*. In: Bernard J. (ed.): *Actualitées Hématologiques*, Masson, Paris, 1969.
33. Goldstein G., Mackay I.R.: *The human thymus*. Heineman, London, 1969.
34. Marmont A.M.: *Pure erythroblastopenia or red cell aplasia: an autoimmune disease responding to immunodepressive therapy*. In: Libansky J., Donner L. (eds.): *Present Problems in Haematology*. Excerpta Medica, Amsterdam, p. 225, 1974.
35. Safdar S.H., Krantz S.B., Brown E.B.: *Successful immunosuppressive treatment of erythroid aplasia appearing after thymectomy*. Brit. J. Haemat., 19, 434, 1970.
36. Marmont A.M., Peschle C., Sanguinetti M., Condorelli M.: *Pure red cell aplasia (PRCA): response of three patients to cyclophosphamide and/or antilymphocyte globulin (ALG) and demonstration of two types of serum IgG inhibitors to erythropoiesis*. Blood, 45, 247, 1975.
37. Peschle C., Marmont A.M., Perugini S., Bernasconi C., Brunetti P., Fontana G., Ghio R., Resegotti L., Rizzo S.C., Condorelli M.: *Physiopathology and therapy of adult pure red cell aplasia (PRCA): a cooperative study*. In: Hibino S., Takaku F., Shaidi N.T. (eds.): *Aplastic anemia*. Proc. 1st Int. Symp. Aplastic Anemia, Kyoto, 3-4 September 1976.
38. Peschle C., Marmont A.M., Marone G., Genovese A., Sasso G.F., Condorelli M.: *Pure red cell aplasia: studies on an IgG serum inhibitor neutralizing erythropoietin*. Brit. J. Haemat., 30, 411, 1975.
39. Gasser G.: *Aplasia or erythropoiesis acute and chronic erythroblastopenia or pure (red cell) aplastic anemia in childhood*. Pediatr. Clin. N. Am., 4, 445, 1957.
40. Fitchen J.H., Cline M.J., Saxon A., Golde D.W.: *Serum inhibitors of haemopoiesis in a patient with aplastic anemia and systemic lupus erythematosus. Recovery after plasma exchange plasmapheresis*. Am. J. Med., 66, 537, 1978.
41. Kelton J.G., Huang A.T., Mold N., Logue G., Rosse W.F.: *The use of in vitro technics to study drug-induced pancytopenia*. New Engl. J. Med., 301, 624, 1979.
42. Burkhardt R., Bartl R., Beil E., Demmler K., Hoffman E., Kroseder S.: *Myelofibrosis-osteosclerosis syndrome. Review of literature and histomorphology*. In: *Dahlem Workshop on myelofibrosis-osteomyelosclerosis syndrome*. Pergamon Press, p. 10, Berlin 1974, Vieweg 1975.
43. *Dahlem Workshop on myelofibrosis-osteomyelosclerosis syndrome*. Pergamon Press, Berlin 1974, Vieweg 1975.
44. Storti E., Perugini S.: *La mielofibrosi idiopatica, aspetti clinici, fisiopatologici e terapeutici*. Atti del 21° Congr. It. Ematol., Modena, 10-11 giugno 1967. Viscontea, Pavia, p. 4, 1967.
45. Jacobson R., Salo A., Fialkow P.J.: *Agnogenic myeloid metaplasia; a clonal proliferation of hematopoietic stem cells with secondary myelofibrosis*. Blood, 51, 189, 1978.
46. van Slyck E.J., Weiss L., Dully M.: *Chromosomal evidence for the secondary role of fibroblast proliferation in acute myelofibrosis*. Blood, 36, 729, 1970.

6
Eosinophils

D. ZUCKER-FRANKLIN

Department of Medicine
New York University, New York, U.S.A.

The chapter on eosinophils in an atlas
on blood cells ought to rank among
the most beautiful of its pages. A century
ago, the provocative staining properties
of the cell's granules caused Ehrlich
to name this leukocyte after the Greek
goddess of dawn, Eos. In more recent
times, ultrastructural studies of eosinophils
have proven aesthetically equally
rewarding. However, the most exciting
era has just begun. This has to do
with the recognition that despite their low
numbers in circulating blood, eosinophils
have many functions that play a crucial role
in the body's defense mechanism.

Detailed descriptions of these newly
defined biochemical and physiologic
processes are not possible within
the confines of an Atlas. These may
be found in a number of comprehensive
up-to-date reviews of this subject [1-5].

The main purpose of this article is to
acquaint the reader with the normal
structure of the cells, with those
physiologic and biochemical features
that can be presented by morphologic
means, and with the alterations seen
in diseases that directly or indirectly
involve eosinophils.

1. NORMAL EOSINOPHILS

1.1. Eosinophil structure and maturation

Eosinophils arise in the bone marrow
where they cannot be distinguished
from other granulocyte precursors before
the promyelocyte stage of development.
This is underscored by current
experience with soft agar cultures
that have been initiated with mononuclear
cells derived from human peripheral
blood [6]. At the outset, such
specimens contain no recognizable
eosinophils. During the first five to seven
days of culture, small colonies of cells
appear which are morphologically
indistinguishable from each other, even
by electron microscopy. By about the 12th
day, characteristic "tight" and "loose"
colonies have developed (**Fig. 1 a-c**).
The former consist of cells with features
of eosinophil promyelocytes; the latter
contain recognizable precursors
of the neutrophil-macrophage series
(**Figs. 1** and **2**). Among other reasons
to believe that neutrophils and eosinophils
arise from different stem cells [1]
is the observation that *in vitro* cultures
yield separate eosinophil and neutrophil
colonies and that mixed colonies are rarely,
if ever, found. With the light microscope,
eosinophil promyelocytes are identified
by virtue of the large size and tinctorial
properties of their granules. Some
of these granules stain basophilic
with the Wright and Giemsa stain,
but the majority are eosinophilic (**Fig. 3**).

Should difficulty in identification arise,
use can be made of the observation
that the peroxidase contained in eosinophils
differs from myeloperoxidase
of the neutrophilic series in substrate
specificity and sensitivity to a variety
of inhibitors (**Fig. 1 c**) [7-11]. As is true
for other promyelocytes, the nucleus
of the eosinophil promyelocyte is round
and may display one or two nucleoli.

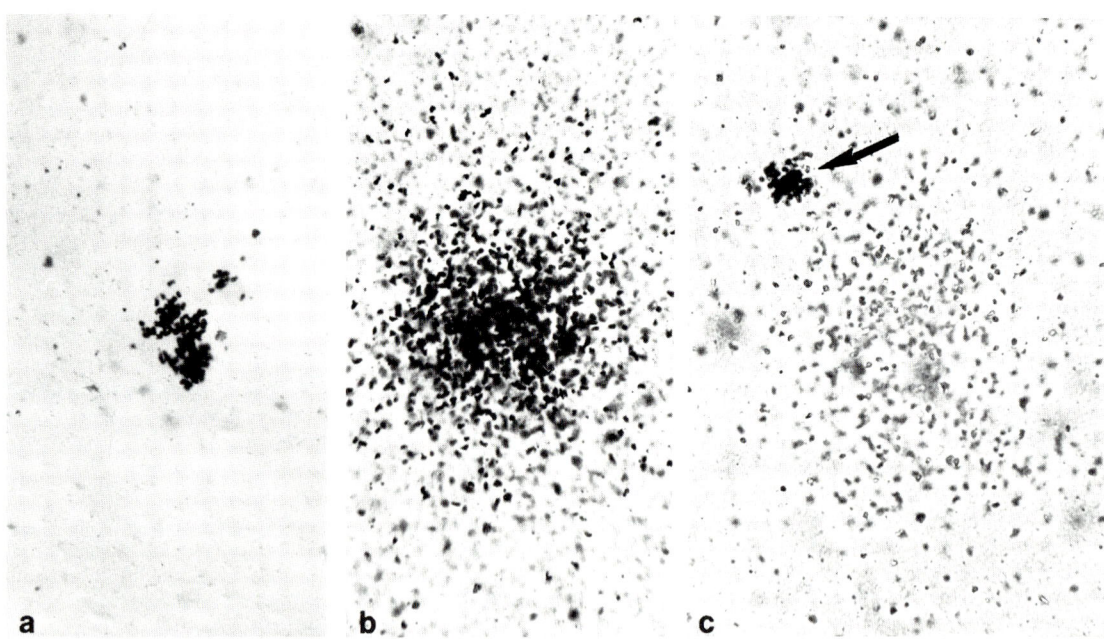

Figs. 1 a-c) Illustrate « tight » (eosinophil) and « loose » (neutrophil/macrophage) colonies grown in soft agar culture. The specimens have been treated with H_2O_2 and benzidine, substrates for peroxidase. The reaction product has rendered both colonies black. The colonies illustrated in **c** were treated with cyanide. Because cyanide inhibits myeloperoxidase, but not eosinophil peroxidase the « tight » eosinophil colony (indicated by an **arrow**) has remained positive whereas the cells in the « loose » colony are now negative for peroxidase ($\times 100$).
Reproduced from ref. 11.

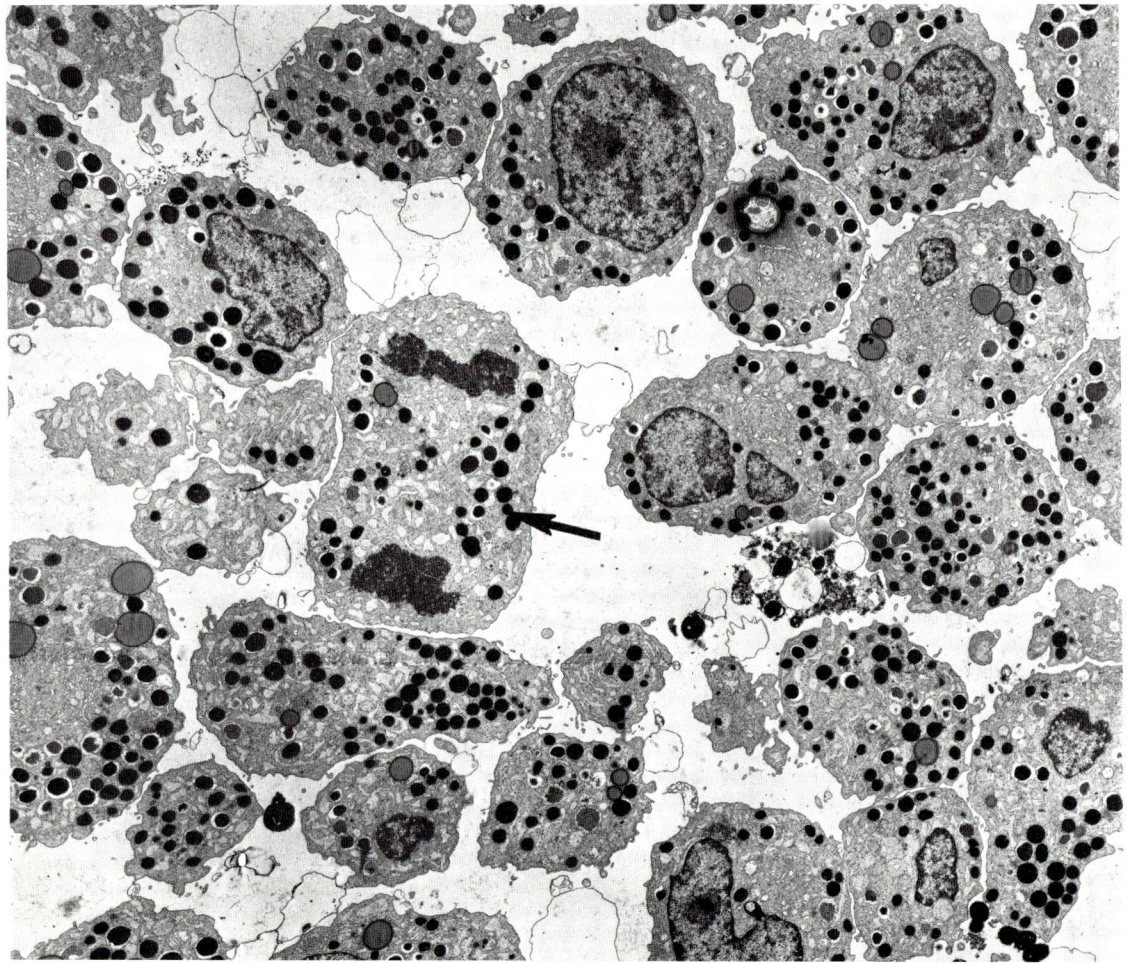

6 EOSINOPHILS

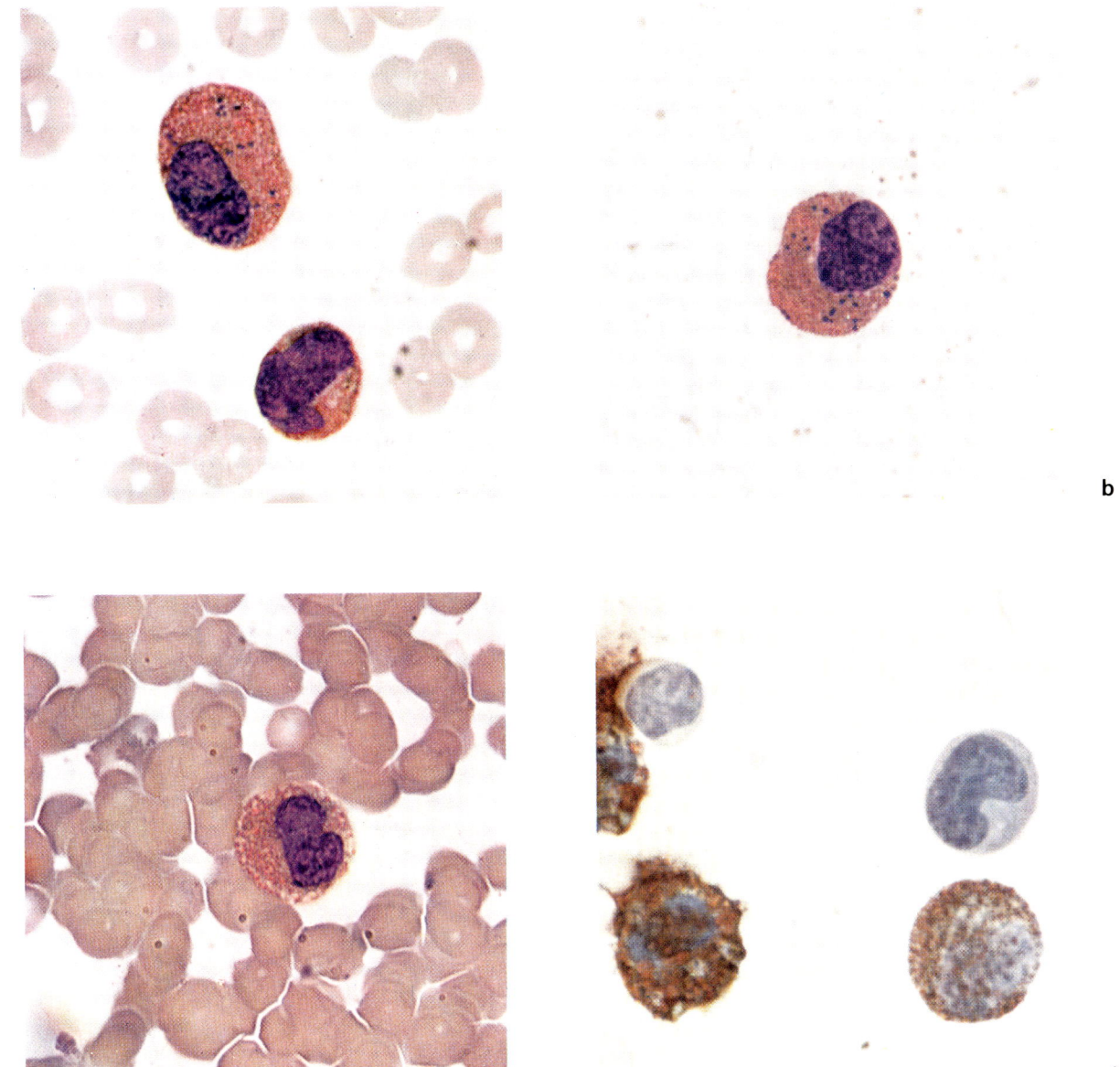

Fig. 3 Eosinophil promyelocyte (**a**), myelocyte (**b**) and metamyelocyte (**c**). Note that some blue-staining, large granules are present in promyelocytes and that these disappear in more mature cells. However, even mature eosinophils remain strongly positive for peroxidase. Eosinophils stained for peroxidase in **d** (method of Dr. J.S. Hanger, University of North Carolina).

Fig. 2 Low power electron micrograph showing a detail of an eosinophil colony grown in soft agar. Most of the cells represent promyelocytes and myelocytes. Note that the granules are round and do not yet possess crystalloids. The **arrow** indicates a promyelocyte in telophase ($\times$ 2400).
Reproduced from ref. 6.

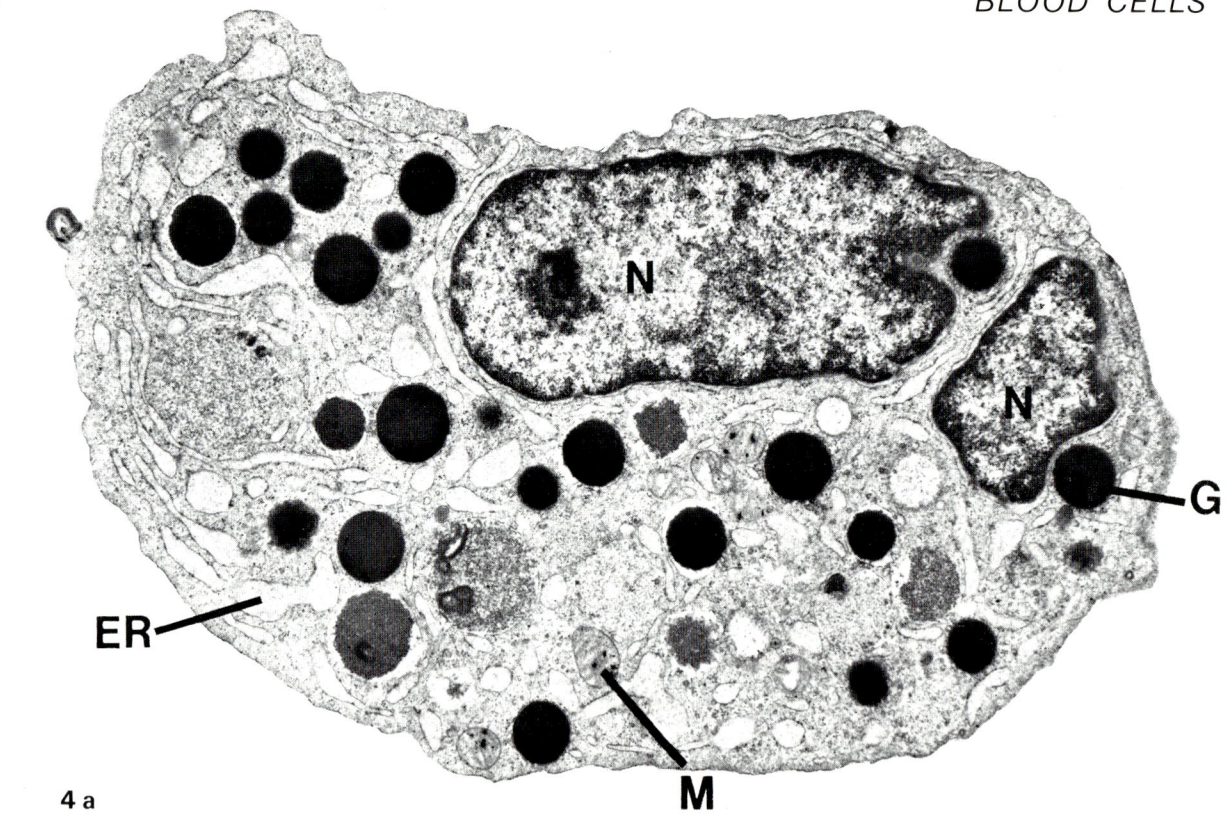

4 a

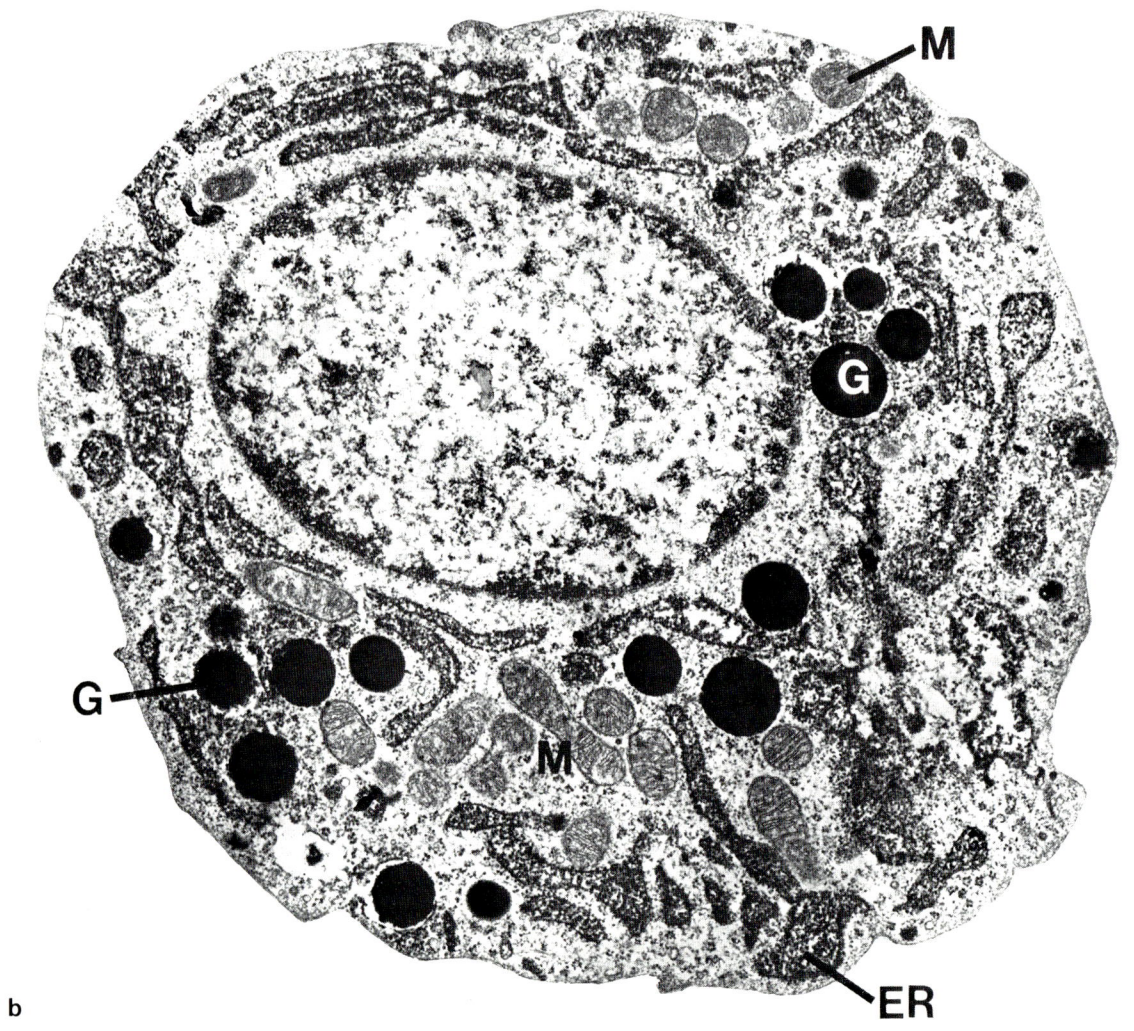

b

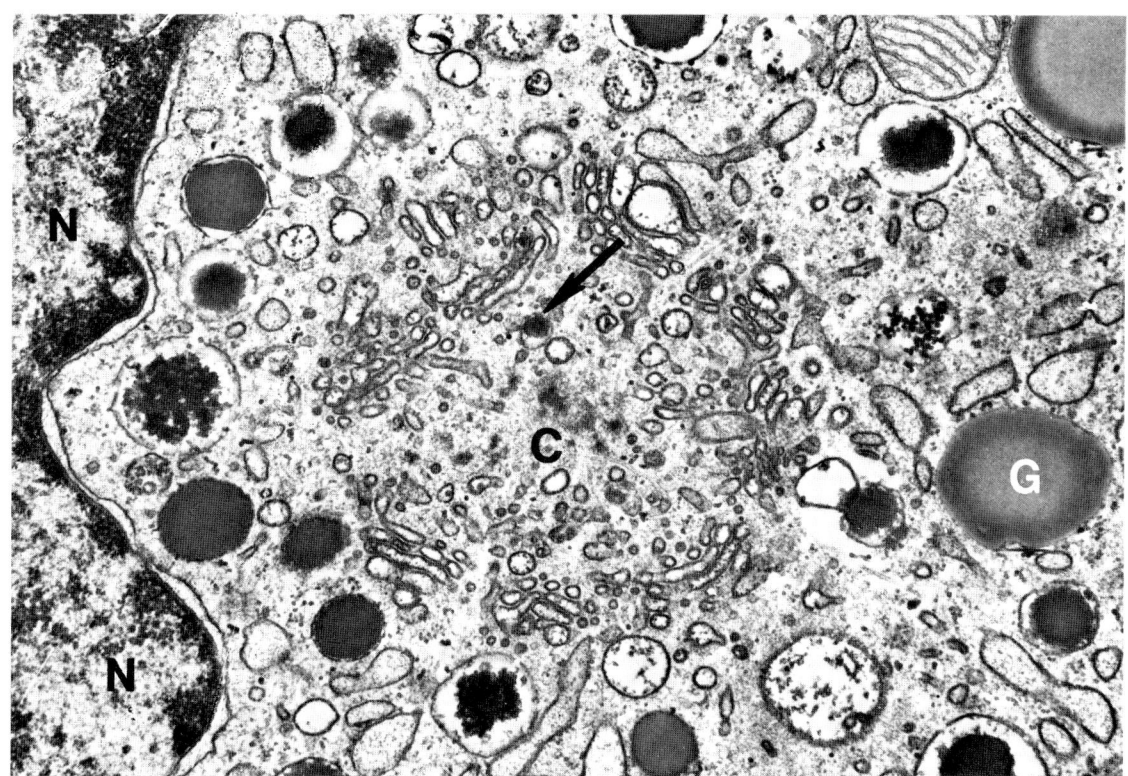

Fig. 5 Detail of an eosinophilic promyelocyte illustrating the Golgi zone to better advantage. In this area the newly synthesized enzymes are believed to be « packaged » by Golgi membranes. The **arrow** indicates the formation of a small granule. The centriole is located in the center of this zone, **C**. **N**, nucleus; **G**, large membrane-bound primary granule ($\times$ 23,000).

The ultrastructural features of the eosinophil promyelocyte are illustrated in **Figures 4 a** and **b**. The granules are round, uniformly electron dense and larger than those of neutrophilic promyelocytes. These so-called primary granules have been shown to contain peroxidase, acid phosphatase, aryl sulfatase, and a number of other lysosomal enzymes [12-16]. As seen in **Figures 4** and **5**, this immature cell still possesses abundant rough endoplasmic reticulum and a large Golgi zone. According to current theory, granule enzymes are synthesized by polyribosomes attached to endoplasmic reticulum which is in continuity with the cisternae of the Golgi apparatus. Here, condensation and final "packaging" takes place, and the membrane-bound granules are released into the cytoplasm (**Fig. 5**). It should be noted that the granules which "bud" off the Golgi apparatus are much smaller (20-30 nm) than the granules seen in the periphery of the same cell (80-120 nm) or in mature eosinophils. To account for the "growth" of the granules, it has been suggested that enzyme-containing vesicles continue to coalesce with them even at sites distant from the Golgi zone. An alternative concept proposed by the author is that there remains physical continuity between the space enclosed by the Golgi vesicles and that of the granules throughout the promyelocyte stage.

Fig. 4 a) Higher resolution of an eosinophil promyelocyte derived from a soft agar colony. Note that the granules (**G**) are round and extremely electron dense. The cytoplasm is still replete with rough endoplasmic reticulum (**ER**). **M**, mitochondrion; **N**, nucleus ($\times$ 11,000).

b) Eosinophil promyelocyte prepared from a bone marrow specimen. The specimen was treated by a method for the detection of peroxidase. The cisternae of rough endoplasmic reticulum (**ER**) contain the electron dense « reaction product » as do the primary granules (**G**). **M**, mitochondria ($\times$ 15,000).

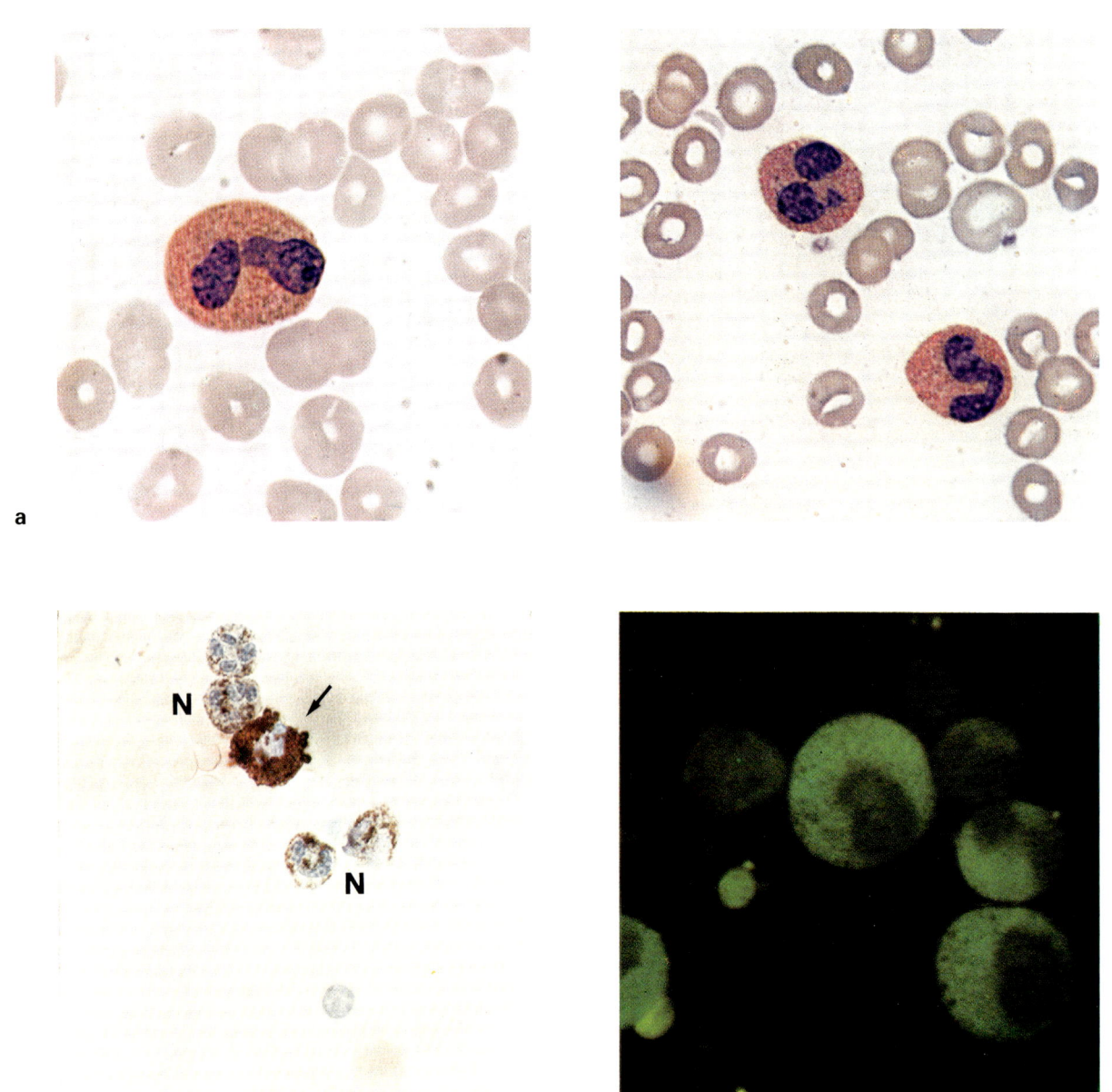

Fig. 6 are a series of light photomicrographs:

a) mature eosinophil with bi-lobed nucleus (Wright's stain);

b) eosinophil from a patient with eosinophilia. Some basophilic primary granules have been retained;

c) blood smear stained for peroxidase. Note remarkable positivity of the eosinophil granules **(arrow)** when compared with neutrophils. Fewer neutrophil granules contain peroxidase **(N)**;

d) treated with fluorescein-labelled antiserum to immunoglobulin showing non specific fluorescence.

d) Courtesy of Dr. G.L. Castoldi, University of Ferrara.

Fig. 7 a) Eosinophil myelocyte treated with substrate for peroxidase. At this stage of development the nucleus is still round and there is a predominance of euchromatin (light staining). The cell has acquired many mature granules as evidenced by the crystalloids that are outlined in negative contrast by the black, peroxidase positive matrix. There is still abundant rough endoplasmic reticulum **(ER)** which also stains positively for peroxidase (black) ($\times$ 13,000).

b) Eosinophil metamyelocyte. As can be seen here the nucleus is indented, almost horseshoe-shaped and contains more heterochromatin than the nucleus of the myelocyte depicted in **a**. Most of the granules are mature. However, a few primary granules remain. This cell was obtained from the same specimen as the cell illustrated in **a**. The granules are positive for peroxidase, but note that profiles of rough endoplasmic reticulum **(ER)** are now devoid of the enzyme ($\times$ 13,000).

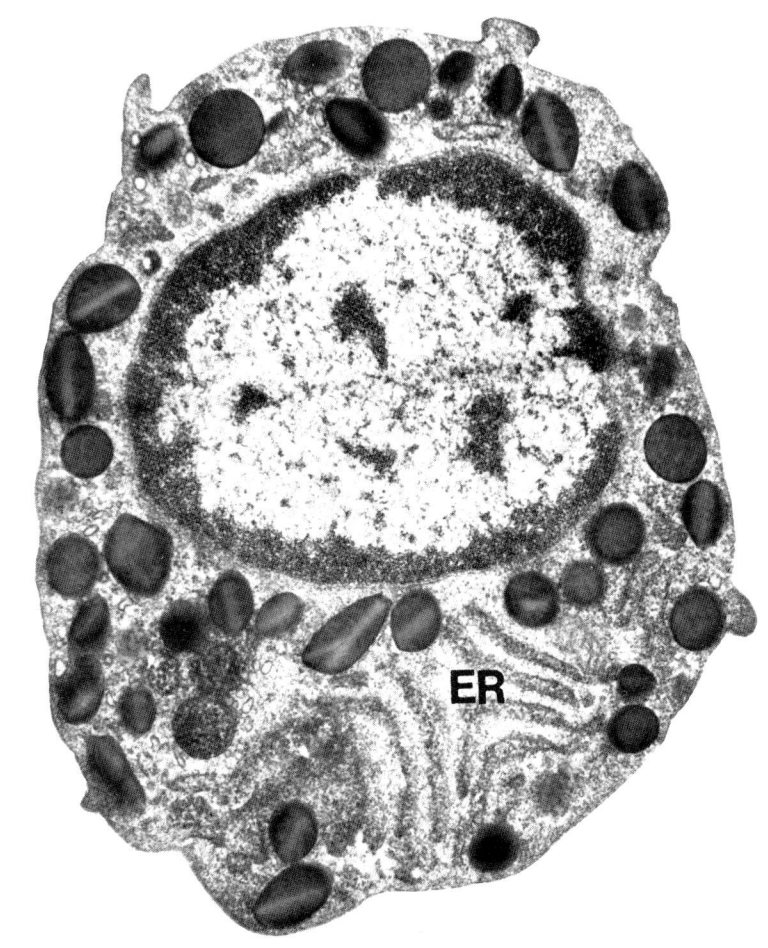

7 a

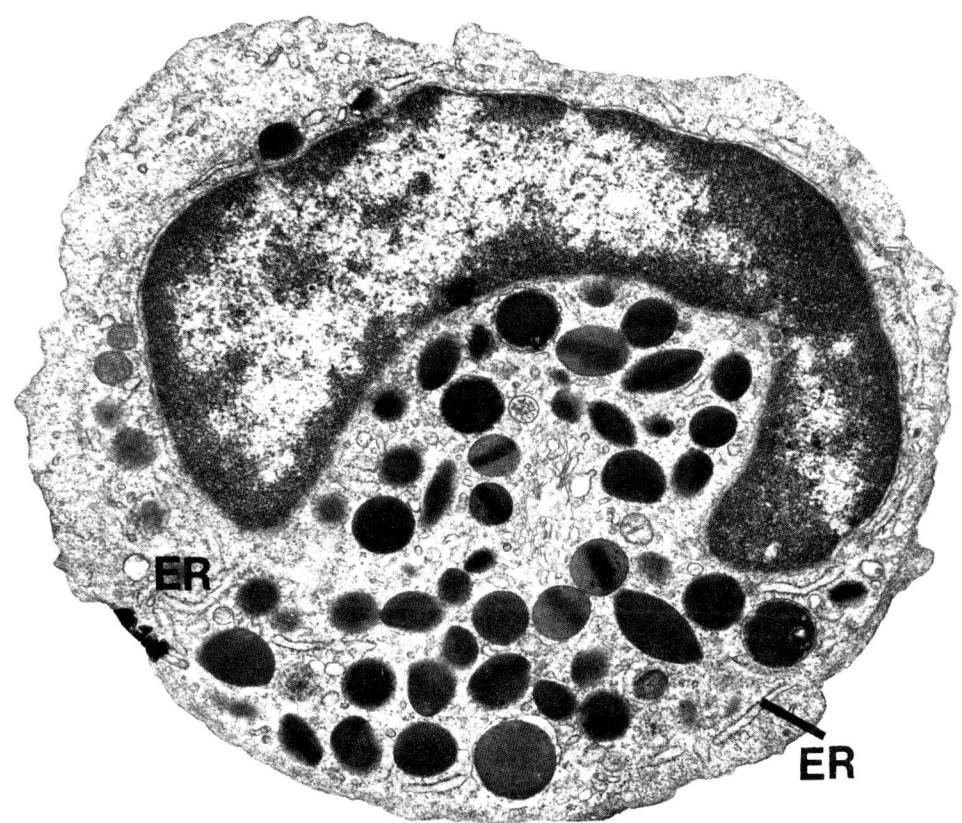

b

This would allow for a continuing flow of newly synthesized protein as well as membranes up to the time when such synthesis ceases, i.e. at the myelocyte stage of development [17]. As a rule, eosinophil promyelocytes are not found in the peripheral blood but they may appear under pathological conditions (vide infra).

At the end of the promyelocyte stage, the nucleus becomes slightly indented (myelocyte) to horseshoe-shaped (metamyelocyte) and the crystalloid-containing granules begin to appear.

These are the "specific" granules that characterize mature eosinophils (**Figs. 6-8**). On light microscopy, they stain orange to deep red with most stains used for routine blood smears. They also can be "stained" by histochemical techniques to reveal a variety of enzymes including peroxidase, acid phosphatase, phospholipase, aryl sulfatase, β-glucuronidase, ribonuclease, and cathepsin. For this reason, they are considered lysosomes. The remarkable refractility and autofluorescence of eosinophil granules is notorious (**Fig. 6 d**) and so is their affinity for most of the fluorescent dyes used to label antisera for immunofluorescent analyses (**Fig. 6 d**) [18]. This should be kept in mind whenever immunofluorescence is employed for the detection of an antigen believed to reside in eosinophils.

1.2. Ultrastructure of mature eosinophils

Nucleus

The majority of human blood eosinophils have bi-lobed nuclei but with eosinophilia, B_{12} or folate deficiency there may be increased nuclear segmentation. As in other granulocytes [19], the dense heterochromatin is distributed mostly in the periphery of the nucleus. The loosely arranged euchromatin believed to be the synthetically active form of chromatin, is found toward the center and in connection with the nuclear pores (**Fig. 8 a**).

In contrast to mature neutrophils which are end stage cells, eosinophils often retain a fairly large nucleolus. Because it has been shown that nucleolar volume is roughly proportional to the amount of ribosomal RNA, the presence of the nucleolus suggests that the cells continue to engage in major synthetic processes even after they have been released from the bone marrow.

Fig. 8 a) *Mature eosinophil. The cell has a bi-lobed nucleus with a small nucleolus (**Nu**). The electron dense heterochromatin is distributed at the periphery whereas the lighter staining euchromatin is seen mostly in the center of the nucleus and in connection with the nuclear pores (**P**). All the granules contain central crystalloids. Small profiles of rough endoplasmic reticulum (**ER**) continue to be present (× 17,500).*
b) *Detail of a mature eosinophil shows the area around the centriole (**C**) to better advantage. Note that the granules appear to radiate out from this zone as though guided by microtubules (**arrowheads**).*
N, *nucleus;* **mg**, *microgranule;* **G**, *Golgi zone (× 25,000).*

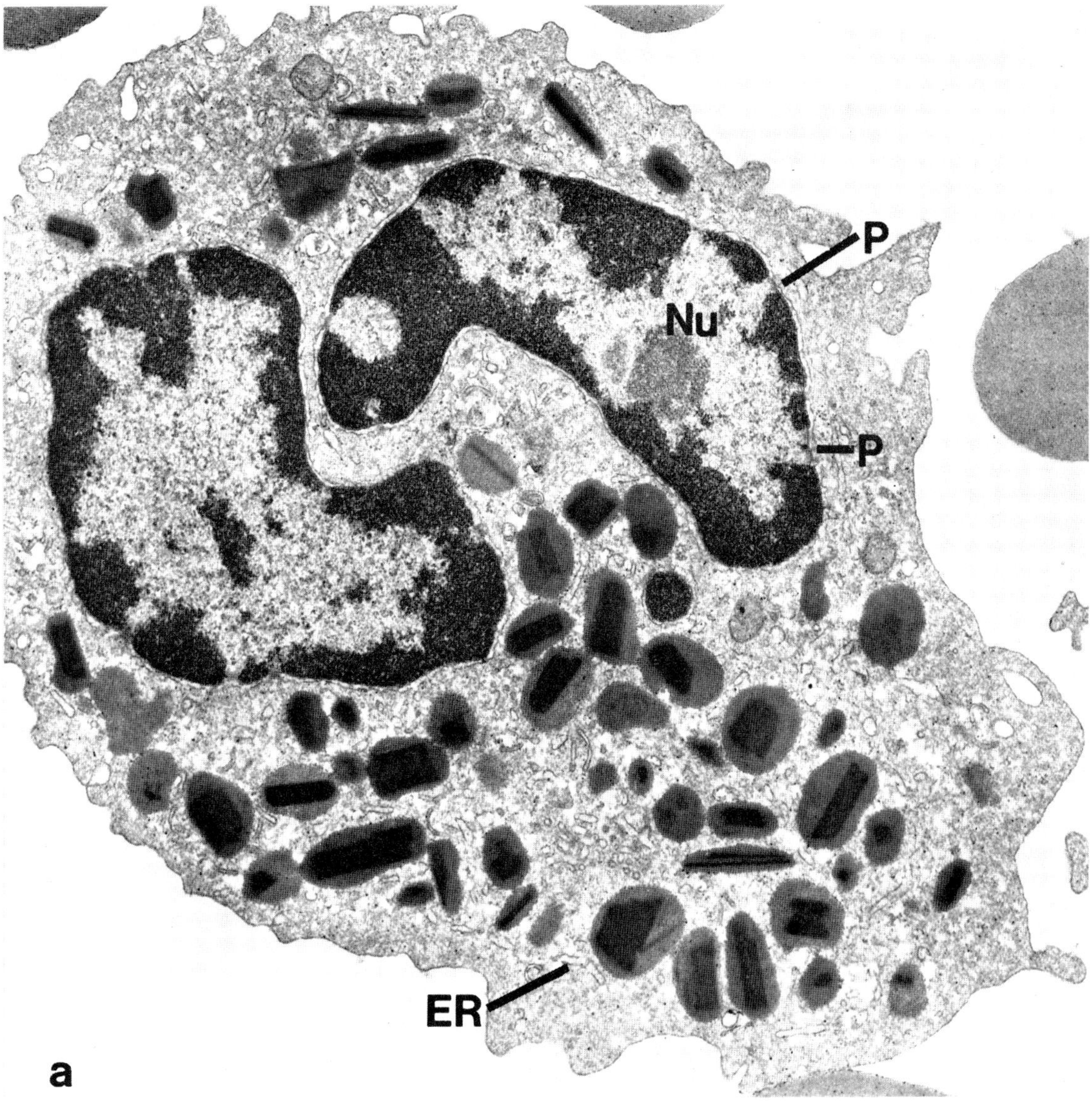

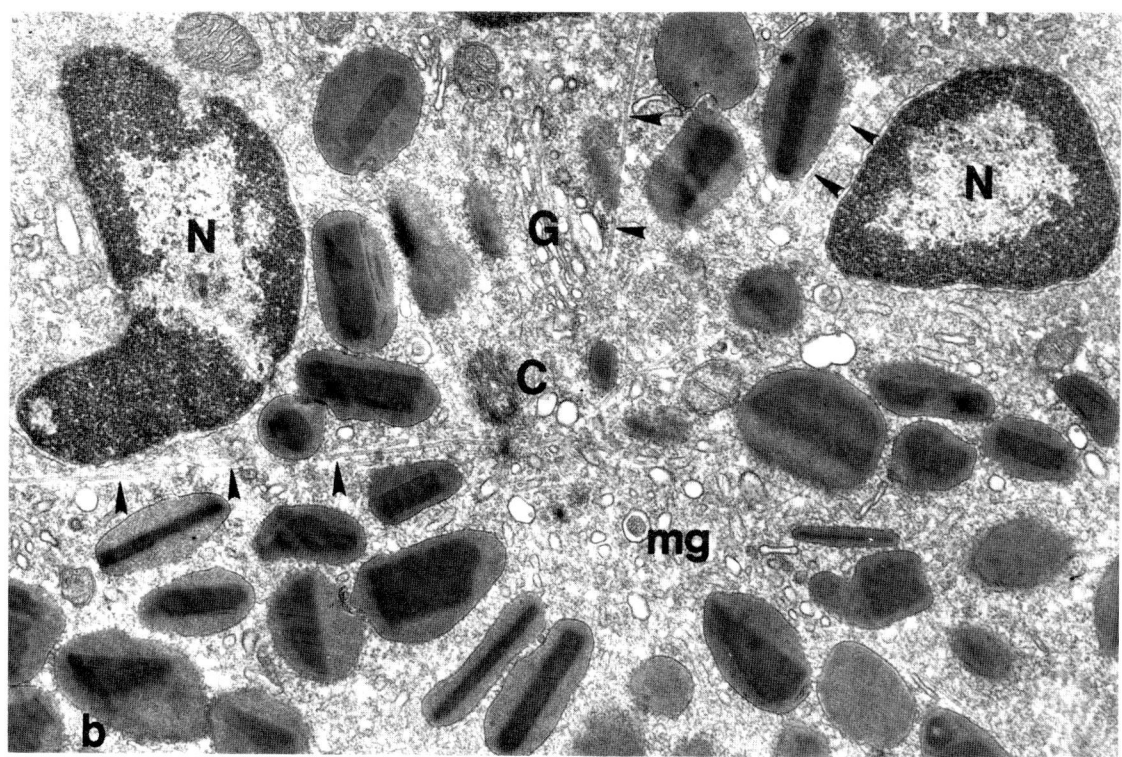

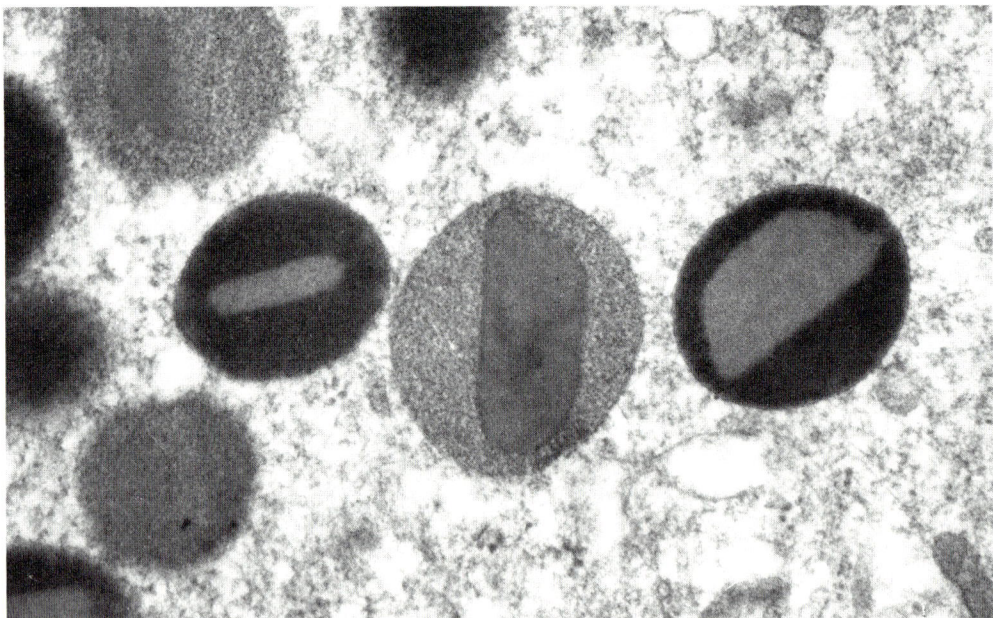

Fig. 9 Detail of an eosinophil obtained from the blood of a healthy subject, selected to illustrate variable electron density of the core and matrix in adjacent granules within the same cell. This may reflect differences in enzyme content. No special staining procedures were used ($\times$ 55,000).

Granules

In mature eosinophils, the majority of the granules are roughly football-shaped, membrane bound organelles measuring 0.15 to 1.5 μm in length and 0.3 to 1.0 μm in their shorter diameter. In most species, including man, they reveal a central bar referred to as the core, crystalloid, or internum that differs in electron opacity from the surrounding matrix. The relative electron density of the core and matrix is to some extent dependent on the fixation and embedding procedures used [20, 21]. Heavy metals precipitate in the matrix and delineate the core by negative contrast. However, reversal of electron density of the core and matrix may even be found among the granules of individual eosinophils (**Fig. 9**). For rat, mouse, guinea pig, and human eosinophils, it has been determined that the core is made up of a crystal (**Fig.10**) consisting of a cubic lattice with a periodicity of 3 nm in rodents, and 4 nm in man [22].

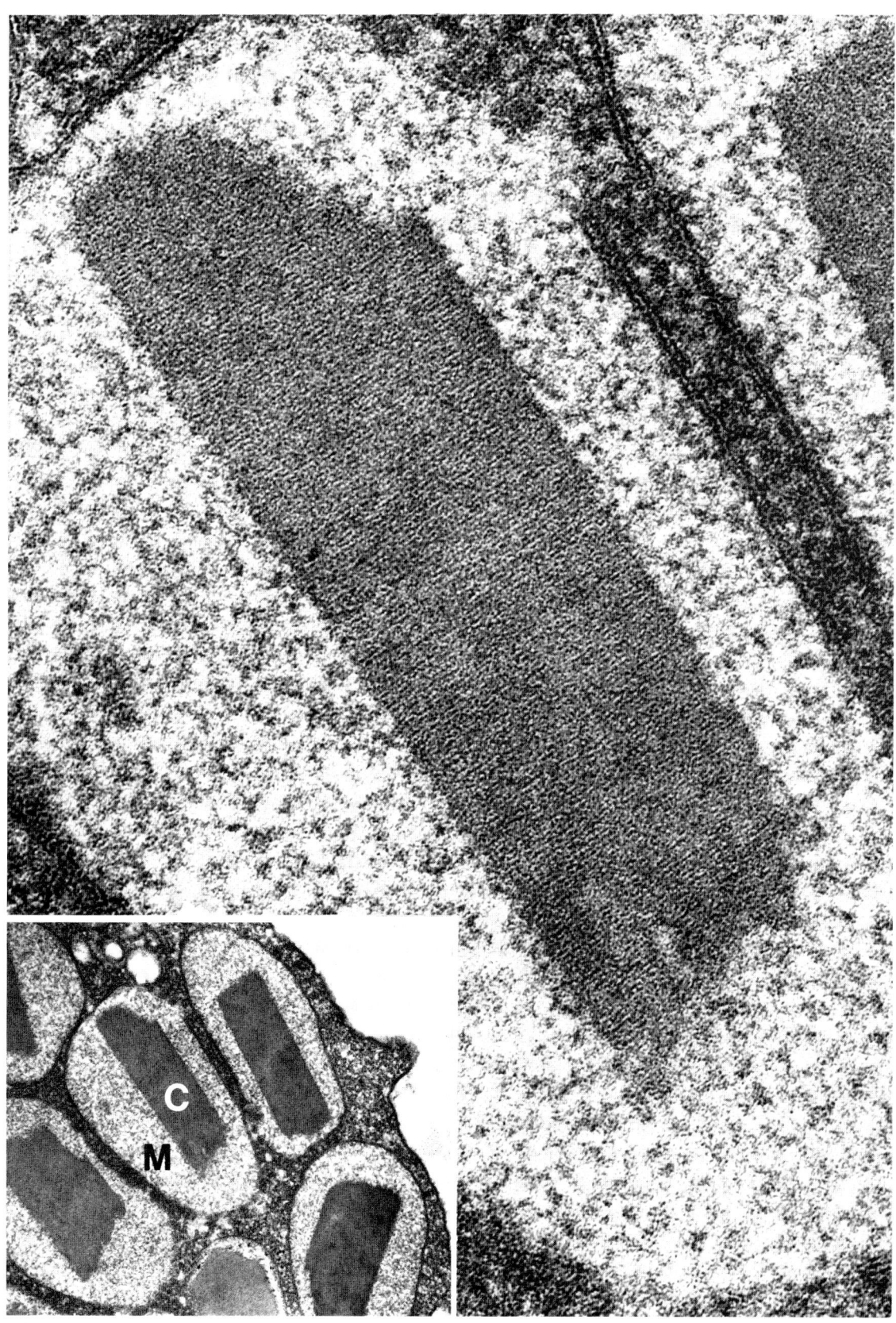

Fig. 10 High resolution electron micrograph of a human eosinophil granule to illustrate the periodic structure of the internum. A detail of the eosinophil from which this granule was obtained is shown at lower left.
M, matrix; C, core (inset, × 48,000; crystal, × 260,000).
Reproduced from ref. 3.

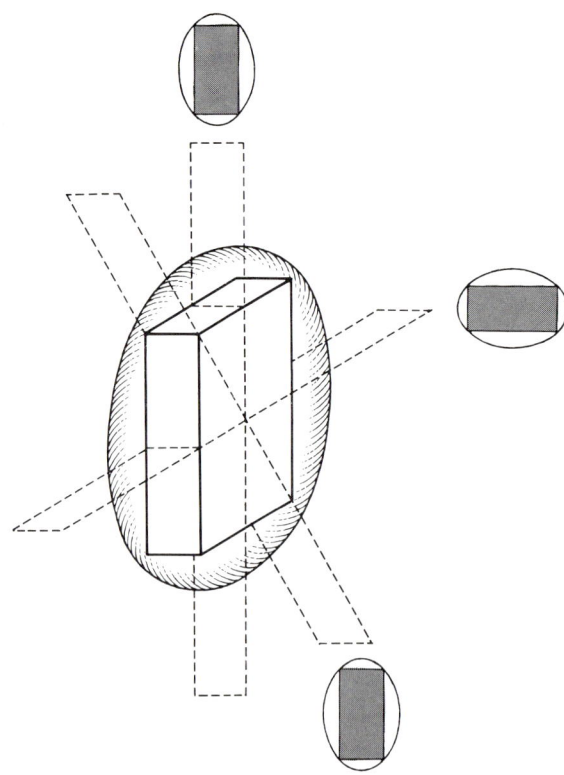

Fig. 11 a) Diagrammatic representation of an eosinophil granule demonstrates how different planes of section through the granule yield similar profiles of core and matrix (drawing contributed by George Grusky, Ph.D., New York University Medical Center).

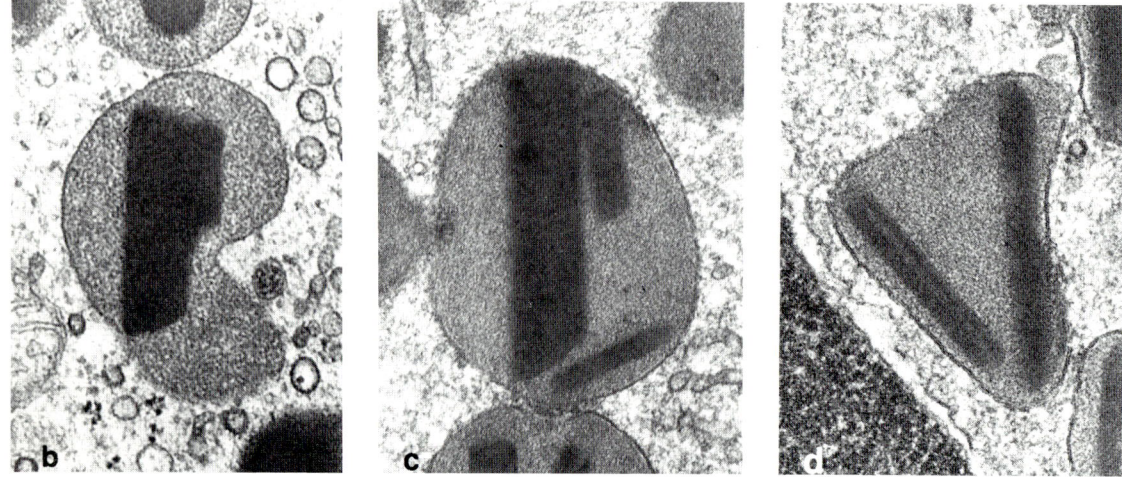

Figs. 11 b, c, d) High resolution of individual granules selected from different eosinophils in blood obtained from healthy subjects. Such granules represent a small percentage, but they are not uncommon. These have been chosen to illustrate the theory that the orientation and shape of the crystals determines to some extent the conformation of the granules (see text) (**b**, × 39,000; **c**, × 44,000; **d**, × 69,000).

The mechanism whereby the "specific" eosinophil granule develops is still under debate. Some investigators have postulated an independent origin for the "primary" promyelocyte granules and those seen in the mature cells. However, the absence of any apparent degeneration of promyelocyte granules and the difficulty of accounting for the loss of such a large number of organelles by mitotic dilution makes this theory difficult to accept. It seems more likely that crystallization occurs within the first-formed granules when the protein that makes up the "core" has reached a critical concentration. An excellent argument in favor of this contention is found in refs. 21 and 23. It should also be noted that despite the random plane of each section, the core almost always occupies the full length of the granule. This leads us to suggest that the crystal takes the shape of a thick domino, the size and rigidity of which determines the size and shape of the granule (**Fig. 11 a**). Supporting this theory is the observation that in some states of eosinophilia when the granules may contain more than one crystal of different size and position, the shape of the granule seems to adapt to that of the crystal (**Fig. 11 b-d**). It should be mentioned, however, that the partition of granule content is not found in all species and that its functional significance has so far escaped definition. For instance, the core of the cat eosinophil granule has a lamellar structure reminiscent of the myelin configuration phospholipids assume in aqueous media (**Fig. 12**).

Biochemical analysis of the granule cores of pig, rat, and human eosinophils has shown them to be insoluble at physiological pH and to consist to a large extent of a basic protein with a high arginine content [24, 25]. Although the core substance appears to be relatively inert, it adsorbs onto membranes and acetic proteins and is able to neutralize heparin. Histochemical methods at the ultrastructural level have localized the hydrolytic enzymes as well as peroxidase to the matrix of the granule and not to its core (**Fig. 7 a**) [16, 26, 27]. In addition to the "specific" granules discussed so far, mature eosinophils possess some smaller granules (0.1-0.5 μm) which have been reported to carry arylsulfatase and acid phosphatase [28]. These smaller structures may play a role in the secretion of aryl sulfatase which is believed to take place in the absence of phagocytosis or degranulation detectable by light microscopy.

Another much ignored organelle which may subserve a secretory function has been named the specific microgranule by Schäffer [29] who has identified this structure in more than 20 mammalian species. The term "granules" may be somewhat misleading since these organelles appear to consist of profiles of smooth endoplasmic reticulum which may assume cup-like, ring or dumbbell-shaped conformations (**Figs. 8, 12, 24**). In eosinophilic states specific microgranules appear to be much more numerous than when the eosinophil count is within normal range.

A glance at **Figures 5**, **8** and **12** will also impress the reader with the abundance of cytoplasmic vesicles, the presence of ribosomes and small profiles of rough endoplasmic reticulum, mitochondria as well as glycogen particles, centrioles and microtubules, all suggesting that the cell remains biosynthetically and metabolically active.
The plasma membrane of the eosinophil is structurally not distinctive from that of other leukocytes. By indirect methods, such as rosetting techniques, the cells can be shown to have membrane receptors for IgG, and complement. It has also been shown that the percentage of cells bearing these receptors and the number of such receptors per cell increase during eosinophilia of diverse causes.

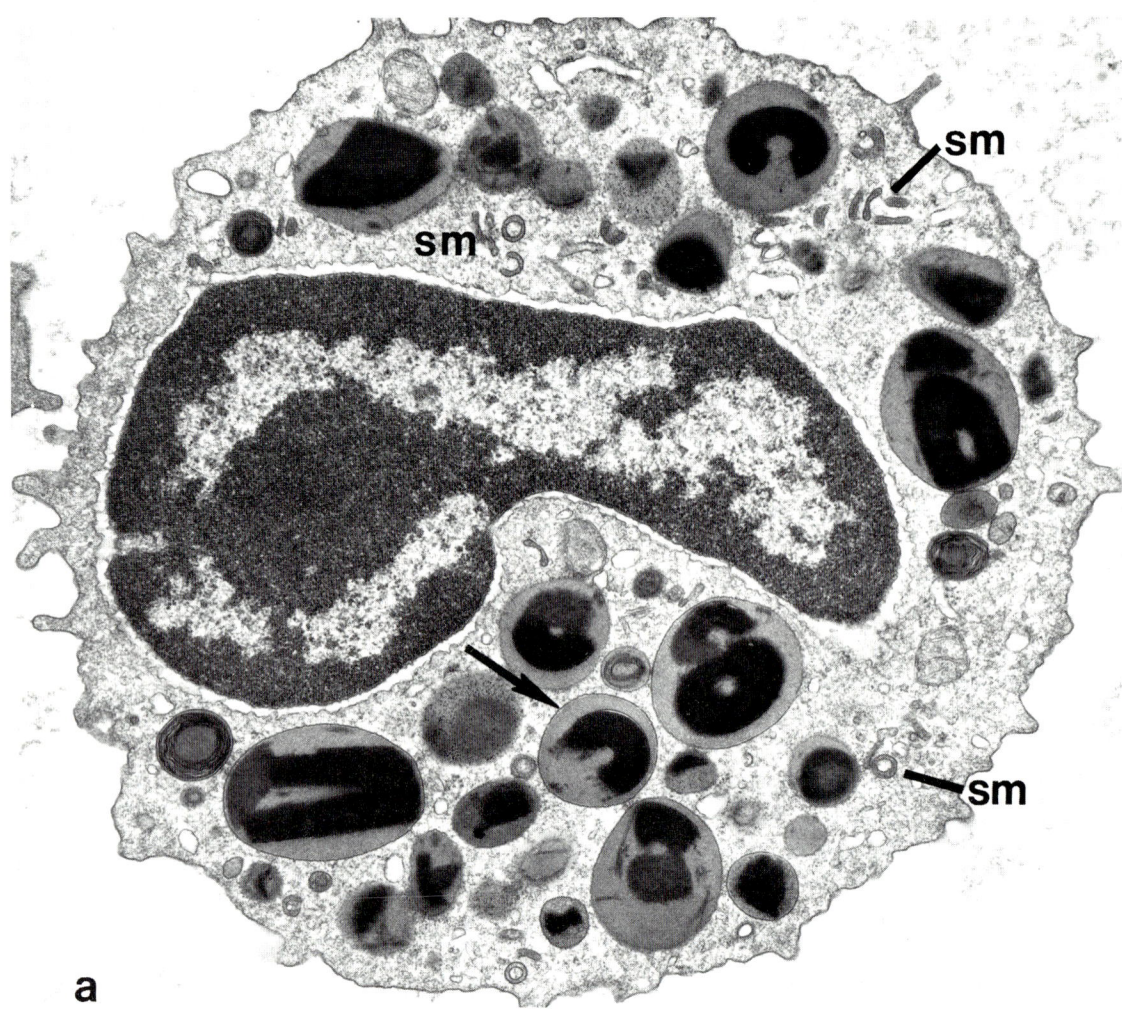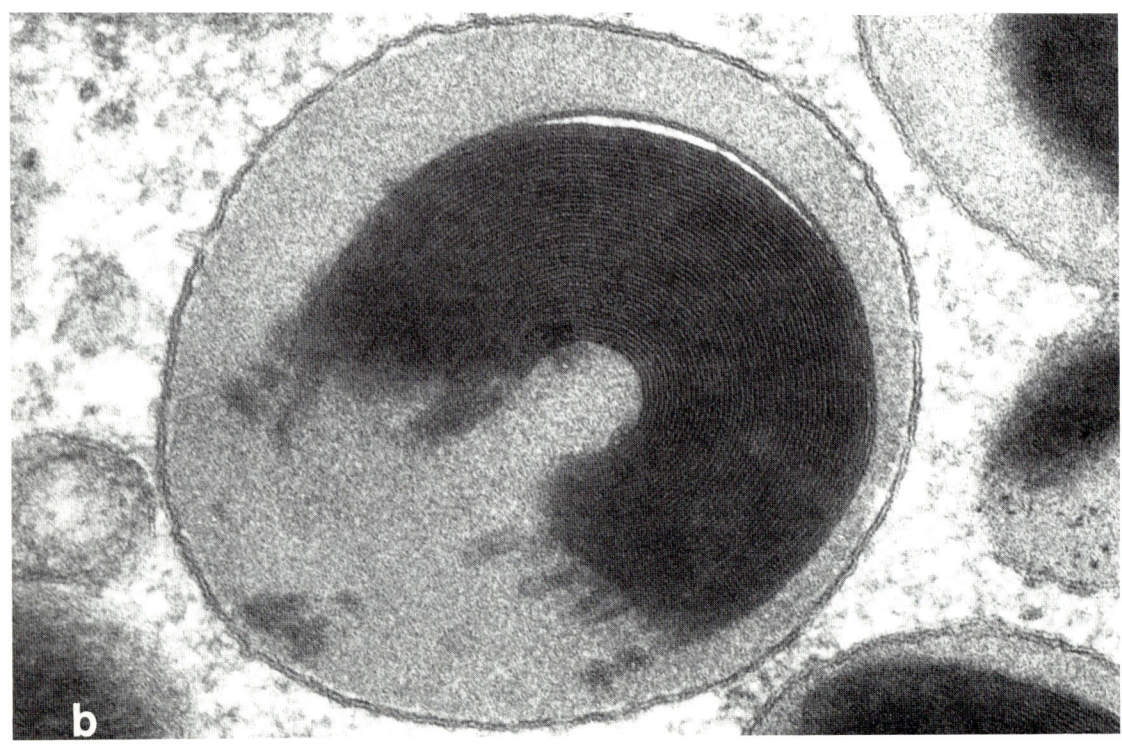

1.3. Morphologic correlates of eosinophil function

Eosinophils function much like neutrophils in that they have amoeboid motion, they phagocytize bacteria, particulates, sensitized erythrocytes (**Fig. 13**) and other antigen/antibody complexes. Their granules coalesce with phagocytic vacuoles [30, 31] and under some conditions they are discharged into the extracellular medium. The cells also respond to chemotaxis by products released from bacteria and components of the complement system [32-33] and they are able to kill microorganisms [34] and parasites [34 a].

Some of these functions are illustrated in **Figures 13-17**. However, other properties, particularly those which distinguish eosinophils from other leukocytes do not lend themselves to visual representation. Among these are: 1) the cell's ability to inactivate slow reacting substance of anaphylaxis (SRS-A) [35]. SRS-A is a potent bronchoconstrictor elaborated by mast cells. It is inactivated by aryl sulfatase, an enzyme with a fivefold higher concentration in eosinophils than in other leukocytes; 2) eosinophils neutralize histamine [36, 37], and 3) the cells elaborate a substance called eosinophil derived inhibitor (EDI) which is purported to inhibit mast cell degranulation [38].

Therefore, eosinophils are likely to play an important, if not a crucial role in abrogating the immediate hypersensitivity response. If this is true the cells must be attracted preferentially to the site where such reactions occur or they must be trapped there while migrating randomly through the tissues. Indeed there is substantial evidence in favor of the view that the chemoattractants responsible are elaborated by antigen sensitized lymphocytes [39, 40] and mast cells [41-43].
With these general concepts in mind, it becomes possible to implicate a variety of mechanisms to explain tissue eosinophilia in many clinical situations. These have been discussed in detail elsewhere [4] and a few examples are provided below.

Fig. 12 *Eosinophil prepared from the peripheral blood of a cat. Note the heterogeneity in granule size (a). The lamellated appearance of the core structure conveys the impression of reduplicated membranes. The granule indicated by the* **arrow** *is shown at higher magnification below (b).* **sm**, *specific microgranules (× 22,000; detail, × 195,000).*

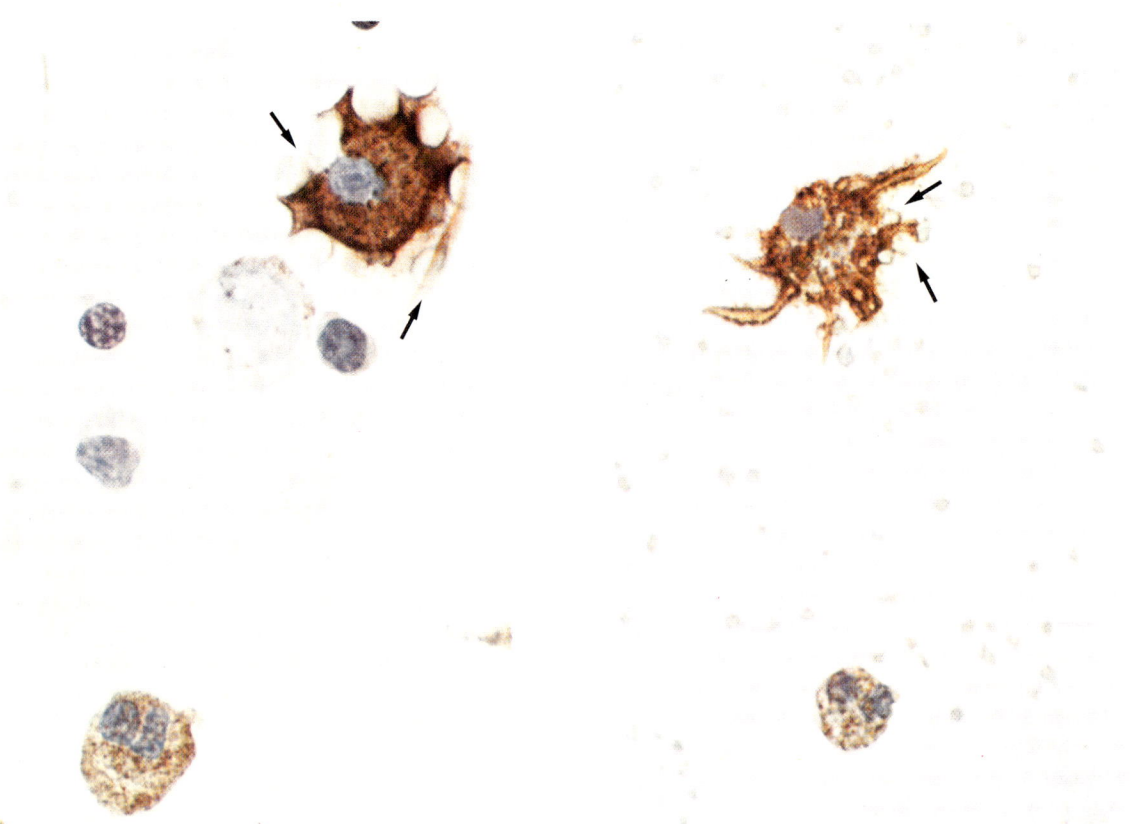

a

b

Fig. 13 Blood smear from a patient with myelogenous leukemia associated with hemolytic anemia and thrombocytopenia. The smears were stained by a special method for eosinophil peroxidase and contributed by Dr. J.S. Hankev, University of North Carolina.

a) The eosinophil on the top is in the process of phagocytosing the sensitized erythrocytes (**arrows**).

b) A large eosinophil with multiple long pseudopods is seen in the process of engulfing platelets (**arrows**).

Fig. 15 Human blood eosinophil from a buffy coat specimen that had been incubated with rheumatoid factor complexed with aggregated gammaglobulin (**RFC**) as an example of an antigen/antibody complex that is readily phagocytosed by the cells. The eosinophil has phagocytosed the immune precipitate which is now seen in phagocytic vacuoles (**PV**). The black material derived from the granules can still be delineated within the phagolysosomes (**PV**) ($\times$ 14,000).
Reproduced from ref. 19.

6 EOSINOPHILS

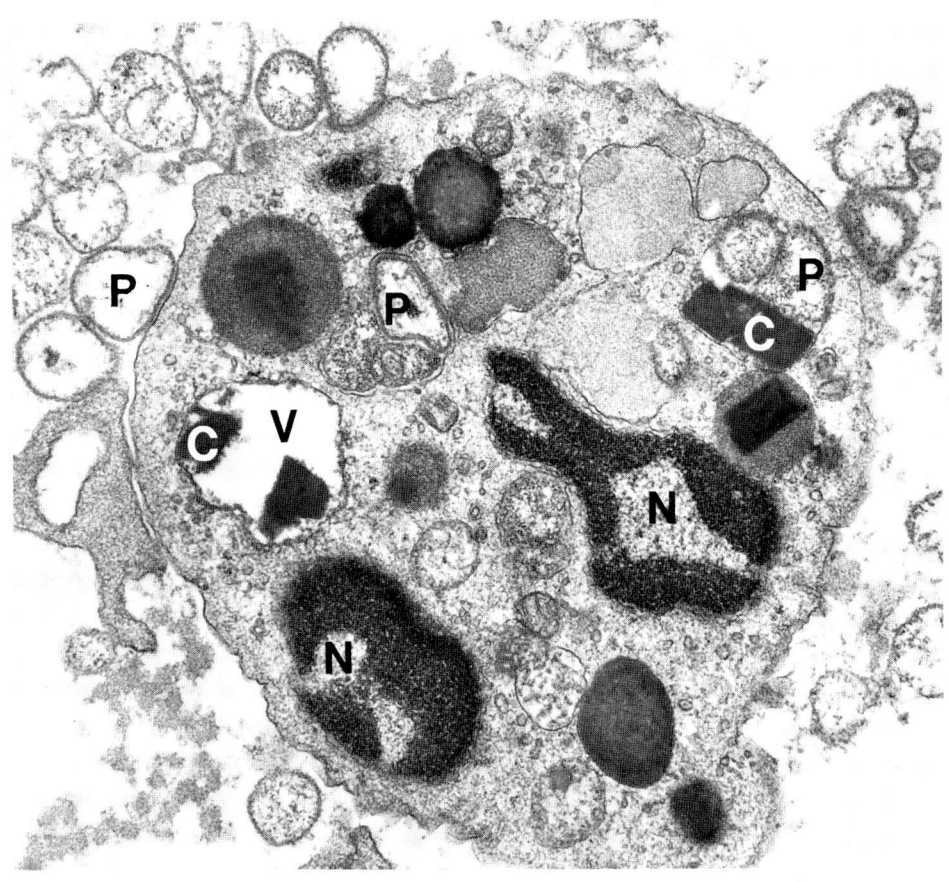

Fig. 14 Human peripheral blood eosinophil from a buffy coat specimen that was incubated with M. pneumoniae (**P**), the organism responsible for atypical pneumonia. Mycoplasmas are avidly phagocytosed by eosinophils. Here they are seen attached to the plasma membrane as well as within phagocytic vacuoles (**V**). Note that in some of the vacuoles the core (**C**) of the granule has not dissolved. **N**, nucleus (× 23,000).
Reproduced from ref. 31.

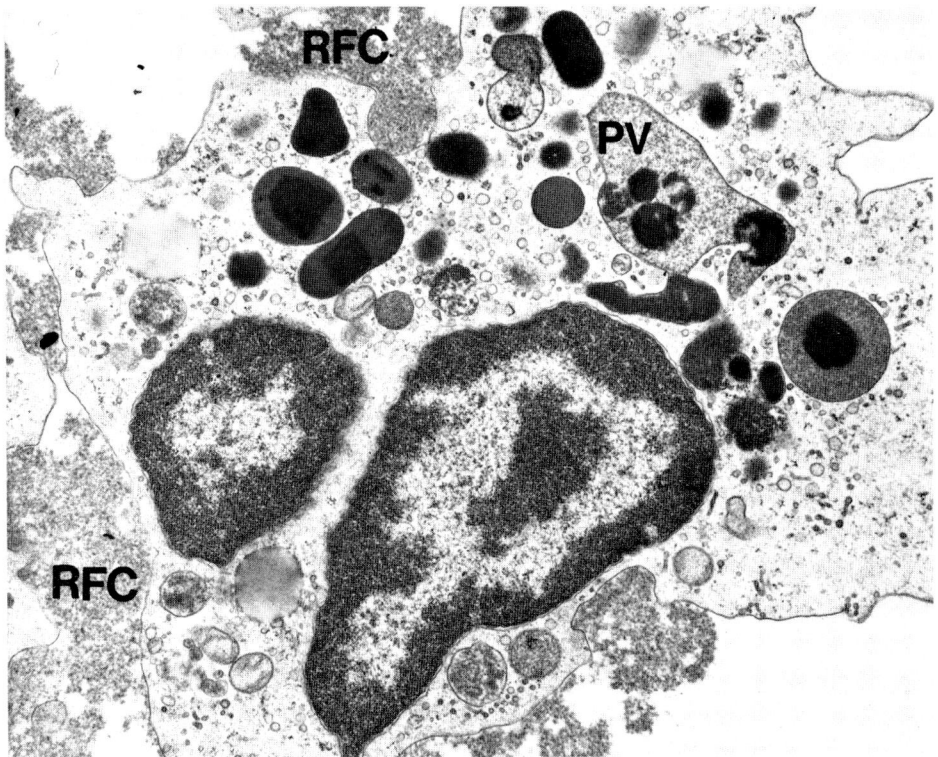

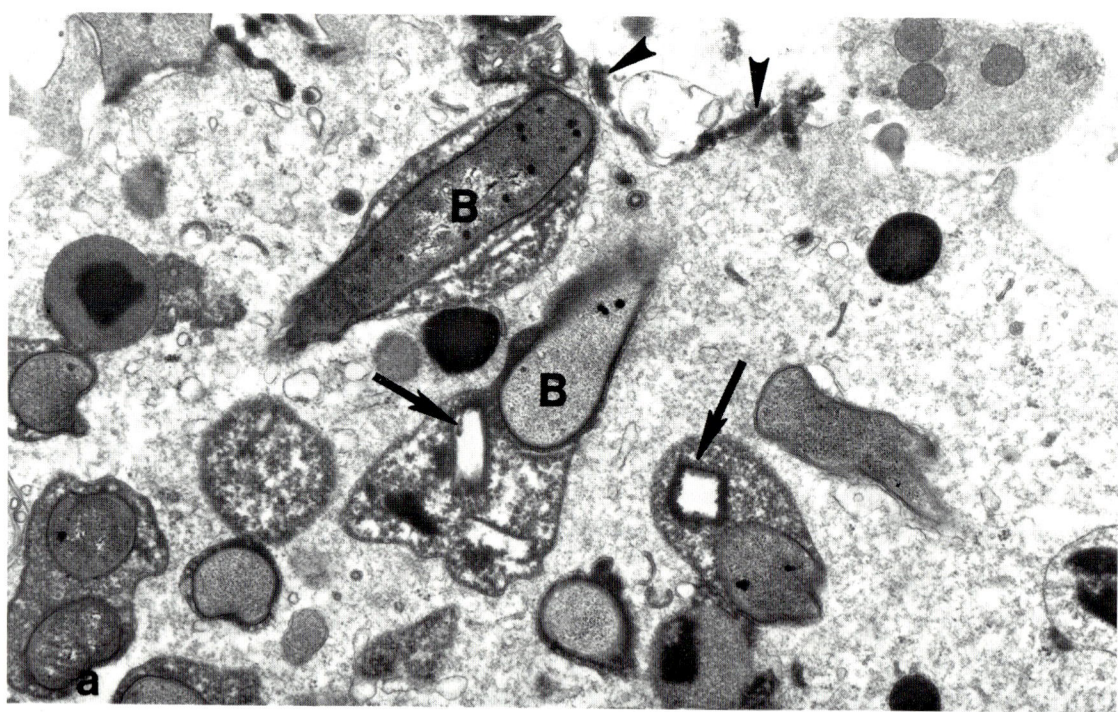

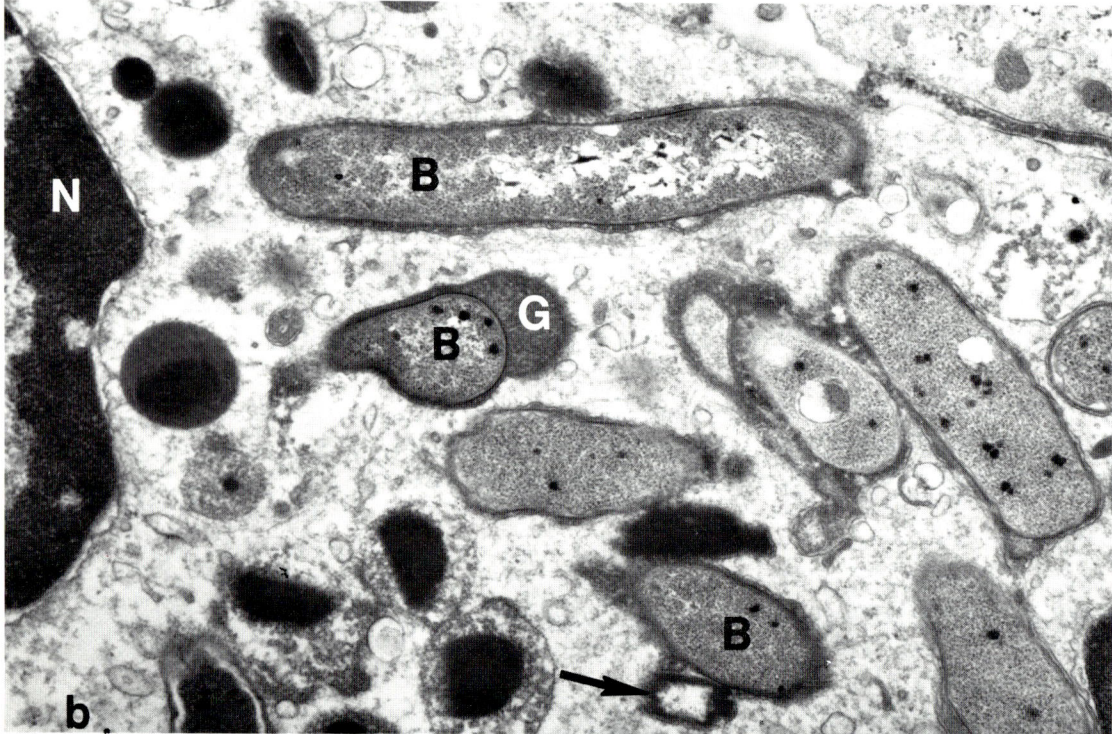

Figs. 16 a, b) Hight magnification details of human blood eosinophils that were incubated with E. coli for 15 min. at 37°C. Innumerable bacteria (B) are seen in phagocytic vacuoles. Coalescence of eosinophil granules (G) with these vacuoles first described in reference 30 is readily apparent. The black material surrounding the microorganisms is also seen on the surface of the cell (**arrowheads** in 16 a). It is known to originate from the granules. Note remnants of crystalline structures within the phagocytic vacuoles (**arrows**). N, nucleus (a, × 22,400; b, × 18,900).

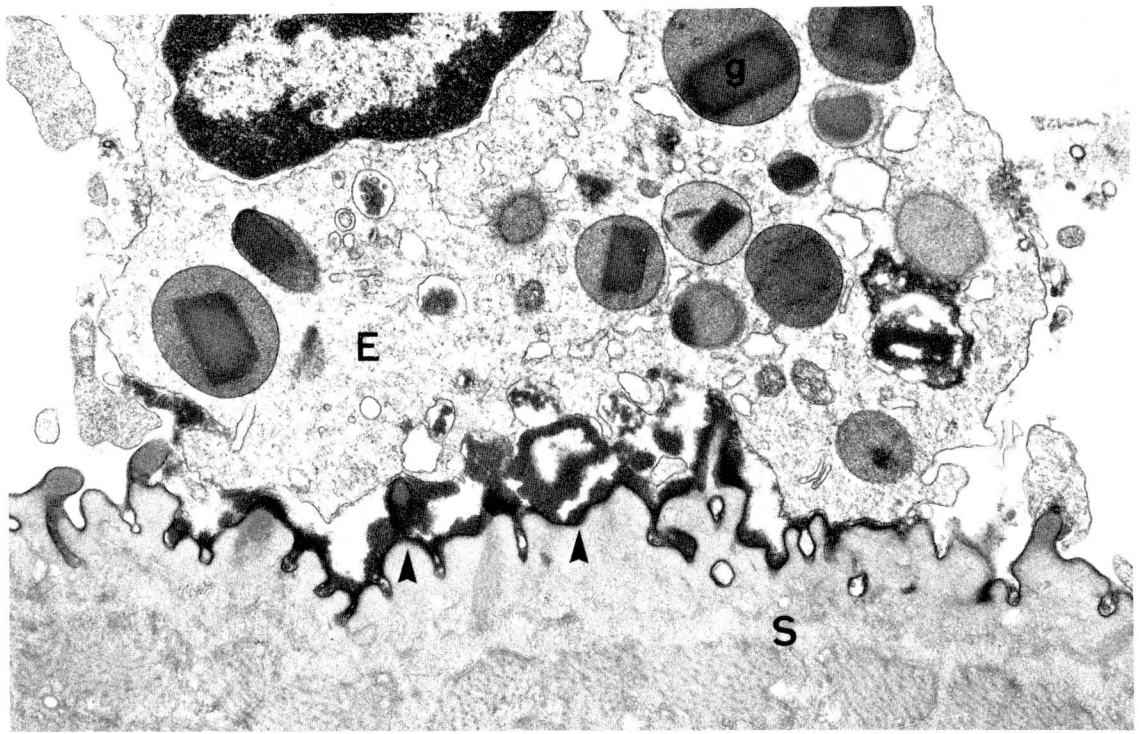

Fig. 17 Detail of a human eosinophil (**E**) adhering to a schistosomulum of S. mansoni (**S**). The parasite has been preincubated in serum from a patient with schistosomiasis in order to coat the schistosomulum with antibody. Note the electron dense material (**arrows**) between the eosinophil and the schistosomulum. This has been discharged by the cell and resembles the material in the dense core of the granules (**g**). It has been shown that a substance isolated from the granules will kill the parasite ($\times$ 19,000).
Courtesy of Drs. G. Korman, A. Butterworth, J. Caulfield, Harvard Medical School.

2. PATHOLOGY OF EOSINOPHILS

The healthy non-allergic subject has an absolute eosinophil count of less than 400/cmm of blood; the mean normal value being about 120/cmm. The cells circulate for an estimated 3 to 8 hours after which they diapedese and migrate into the tissues where their lifespan is not known. It has been suggested that normal levels of eosinophils are maintained by an eosinopoietin analogous to the erythropoietin responsible for the regulation of erythropoiesis [44]. Much work remains to be done in this area to substantiate these preliminary data.

On the other hand, the mechanisms responsible for reactive eosinophilia, i.e. the eosinophilia associated with allergies, infections, inflammatory conditions, parasitic infestation, connective tissue and neoplastic diseases as well as a host of other conditions involving the immune response have been explored more thoroughly [Chapter 11 in ref. 2]. There is compelling evidence in favor of the concept that the stimulus for eosinophilia is dependent on the release of substances elaborated by thymus-derived lymphocytes. This information goes a long way in providing explanations for eosinophilia observed in many conditions involving the cellular immune response or that are otherwise accompanied by lymphoid proliferation of a benign or malignant nature. A few examples are illustrated in **Figures 18 a-d**. To this should be added that eosinophilia is not as much related to the type of antigen as to its tissue location and fixation [45]. Tissues rich in mast cells and basophils, e.g. the lung and gastrointestinal tract represent particularly attractive sites for eosinophil invasion. It has also become clear that immunoglobulin levels *per se* are unrelated to eosinophilia. Even in the case of IgE the level of which tends to parallel the rise and fall of the blood eosinophil count in most (but not all) conditions, no causal relationship appears to exist.

Accelerated proliferation of eosinophils is usually indicated by nuclear immaturity or nuclear hypersegmentation and "blebbing" and what the author likes to call "disorderly" maturation of the granules (**Figs. 19-25**). The immaturity of the cell may also account for the observation that the cells may be less phagocytic (**Fig. 26**). Moreover, massive infiltration of tissues with eosinophils often leads to disintegration of the cells and formation of Charcot-Leyden cystals (**Figs. 27 a-e**). The crystals are believed to consist mostly of the substance that makes up the granule cores [46-48].

They may arise intracellularly as well as in the extracellular milieu wherever degeneration of eosinophils occurs, e.g. in the bronchial or nasal mucus of patients with allergic asthma, the pleural fluid of patients with pulmonary eosinophilic infiltrates or the stools of patients with parasitic infestations (for review, see Chapter 6 in ref. 2). Charcot-Leyden crystals are also subject to phagocytosis by other cells (**Fig. 27 e**).

Fig. 18 *Examples of tissue infiltration with eosinophils. In* **a** *and* **b** *lymphokines released by the lymphoid cells may be responsible for the attraction and/or trapping of eosinophils. In* **c** *substances released by mast cells, such as ECF-A may be implicated. In* **d** *and* **e** *the eosinophils themselves were considered invasive.*
a) *Skin biopsy from a patient with mycosis fungoides. Apart from the large lymphoid cells with convoluted nuclei* (**arrows**) *the tissue is infiltrated with eosinophils.*
b) *Lymph node from a patient with Hodgkin's disease shows Reed-Sternberg cell* (**arrow**) *and infiltration with eosinophils.*
c) *Liver biopsy from a patient with hypereosinophilic syndrome whose blood eosinophil is illustrated in Fig. 28.*
d, e) *Marrow aspiration of an eosinophilic granuloma. Eosinophilic granuloma may be unifocal or multifocal. Usually the lesion exhibits a mixture of histiocytes and eosinophils. In this case, eosinophils at various stages of maturation predominate. In some cases, the cells are very sparse when the term eosinophilic granuloma may even be a misnomer. Unifocal lesions are usually not accompanied by blood eosinophilia.*

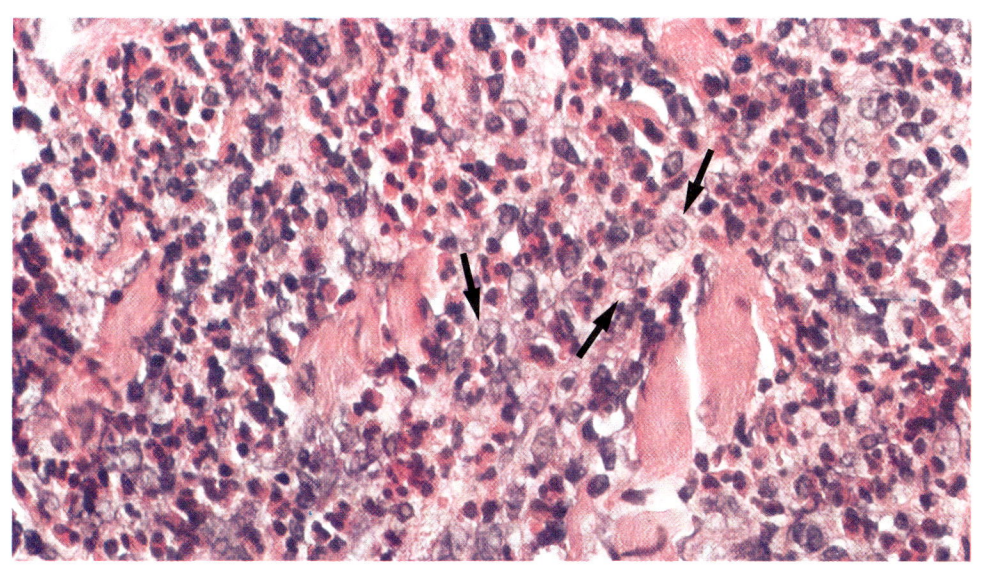
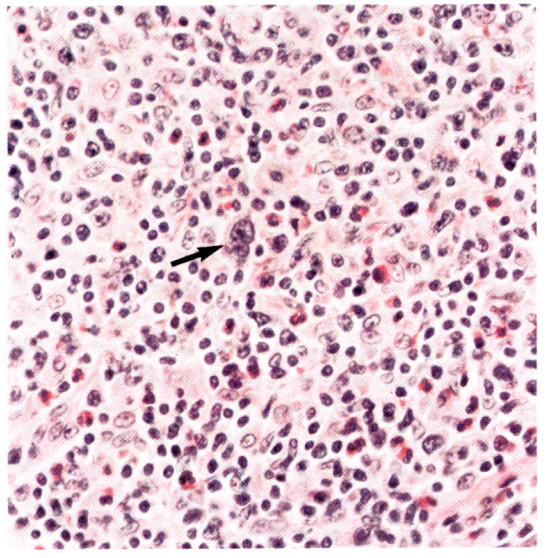
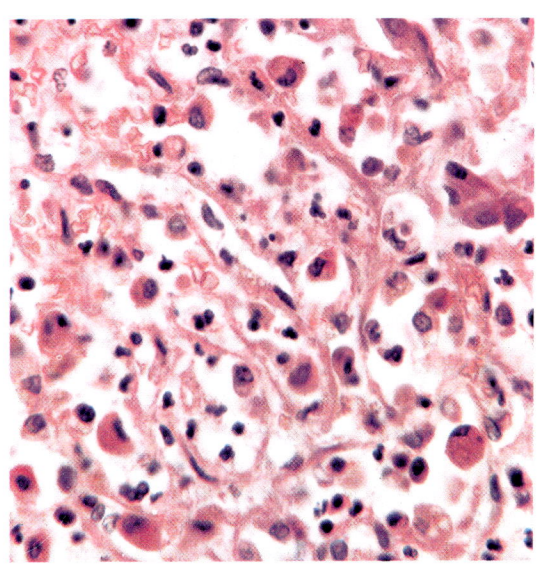
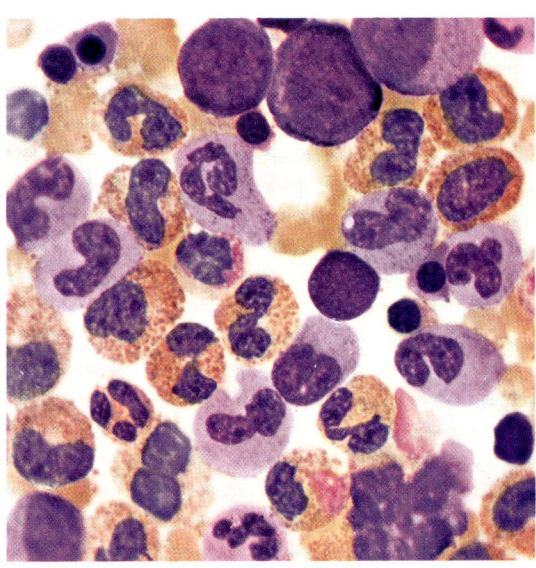
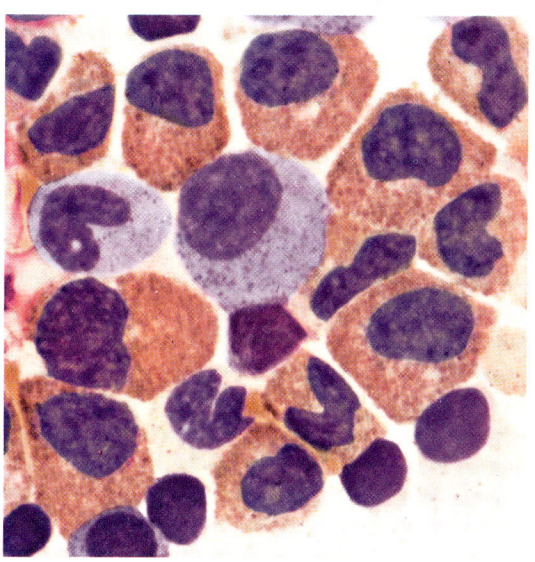

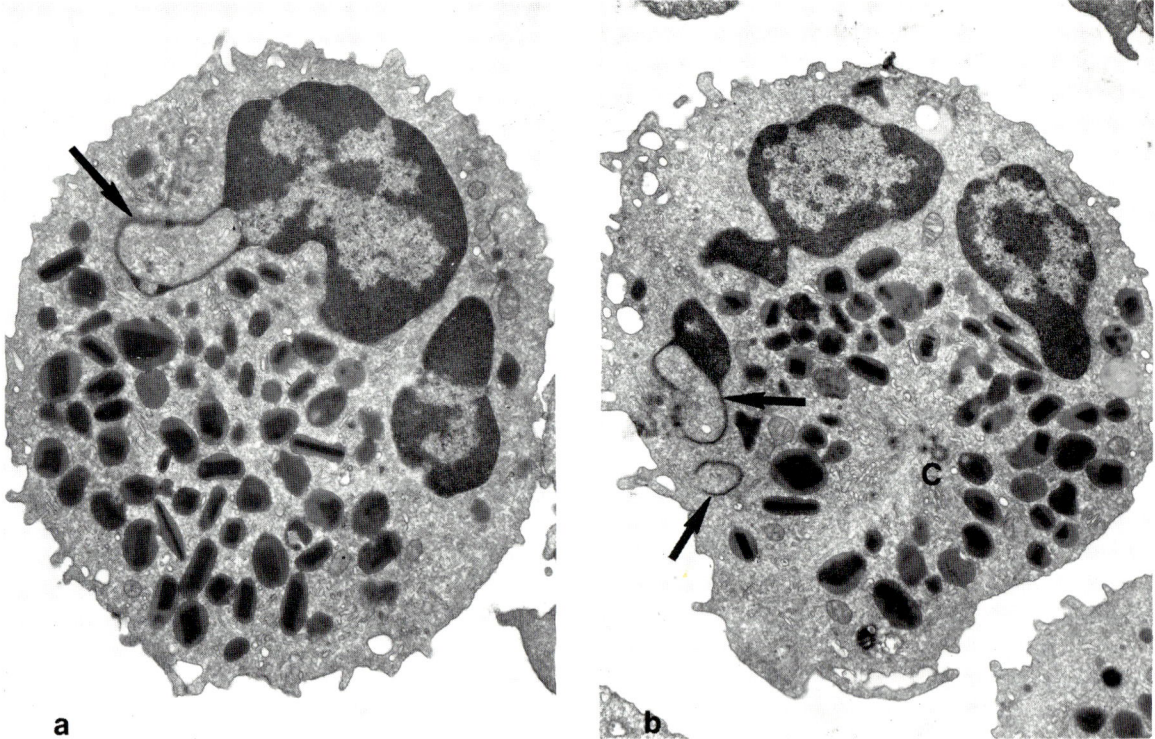

Figs. 19 a, b) Eosinophils obtained from the blood of patients with reactive eosinophilia of diverse etiologies: allergies, dermatitis medicamentosa, parasitic infestations, connective tissue diseases. **C**, centriole. Eosinophils constituted > 25% of the total leukocyte count. Nuclear hypersegmentation and « blebbing » **(arrows)** is common (**a**, × 9,000; **b**, × 8,000).

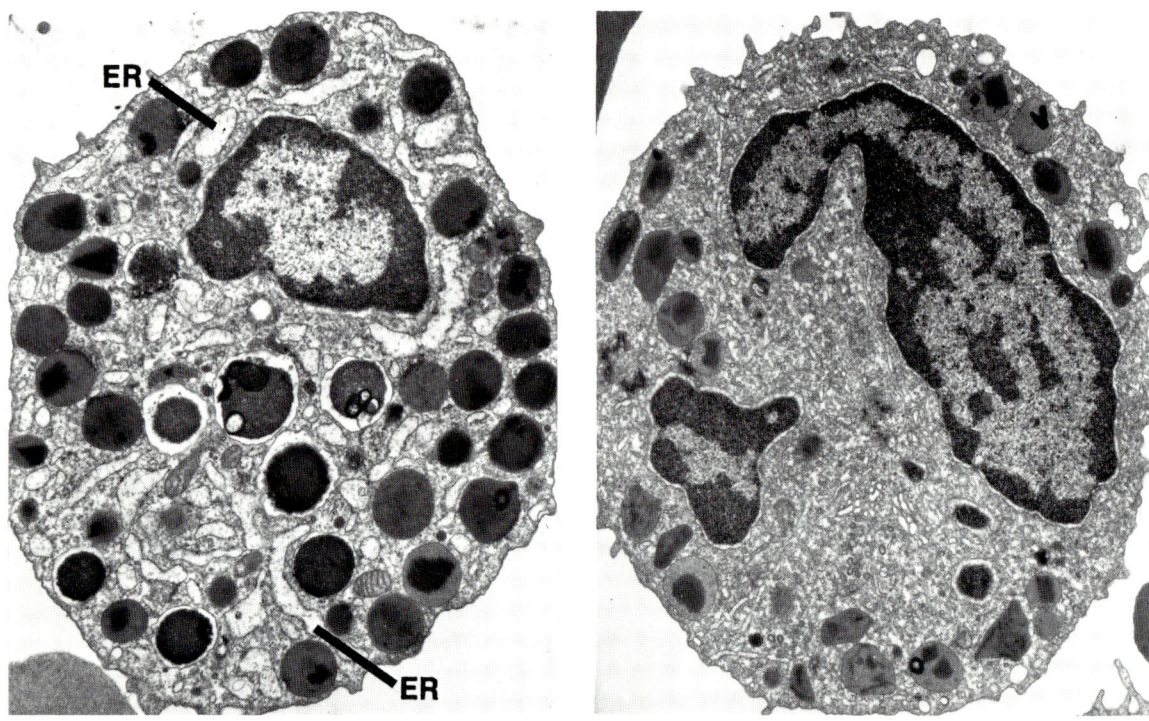

Fig. 20 Peripheral blood eosinophil obtained from a patient with severe eosinophilia associated with lymphoma cutis. Although the nucleus of this cell appears mature, many of the granules have not formed crystalloids. Instead, there are various shapes of electron dense material within the round organelles. Also note that the cell still has an abundance of rough endoplasmic reticulum (**ER**) (× 9,000).

Fig. 21 Eosinophil from the peripheral blood of a patient with an unexplained absolute eosinophil count of 3,000/cmm. The cell depicts sparse abnormal granulations (× 10,000).

Fig. 22 Eosinophil obtained from the blood of a patient with severe reactive eosinophilia illustrates heterogeneity, immaturity, and angularity of the granules. **ER**, endoplasmic reticulum. One of the granules has the appearance of an Auer rod (**arrow**). Eosinophilia subsided without therapy ($\times$ 12,000).

Fig. 23 Eosinophil obtained from the peripheral blood of a patient with cutaneous lymphomatoid granulomatosis. The eosinophils constituted 75% of the peripheral white blood cell count. Note the heterogeneity of the granules and the large lipoid inclusions (**L**). Only one lobe of the nucleus is seen in this plane of section but it has a mature structure ($\times$ 9,000).

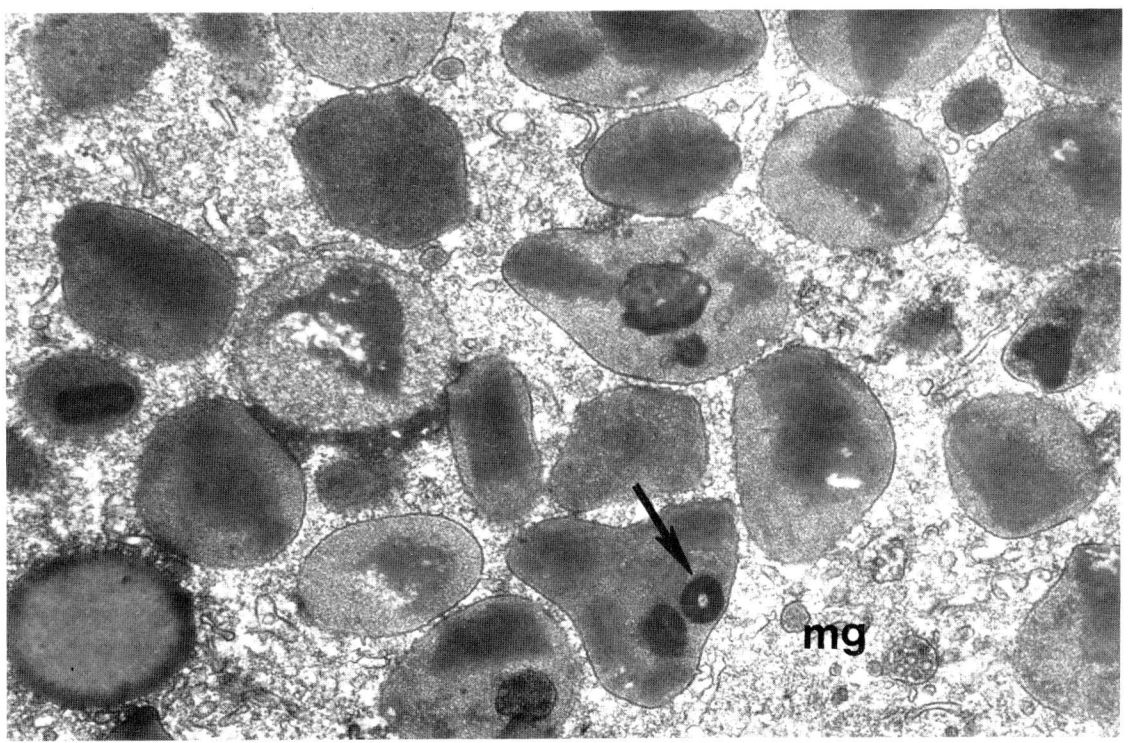

Fig. 24 Detail of a peripheral blood eosinophil obtained from a young woman with a psychiatric disorder. The patient's eosinophil count had risen to 3000/cmm and the cells failed to ingest latex particles. Thorough investigation revealed no underlying disease. The cause of the eosinophilia was attributed to a hypersensitivity reaction to surreptitiously ingested medications. Six months later the eosinophil count, morphology, and function had returned to normal; **mg**, microgranule; the **arrow** indicates a lamellated structure within a granule ($\times$ 37,500).

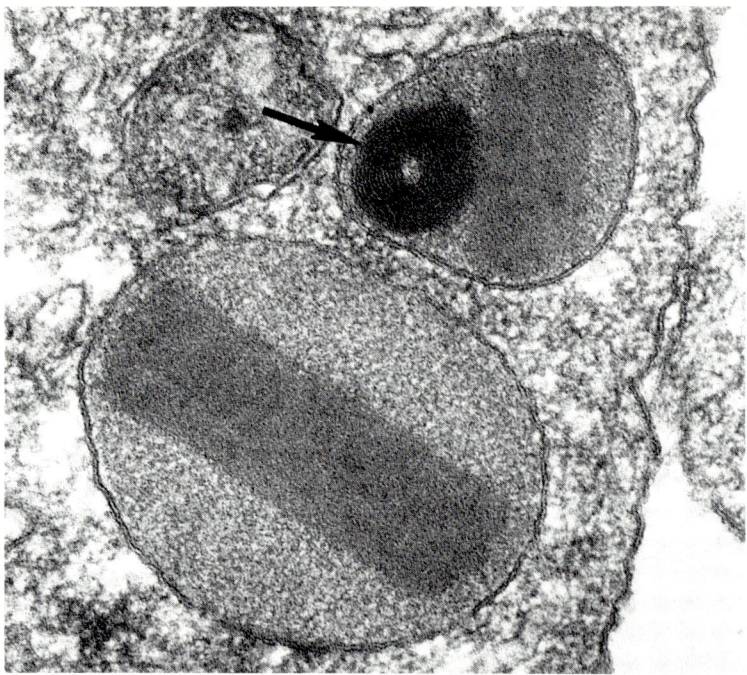

Fig. 25 Detail of eosinophil granules seen in an eosinophil of the patient described in the legend to Fig. 24. Note that one of the granules contains a crystal as well as a lamellated structure (**arrow**) which resembles those seen in cat eosinophils (compare with **Fig. 12**). The high phospholipid content of eosinophil granules has been commented on by many investigators. Phospholipids are known to form lamellated figures in acqueous media ($\times$ 100,800).

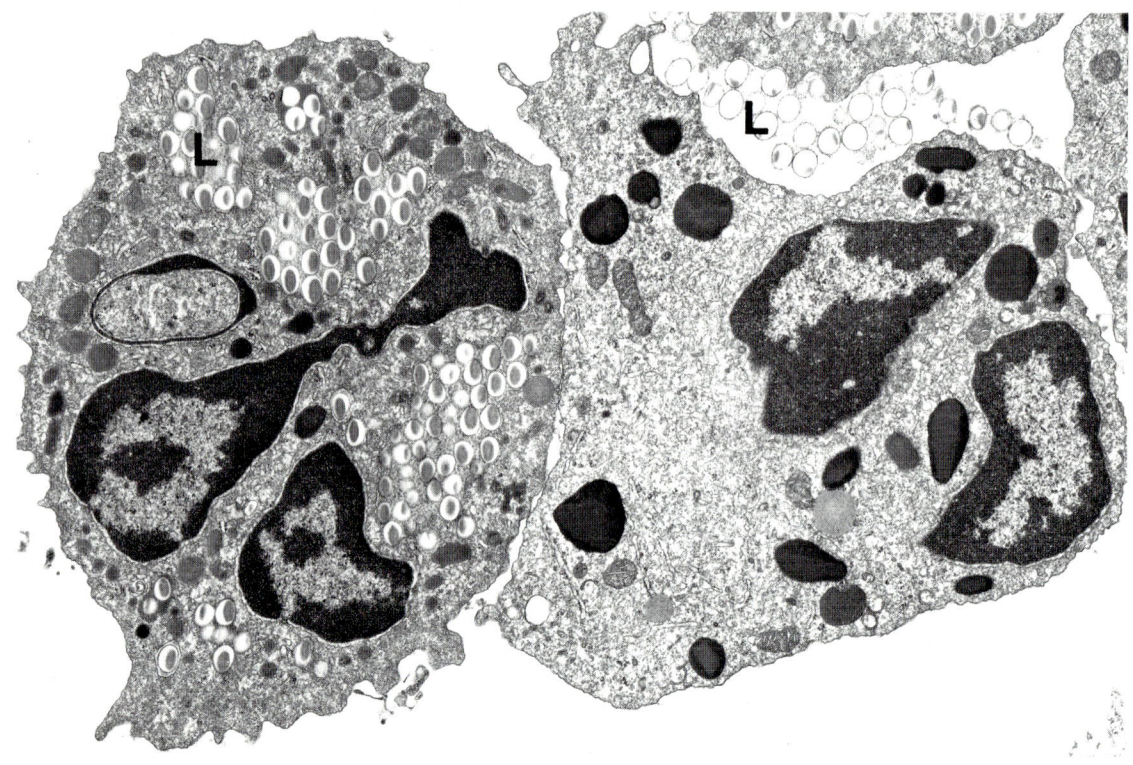

Fig. 26 This electron micrograph was prepared from the buffy coat cells of a patient with severe eosinophilia of unknown etiology. The cells were incubated with latex particles (**L**). The neutrophil (left) has phagocytosed the particles whereas the eosinophil (right) was unable to do so. Note that the eosinophil has a mature appearing nucleus but immature, abnormally-shaped granules ($\times$ 10,500).

Fig. 27 Charcot-Leyden crystals. Figures **a-c** and **e** were prepared from the pleural fluid of a patient with eosinophilic pneumonia. In **a** the needleshaped crystals were found freely among other cellular debris. Figures **b** and **c** illustrate large Charcot-Leyden crystals that have formed within the cytoplasm of immature appearing eosinophils.

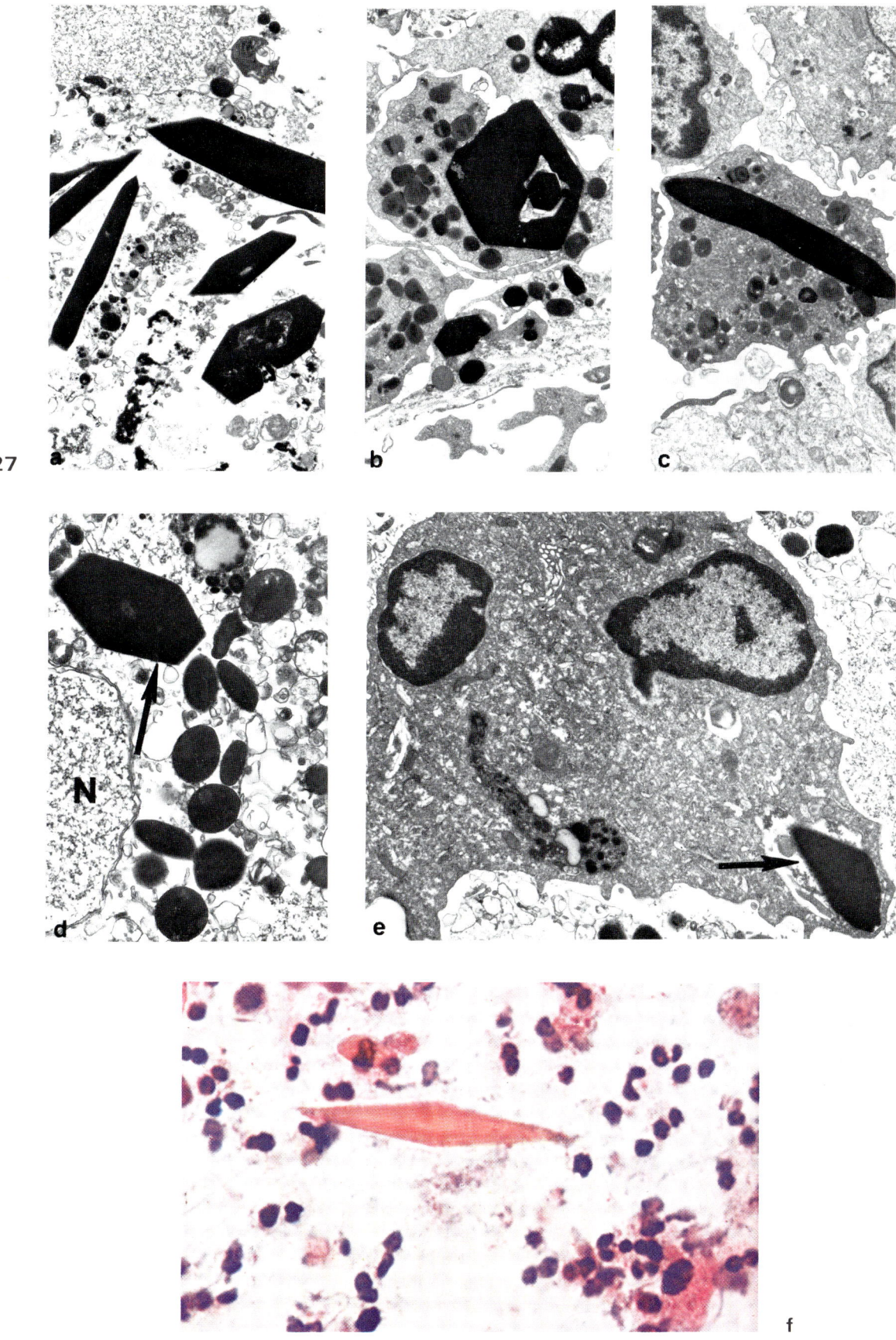

Fig. 27 d) represents a detail of a degenerating eosinophil obtained from the bone marrow of a patient with the hypereosinophilic syndrome. The Charcot-Leyden crystal (**arrow**) is seen within the confines of the degenerating cell. **N**, nucleus.

e) A macrophage in the process of phagocytosing a Charcot-Leyden crystal (**arrow**) as well as other debris found in the bone marrow of a patient with severe eosinophilia of unknown etiology (**a-d**, × ± 5,000; **e**, × 9,000).

f) A Charcot-Leyden crystal from the bronchial secretion of a patient with asthma. Note the eosinophilia of the crystal as seen in light microscopy.

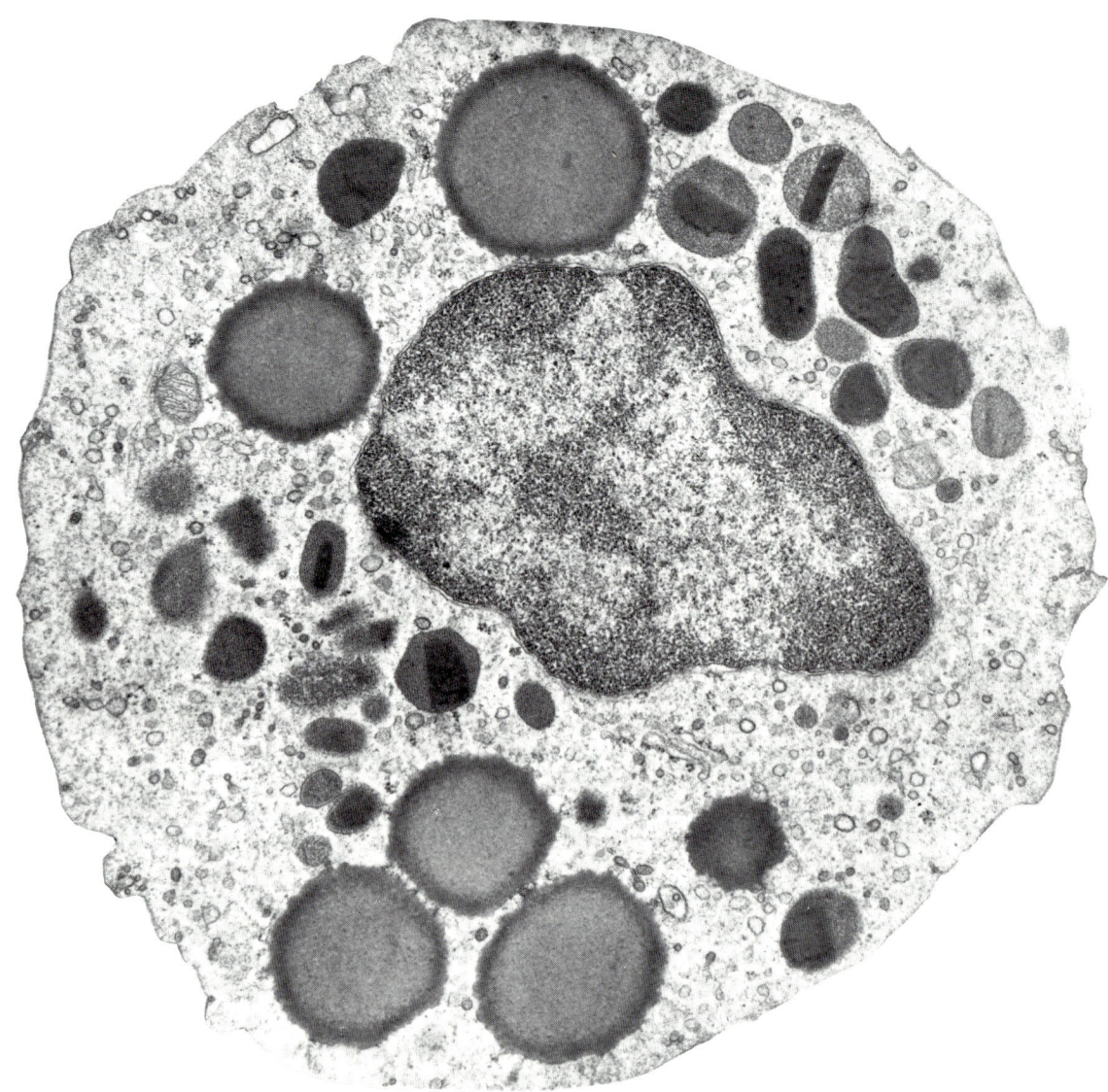

Fig. 28 Eosinophil from the peripheral blood of a 38 year old male with the hypereosinophilic syndrome as defined in references 53 and 54. Total eosinophil count was 20,000/cmm. The patient had pulmonary, neurologic and cardiac manifestations of the disease and succumbed 2 years after diagnosis. Note the heterogeneity of the granules and the large inclusions. These may represent abnormal granules or lipids. However, they are 3-5 times larger than primary granules and a delimiting membrane can not always be resolved ($\times$ 22,000).
Reproduced from ref. 52.

2.1. Malignant or primary eosinophilia

Although there has been an ongoing debate as regards the existence of eosinophilic leukemia as a disease entity [49-52], there is no reason to believe that the eosinophil, in contrast to all other cells, is exempt from neoplastic transformation. The difficulty is to sort out the severe so-called "hypereosinophilic syndromes" (for review, see [53] and [54]) which may be secondary to chronic hypersensitivity of undetermined etiology and the condition in which eosinophilia is autonomous, unremitting, and not responsive to steroids or even chemotherapy. In both situations, the absolute eosinophil count is over 1500/cmm and the total leukocyte count should be well over 20,000/cmm.

At present, there is no way of differentiating these two conditions early in the disease. Clinician and patient must bide their time until improvement, or inexorable deterioration becomes apparent. An example of the morphological abnormalities seen in the hypereosinophilic syndromes is illustrated in **Figure 28**.

Generally, there is evidence of disorderly differentiation and maturation with a greater than normal variation in the distribution, size and shape of the granules. Many of the cells contain lipid inclusions that are not membrane-bound (**Fig. 28**). These should not be confused with primary granules especially because in hypereosinophilic states the promyelocyte granules are often larger and fewer in number than in normal cells. Unfortunately, none of these abnormalities is sufficiently specific to permit far-reaching decisions regarding clinical management.

3. CONCLUSION

One hundred years have passed since Ehrlich recognized the eosinophil as a special type of granulocyte. However, the attention bestowed on this cell became such that by 1914 a review by Schwartz [55] already included more than 2700 references. During the past two decades, the number of articles on the subject of eosinophils has become bewildering. This chapter should not serve as a substitute for these original writings. Rather, the author hopes that it will provide a better understanding of the basic structure of the cell, the morphologic alterations that are associated with its function and the changes that underly its pathology. Such insight is necessary if the biochemical and physiologic data that are currently amassed with such astounding rapidity are to have biological and clinical relevance.

REFERENCES

1. Zucker-Franklin D.: *Eosinophil function and disorders*. Adv. Intern. Med., *19*, 1-25, 1974.
2. Beeson P.B., Bass D.A.: *The eosinophil*. In: *Major Problems in Internal Medicine*. Smith L.H. ed., vol. 14, W.B. Saunders Co., Philadelphia, 1977.
3. Zucker-Franklin D.: *The properties of eosinophils*. In: *Modern Concepts and Developments in Immediate Hypersensitivity*. Bach M.K. ed., Marcel Dekker Inc., New York, pp. 407-430, 1977.
4. Zucker-Franklin D.: *Pathophysiology of eosinophils*. In: *Clinical Immunology Update*. Franklin E.C. ed., Elsevier North-Holland, New York, pp. 227-239, 1979.
5. Mahmoud A.A.F., Austen K.F. (eds.): *Eosinophil*. Centennial publication (in preparation).
6. Zucker-Franklin D., Grusky G., L'Esperance P.: *Granulocyte colonies derived from lymphocyte fractions of normal human blood*. Proc. Natl. Acad. Sci., *71*, 2711-2714, 1974.
7. Archer G.T., Air G., Sackas J., Morell D.B.: *Studies on rat eosinophil peroxidase*. Biochem. Biophys. Acta, *99*, 96-101, 1965.
8. Presentey B., Szapiro L.: *Hereditary deficiency of peroxidase and phospholipids in eosinophilic granulocytes*. Acta Hemat., *41*, 359-362, 1969.
9. Fabian I., Aronson M.: *Deamination of histamine by peroxidase of neutrophils and eosinophils*. J. Reticuloendothel. Soc., *17*, 141-145, 1975.
10. West B.C., Gelbo N.A., Rosenthal A.S.: *Isolation and partial characterization of human eosinophil granules*. Am. J. Path., *81*, 575-585, 1975.
11. Zucker-Franklin D., Grusky G.: *The identification of eosinophil colonies in soft-agar cultures by differential staining for peroxidase*. J. Histochem. Cytochem., *24*, 1270-1272, 1976.
12. Bessis M., Maigne J.: *Le diagnostic des variétés de leucemies äigues par la reaction des peroxydases au microscope electronique. Son interêt et ses limites*. Rév. Franç. d'Etudes Clin. et Biol., *15*, 691-698, 1970.
13. Archer G.T., Hirsch J.G.: *Isolation of granules from eosinophil leukocytes and study of their enzyme content*. J. Exp. Med., *118*, 277-284, 1963.
14. Tanaka K.R., Valentine W.N., Fredricks R.E.: *Human leukocyte aryl sulphatase activity*. Brit. J. Hemat., *8*, 86-92, 1962.
15. Miller F., Herzog V.: *Die Lokalisation von Peroxydase und saurer Phosphatase in eosinophilen Leukocyten während der Reifung*. Z. Zellforsch., *97*, 84-110, 1969.
16. Bainton D.F., Farquhar M.G.: *Segregation and packaging of granule enzymes in eosinophilic leukocytes*. J. Cell Biol., *45*, 54-73, 1970.
17. Zucker-Franklin D.: *Structure and maturation of eosinophils*. In ref. 5.
18. Fuerst D.E., Jannach J.R.: *Autofluorescence of eosinophils: a bone marrow study*. Nature, *205*, 1333-1334, 1965.
19. Zucker-Franklin D.: *Electron microscopic studies of human granulocytes: structural variations related to function*. Semin. Hematol., *5*, 109-133, 1968.
20. Faller A.: *Zur Frage von Struktur und Aufbau der eosinophilen Granula*. Zeitschr. Zellforsch, *69*, 551-565, 1966.

21. Hardin J.H., Spicer S.S.: *An ultrastructural study of human eosinophil granules: maturational shapes and pyroantimonate reactive cation.* Am. J. Anat., *128*, 283-297, 1970.
22. Miller F., de Harven E., Palade G.E.: *The structure of eosinophil leukocyte granules in rodents and man.* J. Cell Biol., *31*, 349-362, 1966.
23. Wetzel B.K.: *The fine structure and cytochemistry of developing granulocytes with special reference to the rabbit.* In: Regulation of Hematopoiesis. Gordon A.S. ed., vol. 2, Appleton-Centruy-Croft, New York, p. 819, 1970.
24. Gleich G.J., Loegering D.A., Mann K.G., Maldonado J.Z.: *Comparative properties of the Charcot-Leyden crystal protein and the major basic protein from human eosinophils.* J. Clin. Invest., *57*, 633-640, 1976.
25. Olsson I., Venge P., Spitznagel J.K., Lehrer R.I.: *Arginine-rich cationic proteins of human eosinophil granules.* Lab. Invest., *36*, 493-500, 1977.
26. Ghidoni J.J., Goldberg A.R.: *Light and electron microscopic localization of acid phosphatase activity in human eosinophils.* Am. J. Clin. Path., *45*, 402-403, 1966.
27. Seeman P.M., Palade G.E.: *Acid phosphatase localization in rabbit eosinophils.* J. Cell Biol., *34*, 745-756, 1967.
28. Parmley R.T., Spicer S.S.: *Cytochemical and ultrastructural identification of a small type of granule in human late eosinophils.* Lab. Invest., *30*, 557-567, 1974.
29. Schaefer H.E., Hubner G., Fischer R.: *Spezifische Microgranula in Eosinophilen.* Acta Hematologica, *50*, 92-104, 1973.
30. Zucker-Franklin D., Hirsch J.G.: *Electron microscope studies on degranulation of rabbit peritoneal leukocytes during phagocytosis.* J. Exp. Med., *120*, 569-576, 1964.
31. Zucker-Franklin D., Davidson M., Thomas L.: *The interaction of mycoplasmas with mammalian cells. I. Hela cells, neutrophils and eosinophils.* J. Exp. Med., *124*, 521-531, 1966.
32. Kay A.B.: *Studies on eosinophil leukocyte migration. II. Factors specifically chemotactic for eosinophils and neutrophils generated from guinea-pig serum by antigen-antibody complexes.* Clin. Exp. Immunol., *7*, 723-737, 1970.
33. Klebanoff S.J., Durack D.T., Rosen H., Clark R.A.: *Functional studies on human peritoneal eosinophils.* Inf. Immunity, *17*, 167-173, 1977.
34. Baehner R., Johnston R.B.: *Metabolic and bactericidal activities of human eosinophils.* Brit. J. Hemat., *20*, 277-285, 1971.
34.a Butterworth A.E., David J.R., Franks D., Mahmoud A.A.F., David P.H., Sturrock R.F., Houba V.: *Antibody-dependent eosinophil-mediated damage to ^{51}Cr-labelled schistosomula of Schistosoma mansoni: damage by purified eosinophils.* J. Exp. Med., *145*, 136-150, 1977.
35. Orange R.P., Murphy R.C., Austen K.F.: *Inactivation of slow reacting substance of anaphylaxis (SRS-A) by aryl sulfatases.* J. Immunol., *113*, 316-322, 1974.
36. Vercauteren R.: *The properties of the isolated granules from blood eosinophils.* Enzymologia, *16*, 1-13, 1953.
37. Kovacs A.: *Antihistaminic effect of eosinophilic leukocytes.* Experientia, *6*, 349-350, 1950.
38. Hübscher T.: *Role of the eosinophil in the allergic reactions. I. EDI- and eosinophil-derived inhibitor of histamine release.* J. Immunol., *114*, 1379-1388, 1975.
39. Colley D.G.: *Eosinophils and immune mechanisms. I. Eosinophil stimulation promoter (ESP): a lymphokine induced by specific antigen or phytohemagglutinin.* J. Immunol., *110*, 1914-1423, 1973.
40. Greene B.M., Colley D.G.: *Eosinophils and immune mechanisms. II. Partial characterization of the lymphokine eosinophil stimulation promoter.* J. Immunol., *113*, 910-915, 1974.
41. Kay H.B., Stechschulte D.J., Austen K.F.: *An eosinophil leukocyte chemotactic factor of anaphylaxis.* J. Exp. Med., *133*, 602-619, 1971.
42. Wasserman S.F., Goetze E.J., Austen K.F.: *Preformed eosinophilic chemotactic factors of anaphylaxis.* J. Immunol., *112*, 351-385, 1974.
43. Clark R.A.F., Gallin J.I., Kaplan A.P.: *The selective eosinophil chemotactic activity of histamine.* J. Exp. Med., *132*, 1462-1476, 1975.
44. Mahmoud A.A.F., Stone M.K., Kellermeyer R.W.: *Eosinophilopoietin: a circulating low molecular weight peptide-like substance which stimulates the production of eosinophils in mice.* J. Clin. Invest., *60*, 675-682, 1977.
45. Schriber R.A., Zucker-Franklin D.: *Induction of blood eosinophilia by pulmonary embolization of antigen-coated particles. The relationship to cell-mediated immunity.* J. Immunol., *114*, 1348-1353, 1975.
46. Samter M.: *Charcot-Leyden crystals. A study of the conditions necessary for their formation.* J. Allergy, *18*, 221-230, 1947.
47. Welsh R.A.: *The genesis of the Charcot-Leyden crystal in the eosinophilic leukocyte of man.* Am. J. Path., *35*, 1091-1103, 1959.
48. El-Hashimi W.: *Charcot-Leyden crystals: formation from primate and lack of formation from non-primate eosinophils.* Am. J. Path., *65*, 311-324, 1971.
49. Bousser J.: *Eosinophilie et leucemie.* Sang, *28*, 553-580, 1957.
50. Odeberg B.: *Eosinophilic leukemia and disseminated eosinophilic collagen disease – a disease entity?* Acta Med. Scand., *177*, 129, 1965.
51. Karle H., Videback A.: *Eosinophilic leukemia or a collagen disease with eosinophilia.* Danish Med. Bull., *13*, 41, 1966.
52. Zucker-Franklin D.: *Eosinophilia of unknown etiology: a diagnostic dilemma.* Hosp. Practice, *6*, 119-127, 1971.
53. Hardy W.R., Anderson R.E.: *The hypereosinophilic syndromes.* Ann. Int. Med., *68*, 1220-1229, 1968.
54. Chusid M.J., Dale D.C., West B.C., Wolff S.M.: *The hypereosinophilic syndrome: analysis of fourteen cases with review of the literature.* Medicine, *54*, 1-27, 1975.
55. Schwarz E.: *Das Wesen der Eosinophilie.* Jahreskurse für ärtztliche Fortbildung. In: Zwölf Monatshäften. Heft 1, pp. 5-22, München, 1914.

7
Basophils

D. ZUCKER-FRANKLIN

Department of Medicine
New York University, New York, U.S.A.

1. INTRODUCTION

It is difficult to find basophils on routine blood smears, but when found they are easily identified. In normal subjects the cells constitute only 0-2% of the white blood cell count (20-60 per cmm of blood), but the deep violet-blue granules make recognition unequivocal (**Fig. 1**). More difficult is an appreciation of various basophil precursors in the bone marrow, particularly because mast cells are often also present at this site. Therefore, it is necessary from the beginning of this chapter to deal with the similarities, differences and inter-relationships of the basophil-mast cell system.

Whereas there is no longer any doubt that basophils arise in the bone marrow, the origin of mast cells has been less firmly established. The genetic independence of the two cells was suggested soon after their discovery by Ehrlich [1] and continued to be claimed until very recently. These claims were based on the distinctive morphology, location and enzyme content of the two cells, though their close functional relationship was never denied.

The properties which distinguish mast cells from basophils are listed in Table 1. While glancing at this table, the reader is reminded, however, that a similar list could be drawn up comparing the properties of monocytes with those of macrophages. Yet, it is known that macrophages differentiate from monocytes and that both cells, no matter what morphology they may assume, are derived from the same bone marrow precursor. Therefore, the concept that cells of similar origin and function may develop diverse morphologic and biochemical properties which are dependent on environmental stimuli is not a novel one.

Table 1 *PROPERTIES DIFFERENTIATING HUMAN BASOPHILS AND MAST CELLS* *
(in addition to the distinctive ultrastructure of their granules)

Basophils	Mast cells
water solubility ++++	water solubility ++
nucleus - segmented	nucleus - round or ovoid
end-stage cell	mitotic potential
peroxidase +	peroxidase −
acid phosphatase −	acid phosphatase +
protease −	protease ++
alkaline phosphatase −	alkaline phosphatase +
LDH +	LDH ?
PAS ++++	PAS +
DPNH diaphorase +	?

* Rat mast cells contain serotonin. This catecholamine has never been demonstrated in human mast cells or basophils.

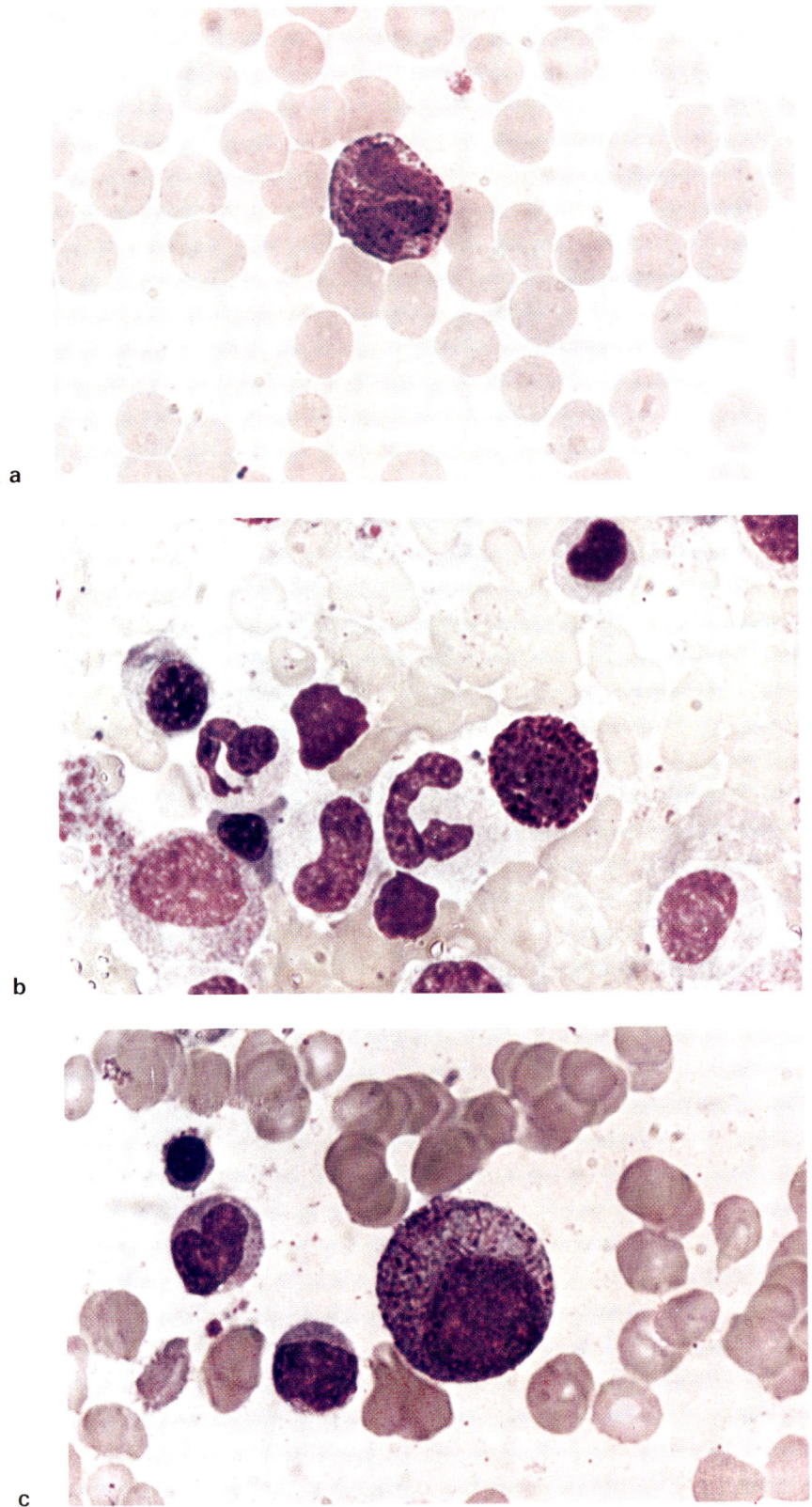

Fig. 1 Basophil/mast cell series in human blood and marrow fixed with alcohol and stained with Wright's except for e.
a) Mature basophil in normal peripheral blood shows segmented nucleus.
b) Mature basophil in normal bone marrow. The granules obscure the nucleus precluding assessment of the degree of nuclear segmentation or distinction between mast cell and basophil.

7 BASOPHILS

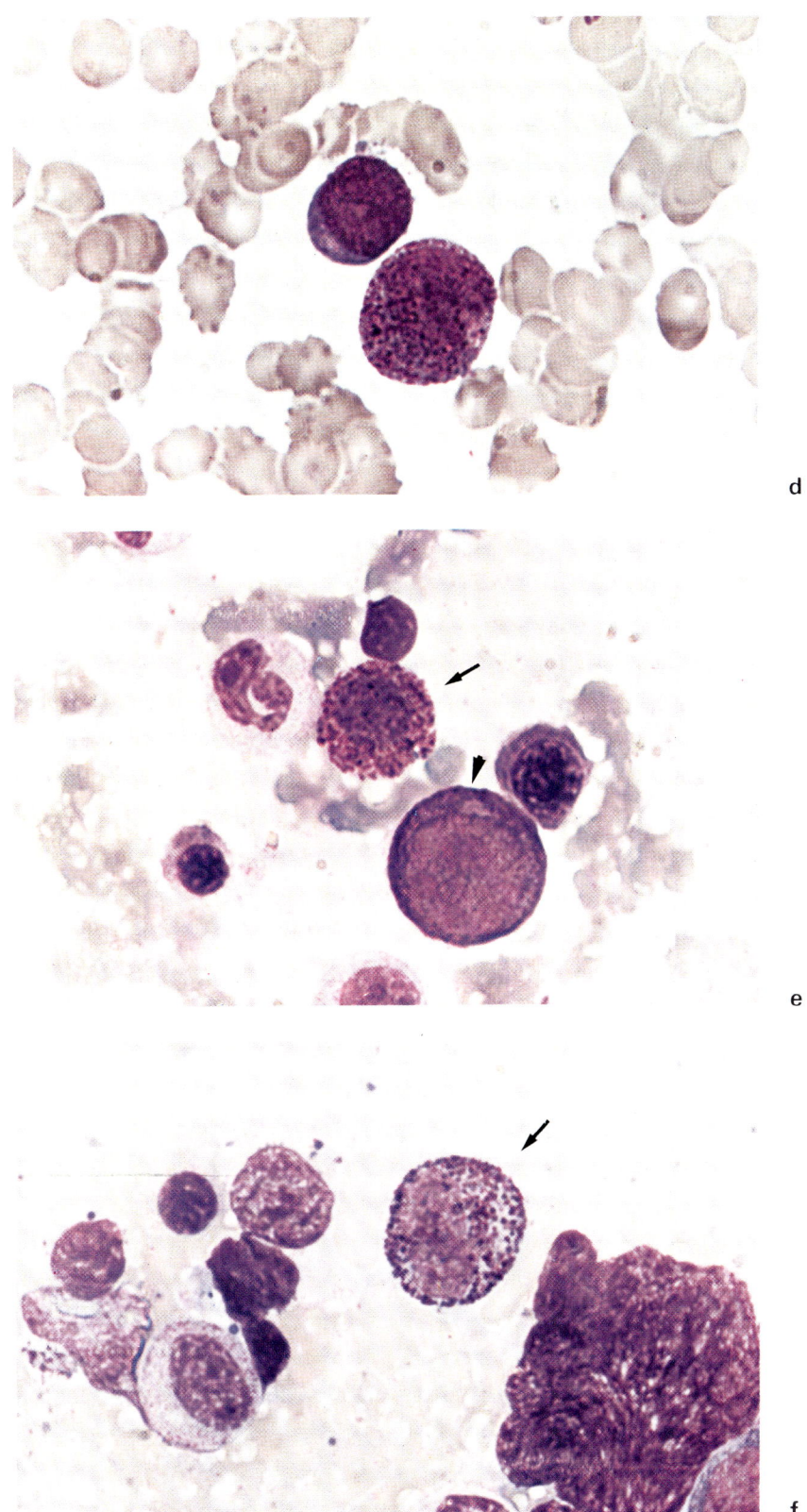

c) Neutrophil promyelocyte with basophilic granules from the bone marrow of a patient with polycythemia vera is presented here for comparison with the basophil cell series.
d) Basophil promyelocyte or early myelocyte.
e) Basophil myelocyte stained with toluidine blue to show metachromasia of the granules (**arrow**). For comparison of size, note the proerythroblast next to it (**arrowhead**).
f) Basophil myelocyte or early metamyelocyte (**arrow**) from a patient with polycythemia vera.

If mast cells like basophils develop from bone marrow precursors, their progenitors would have to look like small undifferentiated cells resembling lymphocytes. In support of this theory is our observation that mast cell colonies in soft agar cultures may be initiated with rat peripheral blood lymphoid fractions [2] (**Fig. 2**) and the reports of many investigators claiming that cultures derived from lymph nodes and thymuses of mice [3, 4] give rise to colonies consisting of cells which look like mast cells or basophils. With the exception of the thymus-derived colonies which have been shown to contain cells with receptors for IgE [5], none of the other studies have included biochemical analyses that would establish the identity of the cells beyond reasonable doubt.

Recently, an entirely different approach, namely the utilization of specific markers on precursor cells in symbiotic rats, also appears to indicate that mast cells are derived from the bone marrow and that these cells in turn have the ability to differentiate into cells with the features of basophils [6-8]. In lower vertebrates [9] and in some pathologic conditions (see below), it may be impossible to distinguish basophils from mast cells morphologically. When this information is added to the widely held view that in most species there is a reciprocal relationship between the numbers of circulating basophils and tissue mast cells, it does not seem amiss to consider the cells simultaneously in the discussion to follow.

2. DEVELOPMENT

2.1. Light microscopy

With some effort, the basophilic granulocyte, like its neutrophilic and eosinophilic counterpart may be identified at the promyelocyte stage of development (**Fig. 1 c, d**). It is smaller ($\pm$ 12 µm) than the eosinophil or neutrophil promyelocyte, has a larger nucleus and thus a higher nucleocytoplasmic ratio. Because with Wright's and Giemsa stains, it is often difficult to distinguish immature basophils from other immature granulocytes, attention to nuclear size may be helpful.

Alternatively, staining with toluidine blue or Alcian blue-safranin [10] will delineate the basophilic cell series to better advantage (**Figs. 1, 2**). Maturation of this cell is not accompanied by a noteworthy change in its size and the terms myelocytic, metamyelocytic and segmented refer primarily to the shape of the nucleus. Little is known as regards the differentiation and maturation of human basophil granules. Although mature basophil granules have been shown to contain histamine [11] and a sulfated mucopolysaccharide with properties akin to heparin [12, 13], it is not certain at what stage of development these substances are synthesized. On the other hand, the differentiation and maturation of mast cells of various laboratory animals have been investigated more thoroughly *in vivo* and *in vitro*. In a classic study, Coombs et al. [14] identified four developmental stages of mast cells in rat embryos based on histochemical analysis and ^{3}H-thymidine uptake. In essence, there is a gradual appearance of Alcian blue positive, Safranin negative granules in stages I, II and III. This is believed to be indicative of increasing amounts of a heparin precursor substance. Stage IV is associated with Safranin positive granules reflecting the presence of a highly N-sulfated polysaccharide likely to be mature heparin (**Fig. 2 a-f**). The appearance of a chymase or trypsin-like enzyme parallels the time of active heparin synthesis, whereas histamine seems to be synthesized and bound to the granule only during the final stage of maturation, stage IV, when mitotic activity has ceased [15]. The PAS reaction also becomes positive during the final stages III and IV, although glycogen is probably extragranular in the cytoplasm [16]. Comparable studies on human mast cells have not yet been carried out.

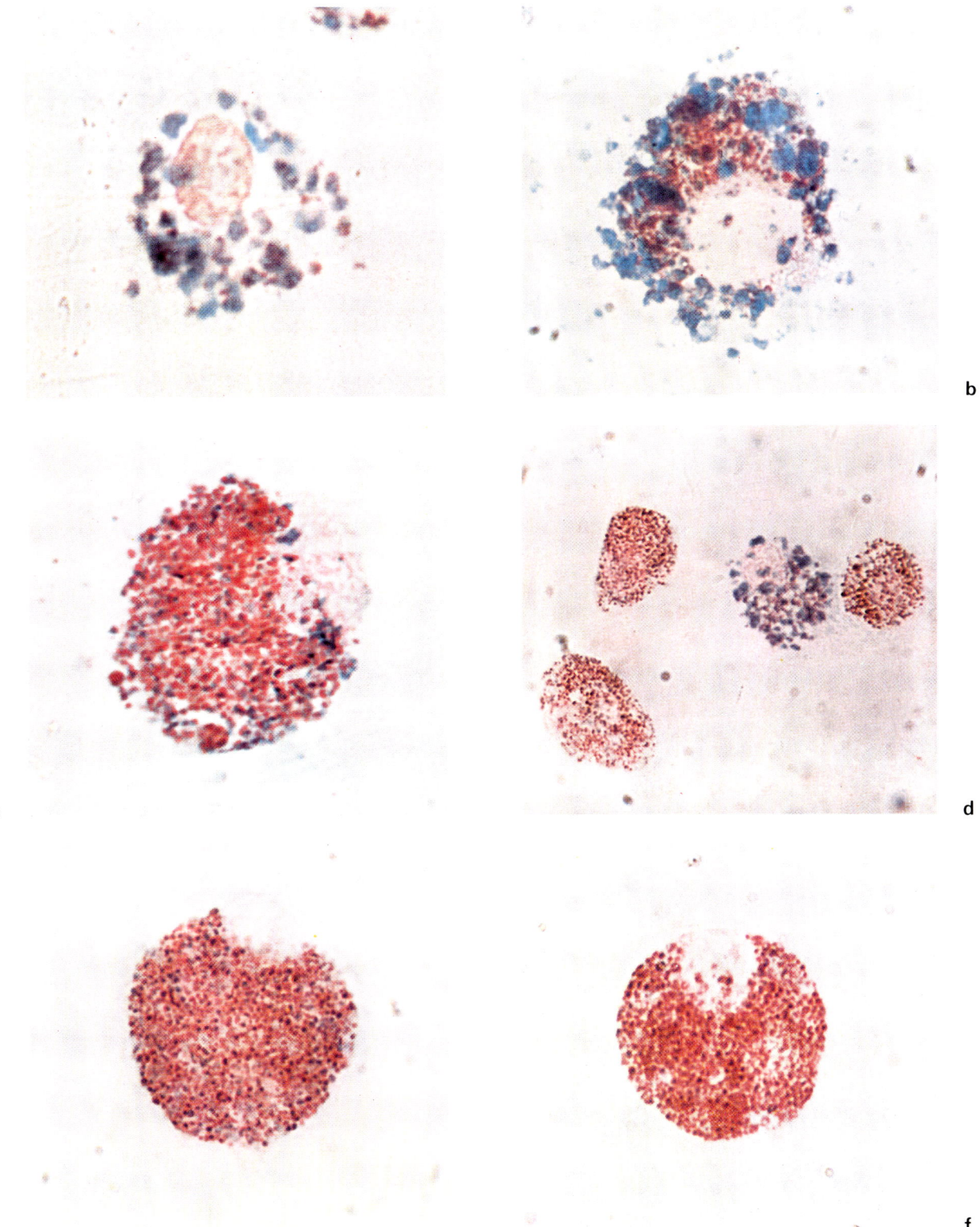

Figs. 2 a-f) Developmental series of basophil/mast cells in soft agar colonies initiated with rat mononuclear blood cells. Colonies were stained with Alcian blue-safranin according to ref. 10 (see text). Gradual increase of safranin-positive granules (red) reflects increasing number of granules containing N-sulfated polysaccharide i.e., heparin. Alcian blue-positive granules are believed to contain a precursor material.

In **a** no red granules are seen, in **b** red granulations begin to appear, in **c** the red, heparin-containing, granules begin to become dominant, in **d** four cells from the same colony show that not all cells are at the same stage of development, in **e** only a few Alcian blue-positive granules have remained, in **f** only "mature stage" stage IV granules are seen.

2.2. Electron microscopy

Analysis of the ultrastructure of human basophils only became possible following the introduction of aldehyde fixatives into electron microscopy [17] whereas the greater availability of mast cells and the lesser solubility of their granules had allowed the ultrastructure of the latter cells to be described much earlier, albeit inadequately by present standards [18-20]. It may be correct to assume that the granules of the basophilic promyelocyte develop like those of other granulocytes at the Golgi zone following synthesis of the granule content by ribosomes on the rough endoplasmic reticulum. On the other hand, the appearance of developing granules in soft agar colonies (**Fig. 3**) may stimulate alternative theories. As illustrated in **Figure 4**, the ultrastructure of promyelocyte granules may be distinguished from eosinophil or neutrophil granules by its fine particulate content. According to Breton-Gorius and Reyes [21], basophilic promyelocyte granules possess peroxidase. Acid phosphatase or other hydrolytic enzymes have not been demonstrated. How the promyelocyte granules "mature" to acquire the morphology characteristic for granules of circulating blood basophils is not known, but inferred from studies conducted on mast cells of rodents [22, 23]. The ultrastructure of mature human blood basophils is illustrated in Figures **5-8**. The granules may vary in size, shape and internal structure. They appear to be devoid of alkaline phosphatase, acid phosphatase and other hydrolytic enzymes, but it is well established that they contain heparin [13] and histamine [24]. Evidence for a peroxidase-like enzyme is also convincing [25]. The ultrastructure of human mast cells is illustrated in **Figures 9** to **12**. In bone marrow, it may be very difficult to distinguish mast cell granules from those of basophilic promyelocytes or myelocytes (see section on basophil/mast cell pathology). Moreover, in many species, basophil and mast cell granules are indistinguishable from each other and may even assume a different structure during fetal, young and adult life of the same animal [26-30]. A description of the morphologic variations in the granules found among basophils and mast cells in species other than man is beyond the scope of this volume.

Fig. 3 *Sparsely granulated basophil from a developing soft agar colony consisting of granulocyte precursors. The culture was initiated with mononuclear cells prepared from the peripheral blood of a healthy subject. Some of the granules are membrane-bound and their content is particulate like that of mature basophils (G). Other granules exhibit reduplication of membranes as well as particles (arrow). There are also aggregates of particles which appear to lie free in the cytoplasm and others that are incompletely surrounded by numerous membranes. To show this to better advantage, the area demarcated by the rectangle is illustrated at higher magnification within the inset at the bottom. There is an abundance of mitochondria (M) and glycogen particles. In the high resolution detail at the bottom, microtubules (T) and filaments are also seen in the cytoplasm (whole cell × 25,000; detail × 61,000).*

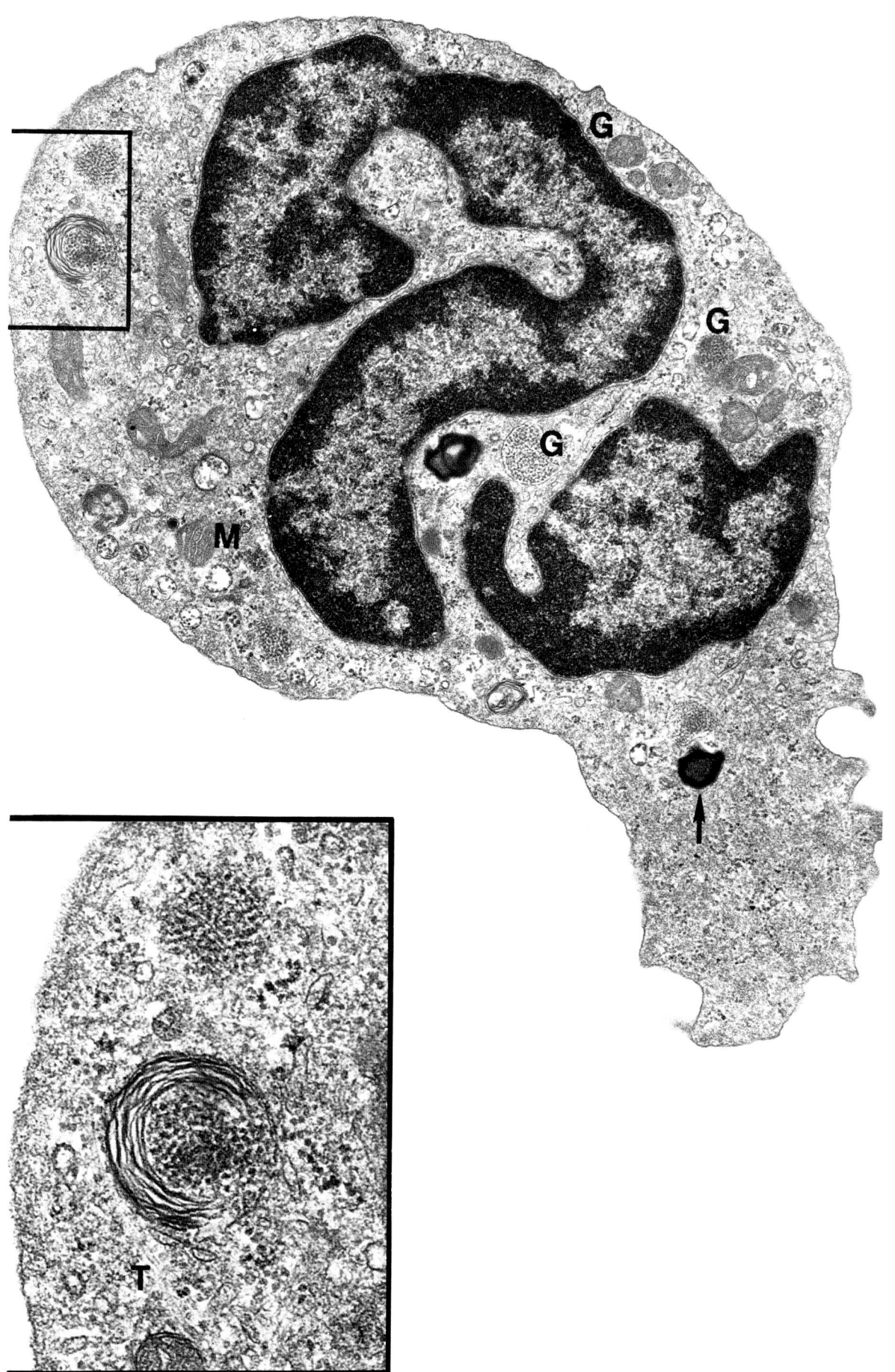

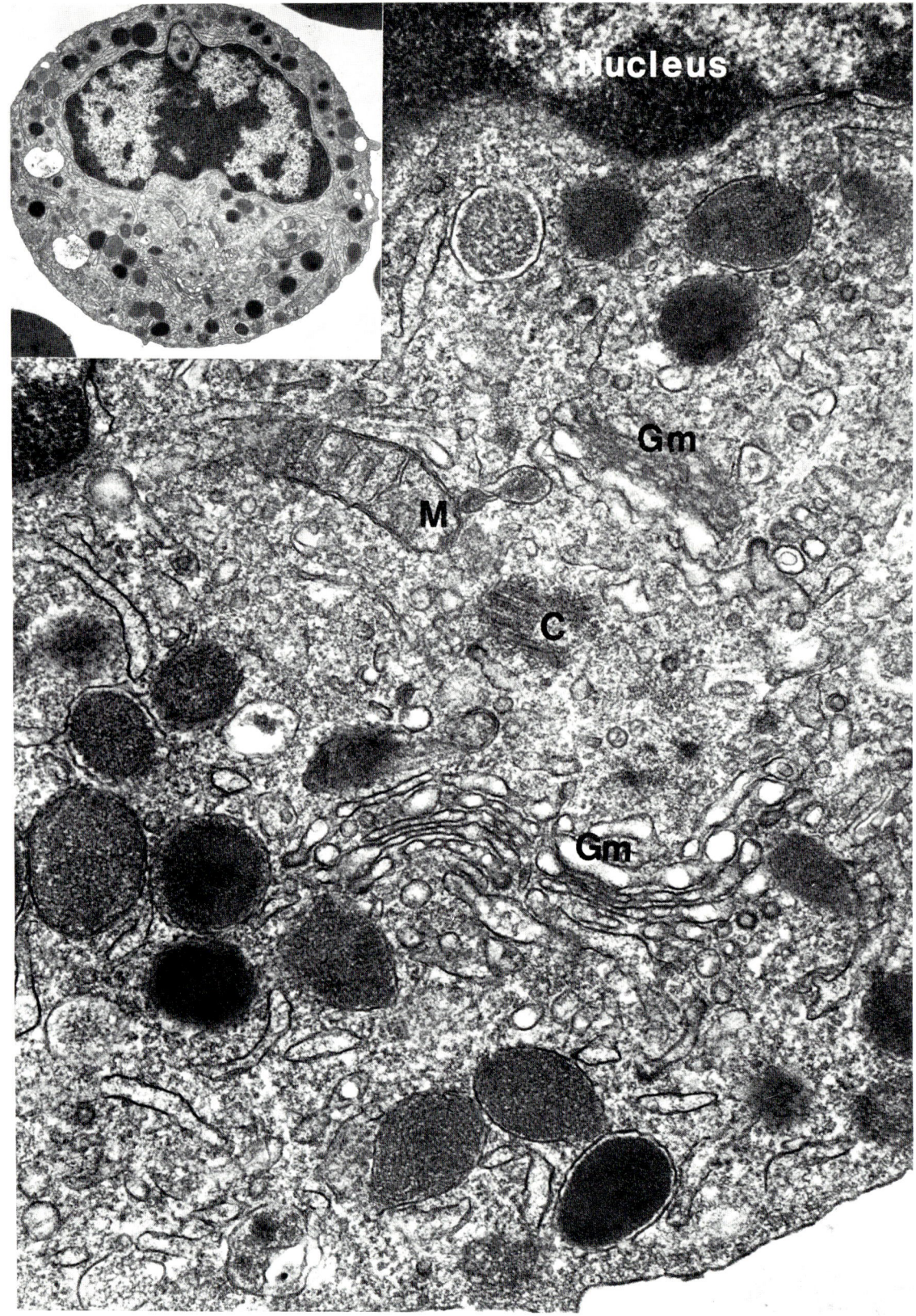

Fig. 4 The cell in the upper left hand corner is a basophilic myelocyte prepared from the bone marrow of a normal subject. The remainder of the illustration represents the Golgi zone of this cell at higher magnification. Note that the content of the granules is not homogenous but finely particulate.
Gm, Golgi membranes; **M**, mitochondrion; **C**, centriole (whole cell × 7000; detail × 49,000).

Fig. 5 Example of a mature blood basophil. The granules are distributed randomly throughout the cytoplasm. Each granule consists of a membrane which surrounds a space that is partially or completely filled with particles of fairly uniform size as illustrated at higher magnification by the three granules below the cell. The size of the particles within each individual granule appears to be uniform, but it may differ from granule

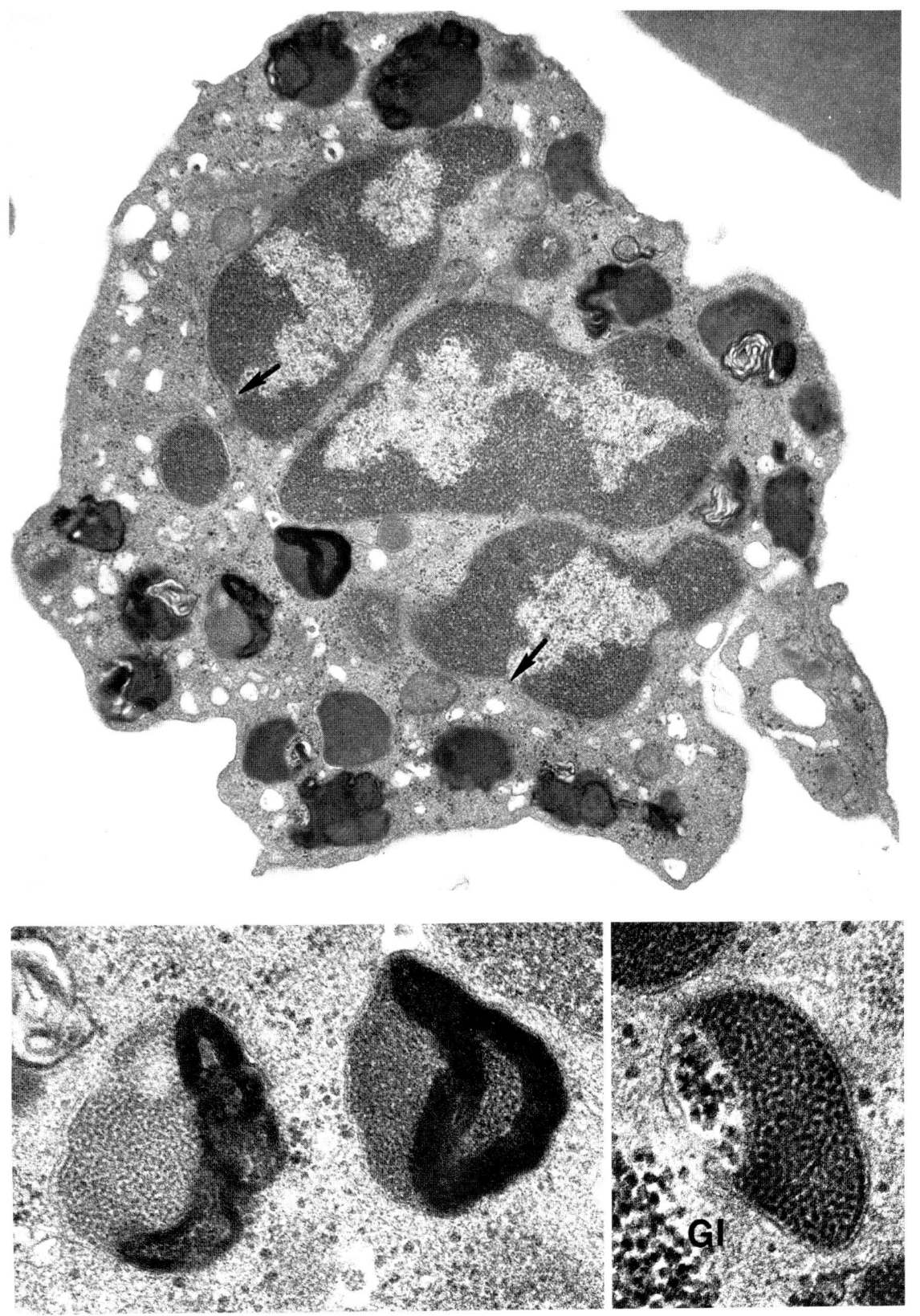

to granule even within the same cell. Reduplication of the granule membrane is often seen and, in some cells, the granules may exhibit a large amount of membrane-like structures reminiscent of myelin figures. Whether there is a sequential change from fine particulate to predominantly membrane-like granule content as the cell ages is open to conjecture. Note that the distribution of chromatin in the multilobed nucleus is identical to that of other mature granulocytes, i.e. neutrophils and eosinophils (see Chapters 4, 6). A nucleolus is only rarely seen and the loosely arranged "euchromatin" appears to be connected with the nuclear pores (**arrows**). The electron dense particles that lie free in the cytoplasm are presumed to be glycogen (**Gl**) (whole cell × 23,000; granules left × 72,000, far right × 78,000).
Reproduced from ref. 17 with permission of the publisher.

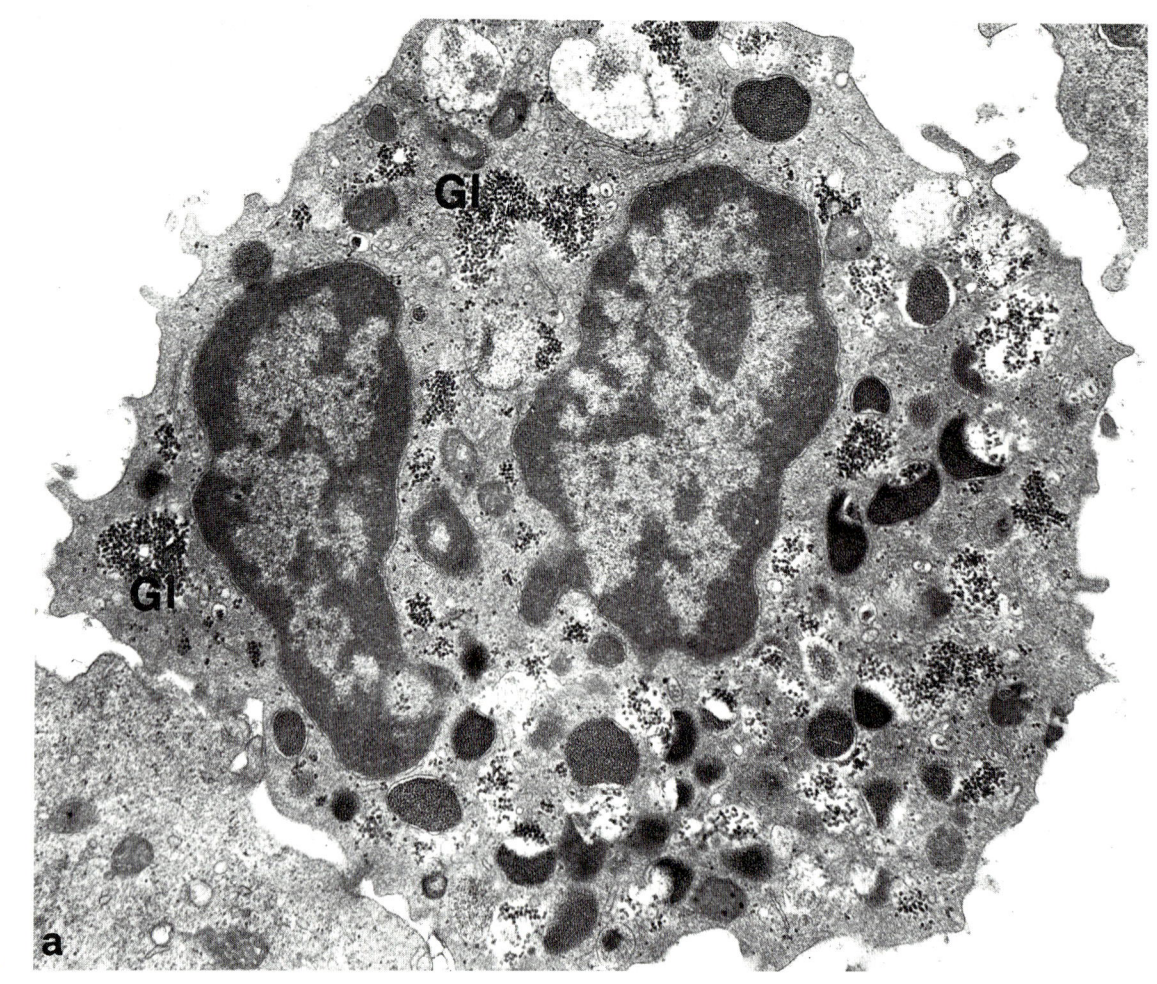

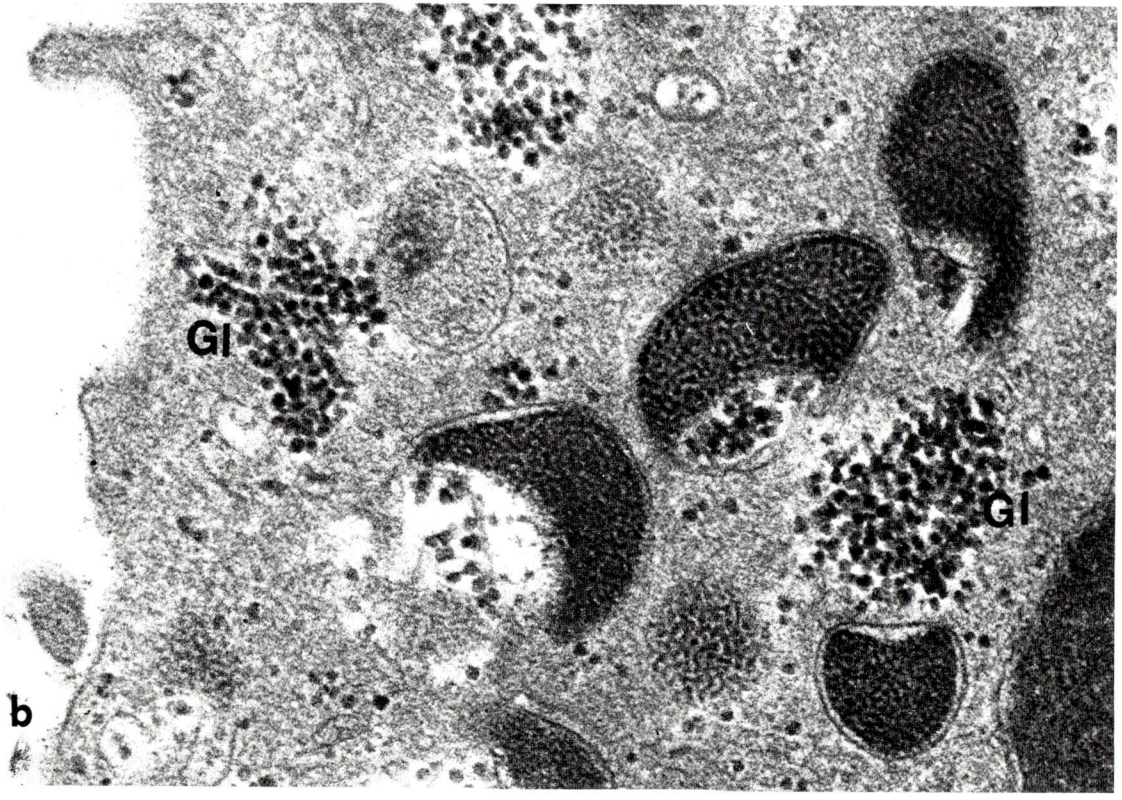

7 BASOPHILS

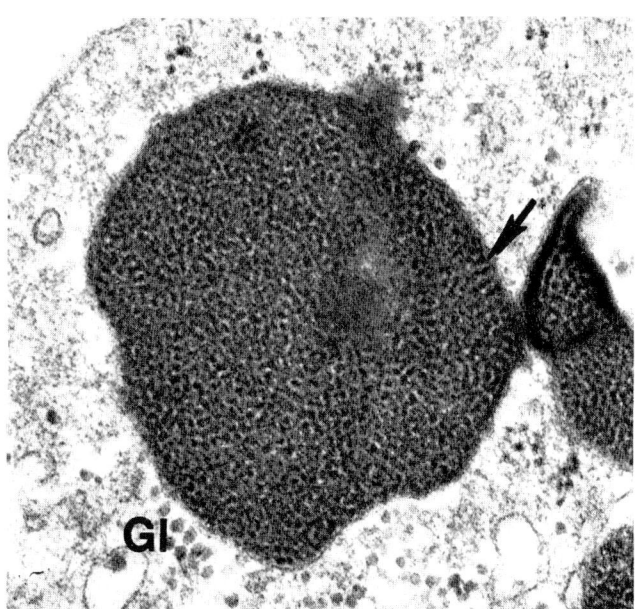

Fig. 7 High magnification of a basophil granule from normal peripheral blood shows how densely the particles are sometimes packed without forming a crystalline pattern. Near the membrane, the particles are often seen in parallel rows (**arrow**). Note presumed glycogen particles (**Gl**) in proximity to the granule ($\times$ 60,000).

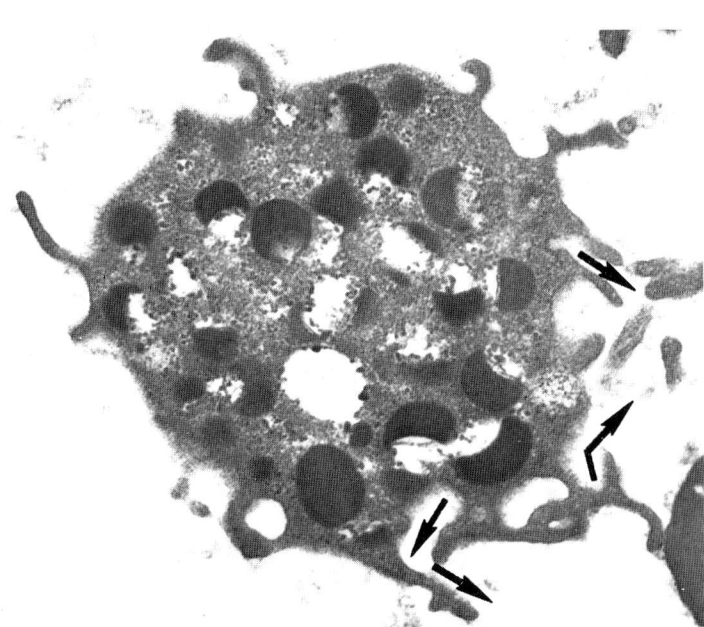

Fig. 8 Section through the pole of a basophil obtained from normal blood. The contour of the cell suggests that some of the granule contents have been discharged e.g. at site where the **arrows** indicate continuity between vacuoles and extracellular space. This is better appreciated in mast cells that have been triggered to degranulate in vitro ($\times$ 12,000).

Fig. 6 Normal blood basophil selected to illustrate the abundance of 25 nm particles presumed to be glycogen (**Gl**). Since most of such particles appear in the vicinity of the granules, it is also conceivable that they represent the heparin precursor, heparin monosulfuric ester which gives a positive PAS reaction. The relationship of the cytoplasmic particles and the particles within the membrane-bound granules, if any, remains to be elucidated (**a** $\times$ 23,000; **b** $\times$ 65,000).

Figure **6 b** reproduced from reference 17 with permission of the publisher.

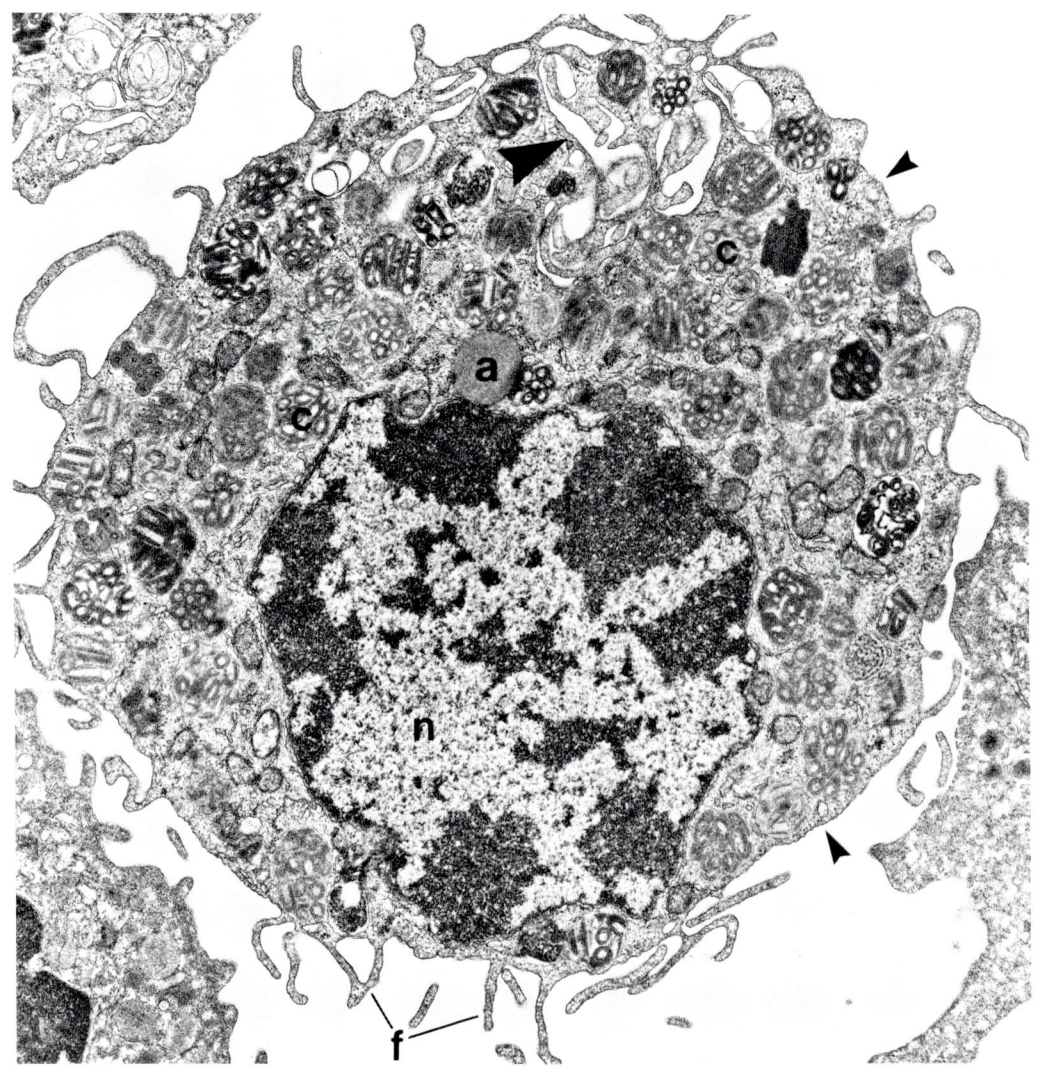

Fig. 9 Low power view of a mast cell dissociated from human lung. Some parts of the membrane appear smooth (**small arrows**). In other areas the plasma membrane seems to have been endocytosed (**large arrow**). Most of the granules contain crystalline scrolls (**c**), but other granules have an amorphous content (**a**). Surface folds, **f** ($\times$ 13,000).

Courtesy of Dr. John P. Caulfield, Harvard Medical School; reproduced from ref. 46 with permission of the publisher.

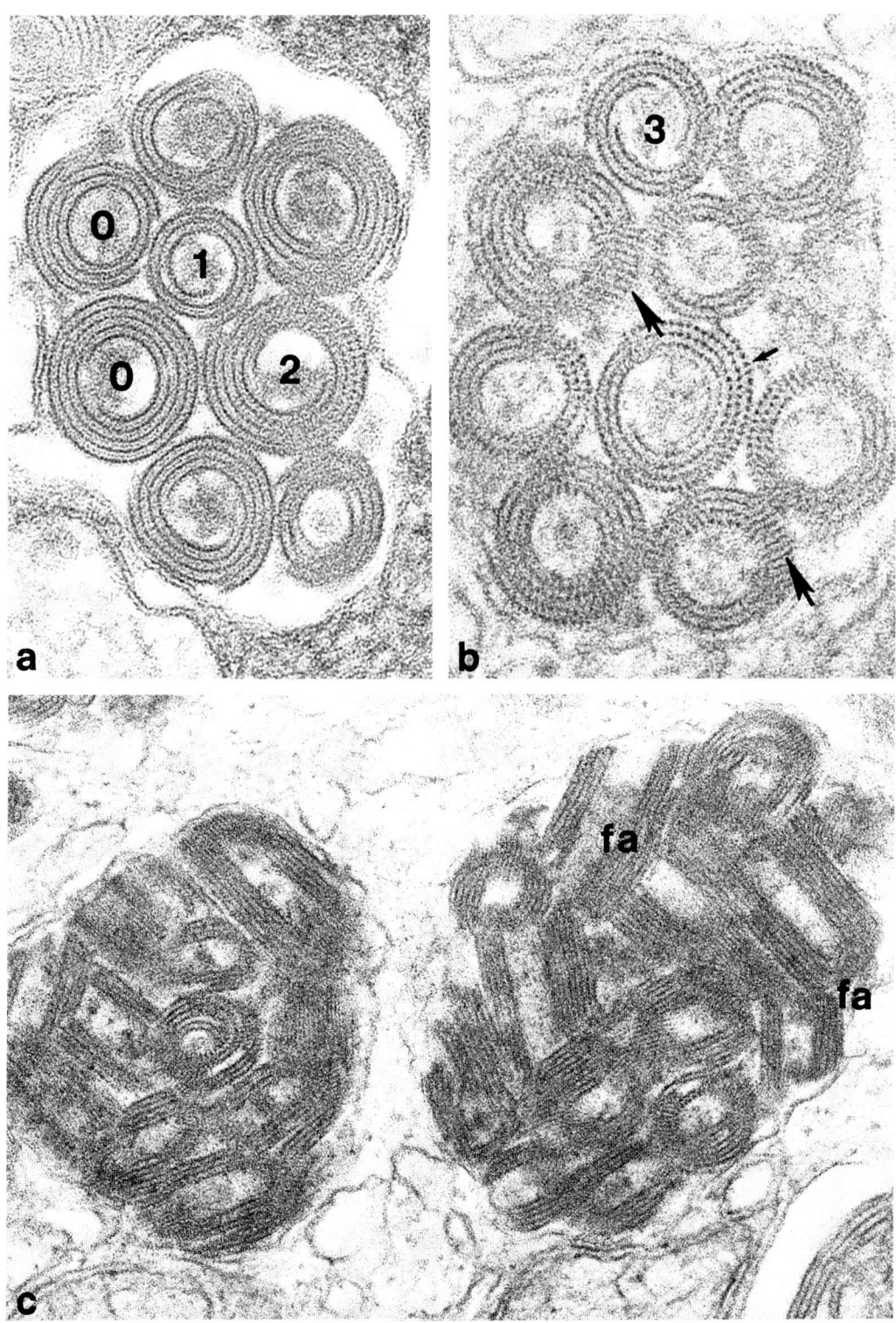

Figs. 10 a-c) High magnification of granules in a mast cell dissociated from human lung. The scrolls are made of concentric layers (**O**) or of 1, 2, or 3 layers coiled within one another (**1**, **2**, or **3** respectively). The structure of the layers is beaded (**small arrow** in **b**) and the spacing in the scroll is nearly at right angles to the spacing between the layers (**large arrow**). In **c**, the scrolls are cut along their long axis and appear as fasciae (**fa**) of electron dense lines separated by electron lucent spaces (**a** × 192,000; **b** × 208,000; **c** × 101,000).
Courtesy of Dr. John P. Caulfield, Harvard Medical School; reproduced from ref. 46 with permission of the publisher.

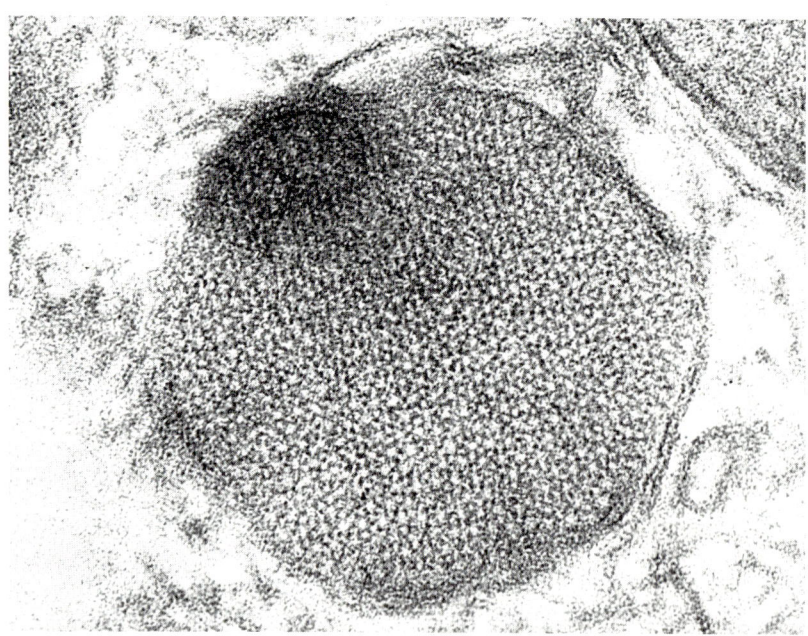

Fig. 11 High resolution of a human mast cell granule which shows a hexagonal crystal lattice pattern. Courtesy of Dr. John P. Caulfield, Harvard Medical School; reproduced from ref. 46 with permission of the publisher.

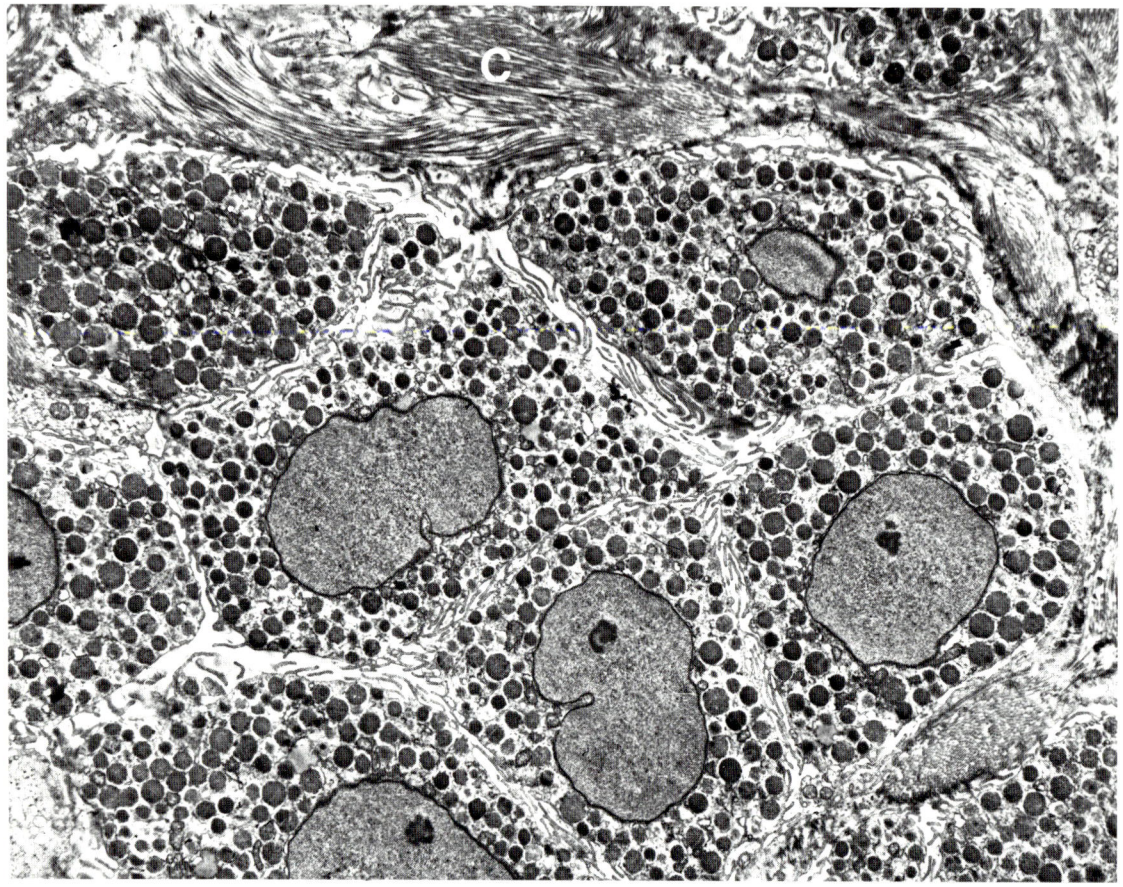

Fig. 12 Low power view of a skin biopsy from a patient with urticaria pigmentosa shows a mast cell infiltrate. Note that the nuclei are round or oval and that they lack heterochromatin (compare with mature basophils, figures **5** and **6**). The conspicuous nucleoli suggest proliferative potential and active protein synthesis. The contour of the cells is marked by numerous villous processes. Collagen, **C** ($\times$ 3,500).

3. FUNCTION

3.1. Secretion - Exocytosis

The major function of basophils and mast cells is secretion. In fact, the cells have been looked upon as unicellular glands. Whereas degranulation of neutrophils, eosinophils and monocytes implies primarily the discharge of granule content into phagocytic vacuoles, degranulation of basophils connotes first and foremost the release of granule content into the cellular environment.
This does not contradict data showing that lysosomal enzymes of other granulocytes may be released extracellularly or that basophil granules may coalesce with endocytic vacuoles. It is merely meant to stress the basic physiological differences among the cells.

The "shedding" of basophil granules concomitant with the liberation of the pharmacologically potent substances, heparin and histamine, is a phenomenon known since the time of Maximov. The interested reader is referred to a vast literature on the subject accumulated by many investigators to whom we are in debt [31-35]. The description presented here will be limited to an illustration of concepts held at the present time.

Once again because of the low numbers of blood basophils, much of our knowledge concerned with the morphologic aspects of the degranulation phenomenon is derived from studies of animal mast cells. However, there is sufficient evidence to suggest that with minor reservations the mechanism is applicable to human basophils as well [36].

In comparison with eosinophils (Chapter 6), basophils are not as susceptible to degranulation by mechanical means [37]. On the other hand, in vitro degranulation of mast cells and basophils is brought about readily by low concentrations of basic polyamines, e.g. compound 48/80 [38], basic polypeptides, e.g. polylysine [39], various lectins, e.g. PHA and concanavalin A [40, 41], the calcium ionophore A 23187 [42] and above all by antiserum to IgE or antigen reacting with IgE to which the cells have been sensitized in vivo [43-46]. Degranulation is energy and Ca^{++} dependent.

On the basis of numerous studies, the following concepts emerge: degranulation begins in the most peripherally located granules [47]. These granules appear to swell just before their perigranular membrane fuses with the plasma membrane when the granule content is extruded.

Almost concomitantly, there is swelling and coalescence of adjacent, deeper situated granules with the former granules. This results in "sets" of granules held by membrane channels that are in continuity with the extracellular environment (**Figs. 13**, **16**, **17** and **18**). It is even likely that degranulation may occur as a focal rather than a global reaction involving the whole cell [48]. Intramembranous alterations in the course of degranulation have been revealed by freeze fracture analysis [59, 50]. However, these images are still subject to definitive interpretation.

In man it is likely that degranulation is mediated primarily by "reaginic" immunoglobulin E. Basophilic leukocytes have receptors for the Fc fragment of IgE which are not present on other leukocytes [51]. It has also been determined that the basophils of normal subjects carry 10-40,000 molecules of IgE on their surface and that additional receptor sites are available to receive additional molecules [52]. In atopic individuals, little IgE will bind to the cells in vitro, suggesting that the membrane of such cells is nearly saturated. Interestingly, the total number of IgE receptors per basophil runs closely parallel to the serum IgE level. Thus, either there is a genetic association between the number of basophil IgE receptors and the level of serum IgE, or the number of IgE receptors on basophils is modulated by the serum IgE concentration [53]. Ordinarily, IgE is bound randomly over the entire basophil surface. However, the receptors are able to move laterally in the plane of the membrane to form "patches" and "caps" [51]. Interaction of an appropriate antigen against which the surface IgE is directed or with an antibody to IgE results in "crosslinking" of membrane sites and degranulation (see **Fig. 18**).

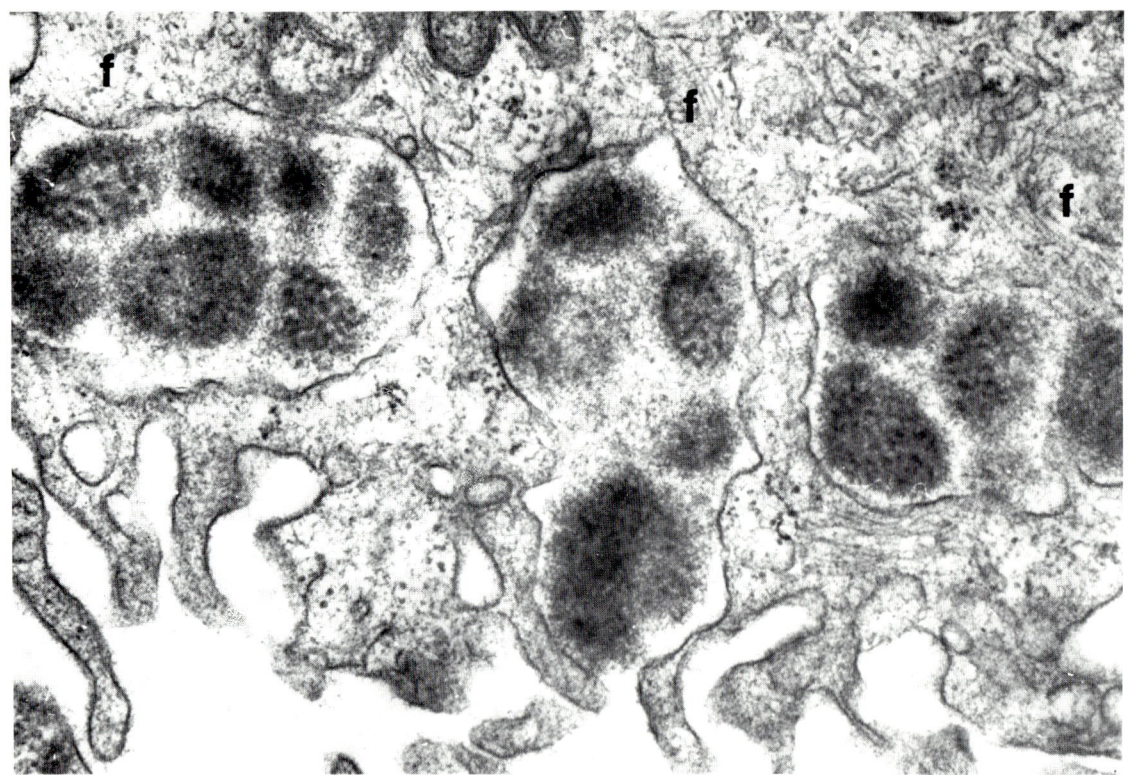

Fig. 13 Detail of the periphery of a mast cell in the process of discharging its granules. The specimen was obtained from the same patient as the one illustrated in figure 12 a few minutes after the patient's skin was irritated. Note that the granules are now devoid of membranes which appear to have been incorporated into the plasma membrane of the cell and that the content of several granules (G) is packed into one space before final discharge. Actin-like filaments discernible in the cytoplasm (f) seem to become more conspicuous during degranulation ($\times$ 47,500).

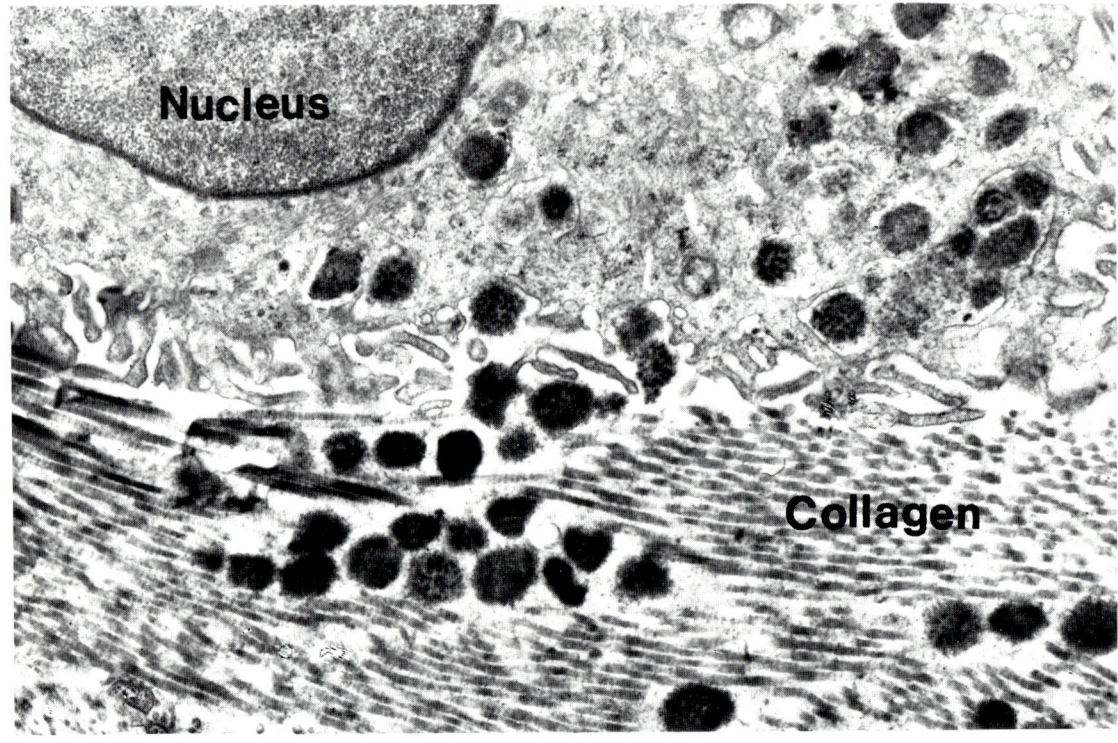

Fig. 14 Periphery of a mast cell from the same specimen as figure 13. Here the cell is almost completely degranulated and the granules which have retained their integrity are seen among collagen fibrils ($\times$ 24,700). Illustrations 12-24 are the courtesy of Drs. George Odland and Frank Parker, and reproduced from ref. 77 with permission of the publisher.

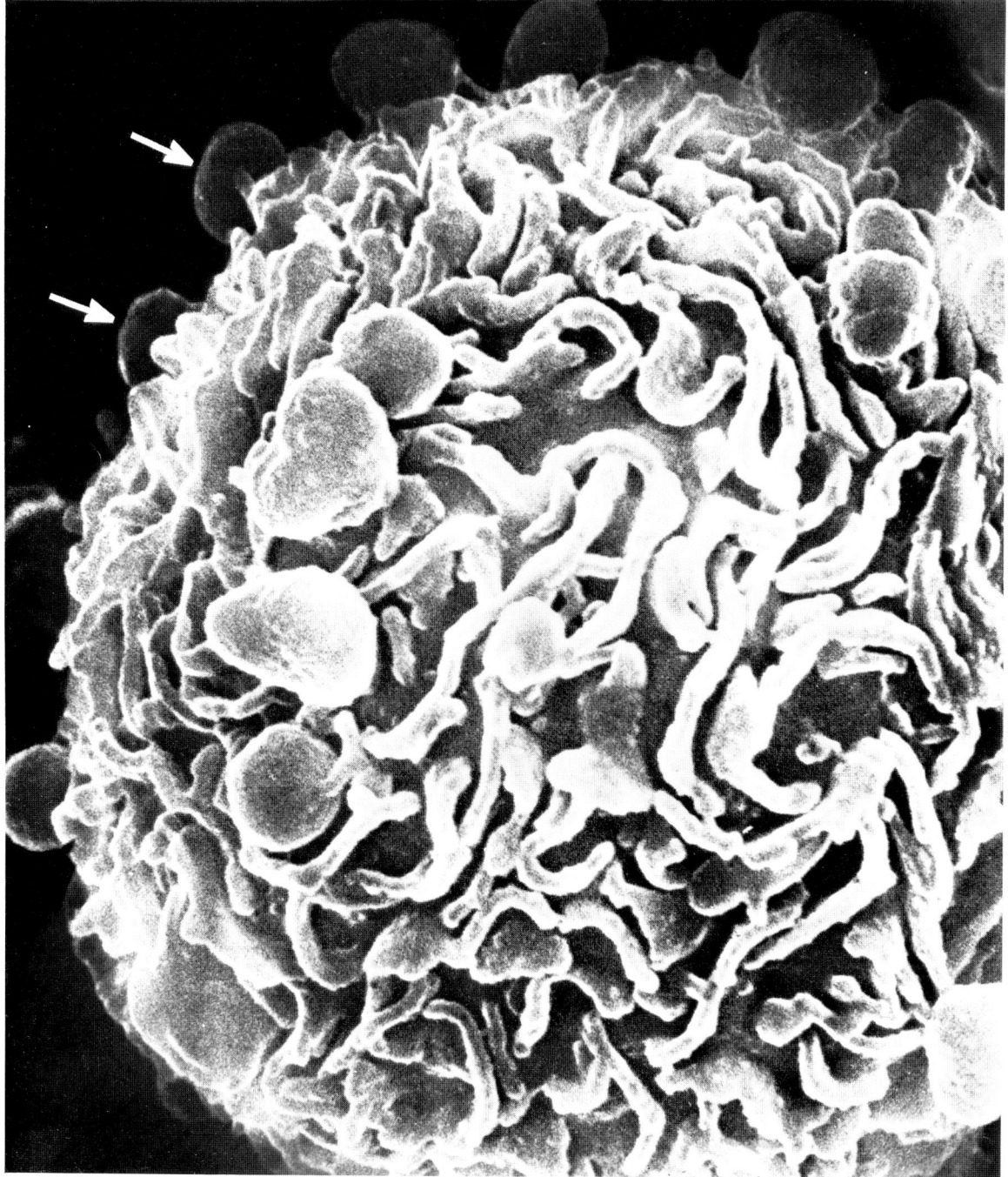

Fig. 15 *Scanning electron micrograph of a secreting mast cell. The round material seen at the periphery (**arrows**) represents the secretion product. Note the abundance of surface processes which are also apparent in sectioned cells examined by TEM ($\times \pm 40,000$).*
Courtesy of Dr. B.H. Satir, Albert Einstein College of Medicine; reproduced from ref. 47, with permission of the publisher.

This can also be achieved with non-specifically aggregated IgE or aggregated Fc fragments of IgE, but not with aggregated F(ab')$_2$ fragments [54]. As in many other cells, the secretory process is modulated by the level of intracellular cyclic AMP. Agents which raise cAMP (isoproterenol and theophylline) inhibit release (for review see refs. 55 and 56). In addition to histamine and heparin, the cells also elaborate a substance which attracts eosinophils, eosinophil chemotactic factor (ECF-A) [57] and slow reacting substance of anaphylaxis (SRS-A), a potent broncho-constrictor which is synthesized by the cell during the course of immediate hypersensitivity reactions (for review see ref. 58). The mechanism by which these mediators are released has not yet been elucidated.

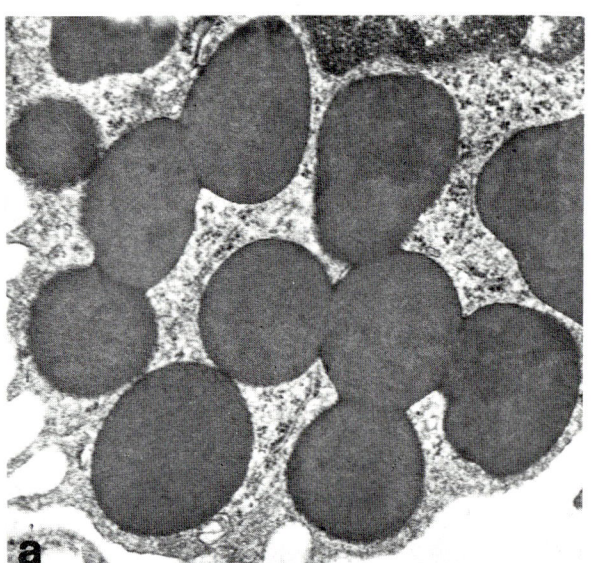
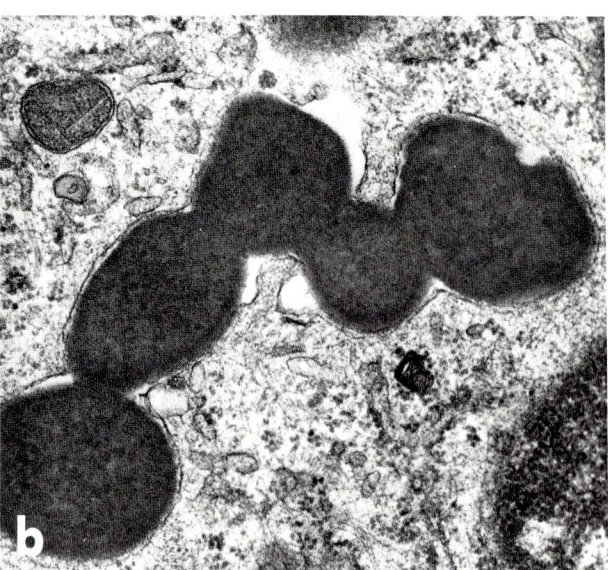
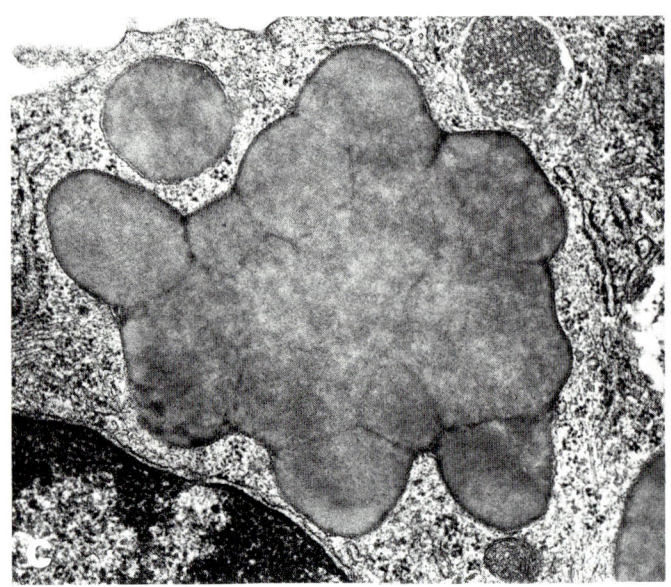

Figs. 16 a-c) Details of rat peritoneal mast cells shortly following the injection of a very small dose of polylysine. The illustrations were selected to show various phases of granule fusion that may take place before as well as during granule discharge. It is believed that mast cell granules may exist as "physiological sets" several being confined to a single membranous compartment in which the spaces constituting the individual granules may be in ready continuity. In **a** the granule membranes are still tightly apposed.
In **b** the perigranular membrane has already separated from the content of the fused organelles.
In **c** a fused granule cluster is seen in a cell 5 days after injection of polylysine. The decreased electron opacity suggests dilution of content, but the granule domains are still visible. It is likely that sets of granules may be discharged in vivo rather than the massive degranulation commonly described under in vitro experimental conditions (see text) (**a** × 24,800; **b** × 31,000; **c** × 17,000).
Courtesy of Dr. Jacques Padawer, Albert Einstein College of Medicine. Reproduced from ref. 39 with permission of the publisher.

7 BASOPHILS

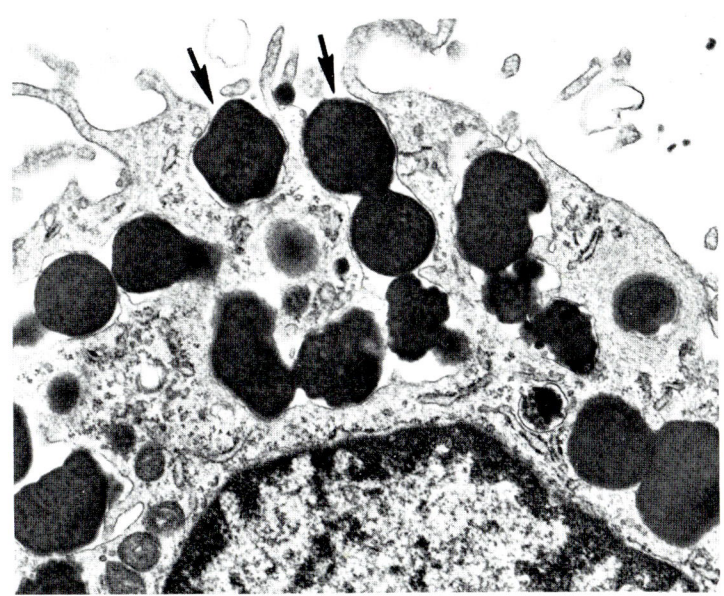

Fig. 17 Periphery of a rat peritoneal mast cell after injection with polylysine. Continuity between fused granule compartments and extracellular space has been established (**arrows**) ($\times$ 5000).
Courtesy of Dr. Jacques Padawer, Albert Einstein College of Medicine. Reproduced from ref. 39 with permission of the publisher.

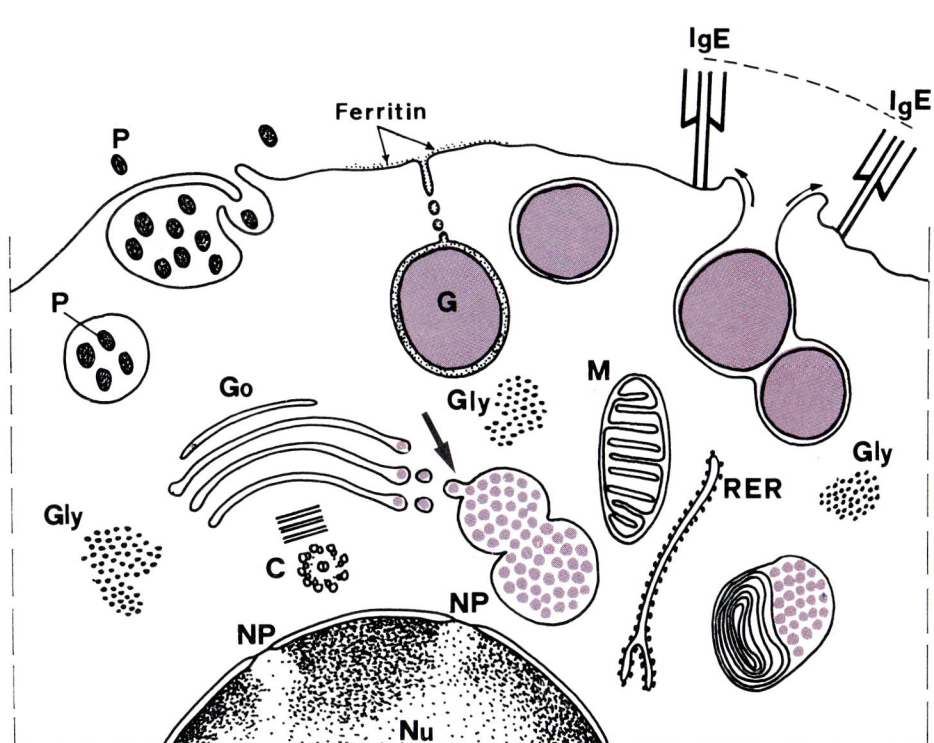

Fig. 18 Diagrammatic representation of basophil function. The cell is able to phagocytose particulates (**P**) which may be found in vacuoles for long periods of time without being degraded. Ferritin and soluble substances may attach to the membrane, be taken up by pinocytotic vesicles which may coalesce with granules (**G**). The plasma membrane has receptors for the Fc component of IgE. Crosslinking of membrane IgE with anti-IgE or other ligands triggers degranulation. The content of new granules is probably synthesized by the RER and packaged by the Golgi membranes (**Go**). Small granules coalesce with large ones (**arrow**). **Gly**, glycogen; **C**, centriole; **NP**, nuclear pore; **M**, mitochondrion; **Nu**, nucleus.

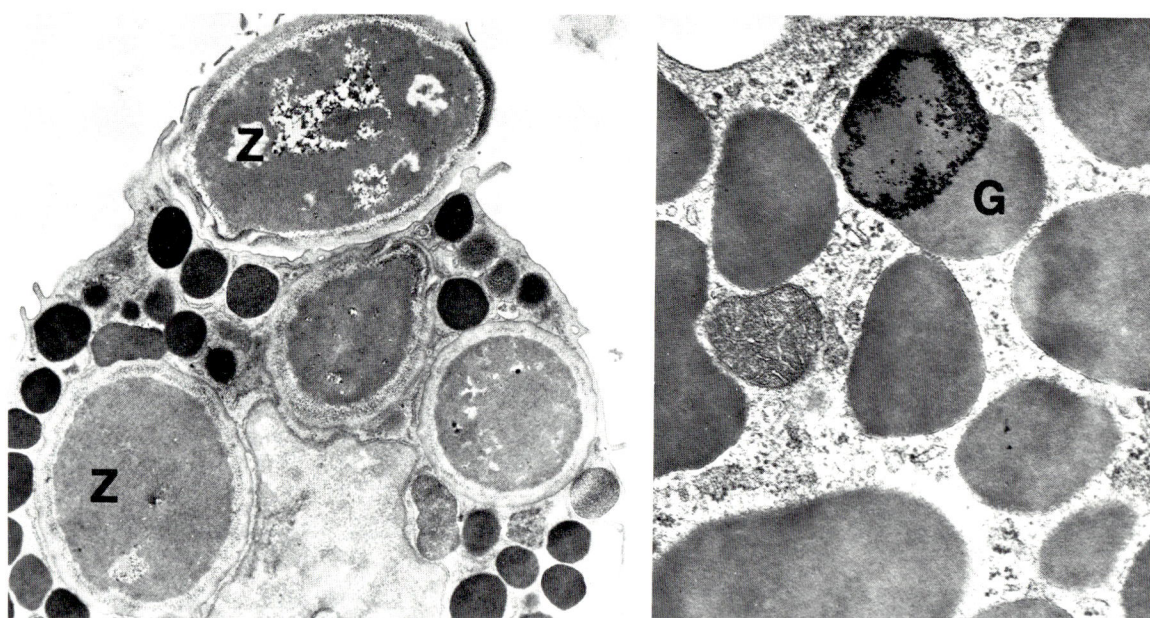

Fig. 19 a) Mast cell from the peritoneal fluid of a rat. The animal had been injected with zymosan particles several hours before the specimen was collected. One zymosan particle (**Z**) appears to be in the process of being internalized. Three zymosan particles are within vacuoles. Note that the mast cell granules have not coalesced with the phagocytic vacuoles. This is in striking contrast to what would be expected in the case of neutrophils or eosinophils.

b) Detail of a mast cell from a rat that had been injected with thorium dioxide 4 months before the specimen was collected. Distribution of colloid in the matrix of the granule (**G**) strongly suggests that fusion of pinocytotic vesicles and granules had taken place ($\times$ 90,000).
Courtesy of Dr. Jacques Padawer, Albert Einstein College of Medicine. Reproduced from ref. 60 and 64 respectively, with permission of the publisher.

3.2. **Endocytosis - Transport - Storage**

Although phagocytosis is not an obvious function of basophils, the cells have been reported to phagocytose sensitized erythrocytes [59], zymosan particles (**Fig. 19 a**), and a host of other particulate substances [60, 61]. Pinocytosis appears to be very active. The solutes are taken up by vesicles which may coalesce with the granules as demonstrated with the help of peroxidase [62], thorotrast or ferritin [63, 64] (**Figs. 19 b and 20**). This is probably the mechanism whereby the cells take up biogenic amines as well as precursor substances (e.g. histidine which they are able to decarboxylate [65]), as well as a variety of mucosubstances, such as heparin. For this reason, it has been suggested that the cells may serve a storage function.

3.3. **Locomotion - Chemotaxis**

Both mast cells and basophils exhibit amoeboid motion which was described as early as 1904 by Maximov [31]. More recently, directed locomotion, i.e. chemotaxis has been observed *in vitro* with basophils responding to a large number of non-specific stimuli. These have included bacterial products, complement components, kallikrein and lymphokines [66]. To account for tissue reactions in which basophils appear to play a prominent role, the existence of substances which attract this class of inflammatory cells preferentially has been postulated. Such factors have recently been described [67, 68].

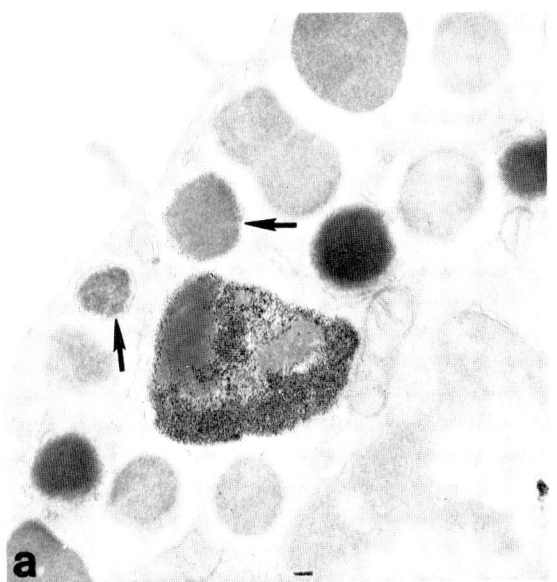 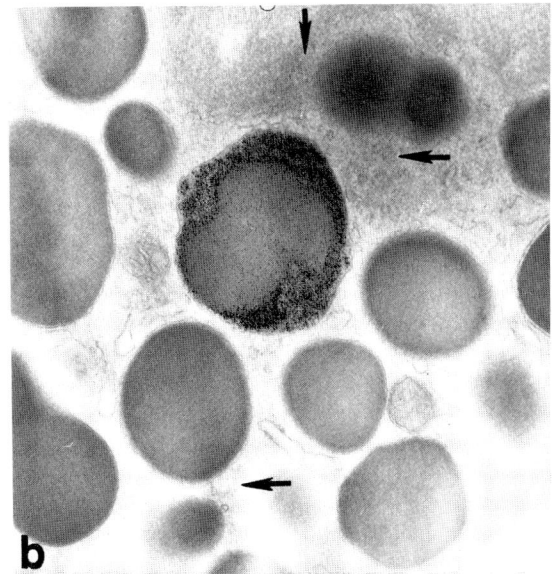

Fig. 20 Details of mast cells from rats that had been injected with ferritin. a) From a specimen collected 24 hours after injection. b) From a specimen collected 7 days after a single injection. The sections are not stained to enhance delineation of smaller aggregates of particles (**arrow**) ($\times$ 32,000).
Courtesy of Dr. Jacques Padawer, Albert Einstein College of Medicine. Reproduced from ref. 61 with permission of the publisher.

4. PATHOPHYSIOLOGY

The pathology of the basophil/mast cell system is considered in two parts:
1) conditions in which basophils/mast cells appear to be intrinsically abnormal, and 2) conditions associated with local or systemic alterations in basophil/mast cell numbers.

4.1. Intrinsic abnormalities

It is generally recognized that the highest blood basophil levels occur in chronic myelogenous leukemia (CML) or other myeloproliferative diseases. When basophilocytosis constitutes over 80% of the white blood cell count, the term basophilic leukemia seems justified [69] (**Fig. 21**).
Indeed, basophilocytosis is often an early manifestation of CML and it is not an uncommon finding in subjects exposed to excessive radiation [70, 71].
As illustrated in **Figures 22-26** the ultrastructure of circulating basophils in myeloproliferative disorders may show many features characteristic of mast cells [72]. Moreover, when lymphoid tumors or lymph nodes of patients with Hodgkin's disease are infiltrated with basophils and/or mast cells, it is often difficult to distinguish one cell from the other [73], even ultrastructurally. The morphologic overlap supports the view that basophils and mast cells are different developmental stages of the same cell.

The tissue counterpart of basophilic leukemia is a mastocytoma or the cutaneous mastocytosis referred to as urticaria pigmentosa. In the latter condition, hyperpigmented skin macules become urticarial when as a result of mild trauma the infiltrating mast cells degranulate and release histamine [74-77] (**Figs. 12-14**). Most patients with urticaria pigmentosa have histaminuria and intermittent symptoms due to high levels of the circulating amine. Because of their invasiveness, the basophils/mast cells in basophilic leukemia and urticaria pigmentosa are considered neoplastic. However, karyotypic abnormalities have not yet been demonstrated.

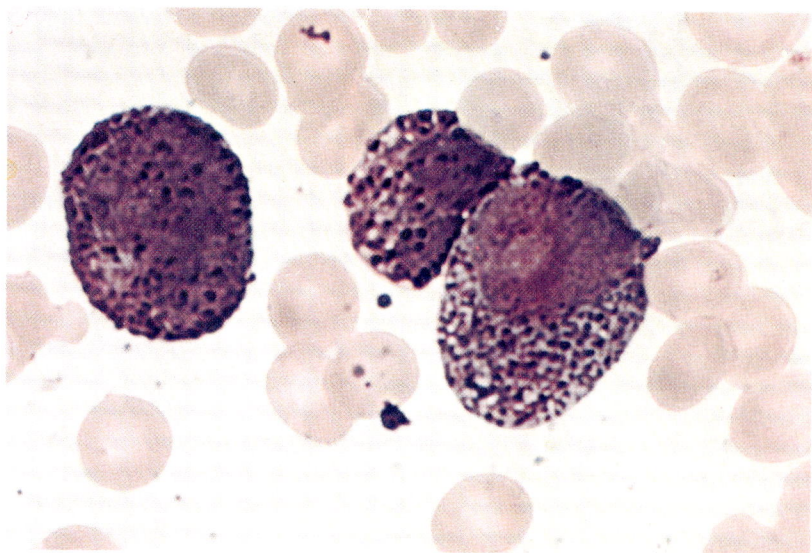

Fig. 21 *Basophilic leukemia. The circulating basophils show distinct granulations, prominent nucleoli and lack of nuclear segmentation.*
Courtesy of Dr. G.L. Castoldi, University of Ferrara.

4.2. "Reactive" changes in basophil numbers

Basophilopenia occurs in practically all conditions associated with eosinophilopenia, and therefore it appears to accompany situations that stress the pituitary-adrenal axis. During leukocytoses accompanying infections, neoplasia or other stress, the basophils all but disappear from the circulation, a helpful variable in the differential diagnosis of myelogenous leukemia versus a leukemoid reaction. An increase in the number of basophils/mast cells in tissues is usually associated with hypersensitivity of the immediate type.

In an elegant series of experiments employing the Rebuck skin window technique (a method whereby a series of coverslips are placed on a cm^2 area of superficially abraded skin and the cellular exudate is sampled at various time intervals) Wolf-Jürgensen and Schwartz [78] noted a high percentage of basophilic leukocytes in exudates of individuals who had been treated with homologous normal lymphocytes. The injected lymphocytes had to be viable in order to elicit the basophil response. Because no mitoses were found among the accumulated basophils, it was postulated that the cells were attracted by a chemotactic factor released by the injected lymphocytes [79].

More recently, Dvorak et al. [80-82] have carried out a large number of experiments demonstrating that not only immediate hypersensitivity, but also cell mediated hypersensitivity of a more delayed type, may be accompanied by tissue infiltration with basophilic leukocytes. The phenomenon appears to be dependent on the mode of sensitization and the type of antigen.
Thus, basophils are characteristically present in allergic contact dermatitis, some types of eczema, and other cutaneous reactions which may have an allergic component [83, 84].

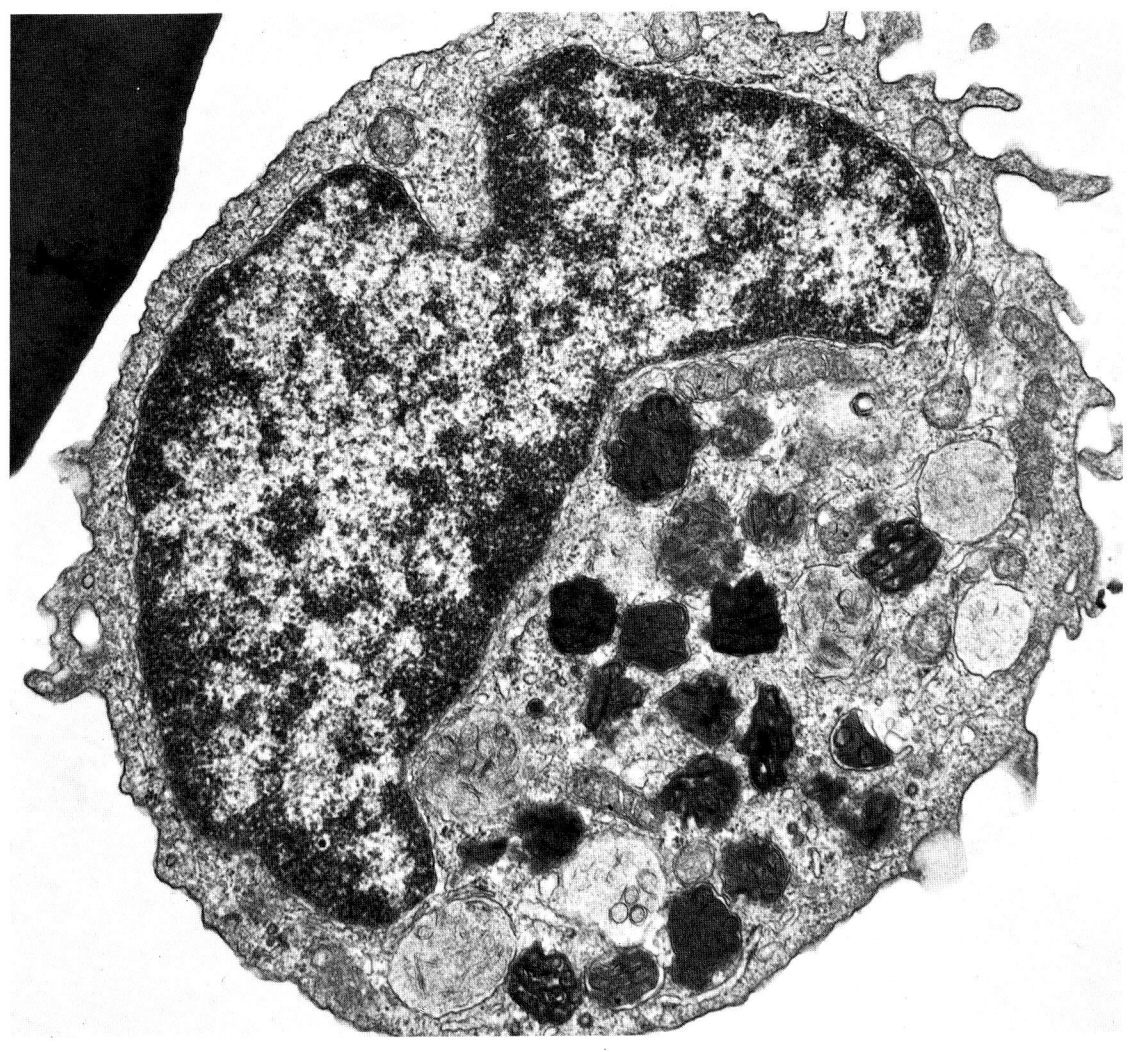

Fig. 22 Peripheral blood cell from a patient with chronic myelogenous leukemia is not distinguishable from a mast cell (compare with fig. 9). The patient had a total leukocyte count of 25,000/cmm with a "basophil" count of 8%. The majority of the granules have "scrolls" and other crystalloid structures. The nucleus is not lobulated like that of a mature basophil and has the chromatin distribution of a less differentiated cell (× 23,000).

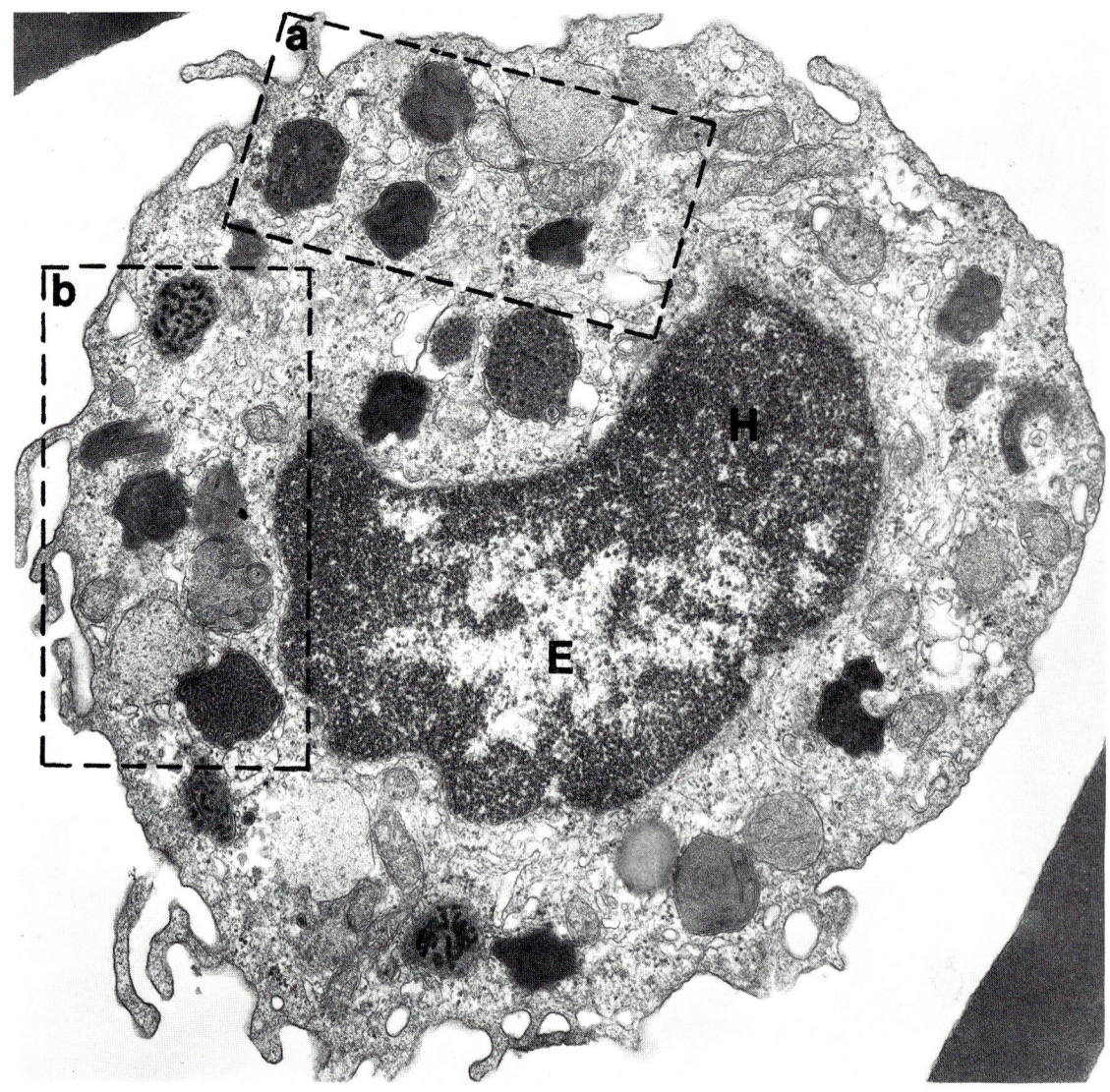

Fig. 23 Cell from the blood of the same patient described in the legend to figure **22**. The nucleous appears more mature than that of the cell illustrated in figure **22** as evidenced by the larger amount of heterochromatin (**H**); **E**, euchromatin. The heterogenous appearance of the granules is noteworthy. Some granules show features characteristic of basophils, others look like mast cell granules. The morphologic overlap supports the view that basophils and mast cells represent different developmental or physiologic forms of the same cell type (see text) ($\times$ 25.000). The areas delimited by the rectangles are shown at higher magnification in figures **23 a** and **23 b**.

a) Note that granule 1 displays particles as well as membrane-like material, granule 2 is partially "solubilized" i.e. the material between the crystalline structures is amorphous, and in granule 3 no structural features are resolved. The cytoplasm is replete with filaments (**f**); **M**, mitochondrion ($\times$ 66,000).

b) The adjacent granules 2 and 3 are particularly noteworthy. Granule 2 shows typical mast cell scrolls, whereas granule 3 shows scrolls as well as the type of particles that are characteristic for basophil granules. Granule 1 exhibits vermiform condensations within an amorphous background substance. This kind of condensation is rarely seen in normal blood basophils ($\times$ 57,000).

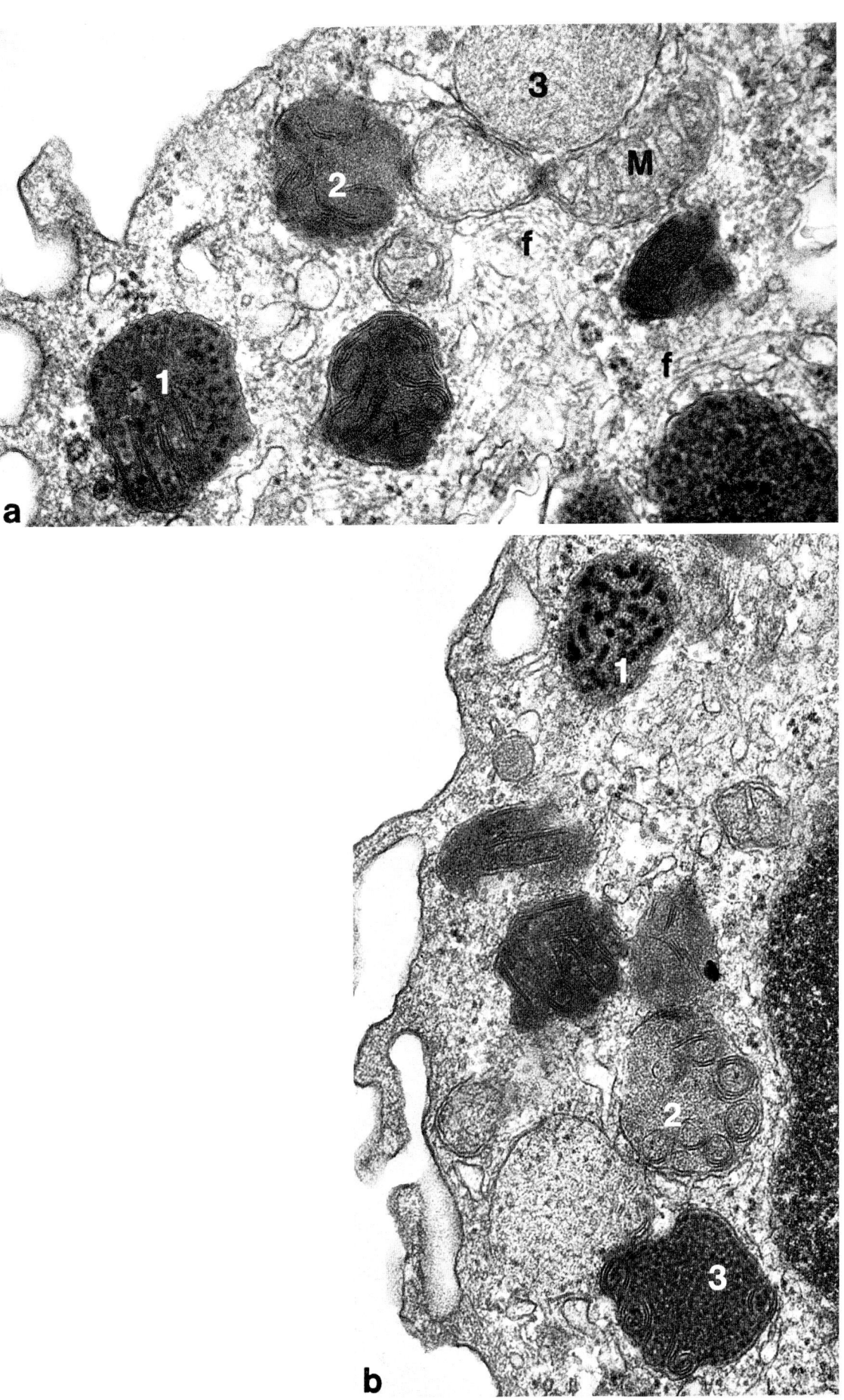

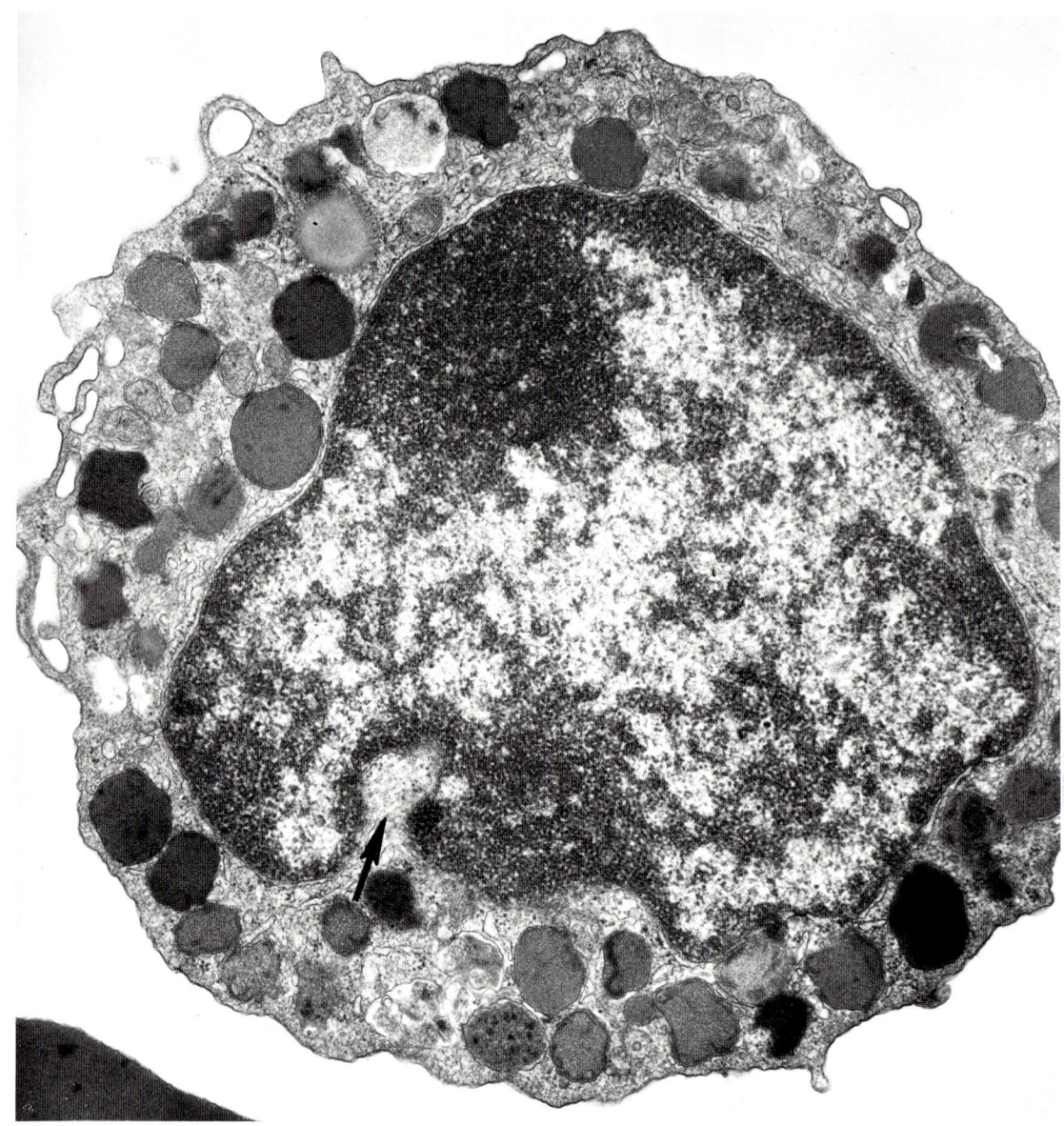

Fig. 24 Circulating mast cell from a patient with a myeloproliferative disorder. The nucleus is not multilobed like that of a normal basophil. Most of the granules have a homogeneous electron dense content as is characteristic for mast cells of many animal species. Similar cells were present in the bone marrow. Such cells are not seen in the blood of healthy subjects and probably present evidence for the disorderly granulopoiesis in myeloid malignancies. **Arrow** indicates microtubules probably associated with the centrosphere ($\times$ 22,500).

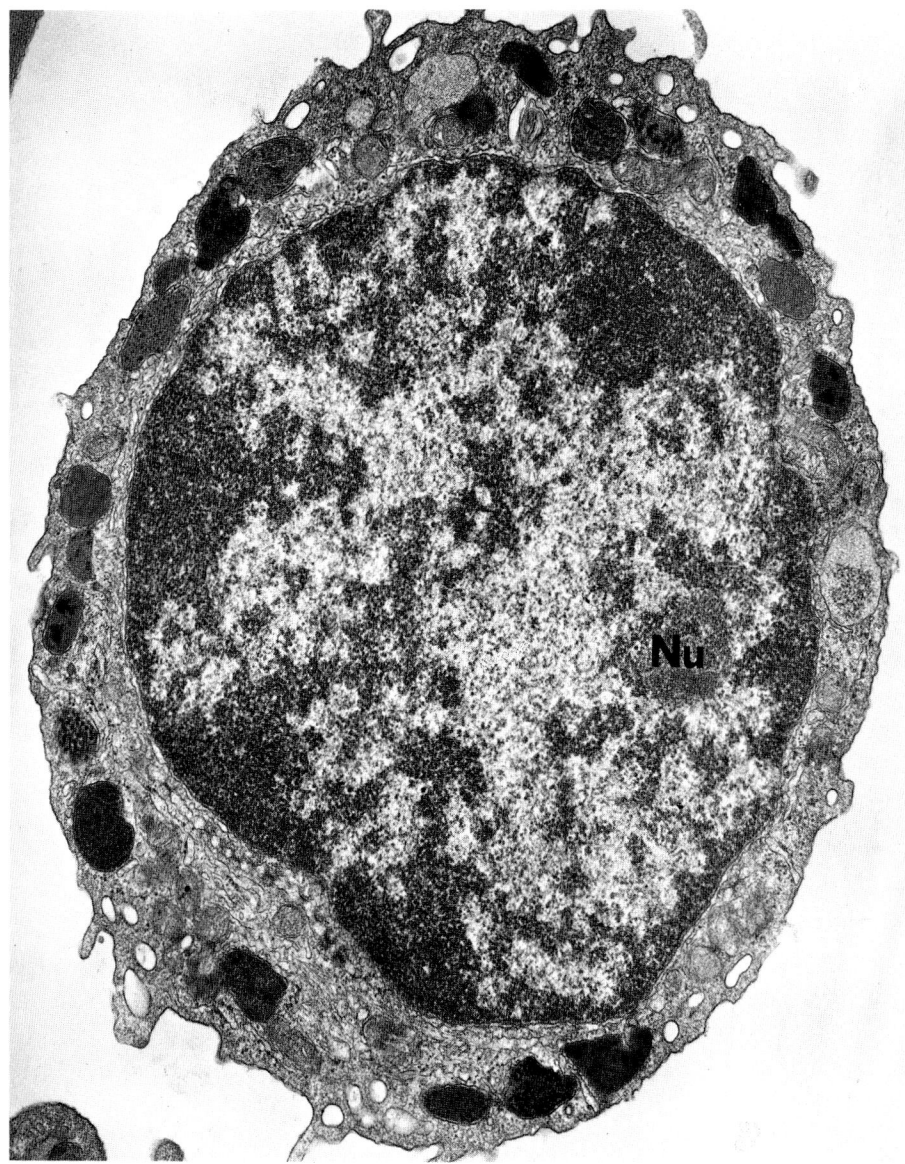

Fig. 25 An unusually small mast cell with a round undifferentiated nucleus and a thin rim of cytoplasm from the blood of a patient with chronic myelogenous leukemia. **Nu**, nucleolus (× 22,000).

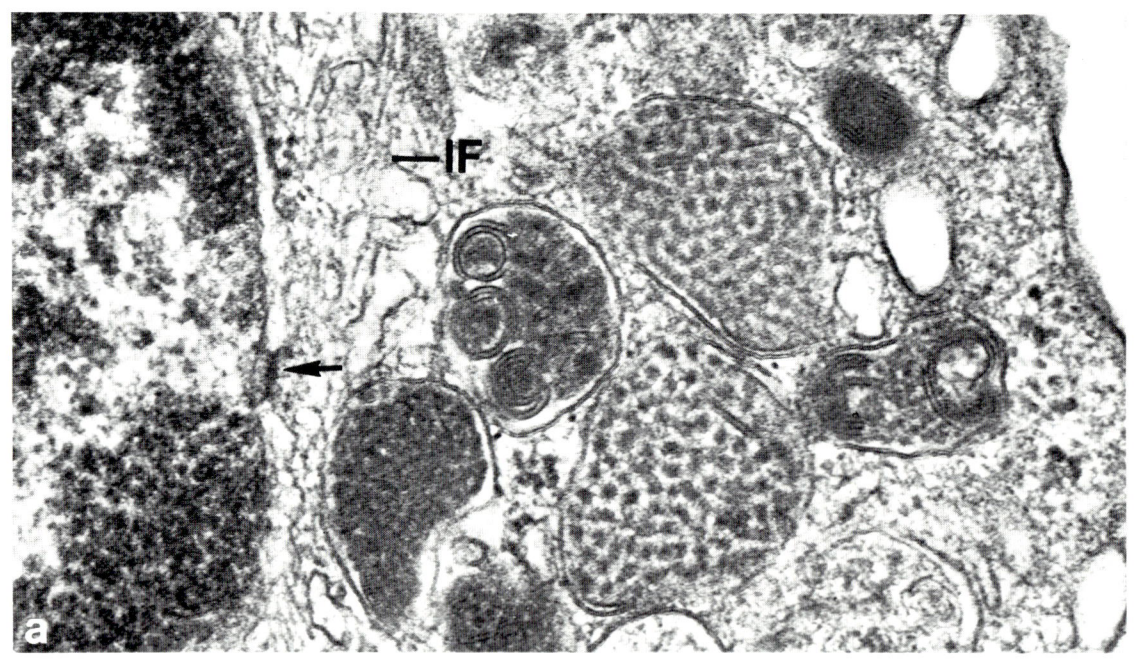

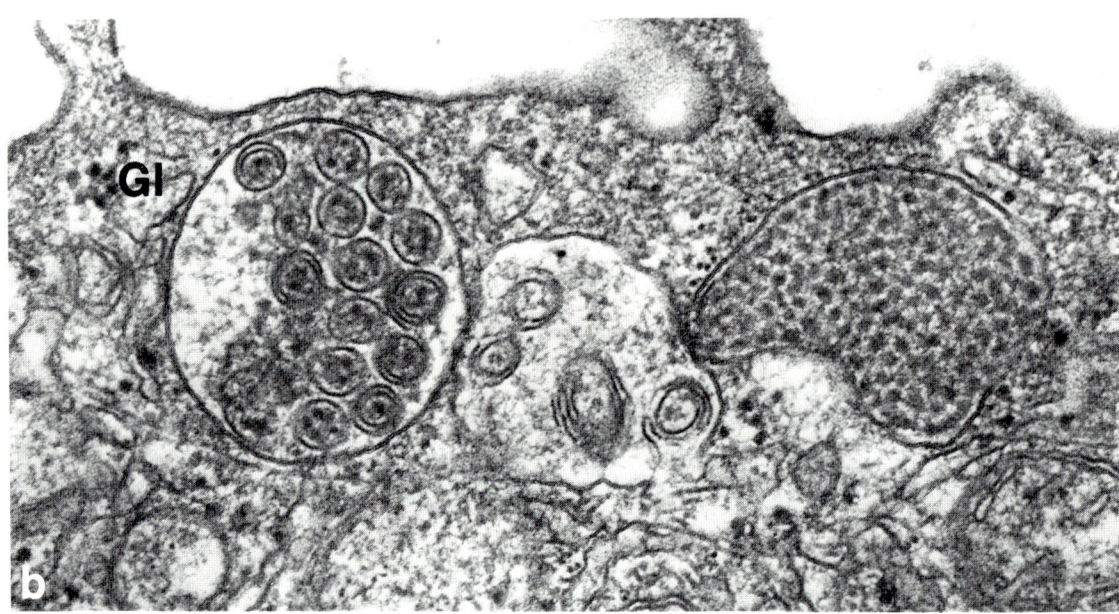

Fig. 26 Details of basophil/mast cells selected to illustrate juxtaposition of particle-filled granules characteristic of basophils and granules containing "scrolls" characteristic of mast cells within the cytoplasm of the same cells. This observation supports the view that the cells belong to the same granulocyte lineage. Figure a exhibits a nuclear pore to good advantage (arrow). IF, intermediate filaments; Gl, glycogen (a × 90,000; b, × 87,000).

As illustrated in **Figures 27** and **28**, when skin is biopsied at a patch test site where a contact allergen had been applied 24-48 hours before, 20-60% of the infiltrating cells may consist of basophils. In all these situations, basophils are probably attracted to the site by products of sensitized lymphocytes. This type of reaction is not limited to the skin, but has also been observed in renal allografts undergoing rejection and in tumor infiltrates [85].

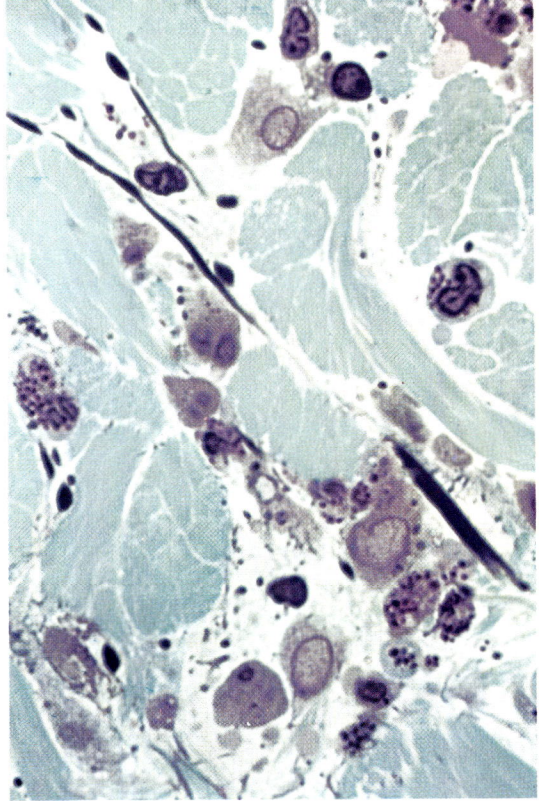 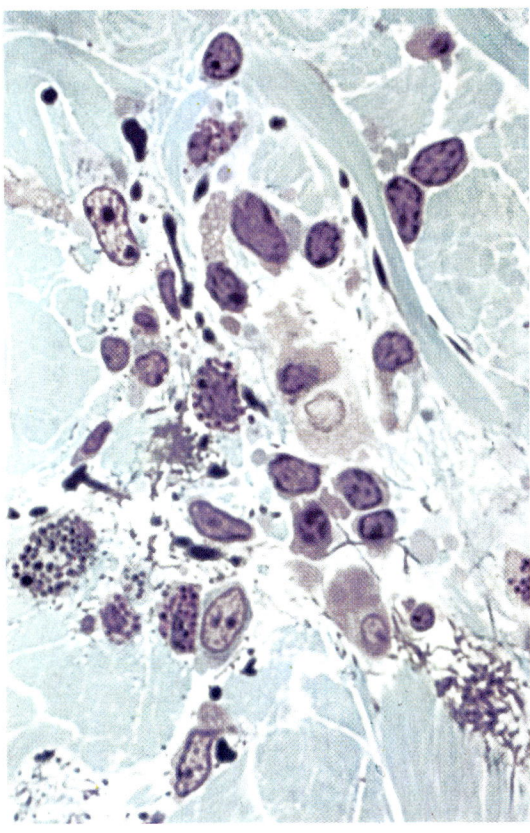

Fig. 27 Skin biopsy of a patient with contact allergy who underwent serial biopsies after patch testing with the allergen. This specimen represents a reaction 50 hours after contact. There are at least 5 basophils. A considerable amount of edema and strands of fibrillar material presumed to be fibrin accompany the reaction. Mononuclear cells are also present.
Courtesy of Dr. Harold F. Dvorak, Harvard Medical School. Reproduced from ref. 80 with permission of the publisher.

Fig. 28 Biopsy of the skin of a patient with a full blown contact allergy reaction. In addition to the conspicuous basophils, the area is also infiltrated by mononuclear cells and eosinophils. Serial biopsies have shown lymphocytes to appear before basophils. These are followed by eosinophils.
Courtesy of Dr. Harold Dvorak, Harvard Medical School.

5. CONCLUSIONS

The relationship of basophils and mast cells is best summarized as follows: basophils seem to participate in the initial response, mast cells partake in more chronic reactions. Both cells originate in the bone marrow from a morphologically unidentifiable precursor that may, however, be the same for mast cells and basophils. Under normal circumstances, the vast majority of mast cell/basophil precursors leave the medullary cavity. They diapedese from the blood into the tissues where they may differentiate and acquire properties characteristic for mast cells.

In a connective tissue environment, the cells may retain their potential for proliferation as evidenced by mitoses seen among mast cells in inflammatory reactions. Whether mast cells may also mature and reach an endstage form which we recognize as basophils is not known. As an alternative to this sequence of events, a small percentage of precursors remain in the bone marrow cavity where, under the influence of this particular microenvironment, they differentiate into basophils. Such cells emerge in the blood as mature, endstage cells that are no longer able to undergo mitosis. It is conceivable that in some conditions specific stimuli accelerate maturation of the marrow pool of precursors causing more basophils to be released into the circulating blood. In myeloproliferative diseases orderly development of various maturation stages is impaired. This may result in the morphologic and biochemical overlap between basophils and mast cells often seen in abnormal clinical states.

REFERENCES

1. Ehrlich P.: *Beiträge zur Kenntnis der granulierten Bindegewebszellen und der eosinophilen Leukocyten.* Arch. Anat. Physiol., *3*, 166, 1879.
2. Zucker-Franklin D.: *Unpublished observations.*
3. Pluznik D.H., Sachs L.: *The cloning of normal "mast" cells in tissue culture.* J. Cell Physiol., *66*, 319-324, 1965.
4. Ginsberg H., Sachs L.: *Formation of pure suspensions of mast cells in tissue culture by differentiation of lymphoid cells from the mouse thymus.* J. Natl. Cancer Inst., *31*, 1-40, 1963.
5. Ishizaka T., Okudaira H., Mauser L.E., Ishizaka K.: *Development of rat mast cells in vitro. Differentiation of mast cells from thymus cells.* J. Immunol., *116*, 747-754, 1976.
6. Kitamura Y., Shimada M., Go S., Matsuda H., Hatanaka K., Seki M.: *Distribution of mast cell precursors in hematopoietic and lymphopoietic tissues of mice.* J. Exp. Med., *150*, 482-490, 1979.
7. Hatanaka K., Kitamura Y., Nishimune Y.: *Local development of mast cells from bone marrow-derived precursors in the skin of mice.* Blood, *53*, 142-147, 1979.
8. Kitamura Y., Hatanaka K., Murakami M., Shibata H.: *Presence of mast cell precursors in peripheral blood of mice demonstrated by parabiosis.* Blood, *53*, 1085-1088, 1979.
9. Michels W.A.: *The mast cells.* Ann. N.Y. Acad. Sci., *103*, 235, 1963.
10. Pretlow T.G., Cassady I.M.: *Separation of mast cells in successive stages of differentiation using programmed gradient sedimentation.* Am. J. Path., *61*, 323-337, 1970.
11. Graham H.T., Lowry O.H., Wheelwright F., Lenz M.A., Parish H.H.: *Distribution of histamine among leukocytes and platelets.* Blood, *10*, 467-481, 1955.
12. Horn R.G., Spicer S.S.: *Sulfated mucopolysaccharide and basic protein in certain granules of rabbit leukocytes.* Lab. Invest., *13*, 1-15, 1964.
13. Amann R., Martin H.: *Blut Mastzellen und Heparin.* Acta Hemat., *25*, 209-219, 1961.
14. Coombs J.W., Lagunoff D., Benditt E.P.: *Differentiation and proliferation of embryonic mast cells of the rat.* J. Cell Biol., *25*, 577-592, 1965.
15. Lagunoff D., Benditt E.P.: *Proteolytic enzymes of mast cells.* Ann. N.Y. Acad. Sci., *103*, 185-198, 1963.
16. Kaung D.T.: *Periodic acid-Schiff reaction in human basophilic leukocytes.* Acta Hemat., *42*, 269-274, 1969.
17. Zucker-Franklin D.: *Electron microscopic study of human basophils.* Blood, *29*, 878-890, 1967.
18. Policard A., Collet A., Prégermain S.: *Etude au microscope electronique des mastocytes des tissus chez les mammifères.* Rév. Hémat., *15*, 374-384, 1956.
19. Winqvist G.: *Electron microscopy of the basophilic granulocyte.* Ann. N.Y. Acad. Sci., *103*, 352-375, 1963.
20. Kobayasi T., Midtgard K., Aboe-Hansen G.: *Ultrastructure of human mast cell granules.* J. Ultrastr. Res., *23*, 153-165, 1968.
21. Breton-Gorius J., Reyes F.: *Ultrastructure of human bone marrow cell maturation.* Internat. Rev. of Cytol., *46*, 251-319, 1976.
22. Coombs J.W.: *An electron microscope study of mouse mast cells arising in vivo and in vitro.* J. Cell Biol., *48*, 676-684, 1971.
23. Terry R.W., Bainton D.F., Farqhuar M.G.: *Formation and structure of specific granules in basophilic leukocytes of the guinea pig.* Lab. Invest., *21*, 65-76, 1969.
24. Prudzansky J.J., Patterson R.: *Subcellular distribution of histamine in human leukocytes.* Proc. Soc. Exp. Biol. & Med., *124*, 56-59, 1967.
25. Ackerman G.A., Clark M.A.: *Ultrastructural localization of peroxidase activity in human basophil leukocytes.* Acta Hemat., *45*, 280-284, 1971.
26. Murata F., Spicer S.S.: *Ultrastructural comparison of basophilic leukocytes and mast cells in the guinea pig.* Am. J. Anat., *139*, 335-352, 1974.
27. Murata F.: *On the fine structure of human basophilic granulocytes and tissue mast cells.* Med. J. Shinshu Univ., *14*, 303-323, 1969.
28. Fedorko M.E., Hirsch J.G.: *Crystalloid structure in granules of guinea pig basophils and human mast cells.* J. Cell Biol., *26*, 973-976, 1965.
29. Vollrath L., Wahlin T.: *Uber die Entstehung von Mastzell-granula.* Z. Zellforsch., *111*, 286-292, 1970.
30. Taichman N.S.: *Ultrastructure of guinea pig mast cells.* J. Ultrastr. Res., *32*, 284-292, 1970.
31. Maximov A.: *Uber entzündliche Bindegewebsneubildung bei der weissen Ratte und die dabei auftretenden Veränderungen der Mastzellen und Fettzellen.* Beitr. Pathol. Anat. Allgem. Pathol., *35*, 93-126, 1904
32. Riley J.F., West G.B.: *The presence of histamine in tissue mast cells.* J. Physiol., *120*, 528-537, 1953.
33. Policard A., Collet A.: *Recherches par microcinématographie en contraste de phase sur le comportement des mastocytes péritoneaux à l'état vivant.* Bull. Micr. Appl., *9*, 81, 1959.
34. Thiéry J.P.: *Etude au microscope électronique de la maturation et de l'excrétion des granules des mastocytes.* J. Microscopie, *2*, 549, 1963.
35. Selye H.: *Experiment und praktische Medizin.* Dtsch. Med. Z., *24*, 717, 1956.
36. Hastie R.: *The antigen-induced degranulation of basophil leukocytes from atopic subjects studied by phase contrast microscopy.* Clin. Exp. Immunol., *8*, 45-61, 1971.
37. Diamant B., Kruger P.G.: *Structural changes of isolated rat peritoneal mast cells induced by adenosine diphosphate.* J. Histochem. Cytochem., *16*, 707-716, 1968.
38. Rohlich P., Anderson P., Uvnas B.: *Electron microscope observations on compound 48/80-induced degranulation in rat mast cells.* J. Cell Biol., *51*, 465-483, 1971.
39. Padawer J.: *The reaction of rat mast cells to polylysine.* J. Cell Biol., *47*, 352-372, 1970.
40. Hook W.A., Dougherty S.F., Oppenheim J.J.: *Release of histamine from hamster mast cells by concanavalin A and phytohemagglutinin.* Infect. and Immunity, *9*, 903-908, 1974.
41. Siraganian P.A., Siraganian R.P.: *Basophil activation by concanavalin A: characteristics of the reaction.* J. Immunol., *112*, 2117-2125, 1974.
42. Lichtenstein L.M.: *The mechanism of basophil histamine release induced by antigen and by the calcium ionophore A 23187.* J. Immunol., *114*, 1692-1699, 1975.
43. Ishizaka T., Ishizaka K., Johansson G.O., Bennich H.:

Histamine release from human leukocytes by anti-IgE antibodies. J. Immunol., 102, 884-892, 1969.
44. Siraganian R.P., Hook W.A., Levine B.B.: *Specific in vitro histamine release from basophils by divalent haptens: evidence for activation by simple bridging of membrane-bound antibody.* Immunochemistry, 12, 149-157, 1975.
45. Ishizaka K., Tomioka H., Ishizaka T.: *Mechanisms of passive sensitization. I. Presence of IgE and IgG molecules on human leukocytes.* J. Immunol., 105, 1459-1467, 1970.
46. Caulfield J.P., Lewis R.A., Hein A., Austen K.F.: *Secretion in dissociated human pulmonary mast cells: evidence for solubilization of granule contents before discharge.* J. Cell Biol. (in press).
47. Burwen S.J., Satir B.H.: *Plasma membrane folds on the mast cell surface and their relationship to secretory activity.* J. Cell Biol., 74, 690-697, 1977.
48. Tasaka K., Endo K., Yamasaki H.: *Degranulation and histamine release in focal antigen-antibody reaction by means of microelectrophoresis in a single rat mesentery mast cell.* Japan. J. Pharmacol., 22, 89-95, 1972.
49. Chi E.Y., Lagunoff D., Koehler J.K.: *Freeze-fracture study of mast cell secretion.* Proc. Natl. Acad. Sci., 73, 2823-2827, 1976.
50. Burwen S.J., Satir B.H.: *A freeze-fracture study of early membrane events during mast cell secretion.* J. Cell Biol., 73, 660-671, 1977.
51. Sullivan A.L., Grimley P.M., Metzger H.: *Electron microscopic localization of immunoglobulin E on the surface membrane of human basophils.* J. Exp. Med., 134, 1403-1416, 1971.
52. Ishizaka T., Soto C.S., Ishizaka K.: *Mechanisms of passive immunization. III. Number of IgE molecules and their receptor sites on human basophil granulocytes.* J. Immunol., 111, 500-511, 1973.
53. Malveaux F.J., Conroy M.C., Adkinson N.F., Lichtenstein L.M.: *IgE receptors on human basophils.* J. Clin. Invest., 62, 176-181, 1978.
54. Becker K.E., Ishizaka T., Metzger H., Ishizaka K., Grimley P.M.: *Surface IgE on human basophils during histamine release.* J. Exp. Med., 138, 394-409, 1973.
55. Plant M., Lichtenstein L.M.: *Pharmacologic control of mediator release.* In: *Immediate hypersensitivity.* Bach M.K. ed., Marcel Dekker, Inc., New York, chapter 17, pp. 503-531, 1978.
56. Morrison D.C., Henson P.M.: *Release of mediators from mast cells and basophils induced by different stimuli.* In: *Immediate hypersensitivity.* Bach. M.K. ed., Immunology series, vol. 7., Marcel Dekker, Inc., New York, pp. 431-502, 1978.
57. Goetzl E.J., Austen K.F.: *Purification and synthesis of eosinophilotactic tetrapeptides of human lung tissue: identification as eosinophil chemotactic factor of anaphylaxis.* Proc. Natl. Acad. Sci., 72, 4123-4127, 1975.
58. Austen K.F., Lewis R.A., Stechschulte D.F., Wasserman S.I., Leid R.W., Goetzl E.J.: *Generation and release of chemical mediators of immediate hypersensitivity.* In: *Progress in immunology, II.* Brent L., Holborow E.J. eds., vol. 2, North Holland, Amsterdam, pp. 61-71, 1974.
59. Ultman J.E., Mutter R.D., Tannenbaum M., Warner R.R.P.: *Clinical, cytologic, and biochemical studies in systemic mast cell disease.* Ann. Int. Med., 61, 326-333, 1964.
60. Padawer J., Fruhman G.J.: *Phagocytosis of zymosan particles by mast cells.* Experientia, 24, 471-472, 1968.
61. Padawer J.: *Phagocytosis of particulate substances by mast cells.* Lab. Invest., 25, 320-330, 1971.
62. Dvorak A.M., Dvorak H.F., Karnovsky M.J.: *Uptake of horseradish peroxidase by guinea pig basophilic leukocytes.* Lab. Invest., 26, 27-39, 1972.
63. Padawer J.: *Uptake of colloidal thorium dioxide by mast cells.* J. Cell Biol., 40, 747-760, 1969.
64. Padawer J.: *Mast cells: extended lifespan and lack of granule turnover than normal in vivo conditions.* Exp. Molec. Path., 20, 269-280, 1974.
65. Heisler S., Uvnas B.: *In vitro studies on the uptake of biogenic amines by rat mast cells.* Acta Physiol. Scand., 86, 145-154, 1972.
66. Kay A.B., Austen K.F.: *Chemotaxis of human basophil leukocytes.* Clin. Exp. Immunol., 11, 557-563, 1972.
67. Boetcher D.A., Leonard E.J.: *Basophil chemotaxis: augmentation by a factor from stimulated lymphocyte cultures.* Immunol. Commun., 2, 421-429, 1973.
68. Ward P.A., Dvorak H.F., Cohen S., Yoshida T., Data R., Selvaggio S.S.: *Chemotaxis of basophils.* J. Immunol., 114, 1523-1531, 1975.
69. Joachim G.: *Uber Mastzellen-leukämien.* Deutsch. Arch. f. Klin. Med., 87, 437-455, 1906.
70. Moloney W.C., Lange R.D.: *Cytologic and biochemical studies on the granulocytes in early leukemia among atom bomb survivors.* Texas Reports Biol. & Med., 12, 887, 1954.
71. Fredericks R.E., Moloney W.C.: *The basophilic granulocyte.* Blood, 14, 571-583, 1959.
72. Zucker-Franklin D.: *Unpublished observations.*
73. Parmley R.T., Spicer S.S., Wright N.J.: *The ultrastructural identification of tissue basophils and mast cells in Hodgkin's disease.* Lab. Invest., 32, 469-475, 1975.
74. Freeman R.G.: *Diffuse urticaria pigmentosa.* Am. J. Clin. Path., 48, 187-199, 1967.
75. Kobayashi T., Asboe-Hansen G.: *Degranulation and regranulation of human mast cells. An electron microscopic study of the whealing reaction in urticaria pigmentosa.* Acta Derm. Venereol., 49, 369-381, 1969.
76. Hashimoto K., Gross B.G., Lever W.F.: *An electron microscopic study of the degranulation of mast cell granules in urticaria pigmentosa.* J. Invest. Derm., 46, 139-149, 1966.
77. Zucker-Franklin D.: *Electron microscope studies of human granulocytes: structural variations related to function.* Sem. Hemat., 5, 109-133, 1968.
78. Wolf-Jürgenson P., Schwartz M.: *Normal-lymphocyte transfer in man: basophil leukocytes in delayed skin reactions.* Lancet, ii, 388-390, 1964.
79. Wolf-Jürgenson P.: *Basophilic leukocytes in delayed hypersensitivity. Experimental studies in man using the skin window technique.* Munksgaard, Copenhagen, 1966.
80. Dvorak H.F., Dvorak A.M., Simpson B.A., Richerson H.B., Leskowitz S., Karnovsky M.J.: *Cutaneous basophil hypersensitivity. II. A light and electron microscopic description.* J. Exp. Med., 132, 558-582, 1970.
81. Dvorak H.F., Mihm M.C.: *Basophilic leukocytes in allergic contact dermatitis.* J. Exp. Med., 135, 235-254, 1972.
82. Dvorak A.H., Mihm M.C., Dvorak H.F.: *Degranulation of basophilic leukocytes in allergic contact dermatitis reactions in man.* J. Immunol. 116, 687-695, 1976.
83. Rorsman H., Slatkin M.W., Harber L.C., Baer R.L.: *The basophilic leukocyte in urticarial hypersensitivity to physical agents.* J. Invest. Dermat., 39, 493-499, 1962.
84. Felarca A.B., Lowell F.C.: *The accumulation of eosinophils and basophils at skin sites as related to intensity of skin sensitivity and symptoms in atopic disease.* J. Allerg. and Clin. Immunol., 48, 125-133, 1971.
85. Colvin R.B., Dvorak A.M., Dvorak H.F.: *Mast cells in the cortical tubular epithelium and interstitium in human renal disease.* Human Path., 5, 315-326, 1974.
86. Asboe-Hansen G.: *The mast cell.* Int. Rev. Cytol., 3, 399, 1954.
87. Braunsteiner H., Zucker-Franklin D.: *The physiology and pathology of leukocytes.* Grune & Stratton, New York, p. 49, 1962.
88. Padawer J. (ed.): *Mast cells and basophils.* Ann. N.Y. Acad. Sci., vol. 103, 1-492, 1963.
89. Selye H.: *The mast cells.* Butterworths, Washington, 1965.
90. Lagunoff D.: *Contributions of electron microscopy to the study of mast cells.* J. Invest. Derm., 58, 296-311, 1972.
91. Dvorak H.F., Dvorak A.M.: *Basophilic leukocytes: structure, function, and role in disease.* Clinics in Hematology, 4, 651-683, 1975.
92. Bach M.K. (ed.): *Immediate hypersensitivity.* Immunology series No. 7, Marcel Dekker, Inc., New York, 1978.

8

The mononuclear phagocyte system
Monocytes and Macrophages

M.J. CLINE

Department of Medicine, University of California
Los Angeles, U.S.A.

1. GENERAL ASPECTS AND DEVELOPMENT

The mononuclear phagocyte system is a complex system of cells widely distributed throughout the body. The earliest members of this cell line are found in the bone marrow and include monoblasts and promonocytes. These mature within the bone marrow to monocytes which leave the marrow and briefly enter the blood. After circulating for only a few hours, monocytes leave the bloodstream and enter the tissues, where they differentiate into macrophages [1, 2]. They form macrophages in many organs: alveolar macrophages, freely wandering pleural and peritoneal macrophages, the Kupffer cells of the liver, and the macrophages that line the sinusoids of the spleen [3]. The term *histiocyte* is often used interchangeably with the term *macrophage*.

A schematic representation of the development of the mononuclear phagocyte system [4-6] is seen in **Figure 1**. It shows progressive development of cells of the mononuclear phagocyte system from monoblast to the mature macrophage.

Examples of bone marrow promonocytes and blood monocytes are seen in **Figures 2** and **3**. With maturation from the monocyte to the macrophage, the cell greatly enlarges and may become multinucleate. It acquires a large number of granules (lysosomes) which are membrane-bound packets containing acid-activated hydrolytic enzymes.

As the cell matures from monocyte to macrophage, its ability to ingest (phagocytize) particles also increases. These cells are avidly phagocytic and can engulf a wide range of organic and inorganic particles. A mature tissue macrophage which has ingested bacteria is shown in **Figure 4**.

The ultimate end-stage of development of this cell line is the multinucleate giant cell seen in granulomatous diseases such as tuberculosis, leprosy or sarcoidosis (**Fig. 5**). Such cells are very large and contain multiple nuclei, abundant cytoplasm and a large store of hydrolytic enzymes packaged in lysosomes.

The kinetics of development of the mononuclear phagocyte system are schematically illustrated in **Figure 6**. This illustrates two mitotic divisions within the promonocyte compartment and then further development of promonocyte to monocyte without further division. The bone marrow stores of monocytes are small, and these cells rapidly leave the marrow compartment to enter the bloodstream. In the peripheral blood monocytes briefly circulate and enter the tissues where they mature to macrophages.
Normally, macrophages never re-enter the blood [1, 2]. From studies in animals and man it is known that the lifespan of the macrophage is at least several weeks and perhaps several months.

In vitro, monocytes undergo the same series of differentiation steps that occur *in vivo*. This process eventuates in the differentiation of precursor cells into macrophages. **Figure 7** shows a recently isolated monocyte from human peripheral blood. It contains a few dense granules (lysosomes). After a few weeks *in vitro* the cell becomes a giant macrophage (**Fig. 8**) demonstrating multiple phase-dense granules and abundant ribbon-like mitochondria.

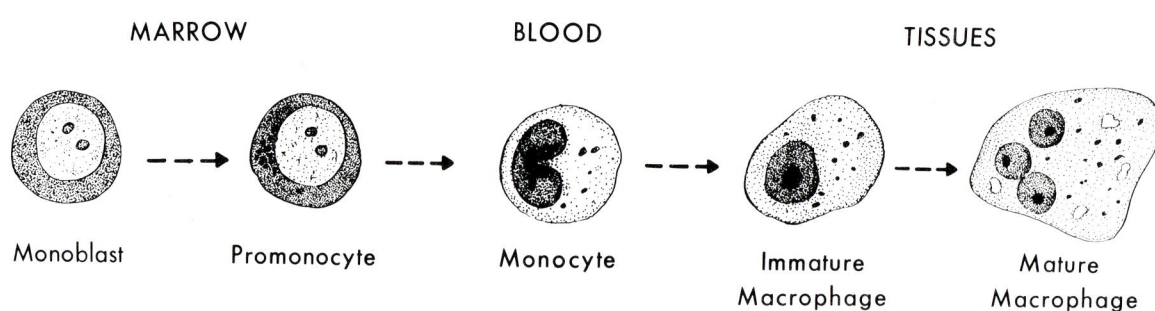

Fig. 1 Sequence of development of cells in the mononuclear phagocyte series. Monoblasts and promonocytes are the least mature cells of the series. Cells through the immature macrophage are capable of division. Reproduced from ref. 3.

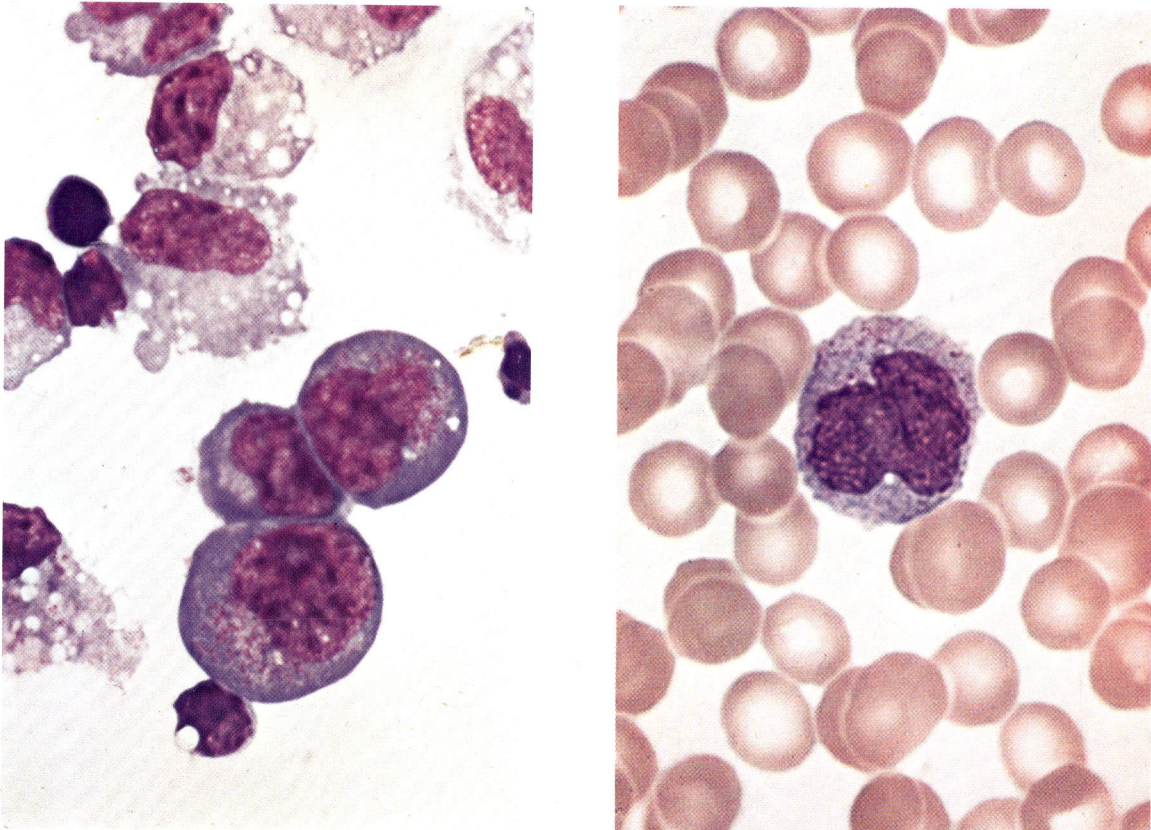

Fig. 2 Promonocytes from the bone marrow of a patient with a monocytic neoplasm. These cells are rather characteristic blast cells with a polar accumulation of granules in a perinuclear clear zone. These granules represent newly formed lysosomes in the Golgi region of the cell. At this stage, the cell demonstrates little phagocytic activity and few of the characteristics of the more mature cell. The promonocyte is characterized by relatively large diameter (10-20 μm), a high nuclear-to-cytoplasmic ratio, a basophilic cytoplasm, some peroxidase activity, glass adherence, and the ability to synthesize DNA.

Fig. 3 A monocyte from the blood of normal man. In conventional Romanovsky-stained preparations, human monocytes appear as large cells, 10-18 μm in diameter, with grayish-blue cytoplasm that frequently contains small numbers of faint azurophilic granules. The centrally located nucleus is indented or horseshoe-shaped and has a fine lacy chromatin structure.

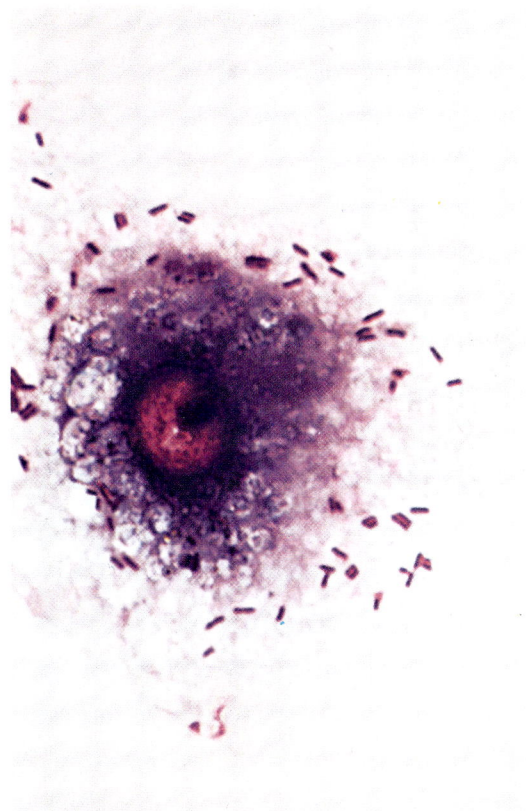
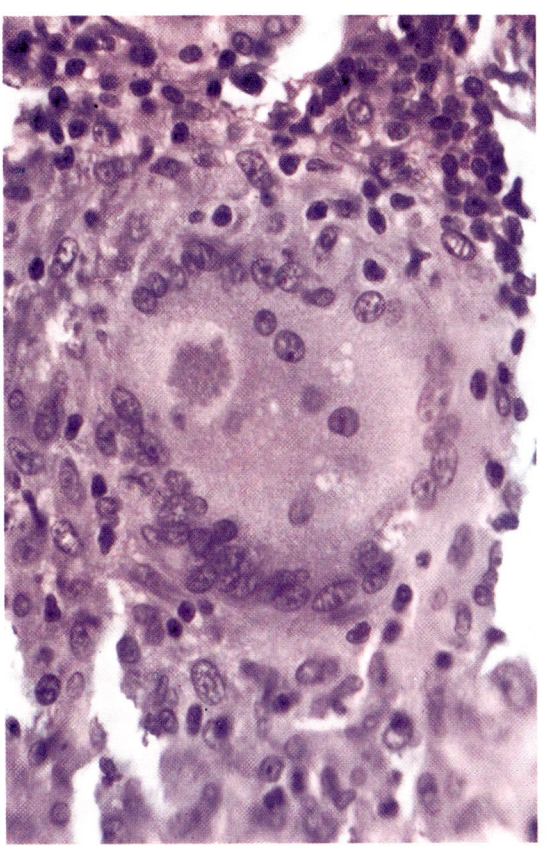

4 5

Fig. 4 *An alveolar macrophage of man. The cell has ingested numerous bacteria. Tissue macrophages are large cells measuring 20-80 μm in diameter. They contain one or more large vesicular nuclei often with prominent nucleoli. Cytoplasmic granules and inclusions are numerous. The cells are motile and phagocytic.*

Fig. 5 *A multinucleate giant cell from a tuberculoid granuloma. These are very large cells with multiple nuclei often demonstrating intracytoplasmic inclusions. They are phagocytic but demonstrate little proliferative activity.*

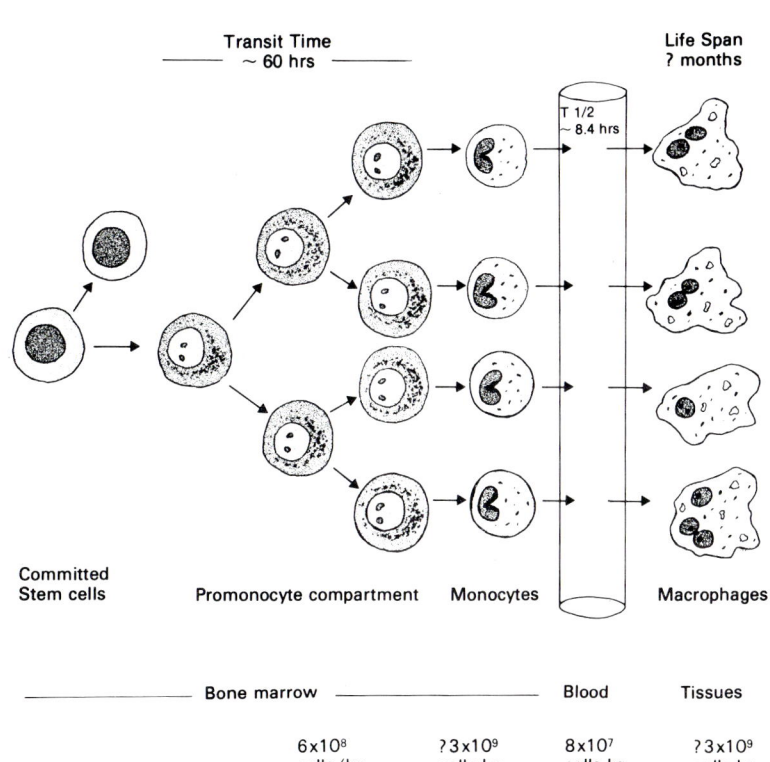

Fig. 6 *Kinetics of the monocyte-macrophage system in man. Promonocytes undergo two divisions before differentiating into monocytes. Monocytes leave the marrow, pass through the blood, and enter the tissues where they mature to macrophages. Macrophages live for many months.*
From Cline, M.J. Production, distribution and fate of monocytes and macrophages. In Hematology, 2nd edition. Williams, W.P., Beutler, E., Erslev, A.J., and Rundles, R.W. (eds.). McGraw-Hill, New York, 1977, pp. 869-874. Reprinted by permission of author and publisher.

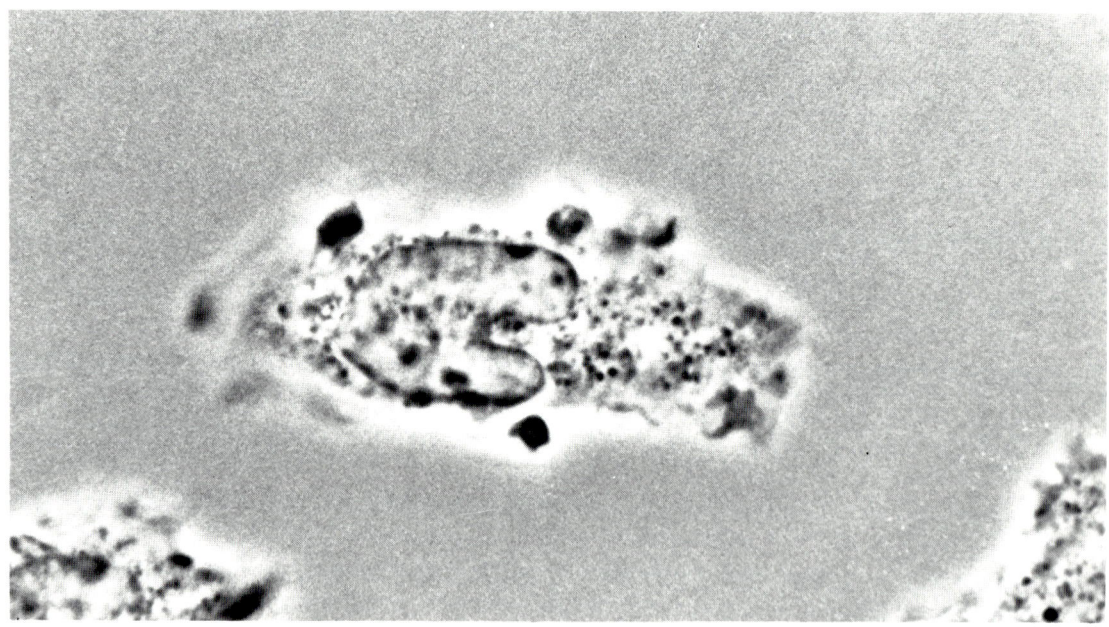

Fig. 7 A human monocyte that has been cultured in vitro for five days. The cell has begun to spread on the surface of the glass coverslip. Cytoplasmic granulation is prominent. These granules represent lysosomes. Reproduced from ref. 3.

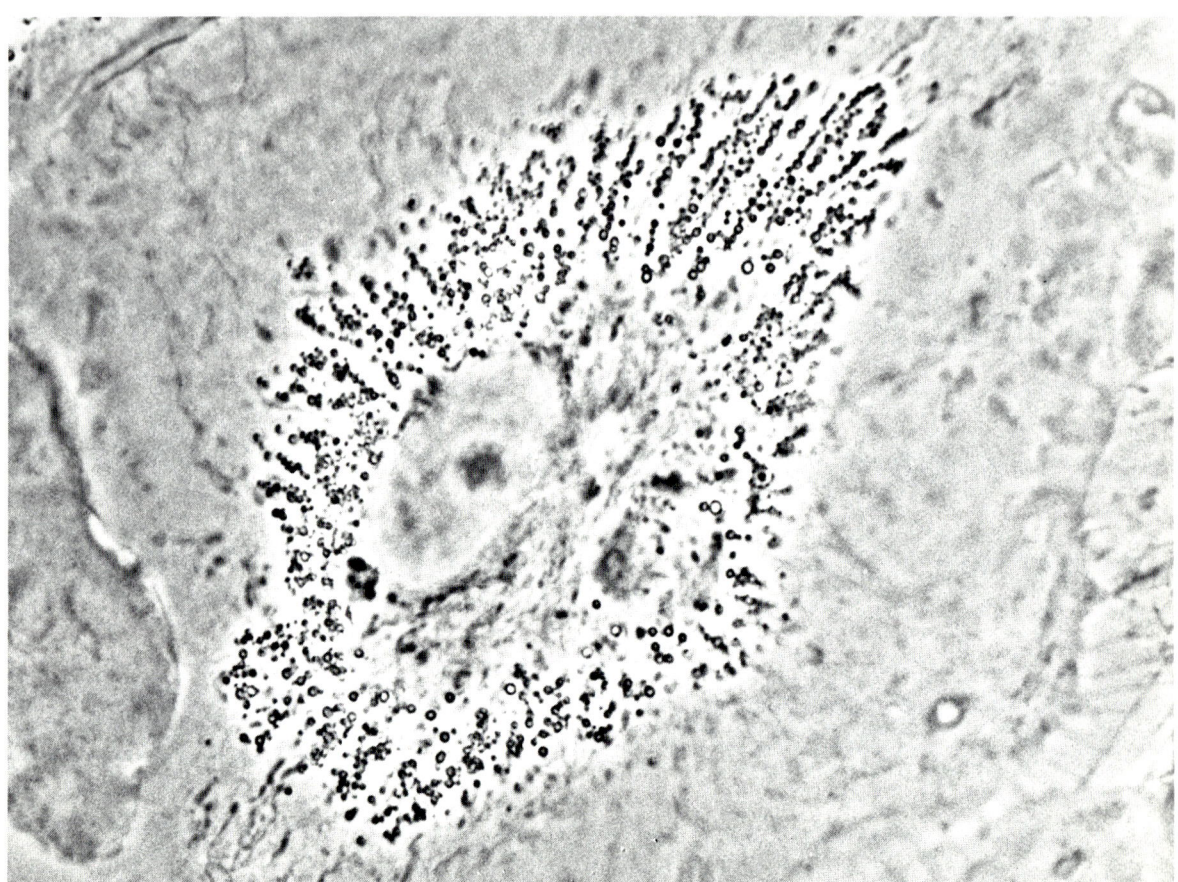

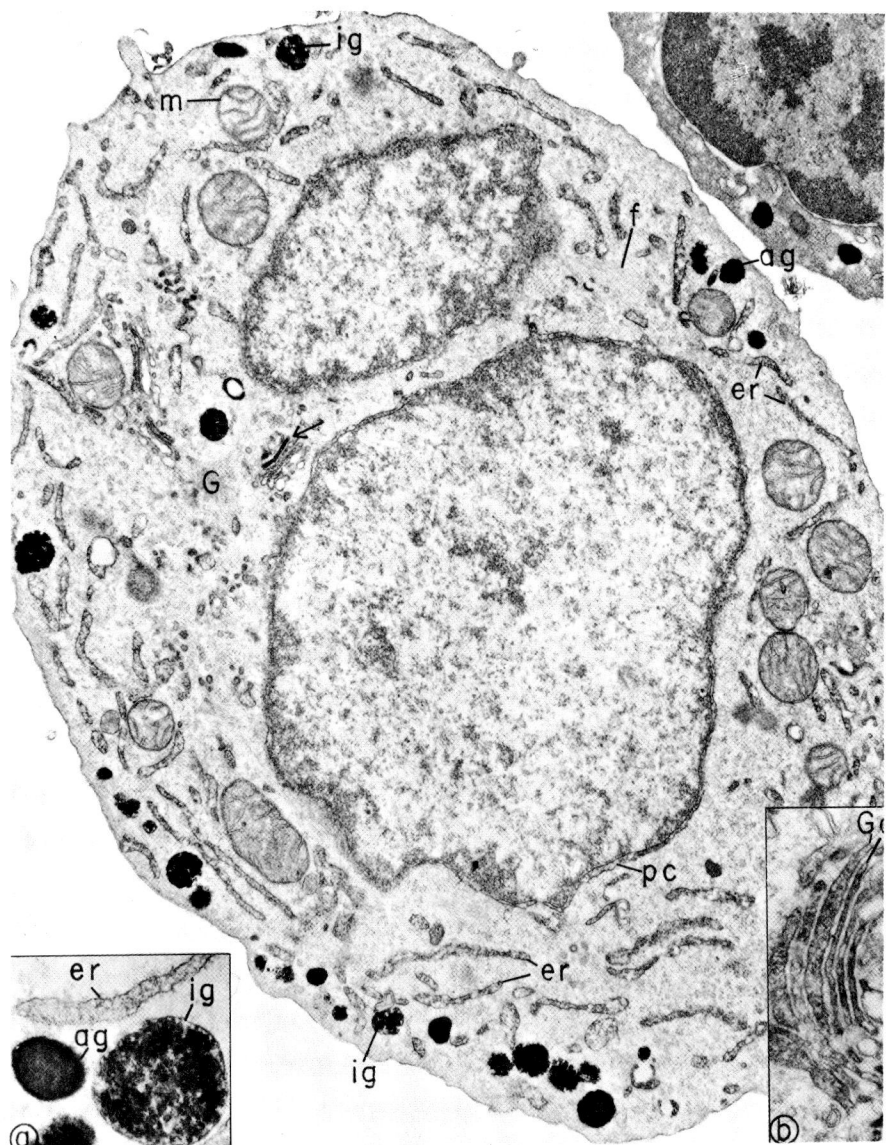

Fig. 9 Promonocyte from human bone marrow reacted for peroxidase. Reaction product is distributed throughout the entire rough endoplasmic reticulum (**er**), including the perinuclear cisterna (**pc**), all Golgi cisternae (**G** and **arrow**), and all immature granules (**ig**) and mature granules (**ag**). It is not found in the mitochondria (**m**). Note that the reaction is more intense in the granules than in the endoplasmic reticulum and that one Golgi cisterna (**arrow**) is more intensely reactive than the others, suggesting that a concentration gradient exists across the Golgi complex. In the human monocyte, clusters of fine filaments (**f**) are common.
Inset **a** is a higher-magnification view showing the dense globular reaction product at low concentration within the rough endoplasmic reticulum and at higher concentration in the immature and mature azurophil granules. In the immature granules, whose content is presumably still undergoing concentration, the aggregates of reaction product are less compact than in the mature granules.
Inset **b** shows reaction product filling six or seven successive cisternae of the Golgi complex of another cell ($\times$ 12,500; **a**, $\times$ 39,500; **b**, $\times$ 34,500).
Reproduced from ref. 5.

Fig. 8 A human macrophage that has developed from a monocyte after culture for 10 days in vitro. This cell is very large with numerous cytoplasmic granules and a readily apparent nucleus with a prominent nucleolus. Ribbon-like mitochondria can be seen throughout the periphery of the cytoplasm.

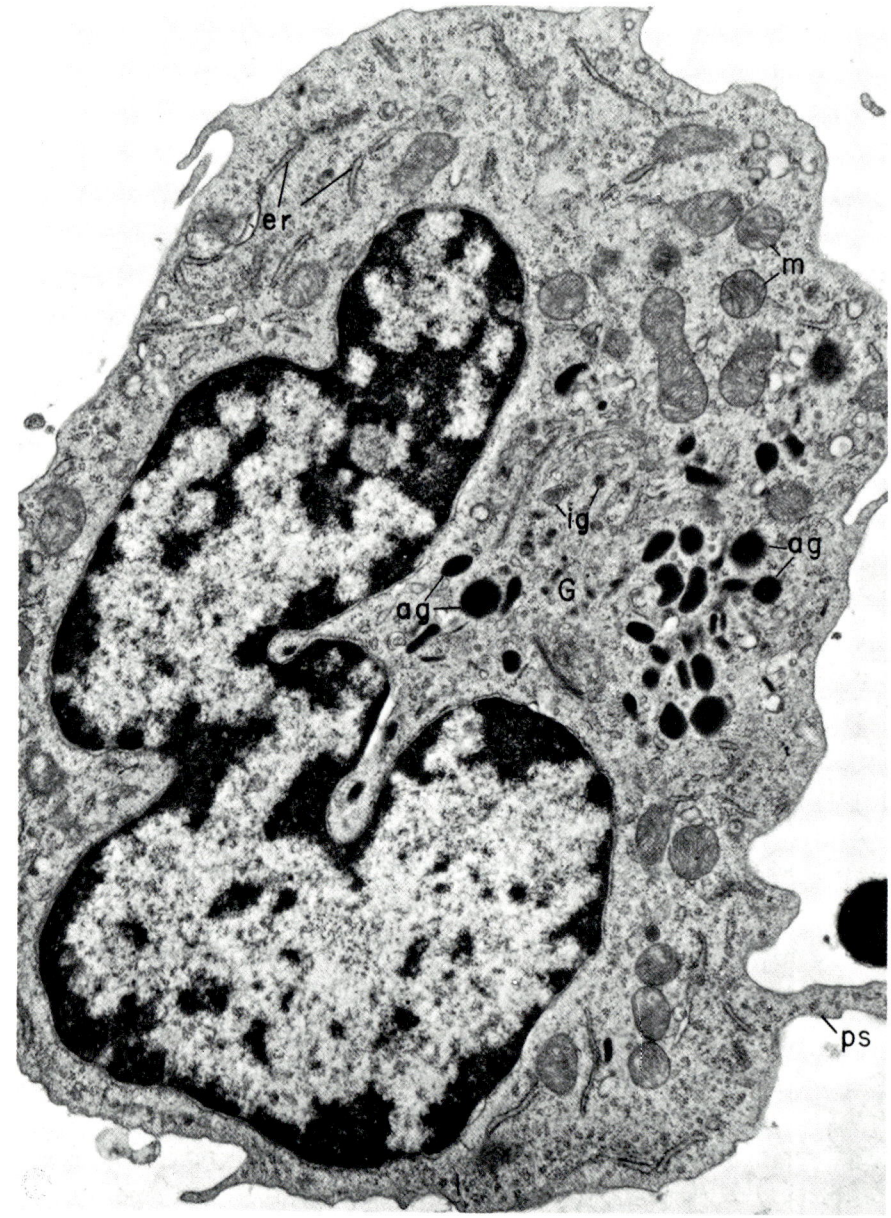

Fig. 10 a) Mature monocyte from rabbit bone marrow, showing its characteristic features: the eccentric, kidney-shaped nucleus with moderately condensed chromatin, and the "rosette" of azurophil granules (**ag**) clustered near the Golgi complex (**G**) at the "hof" of the nucleus. About 30 mature homogeneously dense azurophil granules (variable in shape) can be counted. In addition, numerous small, immature granules (**ig**) are seen in the center of the Golgi region. A few endoplasmic reticulum cisternae (**er**) are present near the cell periphery, and scattered mitochondria (**m**) are seen. Note that a few pseudopodia (**ps**) extend from the surface ($\times$ 16,000).
Reproduced from ref. 5.

Fig. 10 b) Peripheral blood monocyte following incubation with latex particles (**L**) for 20 minutes at 37 °C. The black reaction product indicating peroxidase activity (**arrow**) is seen in only a few granules and vacuoles. Most of the phagosomes are negative ($\times$ 17,150).
Reproduced from Zucker-Franklin, D., Clinics in Haematology 4:485, 1975 with permission of the publisher.

8 MONOCYTES

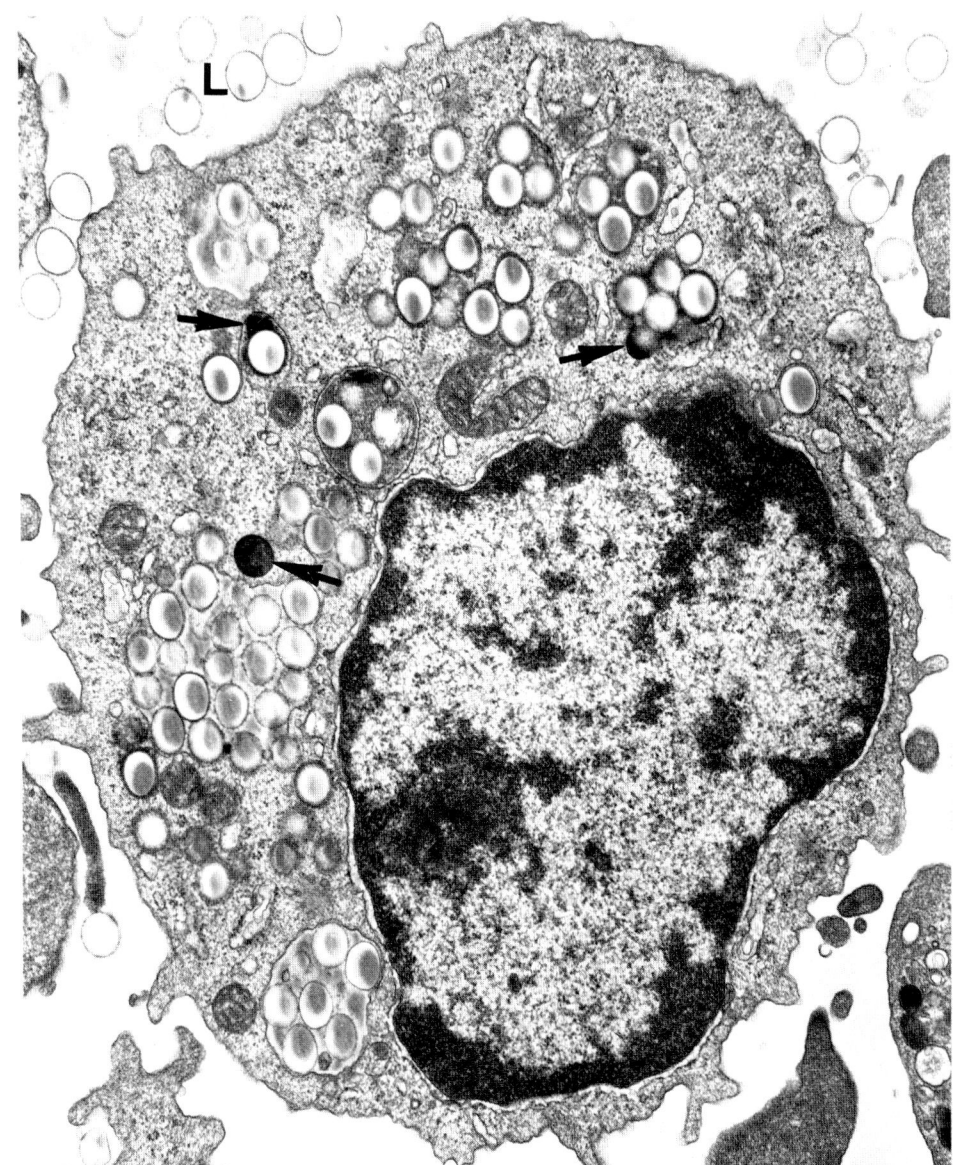

10 b

Macrophage development may also be observed in the transmission electron microscope. The promonocyte (**Fig. 9**) has peroxidase activity in its rough endoplasmic reticulum, in the cisternae of the Golgi apparatus, and in immature granules. With maturation to the monocyte level (**Fig. 10**), peroxidase-positive material decreases, and the mature macrophage has little peroxidase activity (**Fig. 10**). Mature macrophages seen in **Figures 11** and **12** display a cytoplasm containing abundant granules and mitochondria. They may also contain ingested inclusions such as those seen in **Figure 12**.

Mature macrophages that have settled on a surface reveal a thinly spread ruffled cytoplasm when viewed by the scanning electron microscope (**Figs. 13** and **14**). The basal portion of the membrane adheres firmly to the surface on which the cell rests.

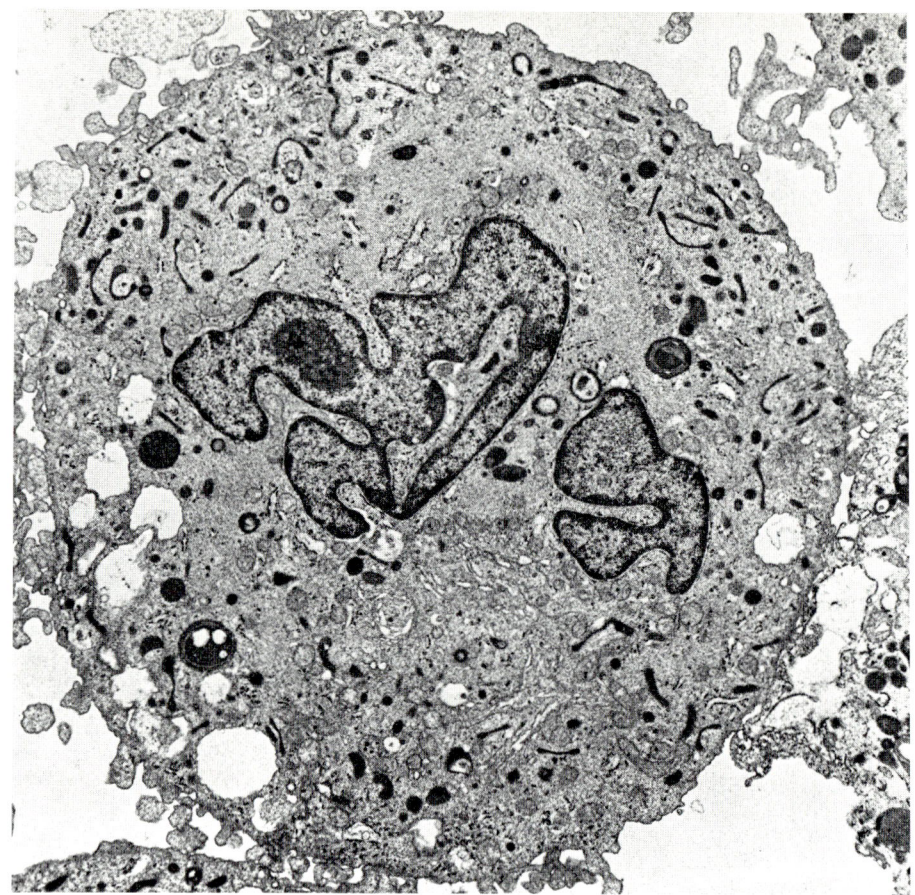

Fig. 11 *Electron micrograph of alveolar macrophage washed from the lungs of a normal, non-smoking subject. Photograph courtesy of Dr. P.E.G. Mann.*

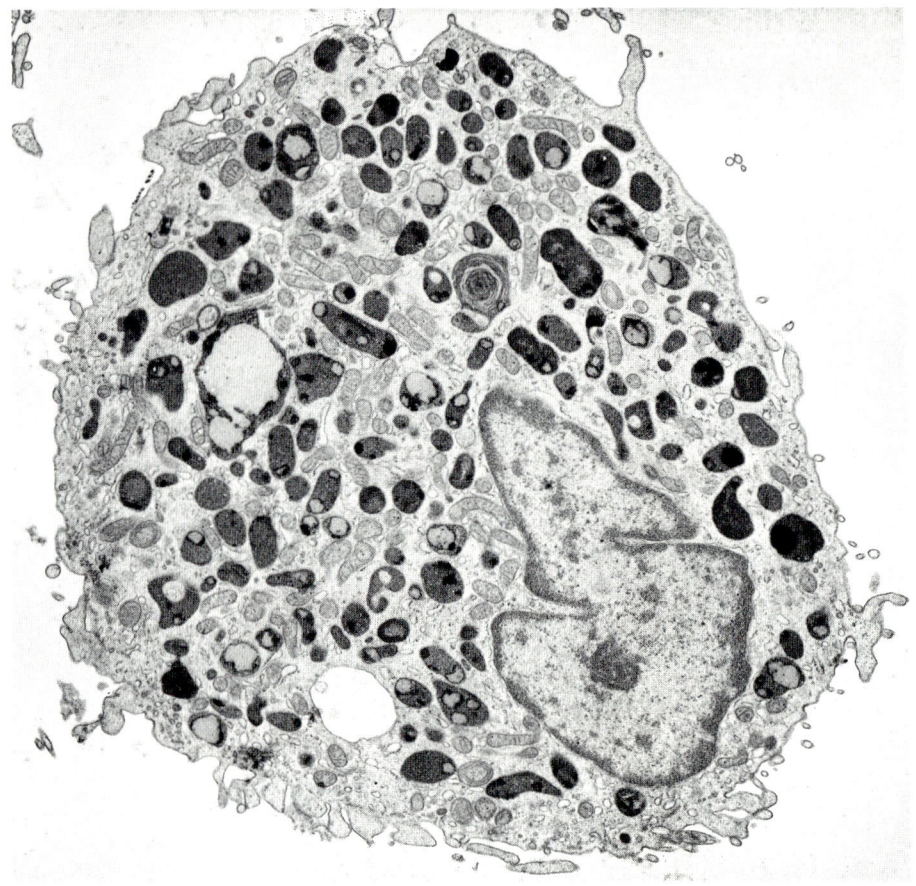

Fig. 12 *Electron micrograph of alveolar macrophage from the lungs of a normal, tobacco-smoking subject. Photograph courtesy of Dr. P.E.G. Mann.*

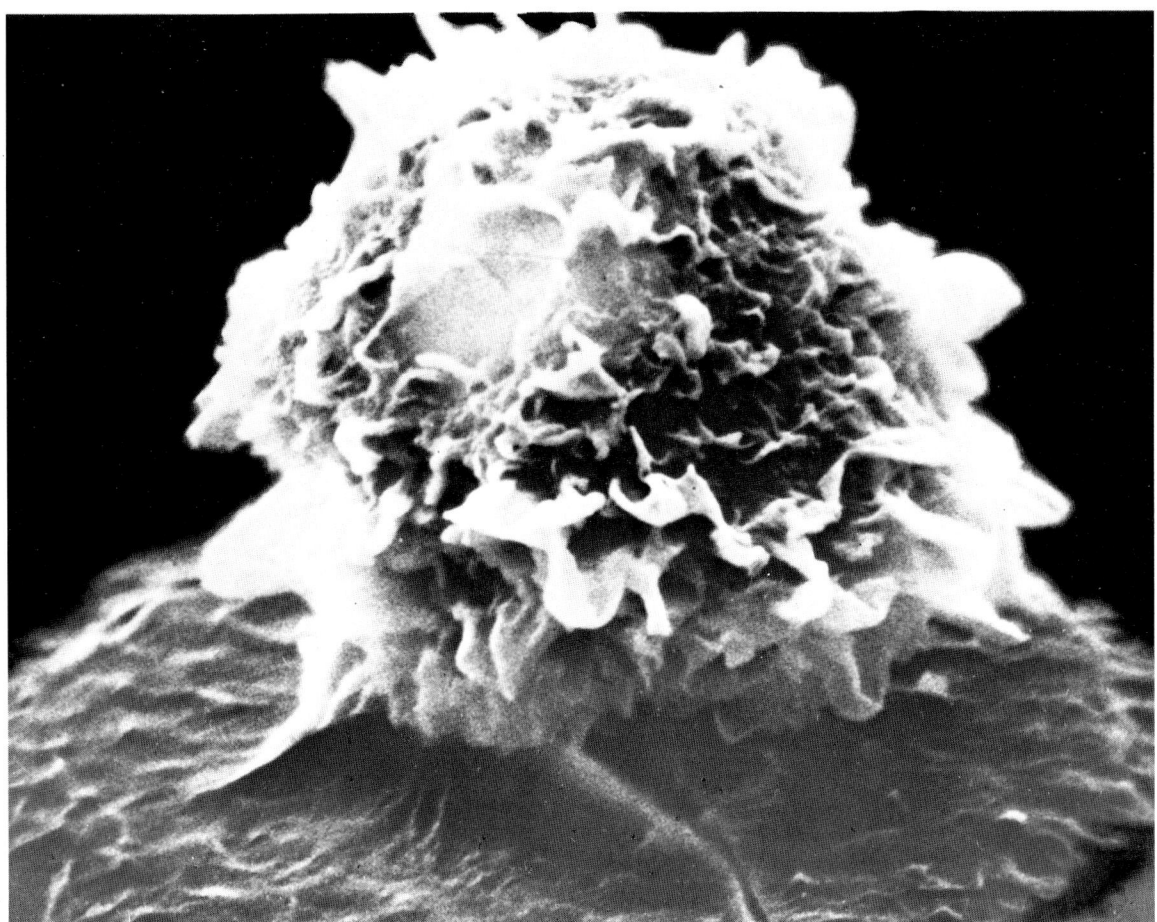

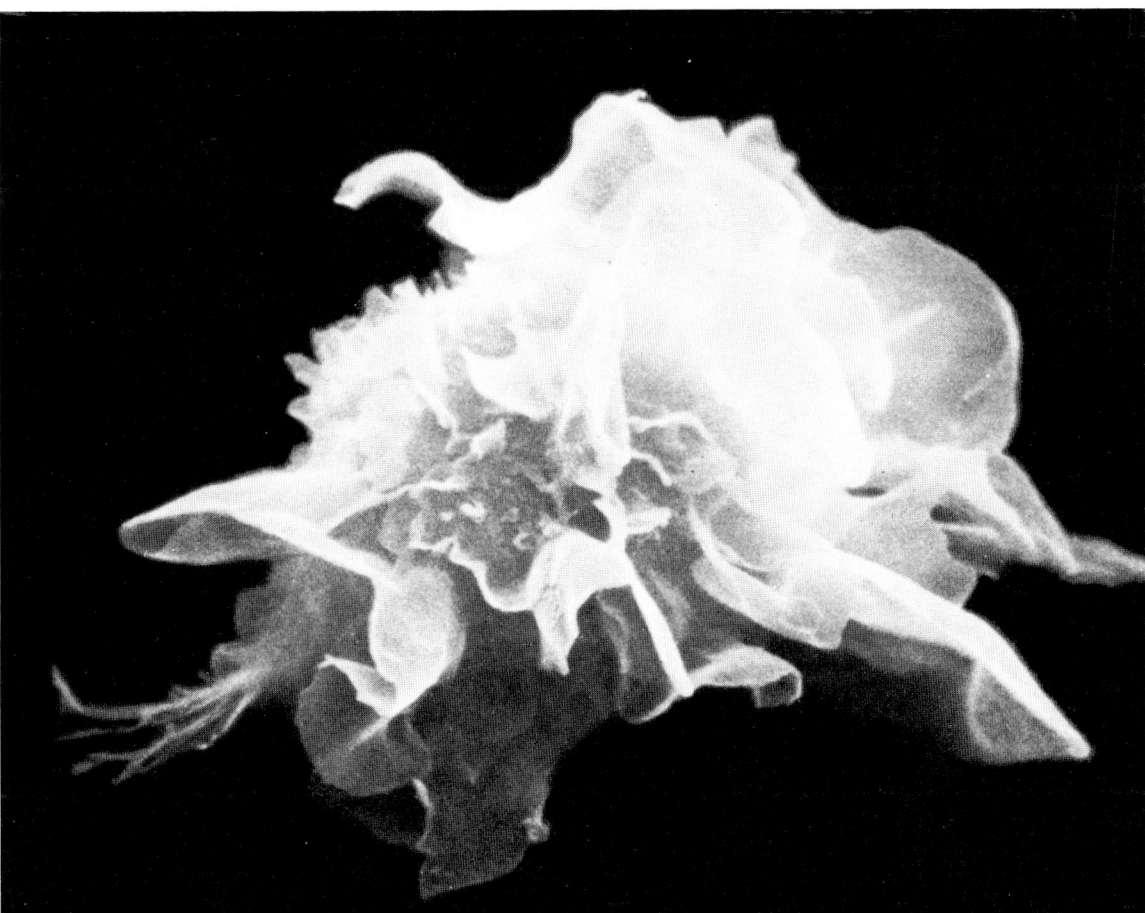

Figs. 13 *and* **14** *Two views of macrophage membranes through a scanning electron microscope. From A.H. Warfel and S.S. Elberg: Science 170:446, 1970. Reprinted by permission of authors and publisher.*

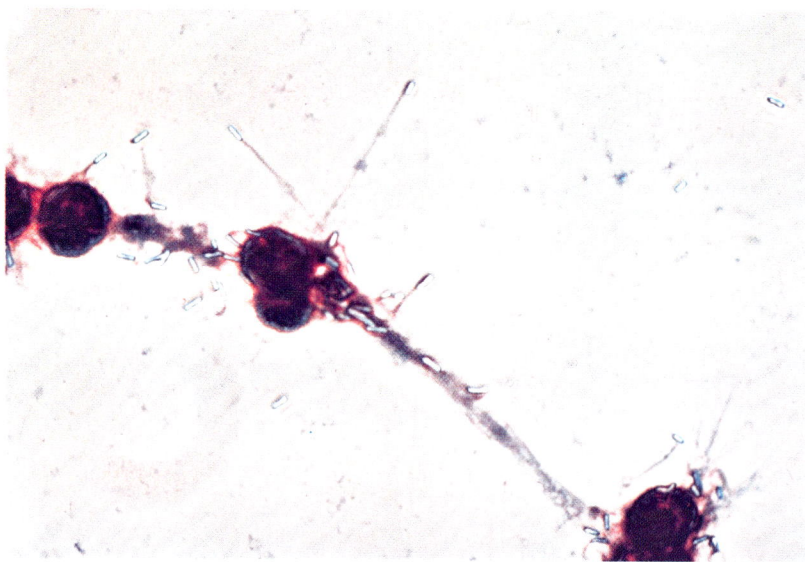

Fig. 15 A cytoplasmic extension from tissue macrophages growing in tissue culture (photographed by phase microscopy). The cytoplasmic extensions contain numerous adherent bacteria. These extensions are drawn into the body of the macrophage during the phagocytic process.

2. FUNCTIONS OF THE MONONUCLEAR PHAGOCYTES

Cells of the mononuclear phagocyte system perform a multiplicity of functions. They form a defense system against microbial invaders. These cells are important in the defense against intracellular parasites, both facultative and obligate. For example, they are important in the control of Mycobacterium tuberculosis, of M. leprae, of Salmonella, and of certain fungal agents [7-9].
The cell line has well-developed phagocytic activity which is most actively demonstrated in the mature macrophages. When living preparations of macrophages are viewed by phase microscopy, they display long sweeping arms of cytoplasm which surround the cell (**Fig. 15**). These cytoplasmic arms come into contact with microorganisms such as bacteria in their environment. They form a firm attachment to the microorganism which is coated with immunoglobulin and/or complement (**Fig. 15**).
The cytoplasmic process is then drawn into the body of the macrophage, and the organism is engulfed into a phagocytic vacuole. Such vacuoles, containing yeast, may occasionally be seen by the light microscope (**Fig. 16**).
The vacuoles are membrane-lined spaces in which the microbe is isolated from the rest of the cell's cytoplasm (**Fig. 16**).

Fig. 16 a) Multiple tissue macrophages which have ingested a yeast, Candida albicans. The yeast are seen to lie within phagocytic vacuoles and cytoplasm. Some of the yeast have been killed and digested and show decolorization; other yeast are living and have prominent mycelial tubes.
b) Electron micrograph of a peripheral blood monocyte from a specimen that had been incubated in vitro with Mycoplasma pneumoniae, the organism responsible for atypical pneumonia. The **arrows** indicate phagocytic vacuoles containing the microorganism. The double **arrow** points to a vacuole in which a lysosome is also evident. Note that this monocyte has an "activated" appearance as suggested by the abundance of lysosomes (**L**) and pinocytotic vesicles. **G**, Golgi. There are also numerous mitochondria, ribosomes and small profiles of rough endoplasmic reticulum ($\times$ 19,000).
Reproduced from Zucker-Franklin et al.: J. Exp. Med. 124:533, 1966.

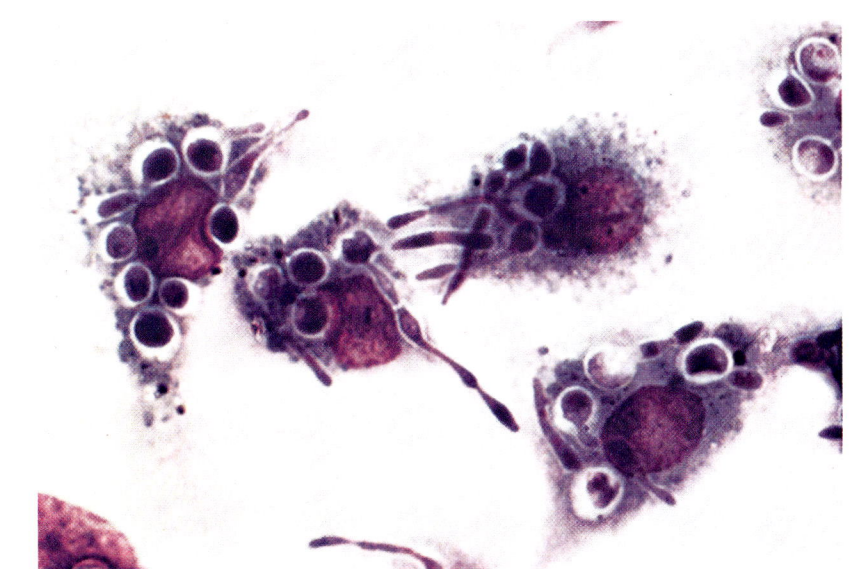

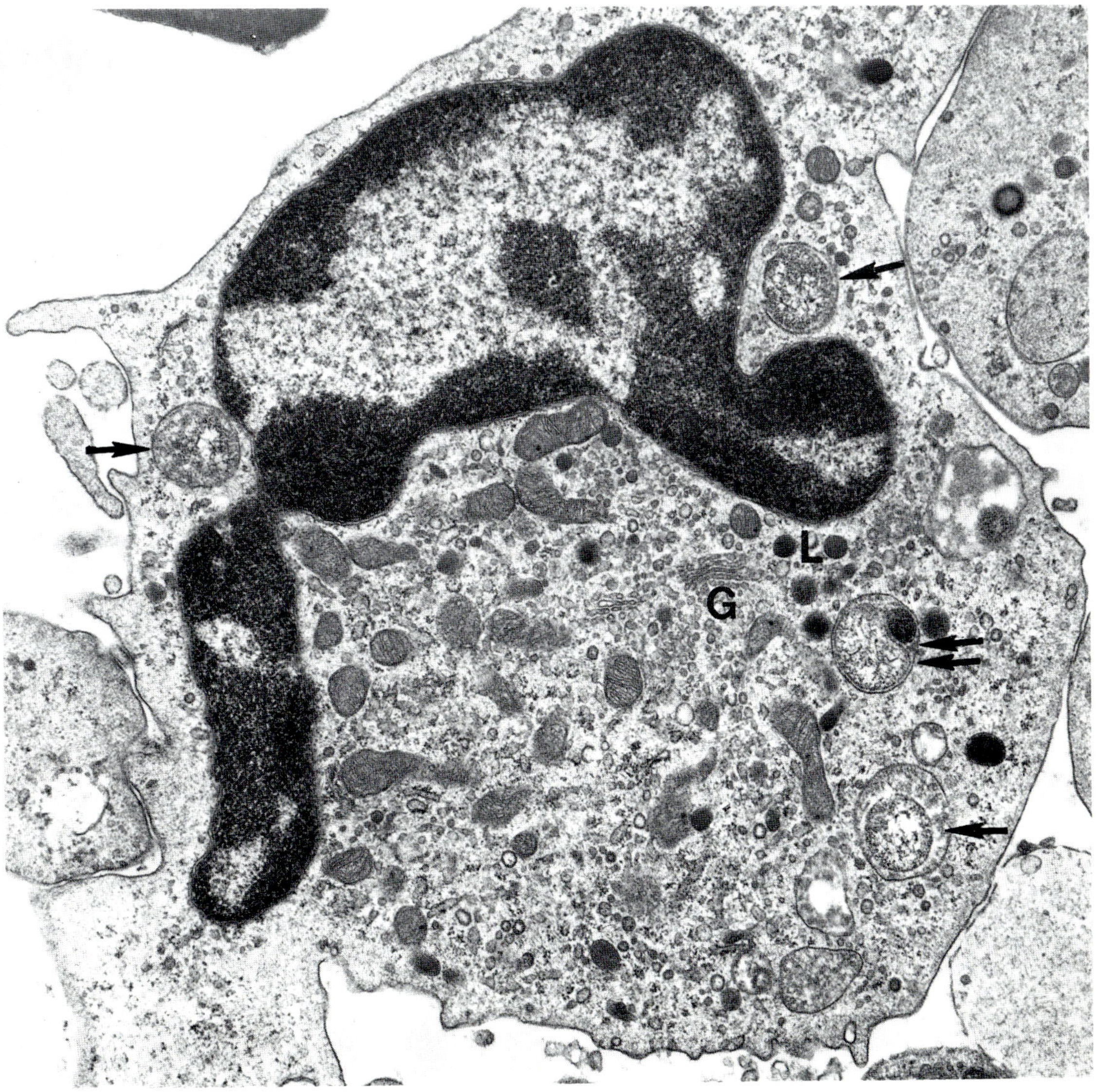

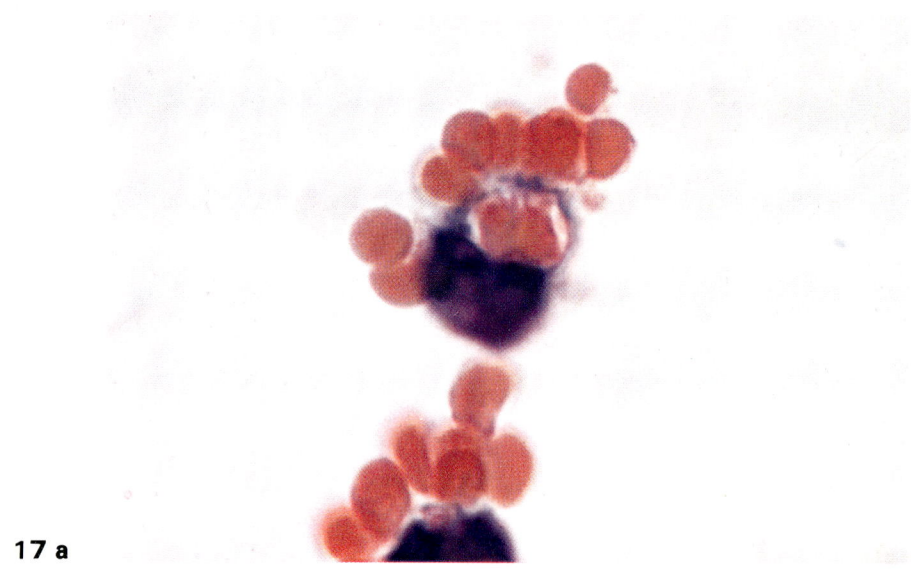

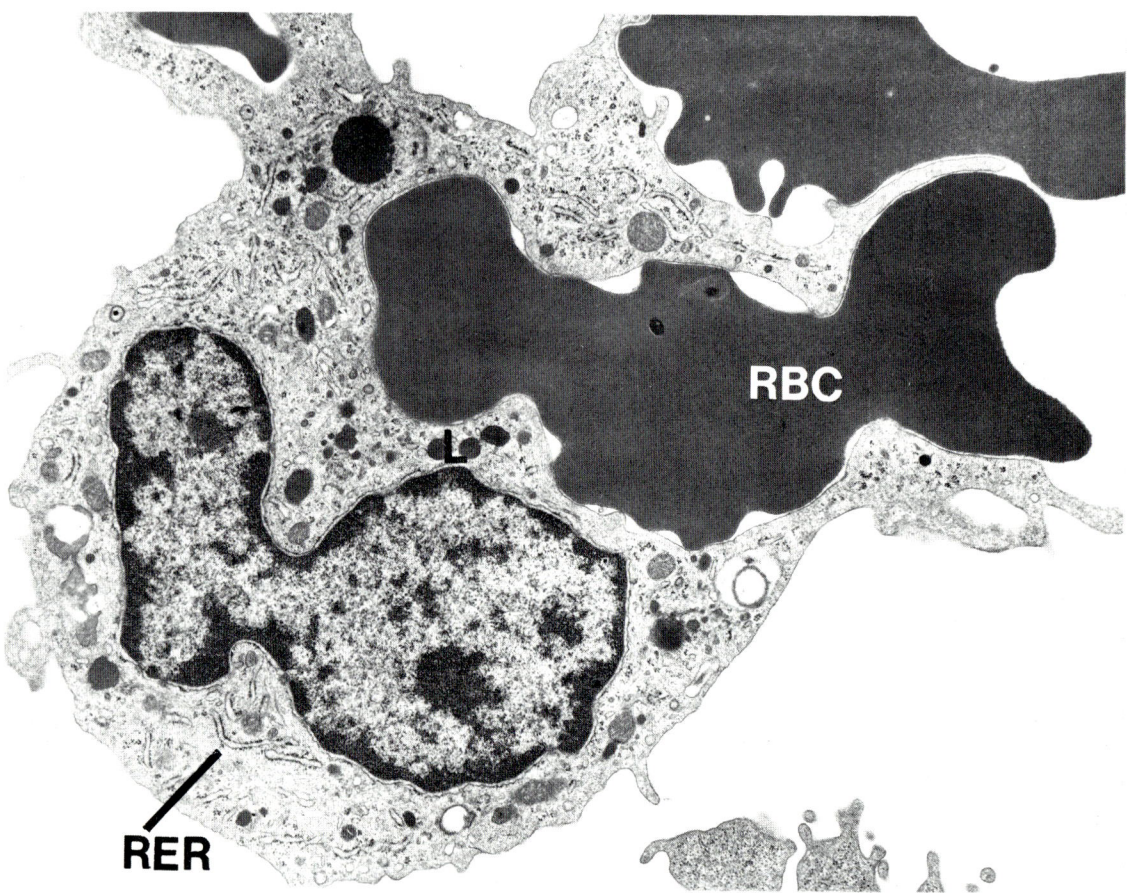

Fig. 17 a) Monocytes and macrophages have membrane receptors for immunoglobulin-G molecules. Red cells coated with immunoglobulin-G can be shown to form a rosette around the macrophages, and some of the cells are phagocytosed by the macrophages. Other red cells will undergo osmotic lysis on the surface of the monocyte. In man this phenomenon probably occurs within the splenic sinusoids where antibody-coated red cells attach to the lining macrophages.

b) Erythrophagocytosis by a monocyte observed in a freshly obtained specimen of human thoracic duct lymph from a patient afflicted with hemolytic anemia. Thoracic duct drainage was carried out to relieve portal pressure. **RBC**, red blood cell; **RER**, rough endoplasmic reticulum; **L**, lysosomes ($\times$ 11,000).

8 MONOCYTES

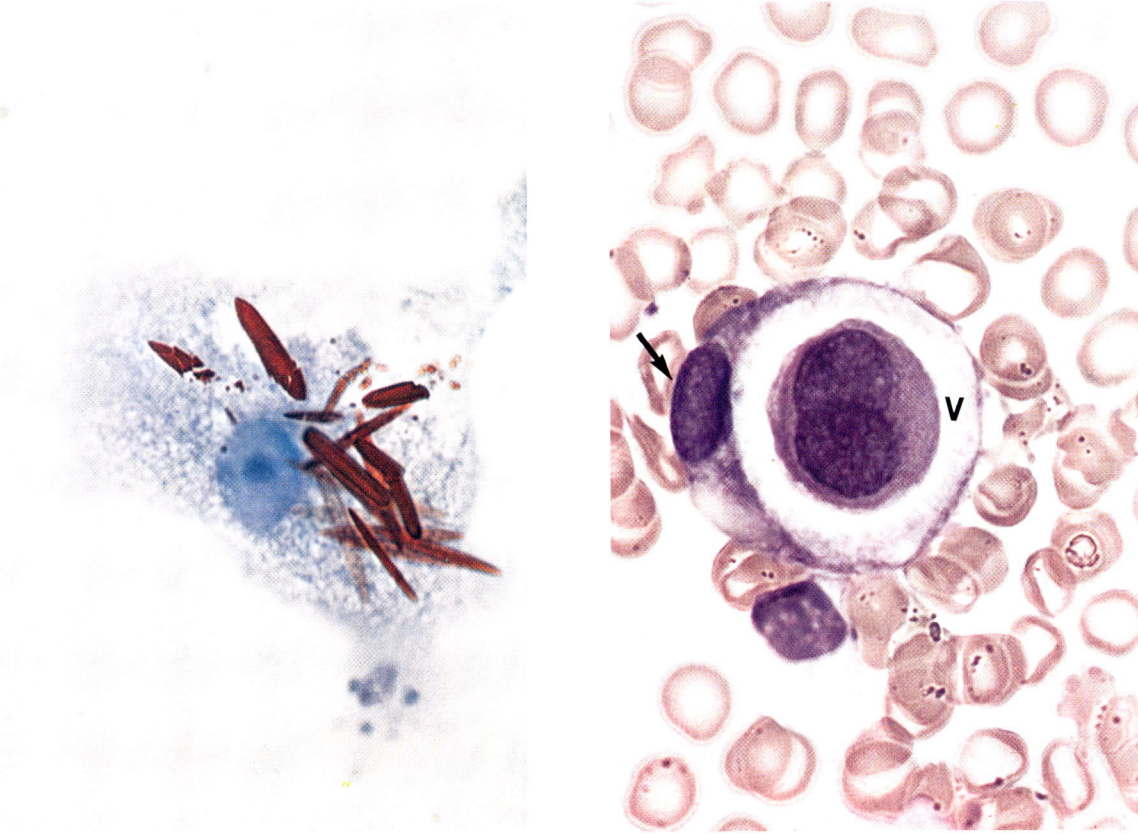

Fig. 18 Macrophages are capable of ingesting a variety of crystalline structures, including silica, beryllium, iron particles, and carbon.

Fig. 19 A breast cancer cell phagocytized by a macrophage from a pleural effusion of a patient with carcinoma of the breast; **V**, vacuole containing the neoplastic cell; **arrow** indicates nucleus of macrophage.

The firm attachment of monocytes and macrophages to microorganisms is achieved through the presence on the surface membrane of receptors for the Fc portion of certain classes of immunoglobulin G molecules, as well as some complement components (especially C′ 3) [10, 11]. Such surface receptors permit the firm attachment of red cells coated with immunoglobulin or complement (**Fig. 17**). Presumably, the receptors are also important in identifying antibody- or complement-coated red cells in hemolytic states.

Another function of macrophages is their ability to dispose of cells that are damaged or dying. Macrophages lining the sinusoids of the spleen can ingest aged erythrocytes [12] (see **Fig. 17**). These mononuclear phagocytes are also involved in removing debris and in the remodeling of tissues and repair of wounds. It is also likely that they function in the removal of debris during the development of embryonic tissues. In addition to their function in removing organic debris, they are important in removing inorganic particles (see **Fig. 18**) which may gain access to the body through the airways or other channels [13]. Thus, alveolar macrophages ingest particulate matter that finds its way into the alveolar spaces such as particles from cigarette smoke (see **Fig. 12**) or bacteria (see **Fig. 4**).

In some instances the phagocytic properties of mononuclear phagocytes can be demonstrated with tumor cells (**Fig. 19**). Mononuclear phagocytes are thought to have a role in controlling the growth of spontaneously arising tumors. This control activity presumably does not involve the phagocytic process; rather, macrophages are thought to kill tumor cells by means of their lysosomal enzymes and only dispose of already killed tumor cells by phagocytosis [14-16].

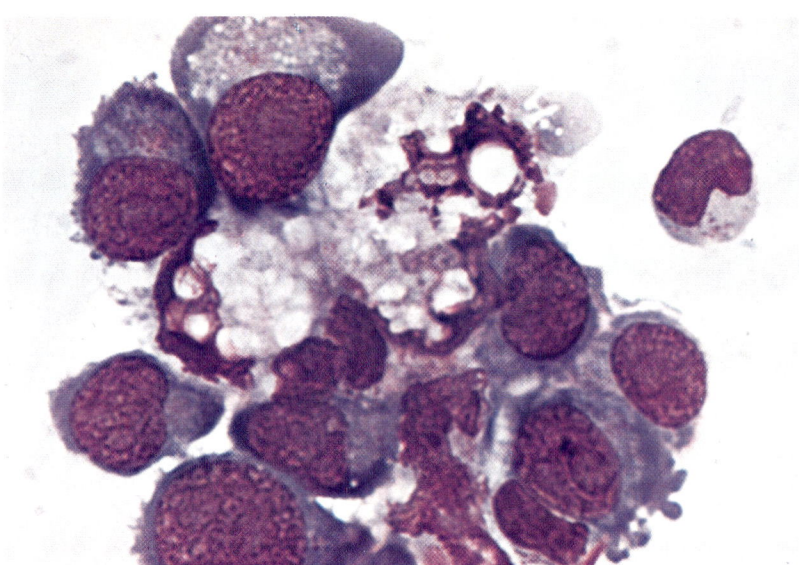

Fig. 20 An "immunologic island" showing lymphoid cells undergoing blastogenic transformation surrounding two light-colored macrophages that have previously been exposed to antigen. The macrophages have been maintained in culture for several weeks and are undergoing degeneration. The lymphocytes demonstrate typical blast cell appearance.

Another well-developed function of the mononuclear phagocyte system is illustrated in **Figure 20**. This function involves macrophage interaction with lymphoid cells in various phases of the immune response. In **Figure 20** is shown an "immunologic island" in which macrophages have been pretreated with antigen and then incubated with lymphocytes from the same individual.

The lymphocytes recognizing antigen associated with the macrophage undergo blastogenic transformation. Macrophages are important in the presentation of certain classes of antigen to lymphoid cells as well as in other aspects of cell-mediated immune reactions [17].

A prototype of a cell-mediated immune reaction is the tuberculoid granuloma (see **Fig. 5**).
Monocytes may be identified among a variety of hematologic cells by certain distinctive histochemical reactions. The cells possess high levels of alpha-naphthyl butyrase and alpha-naphthyl acid esterase and stain richly red in the appropriate histochemical reactions (**Fig. 21**). They are also richly endowed with the lysosomal enzyme acid phosphatase and react strongly in the histochemical reaction for this enzyme (**Fig. 22**). A number of monocyte-macrophage associated surface antigens have been described but these have not been well characterized.

Fig. 21 a) Macrophages have high levels of alpha-naphthyl butyrase. The histochemical reaction for this enzyme stains the cells red-brown. The enzyme is sometimes called macrophage's "lipase" or "esterase".
b) Shows the staining for alpha-naphthyl acid esterase which is localized within the lysosomes.
Courtesy of Dr. G.L. Castoldi, University of Ferrara.

Fig. 22 a) Macrophages have high levels of acid phosphatase, which stains the cell red in histochemical reactions.
b) Shows the localization of leucyl-amino-peptidase in a bone marrow macrophage.
Courtesy of Dr. G.L. Castoldi, University of Ferrara.

8 MONOCYTES

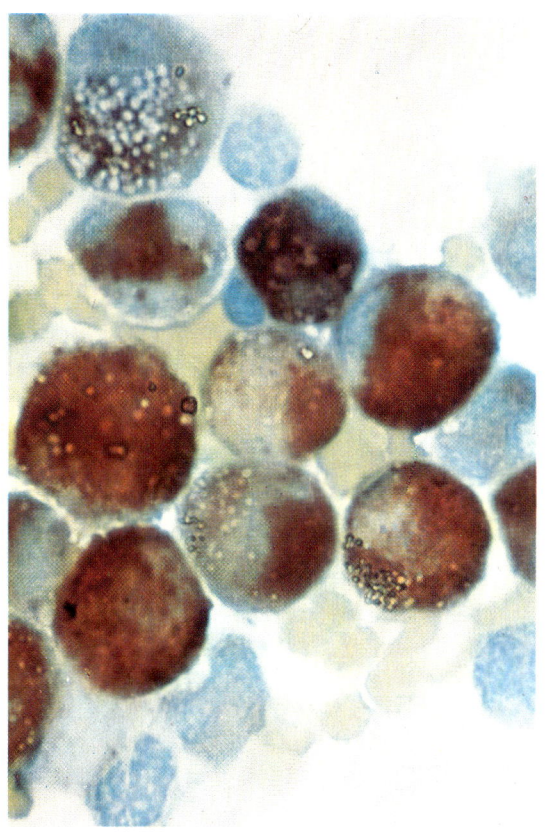

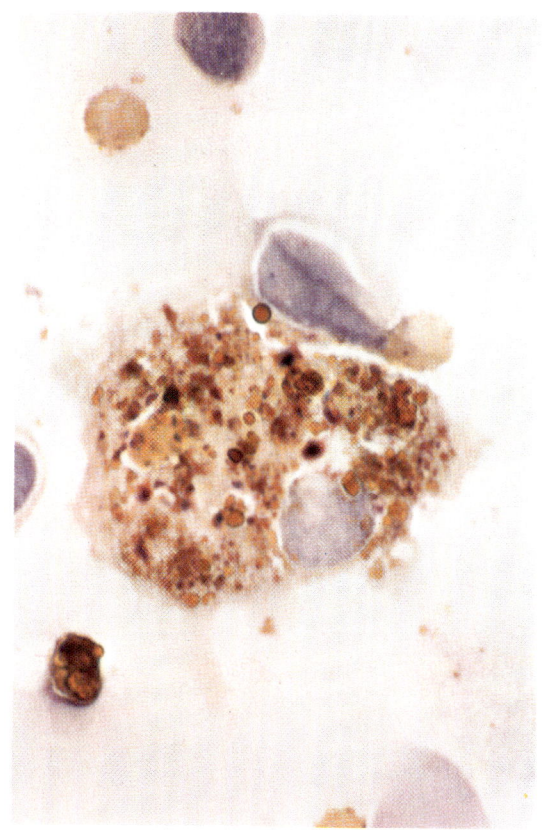

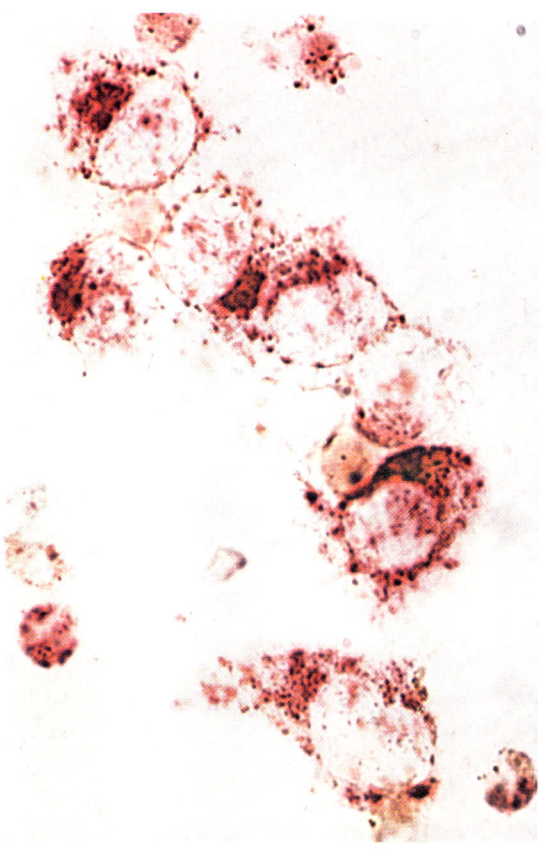

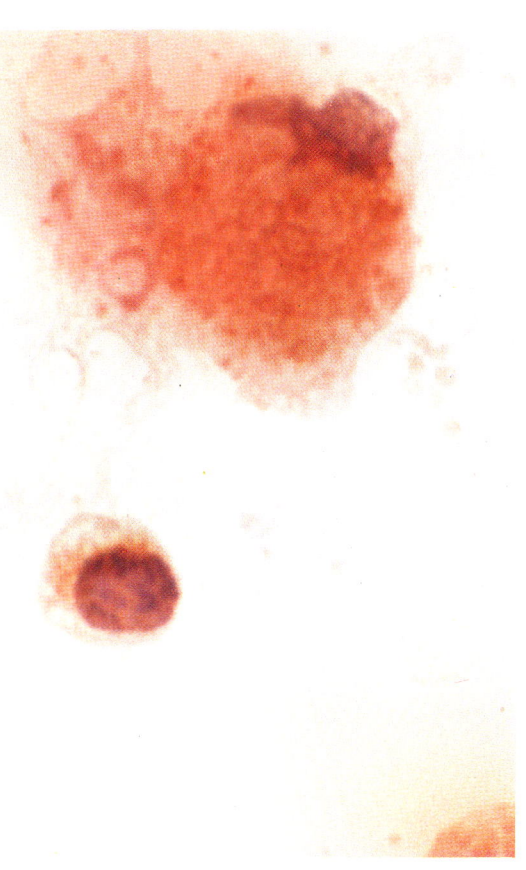

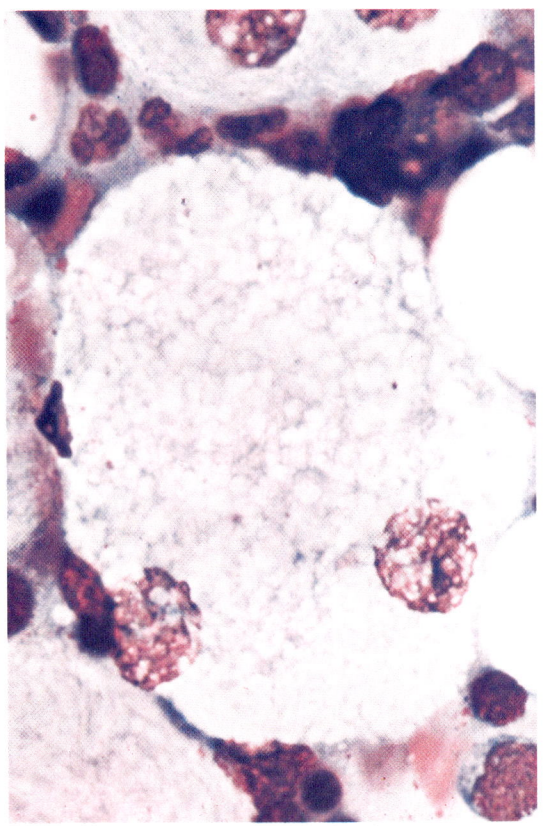 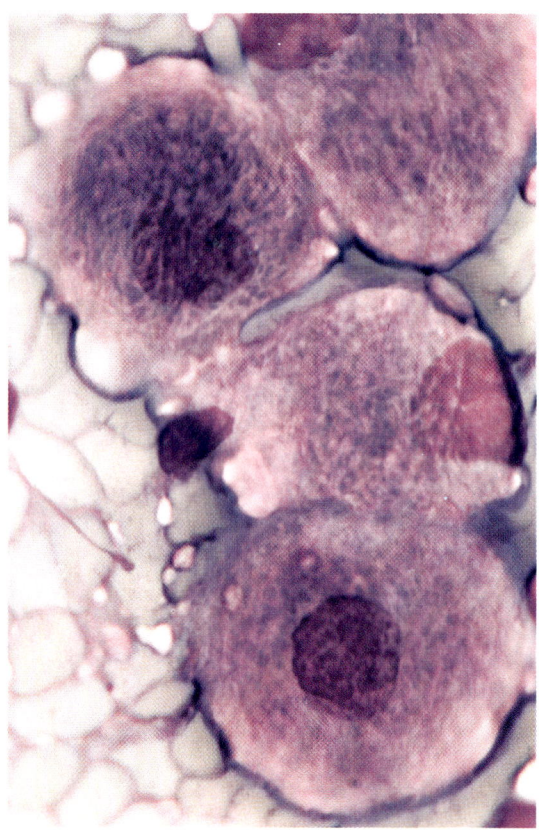

Fig. 23 a) Macrophages from bone marrow of a patient with Gaucher's disease. This binucleate cell is large and foamy and is filled with poorly digested cellular debris.
b) A group of Gaucher's cells from a spleen imprint. The cytoplasm contains undigested material.
Courtesy of Dr. G.L. Castoldi, University of Ferrara.

3. PATHOLOGY OF THE MONOCYTE-MACROPHAGE SYSTEM

A number of diseases of the monocyte-macrophage system have been identified. The first recognized were the "storage diseases" in which macrophages become filled with cell debris. In general, these storage diseases are the result of some abnormality in the macrophage function of debris disposal. Several storage diseases are known to be due to a deficiency in a catabolic enzyme. This results in the inability of the macrophages to catabolize normal cellular components.

Gaucher's disease (**Fig. 23**) is the prototype of these storage diseases. Macrophages in this disorder are deficient in beta-glucuronidase and are unable to catabolize the stroma of ingested cells such as red cells. The consequence is that the macrophages become large and "foamy" and are filled with cellular debris. In this disorder macrophages enlarge and probably increase in numbers, resulting in hepatomegaly and splenomegaly, and encroachment of the marrow space (see also **Figs. 23 c** and **24**). Macrophages encountered in the bone marrow of individuals with intravascular hemolytic disease may demonstrate intracellular pigmentary inclusions (**Fig. 25**). These inclusions reflect an overload of the macrophages' limited digestive capacity.

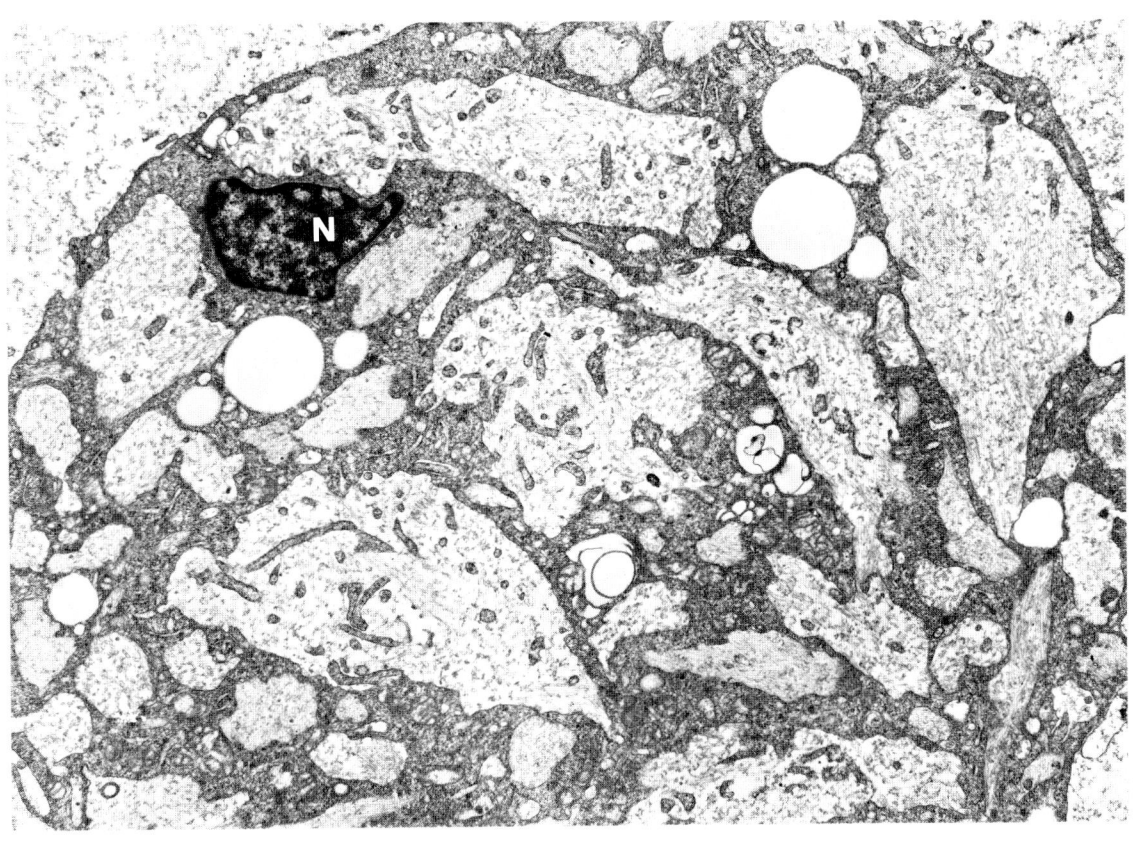
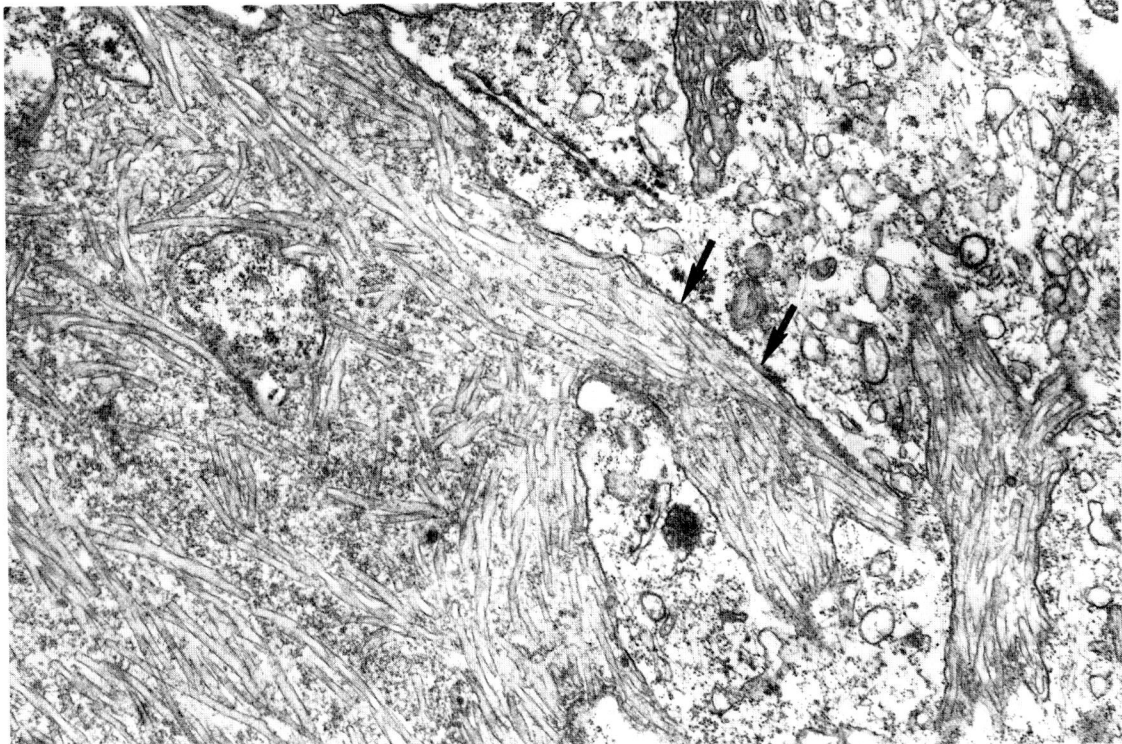

Fig. 23 c) Gaucher's cell. The low power electron micrograph at the top shows the typical relationship of the nucleus (**N**) and cytoplasm distended with membrane-bound spaces containing tubular structures which are seen to better advantage at high resolution (bottom). **Arrows** indicate membrane delimiting inclusion (top × 8,000; bottom × 33,000).
Reproduced from Zucker-Franklin, D., Clinics in Haematol. 4: 485, 1975, with permission of the publisher.

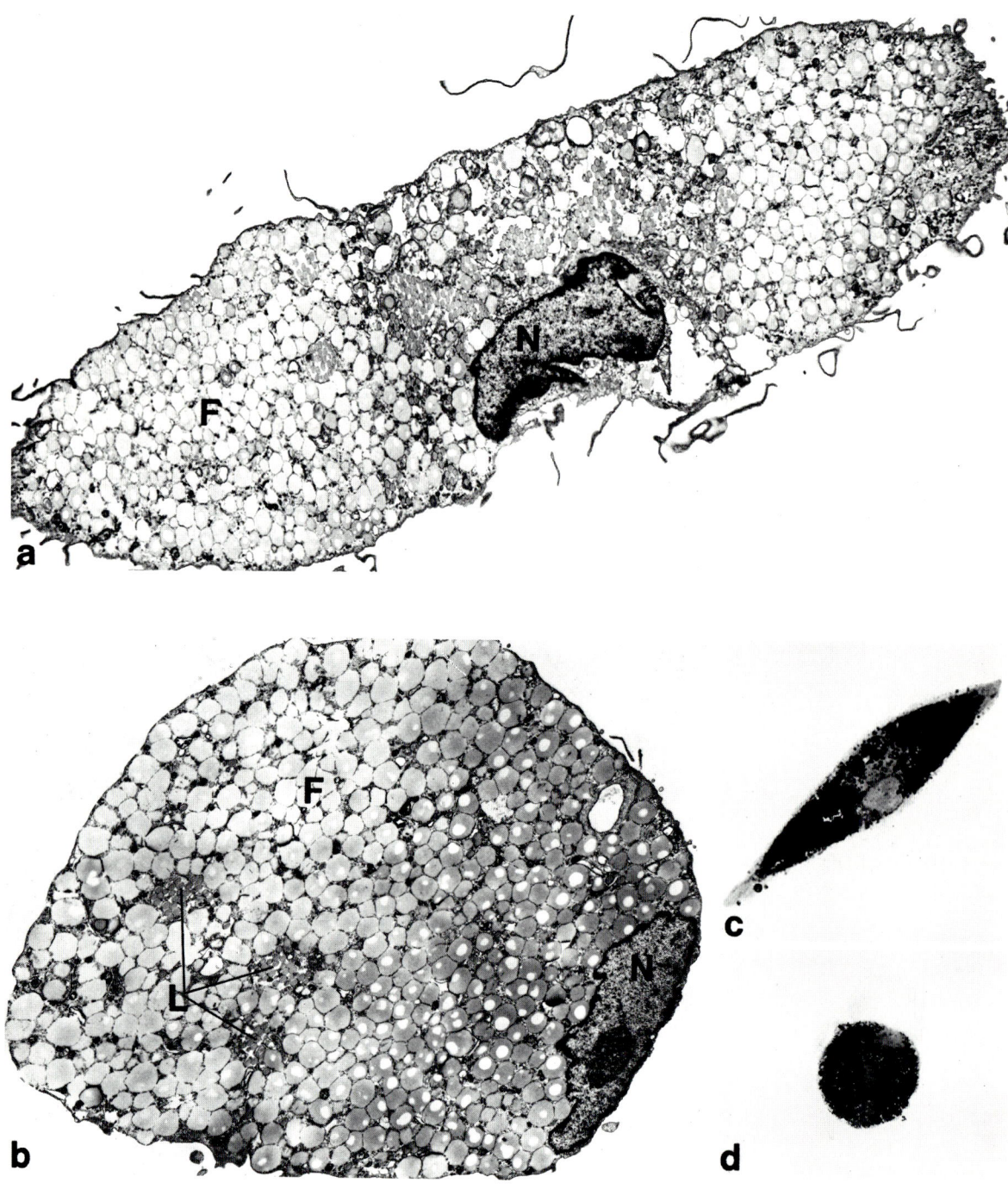

Figs. 24 a, b) When human peripheral blood monocytes are cultured under soft agar, they develop into large "foamy" cells measuring 100 to 500 μm. Histochemical and biochemical analyses proved the inclusions to consist predominantly of neutral fat. Transformation to fat cells occurs in the absence of mitosis.
The cells continue to be phagocytic and bear receptors for complement and immunoglobulin. They may assume a spindle-shaped (**top**) or round (**bottom**) shape. **N**, nucleus; **L**, phagocytosed latex particles; **F**, fat droplets (a × 3,700; b × 4,000).

c and d) Show similar cells stained with Sudan Black, a stain for neutral fat which leaves the nucleus and Golgi zone relatively unstained. It is possible that monocytes play a role in the replacement of hematopoietic tissue by fat in certain hypoplastic states.

Reproduced from Zucker-Franklin et al. Transformation of monocytes into "fat" cells. Lab. Invest. 38:620-628, 1978, with permission of the publisher.

8 MONOCYTES

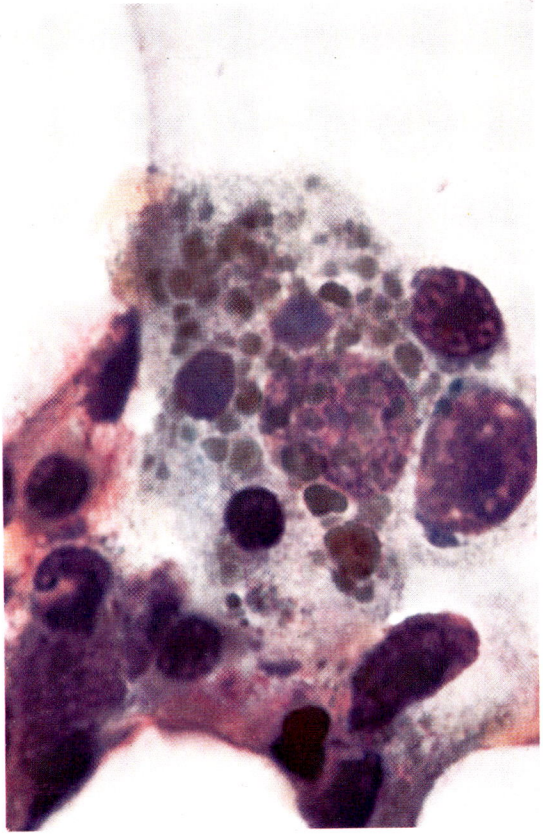
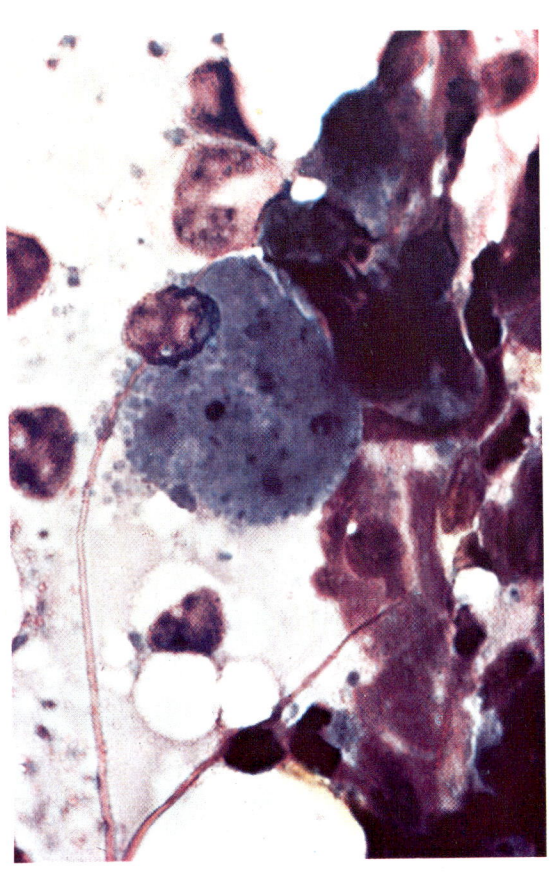

Fig. 25 *A macrophage from the bone marrow of a patient with intramedullary hemolysis of red cells demonstrating numerous inclusions within a macrophage.*

Fig. 26 *A macrophage from a patient with the "sea blue histiocyte syndrome". This patient had a partial deficiency of the enzyme sphingomyelinase.*

A macrophage deficiency of the enzyme sphingomyelinase also results in accumulation of cellular debris within the macrophages. This debris may have a distinctive blue color [19].

The consequence is one of the disorders known as the "sea blue histiocyte syndrome" in which blue-staining macrophages are identified in the bone marrow and spleen of affected individuals (**Fig. 26**).

A spectrum of malignant diseases of the monocyte-macrophage system has been identified [20]. These disorders vary from highly lethal aggressive neoplasms to rather indolent diseases characterized by a protracted course.

Monoblastic leukemia is characterized by primitive mononuclear phagocytes in the peripheral blood and bone marrow [21, 22] (**Figs. 27** and **28**), by tissue infiltration with these cells, and by a variety of clinical abnormalities which reflect the biologic products of the macrophage. These abnormalities include high levels of lysozyme in the serum and urine, proximal renal tubular dysfunction, high fevers, and sometimes susceptibility to infection.

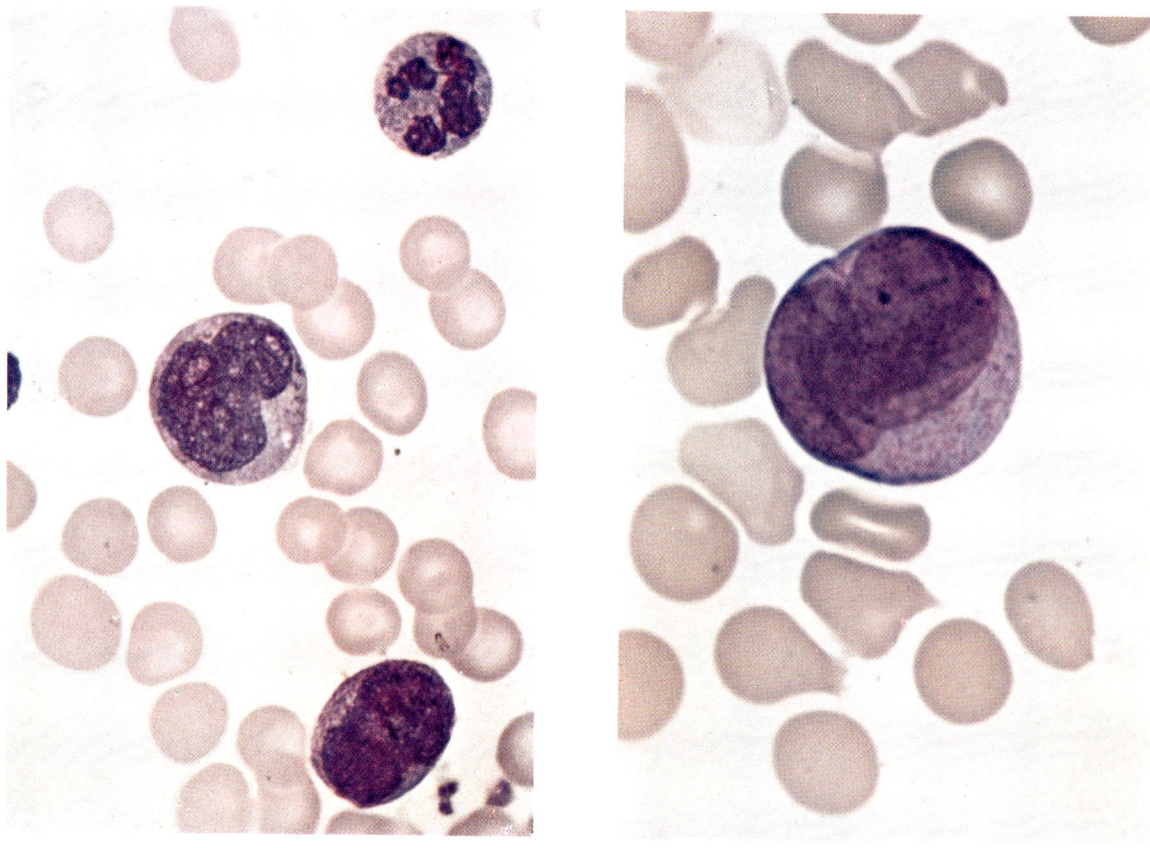

Figs. 27 and **28** *Immature neoplastic mononuclear cells (monoblasts) from patients with acute monocytic leukemia.*

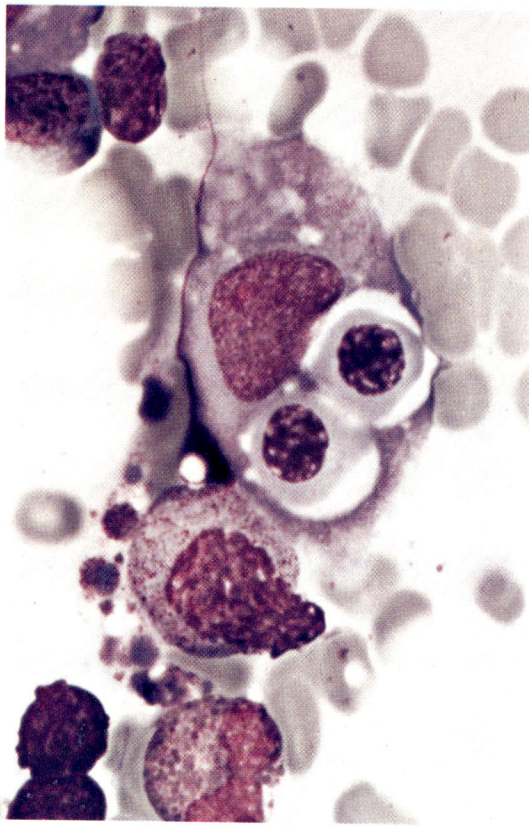

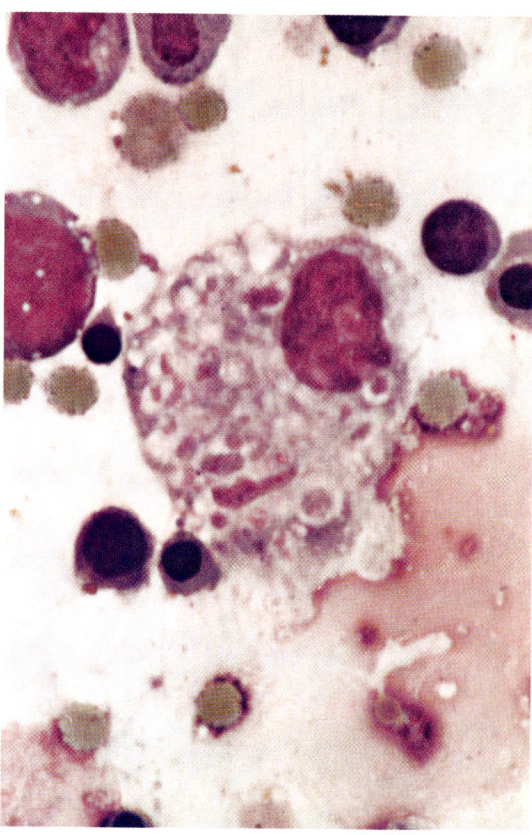

8 MONOCYTES

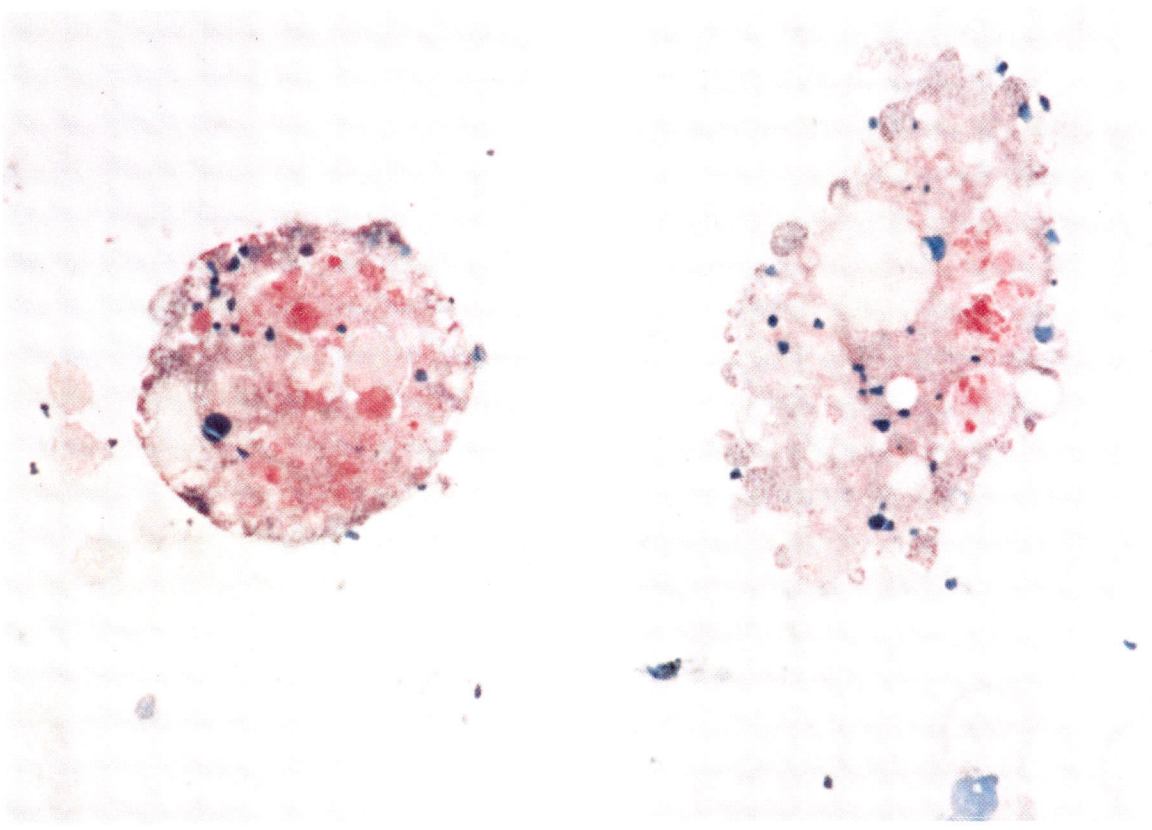

Figs. 30 a, b) *Combined technique for PAS and Prussian blue reaction. Demarcation of large vacuoles containing PAS-positive platelets in the cytoplasm of phagocytes laden with Prussian blue precipitates. Courtesy of Dr. G.L. Castoldi, University of Ferrara.*

Another malignant disorder involving somewhat more mature macrophages is known as histiocytic medullary reticulosis in the adult [3]. It is a disorder characterized by great enlargement of the liver and spleen, minimal lymphadenopathy, debilitating fevers, and a rapidly fatal course. A characteristic finding is phagocytosis of the formed elements of the blood by macrophages in the bone marrow (**Figs. 29** and **30**).

Phagocytosis of red cells, both nucleated (**Fig. 29**) and mature red cells, is a pathognomonic feature of this disease. Macrophages in this disorder retain their phagocytic activity but lose the ability to discriminate between foreign particles and endogenous cells. The resultant clinical manifestations are anemia and sometimes granulocytopenia and thrombocytopenia.

Fig. 29 a) *A neoplastic macrophage from the bone marrow of a patient with histiocytic medullary reticulosis. This macrophage has engulfed two nucleated red blood cells.*
b) *A macrophage from a patient with myelomonocytic leukemia terminated into malignant reticulosis. The cell has ingested several platelets.
Courtesy of Dr. G.L. Castoldi, University of Ferrara.*

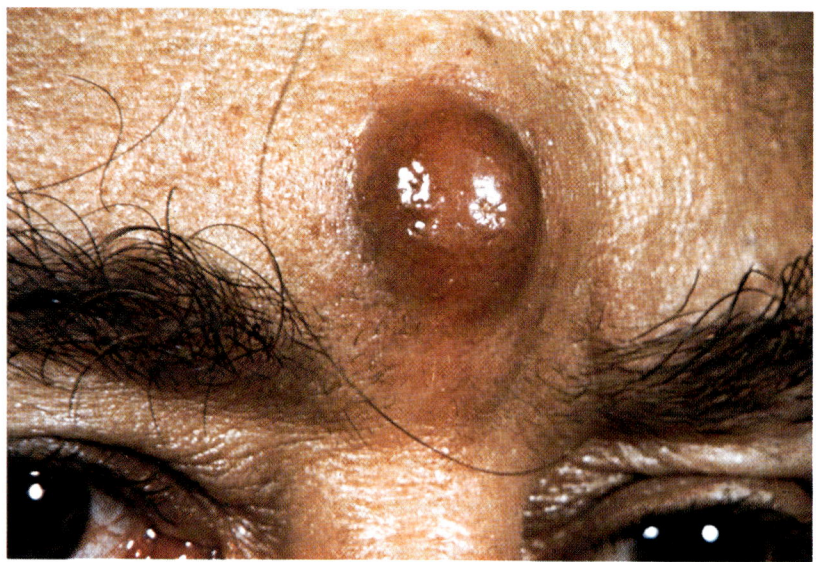

Fig. 31 A skin nodule from a patient with histiocytic medullary reticulosis.

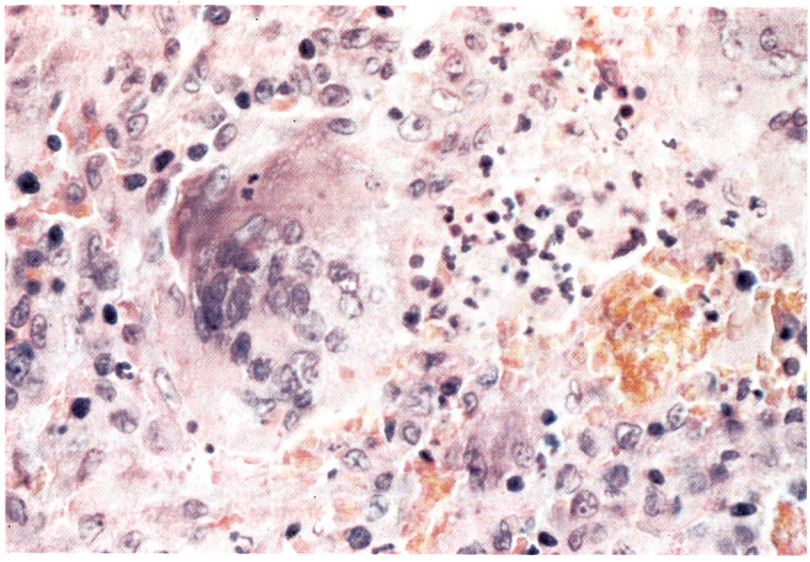

Fig. 32 Tissue infiltration with malignant macrophages in a patient with Letterer-Siwe disease.

Neoplastic macrophages have a propensity to infiltrate the skin and may give rise to a variety of clinical dermatopathies (**Fig. 31**).
Solid cellular infiltrates are an unusual manifestation of these disorders.

The childhood variant of histiocytic medullary reticulosis may be considered to be Letterer-Siwe disease in which skin, lungs, and bone marrow are widely infiltrated with neoplastic macrophages (**Fig. 32**).

More indolent forms of macrophage neoplastic disease include eosinophilic granuloma of bone and Hand-Schuller-Christian disease. These diseases are sometimes designated histiocytosis X [3].

REFERENCES

1. Meuret G., Bammert J., Hoffman G.: *Kinetics of human monocytopoiesis.* Blood, *44*, 801, 1974.
2. Meuret G., Batara E., Furste H.O.: *Monocytopoiesis in normal man: pool size, proliferation and DNA synthesis time of promonocytes.* Acta Haemat., *54*, 261, 1975.
3. Cline M.J.: *The white cell.* Harvard University Press, Cambridge, 1975.
4. Nichols B.A., Bainton D.F.: *Differentiation of human monocytes in bone marrow and blood. Sequential formation of two granule populations.* Lab. Invest., *29*, 27, 1973.
5. Nichols B.A., Bainton D.F., Farquhar M.G.: *Differentiation of monocytes. Origin, nature and fate of their azurophil granules.* J. Cell. Biol., *50*, 498, 1971.
6. van Furth R., Cohn Z.A., Hirsch J.G., Humphrey J.H., Spector W.G., Langevoort H.L.: *The mononuclear phagocyte system: a new classification of macrophages, monocytes, and their precursor cells.* Bull. World Health Org., *46*, 845, 1972.
7. Remington J.S., Krahenbuhl J.L., Mendenhall J.W.: *A role for activated macrophages in resistance to infection with Toxoplasma.* Infect. Immun., *6*, 829, 1972.
8. Mackaness G.B.: *The monocyte in cellular immunity.* Sem. Hematol., *7*, 172, 1970.
9. Territo M.C., Cline M.J.: *Macrophages and their disorders in man.* In: Immunobiology of the Macrophage. Nelson D.S. ed., Academic Press, 1976.
10. Arend W.P., Mannik M.: *The macrophage receptor for IgG: number and affinity of binding sites.* J. Immunol., *110*, 1455, 1973.
11. Roose W.F., de Boisfleury A., Bessis M.: *The interaction of phagocytic cells and red cells modified by immune reactions. Comparison of antibody and complement coated red cells.* Blood Cells, *1*, 345, 1975.
12. Gemsa D., Woo C.H., Fudenberg H.H., Schmid R.: *Erythrocyte catabolism by macrophages in vitro. The effect of hydrocortisone on erythrophagocytosis and on the induction of heme oxygenase.* J. Clin. Invest., *52*, 812, 1973.
13. Golde D.W., Territo M.C., Finley T.N., Cline M.J.: *Defective lung macrophages in pulmonary alveolar proteinosis.* Ann. Intern. Med., *85*, 304, 1976.
14. Evans R.: *Macrophage cytotoxicity.* In: Mononuclear phagocytes in immunity, infection, and pathology. van Furth R. ed., Blackwell Scientific Publications, Oxford, pp. 827-844, 1975.
15. Hibbs J.B. Jr.: *Discrimination between neoplastic and non-neoplastic cells in vitro by activated macrophages.* J. Natl. Cancer Inst., *53*, 1478, 1974.
16. Hibbs J.B. Jr.: *Heterocytolysis by macrophages activated by bacillus Calmette-Guérin: lysosome exocytosis into tumor cells.* Science, *184*, 468, 1974.
17. Unanue E.R., Cerottini J.C.: *The function of macrophages in the immune response.* Sem. Hemat., 7, 225, 1970.
18. Brady R.O.: *Biochemical and metabolic basis of familial sphingolipidoses.* Sem. Hemat., *9*, 273, 1972.
19. Golde D.W., Schneider E.L., Bainton D.F., Penchev P.G., Brady R.O., Epstein C.J., Cline M.J.: *Pathogenesis of one variant of sea-blue histiocytosis.* Lab. Invest., *33*, 371, 1975.
20. Cline M.J., Golde D.W.: *A review and reevaluation of the histiocytic disorders.* Am. J. Med., *55*, 49, 1973.
21. Kass L., Schnitzer B.: *Monocytes, monocytosis and monocytic leukemia.* Charles C. Thomas, Springfield, p. 111, 1973.
22. Miescher P.A., Farquet J.J.: *Chronic myelomonocytic leukemia in adults.* Sem. Hemat., *11*, 129, 1974.

Subject index

Boldface numbers in this index refer to illustrations;
italic numbers indicate the main citation for each subject.

Acanthocyte **68**
Acanthocytosis *124*
- "burr cells" in hepatic disorders 124
- defective synthesis of beta lipoproteins in *124*
- hereditary 124
- in uremia 124
Acetylcholinesterase
  (*see* Erythrocyte membrane)
Acid hydrolases
- eosinophil 269
- lymphocyte *375*, **376**, **377**, **378**, **379**
- monocyte 335
- neutrophil 152
- platelet 576
Acid phosphatase
- in acute lymphoblastic leukemia *425*, **430**
- in chronic lymphocytic leukemia 437
- in lymphoblastic lymphoma 483
- in lymphoid malignancies 412
- lymphocyte **355**, *375*, **379**
- monocyte 335
- tartrate-resistant in hairy cell leukemia 450
Acquired aplastic anemia *241*, **242**, **243**
- bone marrow in 241, **242**, **243**
- bone marrow transplantation in 639
- CFU-C in 243
- congenital 243
- cytotoxic lymphocytes in 241
- dyserythropoiesis in 243
- erythroid dysplasia in **246**
- lymphocytes in 243
- megaloblasts in 243, **247**
- neutrophil counts in 241
- pathogenesis of 241
- plasma cells in 243
- platelet counts in 241
- reticulocyte counts in 241
- suppressor lymphocytes in 241
Actin 54
- erythrocyte membrane 54
- interaction with spectrin 54
- platelet 587, **588**, **589**, 592
Acute lymphoblastic leukemia (ALL) 409, *412*, **413**
- acid phosphatase *425*, **430**
- B-ALL 420
- bone marrow transplantation in 639
- cALL antigen in 425
- chromosome analysis *632*, **632**
- common (c) 420
- cytology **413**, **415**
- FAB classification 412, 415, *420*, 425
- FACS analysis of **421**

- glycogen **414**, **418**
- hexosaminidase isoenzymes *422*, **428**, **429**
- L1 412, **413**, **415**
- L2 412, **413**, **417**
- L3 412, **413**, **419**
- monoclonal antibodies to 657
- morphology **413**
- null *420*
- PAS reaction **414**, 425
- patient's monitoring 433
- phenotype 420
- pre-B ALL 420
- presentation features 434
- prognosis *434*, **435**, **436**
- relapse 434
- remission 434
- surface immunoglobulin in **424**
- T-ALL 420
- T'-ALL 420, 421
- TdT in *422*, **423**, **424**, **426**, **427**
- ultrastructure **415**, **416**, **417**, **418**, **419**
- unclassified 420
Acute myelogenous leukemia (AML) *212*
- as monoclonal disorder 212
- cell proliferation in culture 26
- CFU-GM in 228
- chromosome analysis *612*, **613**, **615**
- classifications *214*
- - FAB *214*
- - - M1 212, **213**, **214**, *214*
- - - M2 *216*, **217**, **218**
- - - M3 *216*, **219**, **220**, **221**, **222**
- - - M4 *222*, **223**
- - - M5 *224*, **224**, **225**, **226**
- - - M6 *227*, **227**
- cytogenetic studies in 212
- G-6-PD isoenzymes in 212
- indolent variant 212
- membrane antigens in 228
- peroxidase in **216**, 228
- Philadelphia chromosome 612
- smouldering variant 212
- - chromosome analysis in **618**
- ultrastructure of 215
Adenosine deaminase
- in lymphoid malignancies 412
- in T cells 375
Agnogenic myeloid metaplasia 27
- cell proliferation in culture 27
- platelets in **598**
Agranulocytosis *250*, **250**, **251**
- infantile genetic 29
- mechanisms of 250
Alkaline phosphatase

- absence in CML 201, **201**
- in neutrophil differentiation 153
- in neutrophils 153, *163*, **165**, 167
- score **165**, **165**
Alder-Reilly anomaly *194*, **195**
Alpha-methyl-dopa 130
Alpha-naphthyl acetate esterase
- erythroblast 91
- in T cell maturation 388
- lymphocyte *375*, **376**, **377**, **378**, **379**
- megaloblast 79
- neutrophil 165
Amino acid
- substitution in abnormal hemoglobins 111
Amyloid *472*
  (*see also* Amyloidosis)
- A protein 472
- birefringence **473**
- phagocytosis **472**, **475**
- structure **473**
Amyloidosis 472
- in familial mediterranean fever 472
- plasma cells **474**, **476**, **477**
- - nuclear inclusions in **476**
- primary 472
- secondary 472
- ultrastructural analysis of **473**, **474**, **475**
Anemia(s)
- acquired aplastic *241*, **242**, **243**
- chemical and drug induced *130*
- congenital dyserythropoietic 92
- due to infection or infestation *126*
- dyserythropoietic *83*
- Fanconi's 243
- hemolytic *123*
- - acquired *126*
- - autoimmune *131*
- - chronic 124
- - hereditary *123*
- - intermittent 124
- hypochromic 99
- iron deficiency 99
- macroblastic 79
- megaloblastic 75, 79
- myelophthisic *134*
- non-addisonian pernicious 75
- pernicious 75, **77**
- - neutrophils in **77**
- - promegaloblast(s) in **76**
- pure red cell aplasia **244**, *245*, **245**
- refractory 84
- refractory with excess of blasts (RAEB) 228, 246, **248**, **249**
- sickle cell *111*, **111**

- sideroacrestic 84
- sideroblastic *84*, **84**, **85**
Angioimmunoblastic lymphadenopathy **520**, *521*
- immunoregulatory failure in 521
- vascular proliferation in 521
Anisocytosis 84
Ankyrin (*see* Erythrocyte membrane)
Anti-antibodies 10
Antibodies
- antinuclear *176*, **178**, **179**, **180**
- as markers 5
- in pure red cell aplasia 245
- monoclonal 6
- to gastric parietal cells **79**
Antibody Dependent Cell Cytotoxicity *402*
Antiserum (a)
- for leukemia cell typing *411*
Aplastic anemia 27
  (*see also* Acquired aplastic anemia)
- cell proliferation in culture 27
- suppressor cells in 27
Arylsulfatase
- eosinophil 269, 271
AS-D-chloroacetate esterase
- in acute erythremic myelosis **117**
Ataxia-Teleangiectasia
- chromosome analysis in 629
Auer body (*see* Auer rod)
Auer rod(s) *228*, **229**
- acid hydrolases in 228
- cytochemistry of 214, **220**
- in acute myelogenous leukemia 214, 216, 228
- phagocytosis **220**
- ultrastructure of **221**, **229**
Autoantibodies
- in acquired aplastic anemia 241
- in autoimmune hemolytic anemia 131
Autoimmune hemolytic anemia (AIHA) *131*, **132**
- and lymphoma 132
- autoagglutination in 132
- cold-reactive autoantibodies in 131
- direct antiglobulin test in 131
- erythrophagocytosis in 131, **132**
- warm-reactive autoantibodies in 131
- with paroxysmal cold hemoglobinuria 131

Babesia microti 128, **130**
Bartonella bacilliformis 128
Basophil(s) *285*
- chemotaxis 306
- contact allergy and 308, *314*, **315**
- count 287
- degranulation **297**, *301*, **302**, **304**, **305**
- - by basic polyamines 301
- - by basic polypeptides 301
- - by lectins 301
- - IgE and 301
- - mechanism of *301*
- development 290
- distinction from mast cells 287
- eosinophil chemotactic factor (ECF-A) 303
- function *301*
- glycogen 290

- granules *287*, **288**
- - Alcian blue staining of *290*, **291**
- - chymase 290
- - heparin 292
- - histamine 290
- - PAS-positivity of 290
- - safranin staining of *290*, **291**
- - sulfated mucopolysaccharides 290
- - ultrastructure of *292*, **293**, **294**, **295**, **296**, **297**, **298**, **299**, **300**
- IgE receptors *301*
- in chronic myelogenous leukemia 205
- in myeloproliferative disorders *307*, **309**, **310**, **311**, **312**, **313**, **314**
- locomotion 306
- metamyelocyte **289**
- myelocyte **289**, **294**
- pathology *307*, **308**
- phagocytosis **305**, *306*, **306**, **307**
- promyelocyte **289**
- relationship with mast cells 287, *315*
- renal allografts 314
- slow reacting substance of anaphylaxis (SRS-A) 303
- skin **300**, *308*, 314, **315**
- thymidine uptake 290
- tissue *308*
- surface morphology **303**
- tumor infiltrates 314
Basophilic leukemia *307*, **308**
  (*see also* Leukemia)
Basophilic stippling
  (*see* Erythrocyte inclusions)
Basophilopenia 308
B-dominant zone(s)
- in lymphoid organs 347
- in lymphomas 481
Bence-Jones proteins 451
Benzene
- anemia 130, **131**
Bernard-Soulier syndrome 597
Beta-glucuronidase
- myeloma plasma cell **453**
- T-cell *375*, **377**
BFU-E *17*, 22, 36, 37
- day 3, 36
- day 8, 36
Blast cell crisis
- chromosome analysis in *611*, **613**
- erythroid precursors in 205
- FACS studies in 205, **208**
- in chronic myelogenous leukemia 205
- lymphadenopathy in 205
- lymphoid 205, **207**
- megakaryocyte precursors in 205
- morphology **209**, **210**, **211**
- myeloid 205, **207**
- phenotype 205, **207**
- pre-B cells in 205
- splenomegaly in 205
- TdT activity 207
Blood group antigens
  (*see also* Erythrocyte membrane)
- and bone marrow engraftment *640*, **641**
- in neutrophils 197
- Kell system 196
Blood island(s) 35
B-lymphocyte(s) 347, *356*
- activation *390*, **391**, **392**, **393**
- complement receptors *366*, **366**
- counts 356

- cytoplasmic immunoglobulin, 356, 357
- EB virus receptors 366, **366**
- enzymes *367*
- Fc receptors *367*
- generation *383*
- HLA-DR membrane antigens *364*, **364**, **365**, **385**
- IgM *383*
- - cytoplasmic 384
- - modulation of 384
- - immature *384*
- markers *357*
- maturation 383
- mature *385*
- morphology *357*
- mouse erythrocyte receptors *367*
- 5'-nucleotidase *367*, **367**, **368**
- phenotype expressions *358*, **383**
- polysomes 357
- specific antigens *357*, **366**
- surface membrane immunoglobulin 347, *356*, *358*, **360**, **361**
- - capping *359*, **360**, **361**, **362**, **363**
- - endocytosis 359
- - resynthesis 359
- surface morphology *358*
- TdT in early **383**
- ultrastructure *357*
Bone marrow
- environment **641**
- in acquired aplastic anemia 241, **242**, **243**
- sinusoids *640*, **641**
- stem cells *639*
- transplantation (*see* Transplantation hematopoiesis)
Boyden chamber 167
BPA (Burst Promoting Activity) 17
Burkitt's lymphoma
- African 514
- and EB virus 514
- chromosome analysis in *622*
- like B-ALL 420, **421**
- like of the adult *552*, **553**
- type lymphoma 546
Burr cells 124

Cabot rings (*see* Erythrocyte inclusions)
Capping
- of lymphocyte Ig **360**, **361**, **362**, **363**
Cathepsin G 152
Cell
- de-differentiation 4
- differentiation 3
- identification *1*
- malignant transformation 4
- maturation 3
Cell-mediated immunity
- monocytes and 334
Centroblast(s) 480
Centroblastic lymphoma *542*, **543**, **545**
Centroblastic-centrocytic lymphoma 488
- ultrastructure **536**, **537**, **539**, **540**, **541**
Centrocyte(s) *478*
Centrocytic lymphoma 487
- ultrastructure *532*, **533**, **535**
Cephalosporins 130
CFU-C
- in aplastic anemia 243

CFU-E 15, *17*, 22, 36, 37
- in null lymphocyte populations 381
- proliferation 27
CFU-EOS *17*, 257, **258**
CFU-GM 15, *17*, 22, 26, 28, 149
- buoyant density 26, 27
- in acute myelogenous leukemia 228
- in null lymphocyte populations 381
- HLA-DR antigens in 149
CFU-MEG 15, *17*, 22
CFU-S 13. 22
Charcot-Leyden crystal(s) *276*, **281**
- in bronchial or nasal mucus 276, **281**
- phagocytosis of 276
Chediak-Higashi-Steinbrink anomaly *188*, **190, 191, 192, 193**
- eosinophils **190**
- in Aleutian mink 188
- in beige mouse 189
- lysosomes in 189, **190**
- neutrophil myeloperoxidase **193**
- oxygen metabolism in 189
Chemical and drug induced anemia(s) *130*
- autoimmune type 130
- - by alpha-methyl-dopa 130
- - by chlorpromazine 130
- - by hydantoins 130
- benzene 130, **131**
- immune complexes in 130
- - by phenacetin 130
- - by quinine 130
- - by stibophen 130
- immunological mechanisms in 130
- lead 130
- passive hemagglutination type 130
- - by cephalosporins 130
- - by penicillin 130
Chemotaxis
- basophil *306*
- eosinophil 271
- neutrophil *167, 168*, **169, 170**
Chlorpromazine 130
Chromosome(s)
- analysis
- - in acute leukemia *612*
- - in acute lymphoblastic leukemia *632*, **632**
- - in acute non lymphocytic leukemia *613*, **614, 615**
- - in acute phase of CML *611*, **613**
- - in myeloproliferative disorders 610
- - - chronic myelogenous leukemia *607, 610*, **611**
- - in polycythemia vera *617*, **618**
- - in preleukemia *620*
- - in promyelocytic leukemia **616**
- - in refractory anemia *620*
- - lymphoproliferative disorders *621*
- - - Burkitt's lymphoma *622*
- - - histiocytic lymphoma *625*, **626, 627, 628**
- - - Hodgkin's disease *622*
- - - malignant lymphoma *621*
- - - poorly differentiated lymphocytic lymphoma *623*, **624, 625**
- - T cell leukemia **629**
- ataxia telangiectasia *629*
- banding **606, 608, 609**
- changes in hemopoietic malignancies 8
- - in hematologic diseases **603**, 605
- identification 607
- - Paris nomenclature for 607, **608**
- in T cell dyscrasias *626*
- marker 13
- multiple myeloma *630*, **631**
- pattern
  (see also Karyotype)
- - normal **606, 608, 609**
- Philadelphia 8, 14, 26, *610*
Chronic granulomatous disease 183, **183, 186**
- NBT test in **183**
Chronic lymphocytic leukemia (CLL) *409, 436*
- acid phosphatase **437**
- cytochemistry **437**
- FACS studies **444**
- immunoglobulin in 492, **442**
- - capping **361**, 444
- - crystals **442**
- - surface **442, 443**
- lymphocyte abnormalities *445*
- morphology **437**
- 5'-nucleotidase 445
- surface markers *443*
- T-cell **437**
- ultrastructure **438, 439, 440, 441**
Chronic myelogenous leukemia (CML) *198*, **198, 199**
- alkaline phosphatase in 200, **201**
- as stem cell neoplasia 198
- basophils in 205
- blast transformation in
  (see also Blast cell crisis) 205
- blue macrophages 201, **205**
- bone marrow morphology in **200**
- cell proliferation in culture *26*
- chromosome analysis *610*
- cytochemistry of **203**
- double peaked myeloid histogram in 200
- eosinophils in 205, **206**
- fibroblast cultures in 198
- G-6-PD isoenzymes 198, **200**
- Gaucher cells in 201, **204**
- megakaryocytes in 205, **206**, 570, **571**
- monoclonality of lymphoid cells in 207
- Pelgeroid changes in **200**
- peripheral blood morphology in **198**, *199*
- Philadelphia chromosomes in 198, **607** *610*, **611**
- secondary myelofibrosis in 201
Chymase
- in basophil granules 290
Clinical applications
of in vitro hematopoiesis *26*
- acute myelogenous leukemia *26*, **27**
- agnogenic myeloid metaplasia *27*
- aplastic anemia 27
- chronic myelogenous leukemia *26*
- myelodysplastic syndromes 28
- neutropenia 28
- polycythemia vera *27*
- stem cell disorders *26*
Clonal expansion
- immunoreactive **410**
- lymphocyte *349, 390*
- malignant **410**
Clostridium welchii 128
Codocyte **68**, *107*
Colchicine 183

Cold agglutinin disease *131*
- during infectious mononucleosis 131
- during Mycoplasma pneumoniae infection 131
- IgM anti-I antibodies in 131
Colony formation in vitro 15, 17
- eosinophils **18, 19**, *257*, **258**
- erythroid cells 22
- granulocytes-monocytes **18, 19, 20, 21, 25**
- mast cells 287, **290, 291**
- megakaryocyte 23, 26, 559
Committed progenitor cells 15
Common ALL antigen *425*
- and patient's monitoring **433**
- expression in hemopoietic malignancies 425
- peroxidase staining of **431**
- positive cells **430**
- ultrastructural localization of **432**
Complement
- erythrocyte lysis by *125*, **126**
- receptors 182
- - B lymphocyte *366*, **366**
- - monocyte 333
Component III
  (see Erythrocyte membrane)
Concavalin A (Con A) 17
Congenital dyserythropoietic anemia 92
- type 1 *92*, **93, 95, 96, 97**
- type 2 *92*, **94, 95, 96, 97**
- type 3 *92*, **94, 95, 96, 97**
Congo red
- staining for amyloid *472*, **473**
Coproporphyria 98, 99
Crithidia luciliae **178**, *180*
CSA 15
CSF 15, 17, 26, 27, 167
Culture of hematopoietic cells *17*, 22
- clinical applications of *26*
- in acute myeloblastic leukemia 27
- in infantile neutropenia
  (Kostman's type) **28**
Cutaneous mastocytosis
  (see Urticaria pigmentosa)
Cytochalasin B 183
Cytological interrelationships
in lymphoid system *481*
Cytomegalovirus
- and lymphoproliferative reactions 514
Cytoskeleton
- erythrocyte 54
- lymphocyte 362, **363**
- neutrophil 183, **232**
Cytotoxic T lymphocytes (CTL) 402
- killing by *402*, **403, 404, 405, 406, 407**
- - target changes during **407**
Cytotoxicity
- antibody dependent cell *402*
- lymphocyte-mediated *402*
- - structural aspects of **403, 404, 405, 406, 407**
- monocyte *333*

Dacryocyte **68**, *70*
Deficiency of
- B_{12} vitamin 79
- folic acid 79
- iron 79
Degranulation
- neutrophil *171*, **173, 175**

Diamond-Blackfan syndrome *245*, **245**
Di Guglielmo syndrome *114*
Discocyte **52**, **65**
Discocyte-echinocyte transition 54
Döhle bodies 188, **188**, **189**
Drepanocyte **68**, **111**, **113**
Drum stick(s) *162*, **162**, **163**
Dutcher's bodies **455**, **468**, **530**, **531**
 (*see also* Plasma cell, nuclear inclusions)
Dyserythropoiesis *83*
- in acquired aplastic anemia 243
- in transplantation hematopoiesis **648**

Echinocyte 64, **64**, **65**, **70**
Echinocytogenetic factors 64
Elastase 152
Ellyptocyte **68**, **70**, **125**
Elliptocytosis *124*, **125**
- hereditary *124*, **125**
Enzymes as markers 4, 5
Eosinophil(s) *255*
- chemotactic factor (ECF-A) 303
-- production by basophils 303
- chemotaxis 271
- colonies *257*, **258**
- counts 276
- derived inhibitor (EDI) 271
- function *271*
- histamine neutralization by 271
- in Chediak-Higashi anomaly **190**
- in chronic myelogenous leukemia 205, **206**
- killing of parasites **275**
- maturation 257
- mature **262**
-- centrioles **265**
-- granule(s)
--- acid hydrolases 269
--- arylsulfatase 269, 271
--- biochemical analysis 269
--- crystals **266**, **267**, **268**
--- development 264
--- disorderly maturation of **278**, **279**
--- membranes **270**
--- peroxidase 269
-- nucleus *264*, **265**
-- peroxidase of **262**, **272**
-- ultrastructure *264*, *266*, **266**, **267**, **268**
- metamyelocyte **259**, **263**
- microgranules *269*, **270**
- myelocyte **259**, **263**
- non-specific fluorescence of **262**
- normal *257*
- pathology *276*
- peroxidase *257*, **259**, **260**, **262**, **263**
- phagocytosis *271*
-- antigen-antibody complexes 271
-- bacteria 271, **273**, **274**
-- platelets **272**
-- sensitized erythrocytes **272**
- promyelocyte *257*, **259**, **260**, **261**
- structure *257*
Eosinophilia *276*
- and basophils 276
- in allergies 276
- in heavy chain disease 469
- in Hodgkin's disease **277**, 504
- in mycosis fungoides **277**, **278**
- in parasitic infestations 276
- lymphokines and 276
- malignant or primary *282*
- reactive **279**
Eosinophilic granuloma **277**
Eosinopoietin 276
Epstein-Barr virus
- and African Burkitt's lymphoma 514
- and infectious mononucleosis 514
- antigens **519**
- cell biology **518**
- receptors on B lymphocytes *366*, **366**
Erythroblast(s) 35
- alpha-naphthylacetate esterase in 91
- basophilic 39, **43**, **44**, **45**
- nuclear extrusion **48**, **49**
- polychromatic 39, **46**, **47**
- primitive 35
- "ragged" 86
- vacuolated 85
Erythroblastic islands 36, *56*, **56**, **57**, **58**
- fetal 36
- in transplantation hematopoiesis **645**, **646**, **647**
- macrophages (histiocytes, reticulum cells) in 56
- nursing cells in 56
Erythrocyte(s) *33*
- destruction 123
-- abnormalities of *123*
- discocyte **52**, **65**
- enzyme deficiencies *124*
- fragmentation syndrome(s) *132*, **133**
-- in uremic hemolytic syndrome **134**
-- keratocytes in 132
-- microangiopathies in 132, **133**
-- schistocytes in 132, **133**
-- spherocytes in **133**
- inclusions *59*, **59**
-- basophilic stippling **60**, **61**
-- cabot rings **60**, **61**
-- Heinz bodies **62**, **63**
-- Howell-Jolly bodies **59**
-- Pappenheimer bodies **60**, **61**
- indices
-- MCV 99
-- MCH 99
-- MCHC 99
- lysis by complement *125*, **126**
- mature **39**, **52**
- membrane, *53*, **53**, **55**
-- particles **55**
-- proteins **53**, *54*
--- acetylcholinesterase 54
--- actin 54
--- ankyrin 54
--- blood group antigens 54
--- component III 54
--- expression during erythropoiesis 54
--- glyceraldehyde-3-phosphate dehydrogenase 54
--- glycosilation of 54
--- HLA antigens 54
--- HLA-DR antigens 54
--- integral 54
--- peripheral 54
--- spectrin 54
--- transmembrane 54
- osmotic fragility 123
- pathological changes in shape *67*
-- acanthocyte **68**
-- annulocyte **99**
-- codocyte **68**, **107**
-- dacrocyte **68**, **70**
-- drepanocyte **68**, **111**, **113**
-- ellyptocyte **68**, **70**, **125**
-- keratocyte **68**, **71**
-- knizocyte **69**, **71**
-- lepto-codocyte **70**
-- leptocyte **71**
-- megalocyte **69**
-- microcyte **69**
-- schizocyte **69**, **71**
-- spherocyte **69**, **71**, **123**
-- target cell **70**
- physiological changes in shape *64*
-- echinocyte 64, **64**, **65**, **70**
-- sphero-echinocyte 64
-- sphero-stomatocyte **66**, **71**
-- stomatocyte 64, **66**, **69**
- proliferation *17*
Erythrogenin 37
Erythroid
- bursts 17, **22**, 36
- clusters 17, **22**, 36
- precursors in blast cell crisis 205
Erythroleukemia *114*, *227*, **227**
- cytochemistry of **227**, **230**
- markers *118*
- ultrastructural features of *118*
Erythron 35
Erythrophagocytosis
- in acute monocytic leukemia **225**
- in histiocytic medullary reticulosis **340**, 341
- in malignant histiocytosis **555**
Erythropoiesis 13, *35*
- abnormalities of 75
- amplification phase of 35, **38**
- enzymes involved in 38
- fetal 35
- general aspects 35
- hepatic phase of *35*, 36, 37
- hyperproliferative *114*
- ineffective **38**, **45**, 103
- in post-natal life 36
- in the yolk sac 35
- macrophages in **37**, **44**
- maturation sequence of **40**
- megaloblastic 13, 36, *75*, 79
- mesoblastic phase of 35
- morphology of *39*
- myeloid phase of 35, 36
- neoplastic 114
- normoblastic 36, 42
- nuclear changes in **43**
- preamplification phase of 35, **38**
- regulation of *37*, **38**
- RNA during *38*, 39
- transplantation *642*, **644**, **645**, **646**, **647**, **648**
- ultrastructure of 39, **41**
Erythropoietin (EP) 15, 17, 36, *37*
- and regulation of erythropoiesis 39
- responsive cells (ERC) 36, **38**
- surface receptors for 38
Esterase(s)
- alpha-naphthyl acetate 165, 375
- granulocyte 165
- in acute monocytic leukemia *224*, **225**, **226**
- in leukemia 165

- lymphocyte 375
- megakaryocyte **573**
- monocyte 165, 334, **335**
- NaF inhibition of 165
- naphthol-AS-D-acetate 165
- naphthol-AS-D-chloroacetate 165, **166**
- Reed-Sternberg cell 498
Exocytosis
- during phagocytosis 172, 182

FAB classification
- of acute lymphoblastic leukemia 415 425
- of acute myelogenous leukemia 214
Familial amaurotic idiocy
- neutrophils in 194
Familial mediterranean fever
- amyloidosis in 472
Fanconi's anemia 243
Fc receptor(s)
- lymphocyte 348, 367
- monocyte **332**, 333
- neutrophil 182
Feeder layer for hematopoietic cultures 22, **24**
Felty's syndrome 29
Ferritin
- in erythropoiesis 40, **44**, **45**
Flow microfluorimetry 6
Fluorescence Activated Cell Sorter (FACS) 5, **6**
- in acute lymphoblastic leukemia **421**
- in blast cell crisis 205, **208**
- in Sézary leukemia **512**
Foamy cell(s) **336**, 338
(see also Macrophages and Gaucher cells)
Folic acid 75
Follicular lymphoma **488**, **489**
Fragmentation syndrome(s)
(see Erythrocyte)

Gammapathies
(see also Heavy chain disease)
- monoclonal 464, **465**
Gaucher
- cells 336, **336**, **337**
- disease 336
Gene expression 3
- for globin synthesis **102**
- for HLA synthesis **364**
- for "Ia" synthesis **364**
- for immunoglobulin synthesis **359**
Germinal center(s) 478, 481
Giant cells 321, **323**
Glanzmann's thromboasthenia 597
- platelets in **599**
Globin
- synthesis 101
- - abnormalities of 101
- - gene expression for **102**
Glucose-6-phosphate dehydrogenase 8
- as marker of monoclonality 8, 14
- in acute myelogenous leukemia 212
- in chronic myelogenous leukemia 198, 200
- in leukemia 8

- in myelofibrosis 252
- isoenzymes 8, **9**
Glutamic acid
- substitution in abnormal hemoglobin 111
Glyceraldehyde-3-phosphate dehydrogenase (see Erythrocyte membrane)
Glycogen
- in acute lymphoblastic leukemia **414**
- in basophils 290
- in neutrophils 158, 163, **164**
- in platelets **574**, **575**
- in T lymphoblasts **401**
Glycophorin (see Erythrocyte membrane)
- antibodies 657, **658**
Gout 181
- crystal phagocytosis in 181, **181**
Graft versus host (GvH) reaction
- in bone marrow transplantation 651
Granulocyte(s)
(see Neutrophil)
- precursors (see CFU-GM)
Granulocyte - Macrophage proliferation 17
Gunther's disease (see Porphyria)

Hairy cell leukemia 445
- acid phosphatase **450**
- cytology **446**
- phagocytosis **450**
- phenotype 445
- ribosome-lamellar inclusions in **448**
- surface morphology **449**
- ultrastructure **447**, **448**
Hand-Schuller-Christian disease 342, **342**
Heavy chain disease(s) 465
- cell ultrastructure **468**, **470**, **471**
- eosinophilia in 469
- immunofluorescence **469**, **472**
Heinz bodies (see Erythrocyte inclusions)
Hematopoiesis 11
- biology of 13
- fetal 13, **14**, **15**
- in long term cultures 22
- in short term cultures 17
- in the bone marrow 13
- in the liver 13
- in the spleen 13
- in the yolk sac 13
- in vitro 13
Hematopoietic islands 13, 15
Hemoglobin 36
- abnormal 111
- amino acid abnormalities 111, 114
- fetal (F) 36
- Gower I 36
- Gower II 36
- Portland 36
- synthesis **83**
- - disturbances of 83
- - in megaloblasts 79
- unstable 114
Hemoglobinuria
- paroxysmal cold 131
- paroxysmal nocturnal 124
Hemolytic anemia(s)
- acquired 126

- autoimmune 131
- chronic 124
- hereditary 123
- intermittent 124
Heparin
- in basophil granules 292
Hermansky-Pudlack syndrome 597
Hexosaminidase isoenzyme(s)
- in acute lymphoblastic leukemia 422, **428**, **429**
- in lymphoid malignancies 412
Histamine
- neutralization by eosinophils 271
- production by basophils 290
Histiocyte(s) (see Macrophage)
Histiocytic lymphoma **496**, **497**
- chromosome analysis **618**, 625, **626**, **627**
- ultrastructure 554, **555**
Histiocytic medullary reticulosis 340, 341, **341**
- childhood variant 342, **342**
- granulocytopenia in 341
- iron in **341**
- phagocytosis of erythroblasts 340, 341
- - platelets 340, 341
- skin infiltrates in 342, **342**
- thrombocytopenia in 341
Histiocytosis X 342
Histaminuria
- in urticaria pigmentosa 307
HLA antigen(s)
- and bone marrow transplantation 639
- in erythrocyte membrane 54
- monoclonal antibodies to 657
- structure **364**
HLA-DR antigen(s)
- B lymphocyte 364, **364**, **365**
- in acute myelogenous leukemia 228
- in lymphocytic leukemia 411
- on CFU-GM 149
- on erythrocyte membrane 54
- regulatory role in hematopoiesis 149
- thymocyte 388
Hodgkin's cell(s)
(see Reed-Sternberg cells)
Hodgkin's disease 498
- chromosome analysis in 622
- eosinophilia in **277**, 504
- histological classification of 504
- - lymphocyte depleted **505**
- - lymphocyte predominant **499**, **502**
- - mixed cellularity **504**
- - nodular sclerosing **502**, **503**
- myelophthisis in 252
- phagocytes in 504
- Reed-Sternberg cells in 498
- Rye classification 504
- sclerosis in 498, **502**, **503**, **505**
Howell-Jolly bodies
(see Erythrocyte inclusions)
Hurler-Pfaundler syndrome
- neutrophils in 194
Hybridoma
- antibodies
- - application of 655
- - B-lineage associated 657
- - cALL associated 657
- - erythroid 657, **658**
- - granulocytic-monocytic 657

- - HLA-associated 657
- - in lymphoid malignancies 412, *659*
- - platelet 657
- - T-lineage associated *657*
- technology *6*, **7**
Hydantoins 130
Hypereosinophilic syndrome 277, **282**
- morphologic abnormalities in **282**
Hypochromia 99, **100**
Hypoxanthine phospho-ribosyl transferase (HPRT) *6*, **7**

Ia antigens (*see* HLA-DR antigens)
Immune complexes
- in chemical and drug induced anemia 130
Immunoblastic lymphoma **490, 491**
- ultrastructure *548*, **549, 550, 551**
Immunofluorescence, indirect *5*
Immunoglobulin 8
- allelic exclusion 8
- allotypes 10
- A on lymphocytes 356
- as marker of monoclonality *8, 9*
- C region **358, 359**
- cytoplasmic, in lymphocytes, 347
- domains *358*
- D on lymphocytes 356
- E and basophil degranulation 301
- E on lymphocytes 356
- E receptors in basophils *301*
- genes 8, *356*, 359
- G on lymphocytes 356
- G receptors
- - on monocytes **332**, 333
- - on neutrophils 182
- - on T lymphocytes *374*
- idiotypes 10
- - in myeloma *452*
- light chain restriction *8, 9*
- light chains on lymphocytes 356
- M on lymphocytes 356
- patches **360**
- restriction 356
- structure **358**
- surface membrane, in lymphocytes 347
- V region **358, 359**
Immunologic islands **334**
Infection or infestation anemia(s) *126*
- by Bartonella bacilliformis *128*
- by Babesia microti *128*, **130**
- by Clostridium welchii *128*
- by Leishmania *128*, **130**
- by Plasmodium falciparum *126*, **127**
- by Plasmodium malariae *126*, **128**
- by Plasmodium vivax *126*
Infectious mononucleosis *514*
- and cold agglutinin disease 131
- atypical lymphocytes in **515**
- EB virus infection and *514*
- lymphoblast ultrastructure in **515, 516, 517, 518**
- Reed Sternberg-like cells in **515**
- T cell function in 514, **518**
Intrinsic factor (IF) 75
Iron
- accumulation
- - in erythroblasts 86, **88, 89**, 90
- - in mitochondria **88, 89**

- - in reticulocytes **91**
- - in reticulum cells **87**
- deficiency without anemia 99
- depletion 99
Iron deficiency anemia 99
- bone marrow in **101**
- complicated 101
- erythrocytes in **100**
- reticulum cells in 101, **101**

Kallikrein
- as basophil chemoattractant 306
Karyotype(s) *605*
- and prognosis of leukemia 614
- in hematologic diseases (*see* Chromosome)
- normal **606, 608, 609**
Keratocyte **68, 71**, 132
Klinefelter's syndrome 162
Knizocyte **69, 71**
Kostman's congenital neutropenia 29, 250
Kupffer cells 321
- iron storage in **87**

Lactoferrin 153
Large granular lymphocyte(s) *369*, **371, 373**
Lead
- anemia 130
Leishman-Donovan bodies *128*, **130**
Leishmania *128*, **130**
LE phenomenon *176*, **177**
Lepto-codocyte **70**
Leptocyte **71**
Letterer-Siwe disease *342*, **342**
Leucyl-amino-peptidase
- monocyte 335
Leukemia
- acute lymphoblastic *412*
- acute myelogenous *212*
- - agranular promyelocytic (M3) *216*
- - hypergranular promyelocytic (M3) *216*
- - myeloblastic with maturation (M2) *216*
- - myeloblastic without maturation (M1) *214*
- - myelomonocytic (M4) *222*
- basophilic *307*, **308**
- chronic lymphocytic *436*
- chronic myelogenous *198*
- hairy cell *445*
- megakaryoblastic *230*, **231**
- megakaryocytic 252
- - in myelofibrosis 252
- monocytic *224*, *339*, **340**
- monoblastic *339*, **340**
- plasma cell *451*
- prolymphocytic *436*
- Sézary cell *506*
- specific antigens 8
Leukemic reticulo-endotheliosis (*see* Hairy cell leukemia)
Lipid inclusions
- in macrophages **338**
- in neutrophils *194*, **195**
Locomotion

- basophil *306*
- neutrophil *167*, **168, 171**
Lupus erythemathosus (LE) *176*
Ly antigens 369
Lymph node(s)
- structure and lymphomas 478, 480
Lymphoblast(s) *390*, **391**
- B *391*, **391, 392, 393**
- - cytoplasmic immunoglobulin *391*
- T **400**, *401*, **401**
- - glycogen in **401**
Lymphoblastic lymphoma **483**
- acid phosphatase in **483**
- Burkitt's type *546*
- ultrastructure *546*, **547**
Lymphocyte(s)
(*see also* B- and T-lymphocytes) *345*
- acid phosphatase 355
- activation *390*
- B (bone marrow-derived) 347, *356*
- binding sites 348
- clones 347, **349**
- cord blood *353*
- cytotoxic 347
- effector 347, *390*
- enzymes 348, **355**
- helper 347
- heterogeneity *347*
- in acquired aplastic anemia 243
- - cytotoxic 241
- - suppressor 241
- interaction with macrophages **348**
- life history 348
- lineages 347, 348
- mediated cytotoxicity *402*
- membrane antigens 348
- microfilaments **362, 363**
- morphology 347, **350, 351**
- normal *347*
- null *380*, **380, 381**
- ontogenesis *382*
- phenotype expressions 348
- physical properties 347, *349*
- proliferation 17
- subsets 347, 348
- suppressor 347
- surface morphology **354**
- T (thymus-derived) 347, *369*
- third population 380
- ultrastructure **350, 351, 352, 353**
Lymphocytic lymphoma **484**
- chromosome analysis *623*, **624, 625**
- ultrastructure *526*, **527**
Lymphocytosis
- in pure red cell aplasia 245
- in virus infections 514
Lymphoid malignancies (*see* Lymphoproliferative disorders)
Lymphoid neoplasms
- in relation to normal lymphocyte differentiation *512*, **513**
- maturation arrest in **513**
Lymphoid system
- cytological interrelationships *481*
Lymphokynes
- and basophil chemotaxis 306, 308
- and basophil degranulation 301
Lymphoma(s)
- chromosome analysis *621*
- Hodgkin's 409, *498*
- non-Hodgkin 409, *478*
Lymphoplasmacytoid lymphoma **486**

- ultrastructure *528*, **529**, **531**
Lymphoproliferative disorders *409*
- application of monoclonal antibodies to *659*
- biological characterization *409*
- chromosome markers in 411, *621*
- classification of *409*
- non-malignant *514*
Lymphosarcoma
  (*see* Lymphoma)
Lysodeikticus lysis
- in acute monocytic leukemia 226
Lysosome(s)
- in Chediak-Higashi anomaly 189, **190**
- monocyte 321, **324**
- platelets 576
Lysozyme 152, 153
- determination by lysodeikticus lysis 226

Macroblast 79
Macroglobulinemia
  (*see* Waldenström's macroglobulinemia)
Macrophage(s) *319*
- alveolar 321
- blue, in chronic myelogenous leukemia 201, **205**
- cytoplasmic extensions **330**
- cytotoxicity 333
- development *321*, **322**
- foamy **336**, **338**, **650**
- function *330*
- Gaucher cells *336*, **336**, **337**
- pathology *336*
- peritoneal 321
- phagocytosis **331**
- - of bacteria **331**
- - of fungi **331**
- - of mineral crystals **333**
- - of neoplastic cells **333**
- - of sensitized erythrocytes **332**
- phagosomes **331**
- pigmentary inclusions *336*, **339**
- pleural 321, **333**
- reactions after bone marrow transplantation *642*, **649**, **650**
- ruffled membranes of **327**, **329**
- scavenger functions **333**, *333*
- sea blue **339**
- surface morphology **327**, **329**
- ultrastructure **327**, **328**
Malabsorption syndrome(s) 79, **80**
Malaria *126*, **127**, **128**, **129**
Malignant Histiocytosis
  (*see* Histiocytic Lymphoma)
Markers
- definition 4
- for cellular identification *1*, 4
- lymphocyte membrane 348, *357*, *358*, *369*
- linked to differentiation 4
- of malignancy 8
- of monoclonality 8, **9**, **10**
Mast cell(s) *287*, **298**, **299**
- colonies 287, 290, **291**
- distinction from basophils 287, 315
- granules *287*
- in myeloproliferative disorders **312**, **313**, **314**

- origin 287, 290
- ultrastructure **298**, **299**
Mastocytoma
  (*see* Urticaria pigmentosa)
May-Hegglin anomaly 188, **189**
Megakaryoblast(s) *559*, **560**, **561**
Megakaryocyte(s) *557*
- colonies 559
- cytoplasm *561*
- demarcation membranes **562**, *563*, **564**
- esterases **573**
- granules *561*, **565**, **566**
- in chronic myelogenous leukemia 205, **206**
- in myelofibrosis-osteosclerosis syndromes **572**
- in myeloproliferative syndromes *570*, **571**
- in pancytopenias **573**
- in polycythemia vera 573
- lymphoid **570**
- marginal zone *567*, **568**
- maturation 559
- mature (*see* stage III)
- microtubules **570**, **571**
- non-producing 567
- normal *559*
- nucleus *561*
- pathology *570*
- peroxidase 561
- ploidy 561
- precursors in blast cell crisis 205
- proliferation 17
- stage I *559*, **560**, **561**
- stage II *559*, **560**
- stage III *559*, **560**
- ultrastructure **561**, **562**, *563*, **564**, **565**, **566**, **567**, **568**, **569**, **570**
- uptake of peroxidase 567
Megakaryoblastic leukemia
  (*see* Leukemia)
Megakaryocytic leukemia
  (*see* also Leukemia)
- and myelofibrosis 252
Megaloblast(s) 75, **76**, **77**
- alpha-naphthyl acetate esterase in 79
- basophilic **76**
- biochemical abnormalities of **81**
- chromosome fragmentation 75
- cytochemistry of *79*
- DNA synthesis in 75, 82
- drug-induced *82*, **82**
- hemoglobin in 79
- in acquired aplastic anemia 243, **247**
- ineffective mitosis of 75, **78**, **82**
- intermediate 79
- kinetics of proliferation 75
- mitotic activity 75, **78**
- polychromatic **76**
- siderotic granules in 79
- transitional 79
- ultrastructure of *79*, **80**
Megaloblastic anemia(s)
  (*see* Pernicious Anemia)
Megalocyte **69**, **76**
Megathrombocyte(s) *567*, **569**, **595**, *595*
Melanosarcoma
- marrow metastases of **136**
Membrane antigens
- acute myelogenous leukemia 228
- blast cell crisis 205, **207**

- lymphocyte 348
Memory lymphocyte(s) **392**, 480
Metamyelocyte(s) *157*
- basophil **289**
- eosinophil **259**, **263**
- giant **81**, *185*, **187**
- "stab" form of nucleus **155**, **157**
Microcyte **69**
Microcytemia **100**
Microenvironment
- bursal **382**
- in aplastic myelopathies 241
- thymic **386**, **387**
Microfilaments
- neutrophil 183
- platelet **575**, **585**, **586**, **591**
Micromegakaryocyte(s) **573**
Microtubule(s)
- megakaryocyte **571**
- neutrophil 183
- platelet **575**, **586**
Mitogen(s)
- responsiveness of T cells 389
Mixed Lymphocyte Culture 389
Modulation
- of surface Ig 345
Monoblast **322**
Monoblastic leukemia **339**, **340**,
  (*see also* Leukemia)
Monoclonal
- antibodies 6
- - application of 655
- - for T cell identification *374*
- B-cell lymphomas **493**, **495**
- proliferations **410**, 411
Monocyte(s) *319*, **322**, **326**
- acid phosphatase **335**
- complement receptors 333
- culture of **324**
- cytochemistry **334**
- cytotoxicity 333
- development *321*, **322**
- esterases 165, **334**, **335**
- - NaF inhibition of 165
- immunological cooperation **334**, *334*
- in cell-mediated immunity 334
- Fc receptors **332**, 333
- functions *330*
- kinetics *321*, **323**
- leucyl aminopeptidase 335
- lysosomes 321, **324**
- monoblasts 322
- pathology *336*
- peroxidase **325**, **327**
- phagocytosis *321*, **327**
- promonocytes 321, **322**, **325**
- surface adhesion of particles **331**, 333
- surface antigens **334**
Monocytic leukemia (*see* Leukemia)
Mononuclear-phagocyte system 319, *321*
  (*see also* Monocyte and Macrophage)
Morquio disease
- neutrophils in 194
Mouse erythrocyte receptors
- in B cell development 385
- in human B lymphocytes *367*, **370**
Mucopolysaccharidoses
- neutrophils in 194
Mycosis fungoides
  (*see also* Sézary syndrome)
- eosinophilia in **277**, **278**

Myeloblast(s) *149*, **150**, **151**
- PAS-negativity of 163
Myelocyte(s) *152*, **155**, **157**
- basophil **289**, **294**
- eosinophil **259**, **263**
- secondary granule formation in 153, **156**
Myelodisplastic syndromes
  (*see also* preleukemic states) 28
- cell proliferation in culture 28
Myelofibrosis-osteosclerosis syndrome *252*, **253**
- chromosome analysis **618**
- G-6-PD isoenzymes in 252
- megakaryocytes in **572**
- megakaryocytic leukemia and 252
- myelofibrosis 252
- osteomyelosclerosis 252
- platelets in **598**
Myeloma(s) 409, *451*
- cytochemistry **453**
- cytology **453**
- flaming plasma cells in **459**
- immunoglobulin
- - crystals in **456**, **462**
- - production in *451*, **459**, **461**
- light chains in 451
- non-secretory 451
- nuclear inclusions in **455**, **462**
- phagocytosis in **458**
- plasma cell
- - chromosome analysis *630*, **631**
- - crystals **456**, **467**
- - polyploid **460**
- - Russell bodies **463**
- - - PAS-positive **463**
- - structure 452
- ultrastructure **454**, **455**, **456**, **457**, **458**
Myeloperoxidase 152, **164**
- in Chediak-Higashi anomaly **193**
Myelophthisic anemia(s) *134*, **135**, **136**, **137**, *252*, **253**
- by metastatic solid tumors *134*, **135**, **136**, *252*, **253**
- in Hodgkin's disease 252
- in primary xanthomatosis 252
- in systemic hematologic proliferations 134
Myelophthisis
  (*see* Myelophthisic anemias)
Myeloproliferative syndromes
- acute erythremic myelosis *114*
- erythroleukemia *114*
- polycythemia vera *118*
Myeloblastic leukemia
  (*see* Leukemia and Acute myelogenous leukemia)
Myelomonocytic leukemia
  (*see* Leukemia and Acute myelogenous leukemia)
Myelopathies
- aplastic 75, *239*
- hypoplastic *239*
- metaplastic *239*
Myelosis
- acute erythremic *114*, **115**
- - AS-D-chloroacetate esterase in **117**
- - PAS-reaction in 116
- - ringed sideroblasts in **117**
- chronic erythremic *114*
- Di Guglielmo syndrome 114
Myosin platelet 587, **588**, **589**, **590**

Naphthol-AS-D-ace tate esterase
- in neutrophils 165
Naphthol-AS-D-chloroacetate esterase
- in neutrophils 165. **166**
Natural killing *402*
NBT test
- in neutrophils *183*, **183**
Neuroblastoma
- bone marrow cells from 385
Neutropenia(s) 28, *194*
- cell proliferation in culture 28
- chronic benign 29
- congenital 29
- drug induced 29
- Felty's syndrome 29
- hereditary autosomal 29
- idiopathic 29
- Kostman's type 29
Neutrophil(s) *147*
- adhesion 196, **197**
- alkaline phosphatase 153, **163**, **165**, 167
- - in chronic myelogenous leukemia 200, **201**
- - in polycythemia vera **201**
- chemotaxis of *167*, 168, **169**, 170
- circulating pool 167
- complement receptors 182
- cytochemistry *163*
- cytoplasmic abnormalities *188*
- - Alder-Reilly anomaly *194*, **195**
- - Chediak-Higashi-Steinbrink anomaly *188*, **190**, **191**, **192**, **193**
- - Döhle bodies *188*, **188**, **189**
- - lipid inclusions *194*, **195**
- - May-Hegglin anomaly *188*, **189**
- - reactive inclusions 188
- - toxic granulations 188
- cytoskeletal proteins 183
- degranulation *171*, **173**, **175**
- differentiation *149*
- esterases 165
- glycogen **158**, *163*, **164**
- granules 149, 163
- - acid hydrolases 152
- - alkaline phosphatase in 153, **163**, **165**, 167
- - as lysosomes 152
- - azurophilic 152, 163
- - cathepsin G 152
- - elastase 152
- - lactoferrin 153
- - lysozyme 153, 183
- - myeloperoxidase 152, **164**, 183
- - origin of 152
- - secondary 152, 153, **156**, **158**, **159**, 163
- - specific (*see* secondary)
- - structural heterogeneity of **158**, **159**
- IgG receptors 182
- kinetics 167
- locomotion *167*, **168**, **171**
- marginated pool 167
- maturation *149*
- mature *157*, **157**, **158**, **159**, **160**, **161**, **162**
- - nuclear swelling of 160, **162**
- - nucleus of 160, **161**
- - protein synthesis in 160
- - thymidine uptake in 160
- metabolism *182*

- microfilaments 183
- microtubules 183
- nuclear abnormalities *185*
- - hypersegmentation 185, **187**
- - - during pregnancy 185
- - - in megaloblastic anemias 185, **187**
- - Pelger-Huet anomaly 185, **186**
- - pseudo-Pelger anomaly **188**
- number, disorders of *194*
- PAS-positivity *163*, **164**, **166**
- pathology *185*
- phagocytosis *171*, **172**, **174**, **176**
- - "frustrated" 171, **175**
- - of nuclei **176**
- - release of hydrolases during 171
- production of 167
- - regulation of 167
- sex chromatins *162*, **162**, **163**
- Sudan Black staining *165*, **166**
- superoxide generation in 182
- surface antigens 149
- surface glycoproteins 149
Non-Hodgkin lymphoma(s) *478*
- B-cell lineage *493*
- - follicular B cell 493
- - immature B cell 493
- - immunoblastic 495
- - plasma cell 496
- - plasma cell precursors 495
- centroblastic centrocytic **494**
- centrocytic **487**
- classifications *478*
- follicular **488**, **489**, **494**, **495**
- histiocytic **496**, **497**
- immunoblastic **490**, **491**
- immunological characterization of *492*
- lymphoblastic **483**
- lymphocytic **484**
- lymphoplasmacytoid **486**, **497**
- monoclonality of **495**
- phenotype *480*, *492*
- receptor silent **496**
- T cell lineage *493*
- T-zone **492**
- ultrastructure *525*
Normoblast(s) (*see* Erythroblast)
Nucleophagocytosis
- in LE *176*, **177**
5'-Nucleotidase
- in B lymphocytes *367*, **367**, **368**, 375
- in CLL lymphocytes 445
Null lymphocytes *380*, **380**, **381**

Opsonin(s) 182
Osteoblasts
- in marrow smears **137**
Osteomyelosclerosis *252*
Osteosclerosis *252*

Pappenheimer bodies
  (*see* Erythrocyte inclusions)
Paraproteinemia(s) *451*
Parasite(s)
- killing by eosinophils **275**
Paroxysmal nocturnal hemoglobinuria (PNH) *124*

- as expression of myeloproliferative disorders 124
- associated to aplastic anemia 124
- cell proliferation in culture 28
- cells 124
- - abnormal sensitivity to complement of 124
- hemosideruria in 124
- PNH I erythrocyte population 124
- PNH II erythrocyte population 124
- PNH III erythrocyte population 124
- Strübing-Marchiafava-Micheli's syndrome in 124
- terminating in myelogenous leukemia 124

Pautrier's microabscess
- in mycosis fungoides 567

Peanut agglutinin
- binding to T lymphocytes *389*, **389**

Pelger-Huet anomaly 185, **186**

Penicillin 130

Periodic Acid Schiff (PAS) reaction
- in acute erythremic myelosis 116
- in acute lymphoblastic leukemia **414**
- in basophils 290
- in neutrophils *163*, **164**, **166**
- in plasma cell Russell bodies **463**
- in thalassemia syndromes 107

Pernicious anemia
- antibodies to gastric parietal cells in **79**
- giant metamyelocytes in **81**
- neutrophil hypersegmentation in 185, **187**
- neutrophils in **77**
- non-addisonian 75
- nutritional deficiencies and 79
- promegaloblasts in **76**

Peroxidase
(*see also* Myeloperoxidase)
- antiperoxidase test
- - for cALL antigen demonstration **431**
- - in lymphoplasmocytoid lymphoma **497**
- eosinophil 262, 269, 272
- in acute myelogenous leukemia **216**, 228
- megakaryocyte *561*, **570**
- monocyte **325**, 327
- uptake by megakaryocytes 567

Phagocytosis 171, 172
- and oxidative phosphorylation 182
- by basophils **305**, **306**, *306*, **307**
- by eosinophils 271
- by hairy cell leukemia cells **450**
- by monocytes-macrophages *321*, **327**
- by neutrophils *171*
- crystal *181*
- - calcium pyrophosphate 181, *182*
- - hydroxyapatite 181
- - in gout 181, **181**
- - monosodium urate 181, **181**, *182*
- erythroblast, in bone marrow transplantation 650
- "frustrated" 171, **175**
- of nuclei *176*
- platelet 597
- release of hydrolases during 171

Phagolysosome(s) **176**
Phagosome(s) 171, **174**, **175**
- macrophage **331**
Phenacetin 130

Philadelphia chromosome 8, 14, 26, 198, *610*
- in acute leukemia *612*
- in blast crisis *611*, **613**
- in chronic myelogenous leukemia **607**, *610*, **611**

Phytohemagglutinin (PHA) 17
- for karyotype analysis 605, **606**
- T cell activation by **400**

Pinocytosis
- by basophils *306*

Plasmablast(s)
- 5'-nucleotidase 368
- immunoglobulin **398**
- structure **392**

Plasma cells(s) 356
- acid hydrolases 367
- amyloidosis **474**, **476**
- crystals **456**, **462**
- fibrils **457**
- immunoglobulin 356, **356**
- in acquired aplastic anemia 243
- membrane phenotype **383**, *385*
- myeloma **453**, **454**, **455**, **456**, **457**, **458**, **459**, **460**, **461**, **462**, **463**
- normal *394*
- nuclear inclusions **455**, **462**, **468**, *530* **531**
- phagocytosis 458
- polyploid **460**
- Russell bodies **394**, **399**, **463**
- structure *394*, **394**, **395**, **396**, **397**
- surface immunoglobulin **399**
- thymidine uptake **398**

Plasma cell leukemia (*see* Leukemia)
- chromosome analysis **618**

Plasmacytoma (*see* Myeloma)

Plasmodium
- falciparum 127
- gametocytes 127
- malariae 128
- merozoites 127, **128**, 129
- schizonts 127
- - anular 127
- - ameboid 127
- trophozoites 127, **128**
- vivax 127

Platelet(s)
- acid hydrolases 576
- actin 587, **588**, **589**, **592**
- and hemostasis 576
- canalicular system 575, **583**, **593**
- contractile system *582*, **585**, **586**
- degranulation 576, **577**
- destruction 597
- dysplasia **598**
- fragmentation 595, **596**
- functions *574*
- giant (*see* Megathrombocyte)
- glycogen **574**, **575**
- granules **574**, **575**, **581**
- in inflammation *587*
- in myelomonocytic leukemia **600**
- in myeloproliferative states 597, **600** **600**
- interaction with cartilage **578**, *579*
- - with collagen 577
- - with thrombogenic surfaces **580**
- interiorization *582*, **583**, **584**
- microfilaments **575**, **585**, **586**, **591**
- microtubules **575**, **586**
- monoclonal antibodies 657

- myosin 587, **588**, **589**, **590**
- pathology *595*
- phagocytosis **597**
- plasma membrane coat **574**, 576
- release from megakaryocytes **569**
- size **595**, **596**, **597**
- storage *582*
- tubulin **581**

Poikilocytosis 84

Pokeweed Mitogen (PWM) 17
- B-cell stimulation by **398**

Polycythemia vera 27, *118*, **119**
- aniso-poikilocytosis in 119
- cell proliferation in culture 27
- chromosome analysis *617*, **618**
- ellyptocytosis in 119
- megakaryocytes in 573
- ovalocytosis in 118
- sensitivity to erythropoietin in 119
- ultrastructural abnormalities in **119**, **120**, **121**

Polymorphonuclear leukocyte(s)
(*see* Neutrophil)

Porphyria(s) 98, **98**
- acute intermittent 98
- congenital erythropoietic 98
- erythropoietic form 98, **98**
- cutaneous-hepatic variant 98
- Gunther's disease 98
- hepatic form 98
- macroerythroblasts in **98**
- nuclear inclusions in 98
- PBG-deaminase deficiency in 99
- "ragged" erythroblasts in 99
- symptomatic 99
- variegate 98

Pre-B cell(s) 383
- cytoplasmic IgM *383*, **384**, **385**
- Ia antigen **383**, 384
- in blast cell crisis 205
- large, *384*, **384**
- small *384*, **384**

Preleukemic states 28
- chromosome analysis in *620*
- in vitro proliferation 28
- platelets in **599**

Progenitor cells 15

Prolymphocytic leukemia **436**, **443**
- morphology **437**
- ultrastructure **438**

Promegakaryocyte(s) *559*, **560**
Promonocyte(s) 321, **322**, 325
Promyelocyte(s) *149*, **152**, **153**, **154**
- basophil 289
- classification *152*
- early (I) 152
- eosinophil 257, *259*, **260**, **261**
- granules 152
- late (II) 152

Promyelocytic leukemia
(*see* Leukemia and Acute Myelogenous leukemia)

Pronormoblast(s) 36, **39**, **42**
Prostaglandins 167
Protoporphyria 98, 99
Pure red cell aplasia **244**, *245*, **245**
- antibodies in 245
- chromosome analysis in **620**
- Diamond-Blackfan syndrome *245*, **245**
- lymphocytosis in 245
- myeloid hyperplasia in **244**, 245

- thymus and 245
Purine nucleoside phosphorylase
- in T cells 375, **377**

Quinacrine
- for chromosome banding analysis 606
Quinine 130

Receptor silent lymphoma *496*
Red cell(s) (*see* Erythrocyte)
Reed-Sternberg cell(s) **499, 500, 501, 502**
- esterases in 498
- origin 498
- ultrastructure **500, 501**
Refractory anemia with excess of blasts (RAEB) 228, 246, **248, 249**
- chromosome analysis in *620*
Renal erythropoietic factor (REF) 37
Reticulocyte(s) 39, **50, 51**
- after bone marrow transplantation **646**
- inclusions 59
Rhopheocytosis 44, 45, 58, 651
Ribosome-lamellar inclusion(s)
- in hairy cell leukemia **448**
Russell bodies **394, 399, 463**
- in lymphoplasmacytoid lymphomas 528, **529**
Rye classification
- of Hodgkin's disease *504*

Schistocyte(s) 132, **133**
Schistosomula 275
- killing by eosinophils 271, **275**
Schizocyte **69, 71**
Severe aplastic anemia
 (*see* Acquired aplastic anemia)
Severe combined immunodeficiency
- bone marrow transplantation in 639
Sex chromatin *162*
- female 162, **162, 163**
- male 162, **163**
Sex-linked agammaglobulinemia
- null cells in 381
Sézary syndrome *506*
- cytochemistry 506, **511**
- FACS studies **512**
- helper cells in 506
- lymphoma **510**
- phenotype 506
- ultrastructure **507, 508, 509, 510**
Sheep erythrocyte receptors *369*, **370**
- in T lymphoblasts 401
Sickle cell anemia *111*, **111**
- intravascular agglutination 111
- retinal vessels in 111, **112**
- ultrastructure 111, **113**
Sickling phenomenon 111, **112**
Sideroblast(s) 84, **86, 88, 89, 90**
- in iron deficiency anemia 101
- in transplantation hematopoiesis **648**
- "ringed" **86, 117**
Sideroblastic anemia *84*, **84, 85**
- hereditary 84
- primary acquired 84, **87**

- reticulum cells in **87**
- secondary acquired 85
Slow Reacting Substance of Anaphylaxis (SRS-A)
- inactivation by eosinophils 271
- production by basophils 303
Spectrin (*see* Erythrocyte membrane)
Spherocyte **69, 71, 123, 133**
Spherocytosis *123*
- hereditary *123*, **123**
- - marrow hyperplasia in 123
- - megaloblastic features in 123
Sphero-echinocyte 64
Sphero-stomatocyte **66, 71**
Sphingomyelinase
- deficiency in macrophages 339
Spleen colony assay 13
Stem cell(s) *13*, 14
- defects in aplastic myelopathies 241
- differentiation *13*, **16**
- disorders 26
- pluripotent 13
- proliferation 14, 22
- reseeding in bone marrow transplantation *639*
Stibophen 130
Stomatocyte 64, **66, 69**
Stomatocytogenetic factors 64
Storage
- diseases *336*
- pool disease 597
Strübing-Marchiafava-Micheli's syndrome 124
Sudan Black
- staining of neutrophils *165*, **166**
- - of monocytes **338**
Superoxide
- generation in neutrophils 182
- - in chronic granulomatous disease 196
Surface antigens
- as markers 4
- lymphocyte *358*, **369**
- monocyte *334*
Surface membrane immunoglobulin *347*
Synartesis *92*, **93**

Target cell(s) **70**
T$_G$ cells *374*
- enzymes 375, **379**
- killing activity *402*
- morphology **373**
- phenotype 375
T$_M$ cells *374*
- enzymes 375, **378**
- morphology **372**
- phenotype 375
T-dominant zones
- in lymphoid organs 347, **377**
- in lymphomas 481
Teratocarcinoma 4
Terminal deoxynucleotidyl transferase (TdT)
- in acute lymphoblastic leukemia *422, 423, 424, 426, 427*
- in blast cell crisis 207
- in chronic myelogenous leukemia 228
- in lymphoid malignancies 412
- pre-B cell *383*, **383**
- thymocyte 388, **389**

Thalassemia syndromes *101*
- alpha 102
- beta 103, **103, 104, 105, 106**
- codocytes in **107**
- erythrocyte inclusions in 105
- foamy cells in **110**
- ineffective erythropoiesis in 103
- intermedia 102
- major 102
- marrow hyperplasia in 105, **106**
- minor 102
- morphological features of *103*
- homozigosity in 103, **106**
- PAS-positive erythroblasts in 107
- ultrastructure of
- - erythroblasts in **107**
- - erythrocytes in **107, 108, 109**
- - macrophages in **110**
Third population cells *380*
- enzymes *379*
- markers 380
- morphology **380, 381**
Thrombocyte(s) (*see* Platelets)
Thrombocytopenic purpura *595*, **596**
Thrombocytosis
- essential
- - chromosome analysis in *619*
Thrombopoietin 17, 567
Thrombus **594**
Thy 1 antigens 369
Thymocyte(s)
- antigens *389*
- HLA-DR antigens 388
- phenotype *388*, **388, 389**, *389*
- TdT *388*, **388**
Thymus
- and pure red cell aplasia 245
- structure *386*, **386, 387**
TL antigen(s) 369
- thymocyte 388
T-lymphocyte(s) 347, *369*
- acid phosphatase 375, **379**
- activation **400, 401**, *401*
- antigens *389*, **389**
- counts 369
- cytotoxic *402*
- distribution in lymphoid organs *374*
- E rosettes *369*, **370**
- enzymes *375*
- - ANAE 375, **376, 377, 378, 379**
- - beta-glucuronidase 375, **377**
- - PNP 375, **377**
- generation *386*
- identified by monoclonal antibodies *374*
- immunoglobulin receptors *374*
- - IgA *374*
- - IgG *374*
- - IgM *374*
- maturation *386*
- membrane antigens 369
- morphology *369*, **371, 372, 373**
- phenotype expressions 369
- surface markers *357*, *369*
- T$_G$ cells *373*, 374
- T$_M$ cells *372*, 374
Transplantation hematopoiesis *637*
- blood group antigens in *640*, **641**
- conditioning before 639
- dyserythropoiesis in **648**
- erythroblastic islands in **645, 646, 647**

- erythropoiesis in *642*, **644, 645, 646, 647, 648**
- evidence of engraftement *640*
- graft versus host reaction in 651
- granulocyte production in 642, **643**
- HLA antigens in 639
- immunodeficiency after *651*
- immunoreconstitution after *651*
- macrophage reactions *642*, **649, 650**
- megakaryocyte production in *642*
- morphology of *642*
- rejection in 640
- reticulocytes after **646**
- sideroblasts in **648**
- stem cell reseeding in 639
T-zone lymphoma **492**
Trypanosoma lewisi **180**
Tuberculoid granuloma 323
Turner's syndrome 162

Uremic hemolytic syndrome **134**
Uropod
- lymphocyte **362, 363**, 390
Urticaria pigmentosa *307*
- basophils in **300**
- histaminuria in 307

Vitamin(s)
- B_{12} 75
- - deficiency 75

Waldenström's macroglobulinemia 411, *464*, **464, 465, 466, 467**
- erythrocyte agglutination **466**
- lymphoplasmacytes **464**
- - immunoglobulin **465**
- - ultrastructure **466, 467**
Wiskott-Aldrich syndrome 597
- bone marrow transplantation in 639

Xanthomatosis
- myelophthisis in primary 252
X-ray crystallography
- studies for amyloid 472

Y-chromatin body *162*, **163**
- and bone marrow engraftment *640*